AF393581

Corey S. Scher

Editor

Anesthesia for Trauma

New Evidence and New Challenges

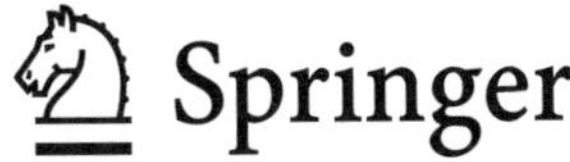 Springer

Editor
Corey S. Scher
Bellevue Hospital Center
New York University
New York, NY, USA

ISBN 978-1-4939-4791-1   ISBN 978-1-4939-0909-4 (eBook)
DOI 10.1007/978-1-4939-0909-4
Springer New York Heidelberg Dordrecht London

Preface

I keep time through a conglomeration of the media, the music industry, and film. My first exposure to trauma was through the nightly telecasts of the war in Viet Nam by the partnership of Chet Huntley and David Brinkley of NBC news. Walter Cronkite was a legend at the same time period and represented CBS. Both were responsible for the graphic images of the war; Night night after night, for years, I was mesmerized by the images of the wounded and dead. The film industry joined in, taking advantage of the politics of the war and the staggering number of the injured and dead to make *Apocalypse Now*, *Born on the fourth of July*, *Platoon*, *Good Morning Viet Nam*, and so on. Although these were just films, their closeness to reality put the trauma patients in my face. With the music and festival of Woodstock, I have never been able to turn back.

Trauma was again brought front and center as the seed of medical school was planted in my mind. Trauma was clearly a specialized field of medicine. Like many fields of medicine, there is little consensus on what to do with the trauma patient. In our recent history, other causes of trauma such as 9/11, Hurricane Katrina, the Haitian Earthquake, and the Tsunamis of Thailand and Japan have challenged trauma providers. Each one of these disasters presented trauma providers new sets of problems never seen before. The ongoing and complex conflicts in the Middle East (*The Hurt Locker*, *The Lone Survivor*, *Argo*, and *Zero Dark Thirty*) brought explosive devices, rocket-propelled grenades, and suicide bombers that created injuries we have never seen and challenged us to the highest level in terms of prevention and treatment.

Readers in professional fields look at textbooks seeking recipes to handle defined medical or legal problems. The initial intent of this book was to offer recipes to the anesthesiologist for each type of trauma. As all authors describe in this book, no two traumas are alike, most traumas include multiple sites that change the rules for one site. From a clinical research perspective, it is almost impossible to find a cohort of patients that match one another. Simply stated, a consensus of practice is offered in each chapter, but the scientific evidence may not be strong. The massive transfusion protocol in Dr. Dutton's chapter is well subscribed to by clinicians throughout the country with questionable evidence.

We break trauma down into anatomical parts and try to offer consensus. The book starts off with one of the most important topics: assessment of the trauma patient. Dr. Wilson's systematic examination of the patient and gathering of data is the standard approach to the trauma patient (Advanced Trauma Life Support). Dr. Dutton's chapter on blood and blood products is in alignment with the recommendations of American Society of Anesthesiologists. That said, many trauma centers have not adopted these recommendations for complex reasons. My chapter offers a consensus on how to take care of the multitrauma patient. The evidence is strong but goes against the grain of an approach that dates back to the Civil War (Lincoln 2013). There will be many naysayers who will keep to the current paradigm they practice from. Simply stated, trauma providers may not buy into what is now new evidence.

At every national anesthesia meeting, exhibitors demonstrate the latest difficult airway device. Dr. Capan has an international reputation for airway management. This is an area of enormous research and development in devices that deal with the difficult and traumatized airway. It is conceivable that the conventional laryngoscope's life span can now be measured. Dr. Capan fills in any possible deficit in the understanding of the challenging airway in his chapter keeping in mind new ways to assess the bad airway with new devices.

It is difficult to separate the traumatized airway from cervical spine injuries. Dr. Abramowicz, a national expert on neuroanesthesia, links the two while Dr. Frost, a well-known name in the field of anesthesia and brain science, covers the brain and the spinal cord. It would be unusual if an airway trauma did not include the brain and the spinal cord. Dr. Frost offers the newest evidence on the brain, a subject that seems to be waxing and waning each year.

Dr. Wang wrote two crucial chapters on burns. Many level I trauma centers may not take care of severely burned patients. The criteria for a hospital to have a burn center are different from a level I trauma center. It is not unusual that trauma centers do not provide burn skills; I have read it several times to gain another skill that I am missing in my trauma repertoire. It is the largest topic as it makes up what is missing in the anesthesiologist's literature.

There are several chapters, which I call foundation chapters for clinicians, that describe the physiological changes in the body with severe trauma. Dr. Liu et al. have written a comprehensive piece on the physiological derangement of the trauma patient. In his chapter on trauma simulation, civilian trauma systems, Dr. Choi has presented the emerging world of simulation for the clinician so that critical advanced trauma life support steps are not missed during the assessment and initial treatment.

There are three patient populations that get special attention: the pediatric trauma (Dr. Fox), the pregnant (Dr. Fedson-Hack) trauma patient, and the complex geriatric patient, whose number increases (Dr. Alrayshi). In all the three chapters, we see a long stream of patients flowing into the trauma bay. The endless lineup of these three groups of patients makes these chapters a vital and wonderful welcome to this book.

The persistent Middle East wars have exposed anesthesiologists to blast injuries from suicide bombers, rocket-propelled grenades, and a wide array of explosive devices. The medical corps of our armed services have outfitted our soldiers with Kevlar vests, and a medical pack that soldiers wear. Dr. Field's chapter on trauma on the military might be the most compelling in the book as new treatments for severe trauma to the arms and legs are discussed. Dr. Boldt's chapter on microvascular surgery on extremities and wound from war complement Dr. Field's work. These all tie in well with the 2013 Boston Marathon attack when two pressure cookers exploded and killed 3 and wounded over 260 civilians. These events resulted in multiple amputations and leg-sparing operations.

From terrorist blast injuries to motor vehicle accidents to bar fights, facial trauma is almost always involved. Dr. Clebone's comprehensive chapter on facial trauma breaks down a very complex topic into a systematic mode of making a comprehensive diagnosis and its invariable relationship to airway trauma. The chapter moves the anesthesiologist to securing the airway in manners not usually performed, which makes this chapter essential for all members of the trauma team.

Most of our penetrating trauma patients either are inebriated or test positive for an illicit substance like cocaine and heroin. Prescription pain killers, benzodiazepines and countless other possible substances. Dr. Bryson's chapter on substance abuse is enlightening as the initial assessment is masked by these substances. There is a strong link between trauma and this chapter is eye-opening to the clinician. The anesthesiologist must consider the patient as abusing substances until the toxicology screen comes back. Treating for withdrawal must also be considered. The chapter is the most comprehensive I have seen on the subject.

There is rarely a night that a national news station is not reporting on trauma whether from conflict or by accident. Dr. Kaye, a popular name in pain management, addresses pain in his superbly written chapter. There are recipes in his chapter that are evidence based and can be followed.

Dr. Roccaforte ties many of the themes of the book together with Civilian Trauma Systems, Disaster Management and Critical, How do we organize if another large-scale attack hits the United States. How are resources distributed and what is new in critical care for these patients?

The title of the book restates one of the oldest themes in medicine. New evidence asks the clinician to step away from concepts ingrained in their practice and change it. Often, change is made, and new evidence turns out to be false. The reader of this book is asked to step back and consider those clinical changes that may improve their practice. The more the clinicians change their practice, the more likely that the evidence has staying power.

New York, NY   Corey S. Scher

Contents

List of Contributors

Apolonia E. Abramowicz, M.D. Department of Anesthesiology, Montefiore Medical Center, Albert Einstein College of Medicine, New York, NY, USA

Walid Alrayashi, M.D. Department of Anesthesiology, New York University Medical Center, New York, NY, USA

Zarah D. Antongiorgi, M.D. Department of Anesthesiology, UCLA David Geffen School of Medicine, Ronald Reagan UCLA Medical Center, Los Angeles, CA, USA

David W. Boldt, M.D., M.S. Department of Anesthesiology and Critical Care, UCLA David Geffen School of Medicine, Ronald Reagan UCLA Medical Center, Los Angeles, CA, USA

Whitney K. Braddy, M.D. Department of Anesthesiology, Tulane University Medical Center, New Orleans, LA, USA

Ethan O. Bryson, M.D. Department of Anesthesiology and Psychiatry, Icahn School of Medicine at Mount Sinai, New York, NY, USA

Maria Bustillo, M.D. Department of Anesthesiology, Montefiore Medical Center, Albert Einstein College of Medicine, New York, NY, USA

Levon M. Capan, M.D. Department of Anesthesiology, New York University School of Medicine, Bellevue Hospital Center, New York, NY, USA

Mingbing Chen, M.D., Ph.D. Department of Anesthesiology, Wuhan Tongji Hospital, Wuhan, China

Lynn Choi, M.D. Department of Anesthesiology, Bellevue Hospital—NYU, New York, NY, USA

Seth Christian, M.D. Department of Anesthesiology, Tulane University Medical Center, New Orleans, LA, USA

Inca Chui, M.D. Department of Anesthesiology, New York University Langone Medical Center, New York, NY, USA

Anna Clebone, M.D. Department of Anesthesiology and Perioperative Medicine, Case Western Reserve University, University Hospitals, Cleveland, OH, USA

Richard P. Dutton, M.D., M.B.A. Department of Anesthesia and Critical Care, University of Chicago, Chicago, IL, USA

Aaron M. Fields, M.D. Department of Surgery, Tripler Army Medical Center, Honolulu, HI, USA

L. Yvette Fouché-Weber, M.D. Department of Anesthesiology, University of Maryland Shock Trauma Center, Baltimore, MD, USA

Charles J. Fox, M.D. Department of Anesthesiology, LSV–Health–Shreveport, Shreveport, LA, USA

Elizabeth A. M. Frost, M.B., Ch.B., D.R.C.O.G. Department of Anesthesiology, Icahn Medical Center at Mount Sinai, New York, NY, USA

Santiago Gomez, M.D. Department of Anesthesiology, Tulane University Medical Center, New Orleans, LA, USA

Anjali K. Fedson Hack, M.D., Ph.D. New York, NY, USA

Lindsay R. Higgins, M.D., M.P.H., B.S. Department of Anesthesiology, Tulane University, New Orleans, LA, USA

Michael S. Higgins, D.D.S. Department of Anesthesiology, University of Illinois Medical Center, Chicago, IL, USA

Jacob C. Hummel, M.D., M.S.B.S. Department of Anesthesiology, Tulane Hospital, New Orleans, LA, USA

Alan David Kaye, M.D., Ph.D., D.A.B.A., D.A.B.P.M., D.A.B.I.P.P. Department of Anesthesiology, LSU School of Medicine T6M5, New Orleans, LA, USA

Henry Liu, M.D. Department of Anesthesiology, Tulane University Medical Center, New Orleans, LA, USA

Christopher K. Merritt, M.D. Department of Anesthesiology, LSU Health Sciences Center, New Orleans, LA, USA

Sanford M. Miller, M.D. Department of Anesthesiology, Bellevue Hospital Center, New York, NY, USA

J. David Roccaforte, M.D. Department of Anesthesiology, New York University, Bellevue Hospital, New York, NY, USA

Frank Rosinia, M.D. Department of Anesthesiology, Tulane University Medical Center, New Orleans, LA, USA

Orlando J. Salinas, M.D. Department of Anesthesiology, LSU Health Sciences Center, New Orleans, LA, USA

Corey S. Scher, M.D. Department of Anesthesiology, NYU/Bellevue Hospital Center, New York, NY, USA

Moises Sidransky, M.D. Department of Anesthesiology, LSU HSC New Orleans, New Orleans, LA, USA

Juan Tan, M.D., Ph.D. Department of Anesthesiology, Wuhan Tongji Hospital, Wuhan, China

Cynthia Wang, M.D. Department of Anesthesiology, Ronald Reagan UCLA Medical Center, Los Angeles, CA, USA

Chad T. Wilson, M.D., M.P.H. Department of Surgery, New York University School of Medicine, New York, NY, USA

Hong Yan, M.D. Department of Anesthesiology, Wuhan Central Hospital, Wuhan, China

Initial Assessment and Management of the Trauma Patient

Chad T. Wilson and Anna Clebone

On arrival to the hospital, the injured patient requires immediate attention. Severely injured patients often have dramatic presentations, and chaos is apt to ensue among providers if they are not well prepared. A rational and predefined plan for diagnosing and treating the trauma patient is necessary. The standard approach of performing a full history and physical exam, ordering tests, and then providing treatment is not appropriate, as some patients will have succumbed to their injuries during that time. Instead, the initial assessment and management of the trauma patient needs to be expedient, highly ordered, and prioritized to rapidly and reliably diagnose and treat the most immediately life-threatening problems, but also evaluate for occult injuries that could cause major morbidity and mortality if not identified early.

The Advanced Trauma Life Support (ATLS) training program was developed to provide uniformity in the assessment and management of trauma patients. ATLS was first utilized to teach trauma management to rural doctors in the late 1970s [1]. The program was adopted nationally by the American College of Surgeons Committee on Trauma (ACSCOT) in 1980 and has since been taught worldwide and updated to reflect the latest evidence in trauma care [2]. ATLS, now in its 9th edition, is taught to surgeons, emergency medicine physicians, anesthesiologists, nurses, and advanced care providers. This chapter largely reviews the approach taught in ATLS (now in it's 9th edition) [3].

Pre-hospital and Triage

In many communities, information is provided by emergency medical personnel about a trauma patient prior to arrival to the hospital. Pre-hospital notification allows team members to be alerted, including the trauma surgeon, anesthesiologist, nursing team, and radiology and operating room staff. A team meeting can be held, and preparation can be tailored to specific information provided about a patient. For example, pre-hospital notification regarding a patient with a gunshot wound to the chest and labored breathing would prompt the team to prepare and open a chest tube insertion kit. Finally, pre-hospital notification allows the trauma team to put on personal protective equipment (gloves, gowns, and masks) before the patient arrives. A combative patient can expose providers to substantial amounts of bodily fluids, and the incidence of blood-borne

C.T. Wilson, M.D., M.P.H. (✉)
Department of Surgery, New York University School of Medicine, 550 First Avenue, NBV 15s5, New York, NY 10016, USA
e-mail: Chad.wilson@nyumc.org

A. Clebone, M.D.
Department of Anesthesiology and Perioperative Medicine, Case Western Reserve University, University Hospitals, 11100 Euclid Avenue, LKS 5007, Cleveland, OH 44106, USA
e-mail: Anna.Clebone@UHhospitals.org

C.S. Scher (ed.), *Anesthesia for Trauma*, DOI 10.1007/978-1-4939-0909-4_1,
© Springer Science+Business Media New York 2014

Table 1.1 Example of tiered trauma team activation criteria for trauma patient triage

Level 1	*Physiologic criteria:*
	• Impending respiratory failure or intubated
	• Systolic blood pressure $\leq$ 90 mmHg
	– Systolic blood pressure $\leq$ 20 mmHg below age appropriate blood pressure in pediatric patients (age < 15 years)
	• GCS < 10
	• HR > 120
	Anatomic criteria:
	• All penetrating injuries to the head, neck, torso, or extremities proximal to the elbows or knees (excluding minor lacerations)
	• Any penetrating injury with hemodynamic instability
	• Any extremity amputation proximal to the wrist or ankle
	• Crushed, mangled, degloved, or pulseless extremity
	• Pelvic fracture (excluding falls from standing)
	• Two or more long bone fractures
	• Suspected spinal cord injury/paralysis
	• Motor vehicle crash with:
	– Ejection or death of a passenger
	– Intrusion > 12 in. into passenger area
	• Falls > 20 ft (>10 ft or 2 × height in age < 15)
	• Inhalation injury or second- and third-degree burns involving >20 % body surface area
	• Transfers from other hospitals receiving blood
	• Discretion of attending physician or nursing
Level 2	*None of the above, and any of the following:*
	Physiologic criteria:
	• GCS < 13
	• HR 100–120
	Anatomic criteria:
	• Any fall above standing height with loss of consciousness or falls >10 ft
	• Substantial (>20 mph impact) auto-pedestrian, auto-bicycle, motorcycle crash
	• Pregnancy beyond 20 weeks and significant mechanism of injury
	• First- and second-degree burns $\geq$5 % and $\leq$20 % body surface area
	• Discretion of attending physician or nursing
	• Age > 70 years or anticoagulation
Level 3	*None of the above, and any of the following:*
	• Non-emergent consults for trauma not meeting activation criteria
	• Trauma patients with substantial mechanisms being admitted to other services
	• Trauma patients > 24 h
	• Trauma patient transfers not meeting level 1 or 2 criteria

disease is higher in trauma patients than in the general hospital population [4].

Triage of trauma patients is critical to ensure appropriate resource utilization and to decrease morbidity and mortality. When data is available, either pre-hospital or on arrival, patients are typically classified into a three-tiered system of resource utilization, from Level 1 (highest acuity) to Level 3 (lowest acuity) (Table 1.1). Level 1 activation triggers a high resource emergency trauma team reaction, a Level 2 activation results in a moderate resource urgent trauma team response, and Level 3 activation receives a routine trauma team consult. The tiered activations result in greater resources being made available more rapidly when needed. A tiered system of triage and trauma team activation results in better resource utilization and decreased mortality compared to systems where triage triggers do not exist [5].

Triage of trauma patients can occur based on clinical condition, mechanism of injury, age, or comorbid conditions. Clinical criteria such as vital signs, consciousness level, and ventilation assistance are validated as predictive of mortality [6]. A mechanism of injury such as penetrating trauma to the neck or torso justifies a high level of triage even in the presence of normal initial vital signs and mental status. Variation exists in mechanism criteria among trauma centers. For example, a motor vehicle accident would be considered more concerning in a rural trauma center near several major interstate high-speed highways than in an urban setting where driving occurs at lower speeds on congested local streets. Due to their vulnerability, pediatric and elderly patients warrant special consideration during triage. Patients benefit from appropriate triage and prompt evaluation using the ATLS system.

Primary Survey

Every trauma patient is evaluated using the primary survey, a rapid, reproducible physical exam designed to diagnose and treat immediately life-threatening conditions first. All patients are evaluated for physiologic or anatomic derangements that could lead to early mortality and morbidity. Treatment of problems identified during the primary survey begins without delay, before the survey is completed. The sequence of the primary survey can be remembered with the following mnemonic: "A.B.C.D.E."

Airway (Maintain a patent airway with cervical stabilization)

Breathing (Ensure oxygenation and ventilation)

Circulation (Fluid resuscitation and identify and control hemorrhage)

Disability (Identify any gross neurologic deficits)

Exposure/Environment (Undress patient for complete exam, then prevent hypothermia)

Keep in mind that while the primary survey has a clear order to *priority*, the assessment and treatment of problems identified in the primary survey can and should happen in parallel. If an airway problem is identified at the beginning of the survey, and a decision is made to obtain a secure airway for the patient, the rest of the primary survey should continue while the airway is secured. This is accomplished with a team approach to the primary survey, where multiple care providers perform different parts of the primary survey and report to a team leader who "runs the trauma" by coordinating the effort. This team approach reduces resuscitation time significantly (Fig. 1.1) [7].

Full monitoring of the patient, including an electrocardiogram (ECG) if indicated, as well as the administration of oxygen, intravenous fluid, blood products, or medications as warranted should occur in parallel with the primary survey. This can only be accomplished with a team approach to the primary survey.

The elements of the primary survey must be continually reevaluated in a sequential manner due to the fact that a trauma patient's condition can evolve and deteriorate rapidly. This is especially true if at any point a patient is not responding in an expected manner to resuscitation efforts. Consider this scenario: A patient with a head injury secondary to a high fall is intubated on arrival for poor mental status and an inability to protect his airway. Subsequently, the patient was found to have good breath sounds bilaterally with manual ventilation, as well as normal vital signs and circulatory assessment. Ten minutes later, just prior to CT scan, he becomes progressively hypotensive. The astute clinician returns to the primary survey and notes that the endotracheal tube is still in the same position; however, breath sounds are absent on the right side, and new subcutaneous emphysema has appeared over the right chest wall. On closer examination, the patient's neck veins are now distended, and the trachea appears to be shifted to the left. A right-sided chest tube is inserted to relieve a tension pneumothorax that was exacerbated by positive pressure ventilation after intubation. This example highlights the rapid evolution of a trauma patient's condition

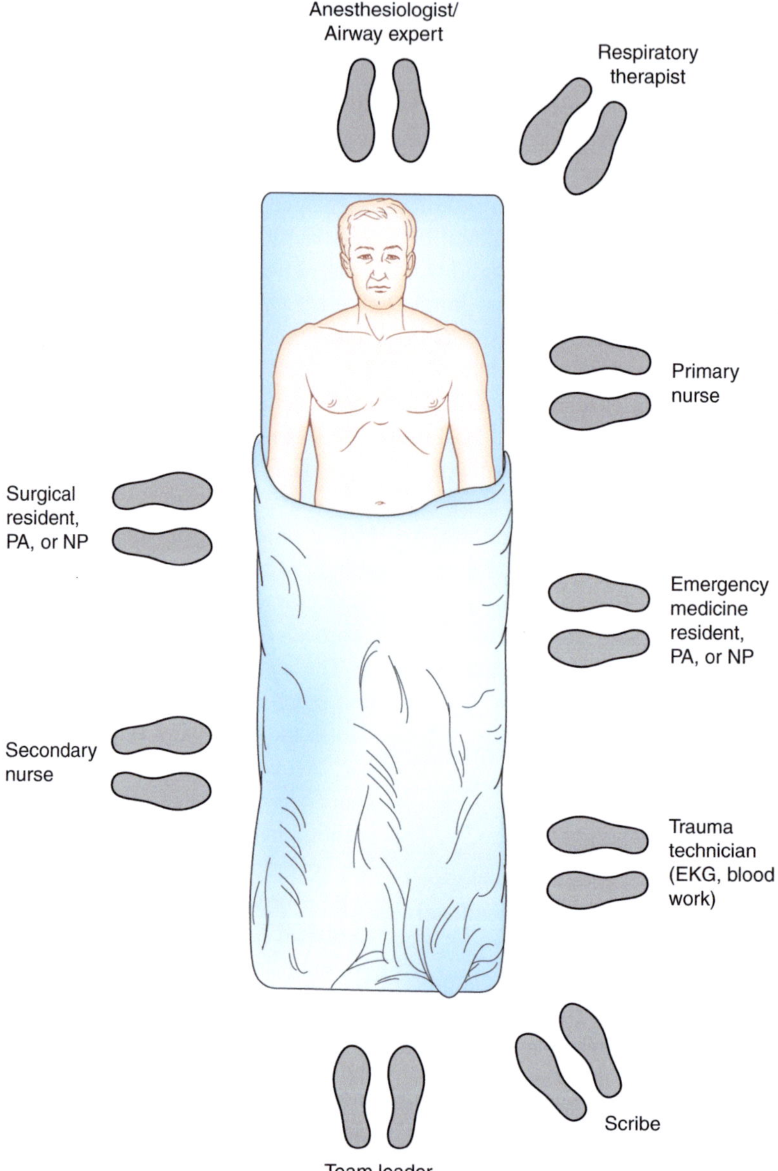

Fig. 1.1 Example of trauma team personnel placement around the bedside of a trauma patient

and the importance of returning to "A, B, C, D, and E" repeatedly during initial management.

Airway

The first priority in the primary survey of the trauma patient is a rapid, but accurate assessment of the airway. Typically, little information is available about a patient's medical history and previous airway management. Trauma patients may have unstable cervical-spine injuries that cannot be immediately evaluated. As a result, any manipulation of the cervical spine may be unsafe. Tilting the head into "sniffing position" to improve airway patency is therefore often contraindicated. Considering the often spectacular presentation of the most severely injured patients, typically with an unknown medical history, occult injuries, and little time to establish an airway (all while maintaining cervical spine precautions), managing the airway in the trauma patient presents a challenge which requires a specialized skill set.

Some patients will arrive with an advanced airway placed in the field, which may be an endotracheal tube, supraglottic airway (such as a laryngeal mask airway "LMA"), or duel lumen esophageal tube (Combitube™). It is paramount that this airway be assessed by confirming position, effective ventilation, and adequate airway protection. A supraglottic airway or dual lumen esophageal tube is less secure than an endotracheal tube, and possibly ineffective with regard to ventilation and airway protection. In some cases, an airway placed in the pre-hospital setting will need to be replaced with an endotracheal tube, depending on the provider's assessment of the situation and accompanying risks and benefits.

In the conscious trauma patient, the best means of assessment is to simply ask, "what is your name?" A response given in a normal voice is indicative of a currently intact airway. If the patient is unable to speak, or his or her voice sounds altered, then airway compromise may be present, and more investigation is warranted. Keep in mind that some patients are unable to verbalize for reasons unrelated to airway compromise, such as a language barrier, mental disability, or psychiatric illness. Additionally, some injuries, such as burns, cause progressive airway swelling which can lead to progressive airway compromise even in the presence of an initially normal exam.

In an apparently unconscious or severely intoxicated patient, assessment of the airway starts with a chin lift and jaw thrust to open the pharynx while avoiding manipulation of the cervical spine. The oropharynx should then be examined and cleared of blood, vomitus, and debris by suctioning. A patient who responds vigorously to attempted suctioning may be able to protect his or her own airway. If obstruction is relieved via these simple maneuvers and airway protection is intact, an advanced airway may not be required, and supplemental high flow oxygen via face mask should be provided. In contrast, patients with obvious hoarseness, stridor, retractions, or respiratory distress may need further airway management, and patients with a Glasgow Coma Score of less than 8 or persistent airway obstruction require endotracheal intubation or a surgical airway.

Rapid sequence induction (RSI) and intubation with a cuffed endotracheal tube is the most commonly employed method of securing an advanced airway in a trauma patient. The goal of RSI is to decrease the risk of aspiration. The time between complete loss of airway reflexes and obtaining a secured airway is minimized by simultaneously administering a fast acting sedative/hypnotic agent and a muscle relaxant. When possible, bag mask ventilation is not performed due to the potential for insufflating the stomach and causing aspiration of gastric contents. The benefits of an RSI must be balanced with the risks. In a patient who may be difficult to mask ventilate or intubate, securing the airway after applying topical local anesthetics and using minimal sedation (an "awake intubation") is indicated. Hypotensive patients may not tolerate the loss of sympathetic tone and myocardial depression that accompanies the administration of sedative/hypnotic medications. Comatose patients often do not require additional sedation for laryngoscopy to be performed. In patients with head and neck trauma, visualization of the glottis and establishment of an airway may be impossible via direct laryngoscopy, and use of a specialized device such as a fiberoptic bronchoscope, video laryngoscope, or rigid bronchoscope or emergent placement of a surgical airway such as a tracheostomy or cricothyroidotomy may be necessary. An alternate plan for ventilation should exist for cases in which direct laryngoscopy fails. Agents for blood pressure support should be immediately available.

In the trauma patient, coexisting injuries must be considered. Importantly, cervical spine precautions must be maintained at all times. This is usually accomplished by placing the patient in a rigid cervical collar during or prior to the initial assessment. This collar is often removed for airway management to provide room for mouth opening during laryngoscopy. When this collar is off of the patient, an individual must be assigned to maintain manual in-line cervical immobilization at all times until the airway is secured and the collar is replaced.

Breathing

Next, the patient's breathing, ventilation, and oxygenation should be assessed, and any life-threatening derangements must be treated. Physical exam, pulse oximetry, and continuous end-tidal carbon dioxide monitoring should be used. Inspection involves noting if breathing is comfortable or labored. Hypoxia can be a cause of confusion and combativeness in a patient. The patient's color is noted (normal, cyanotic, or pale) and the chest wall is observed for normal motion. The chest should be palpated for unstable segments and crepitus. Finally, bilateral auscultation should be performed to determine the presence, symmetry, and quality of breath sounds. Diminished or absent breath sounds on one side is a cause for concern. If the patient is unstable in any way, intervention is warranted emergently.

The most common interventions performed during the primary survey to support breathing are supplemental oxygen delivery, assisted or mechanical ventilation, and tube thoracostomy or chest tube insertion. Supplemental oxygen by face mask is used liberally during the primary survey in spontaneously breathing patients until normal oxygenation can be ensured. Common causes of hypoxic respiratory insufficiency in trauma patients are pulmonary contusion and aspiration pneumonitis. A patient who is hypoventilating can be assisted by bag mask if the patient is able to maintain airway protection. Common causes of impaired ventilation in trauma patients are rib fractures/flail chest, intoxication/drug overdose, and severe head injury. A more definitive airway may be needed in those patients with more profound hypoxic or hypoventilatory respiratory failure. Tube thoracostomy is indicated in patients with decreased or absent breath sounds and hypotension or severe respiratory distress due to a hemothorax or tension pneumothorax.

A hemothorax is the accumulation of blood in the pleural cavity around the lung, which can occur in either blunt or penetrating trauma. The diagnosis is suspected in a patient with diminished or absent breath sounds. In the stable patient, the presence of a hemothorax may be confirmed with a portable chest radiograph. For the patient in distress, a large bore (at least 28 French) chest tube is inserted on the side with diminished breath sounds. Hemodynamic instability or massive hemothorax (an output of greater than 1,500 cm^3 of blood from the chest, less in small or pediatric patients) are indications for an operative exploration to control the source of bleeding. In addition to being diagnostic, chest tube insertion is therapeutic via improving ventilation, relieving tension, and collecting blood that can be autotransfused. Autotransfusion of filtered blood in trauma patients can be a safe alternative to transfusing banked blood [8]; however, filtered blood is inherently depleted of clotting factors and platelets, which may also need to be replaced [9].

A pneumothorax is the presence of air in the pleural cavity around the lung, which can also occur in both blunt and penetrating trauma. The diagnosis and symptoms can be subtle on physical exam if the pneumothorax is small and is often only revealed on chest radiograph or computed tomography scan. Of greatest concern during the primary survey is the presence of a *tension* pneumothorax. Air under pressure in the pleural cavity causes the mediastinum and its contents to shift away from the ipsilateral side of injury towards the contra-lateral side of lower pressure. This can be immediately life-threatening by causing obstruction of venous return to the heart and cardiovascular collapse. While the diagnosis of small (or occult) pneumothorax is difficult on physical exam, the diagnosis of tension pneumothorax should be able to be made at the bedside without imaging. If a patient is experiencing acute respiratory failure or hemodynamic instability with hypotension and has unilateral diminished breath sounds, one should strongly suspect a tension pneumothorax, and a chest tube should be placed immediately to alleviate the pressure. Other physical exam findings that are suggestive of tension pneumothorax are distended neck veins, subcutaneous emphysema, and tracheal deviation. If a chest tube cannot be safely placed in an expeditious manner, needle thoracostomy is an acceptable alternative, which is performed by inserting an angiocatheter (usually 14 gauge) between the ribs, into the second intercostal space in the mid clavicular line. Although technically simple, needle thoracostomy can cause a puncture of the lung or laceration of a blood vessel (such as the internal mammary artery), therefore it should only be employed in an emergency situation.

An open pneumothorax ("sucking chest wound") is an injury to the chest wall that communicates freely with the pleural space. Inspiration generates negative pressure, pulling air into the pleural space through the wound, potentially causing lung collapse and acute respiratory failure. The definitive treatment is tube thoracostomy (a "chest tube") and repair/dressing of the wound. If a chest tube is not available, however, an alternate treatment is to place a partially occlusive dressing over the wound. The goal of the partial occlusion is to achieve a one-way valve to avoid pulling in air through the wound while allowing an opening for pressure to be relieved, in order to decrease the risk of a tension pneumothorax. This is classically achieved by taping the dressing on three sides to hold the dressing over the wound, but leaving the fourth side free so that air can escape from that side of the dressing (Fig. 1.2).

Circulation

After addressing the highest priorities in the primary survey (airway and breathing), circulation must be assessed to determine the presence or absence of shock. Shock is defined as inadequate organ perfusion and tissue oxygenation. In the trauma patient, shock is assumed to be hypovolemic/hemorrhagic and

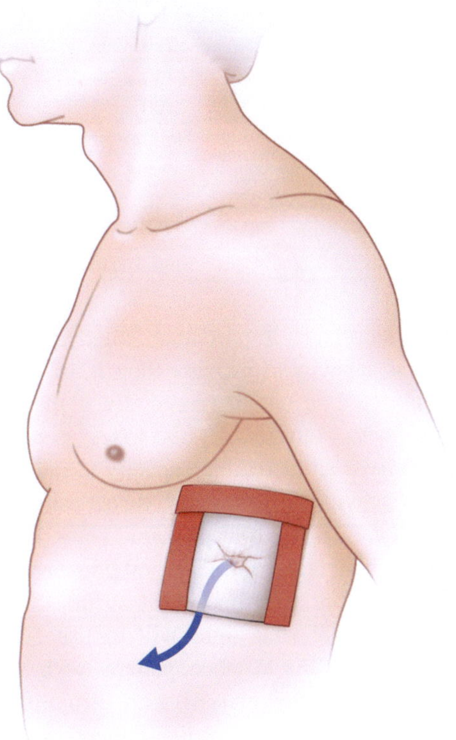

Fig. 1.2 Partially occlusive dressing (taped on three sides only) for open pneumothorax functions as a one-way valve, to relieve any tension, but not allow air to be sucked into the wound

resuscitation begins as soon as vascular access can be obtained. The possibility of neurogenic shock (e.g., spinal cord injury) or cardiogenic shock (e.g., pericardial tamponade) should also be considered. The focus of this segment of the primary survey should be assessing for the presence of shock, determining the cause (usually blood loss) and beginning resuscitation.

Assessment of shock begins with performing a physical exam and evaluating a patient's vital signs. Patients with hemorrhagic shock typically develop derangements in their blood pressure and heart rate that are proportional to the amount of blood loss and degree of shock (Table 1.2). Hemorrhage will lead to a decreased preload, which triggers a compensatory increase in heart rate to maintain cardiac output. Blood pressure will fall as hypovolemia worsens. These changes

Table 1.2 Classes of hemorrhagic shock by ATLS designation for a 70 kg patient [3]

	Class 1	Class 2	Class 3	Class 4
Blood loss (mL)	<750	750–1,500	1,500–2,000	>2,000
Blood loss (%)	<15	15–30	30–40	>40
Heart rate (bpm)	<100	>100	>120	>140
Systolic blood pressure	Normal	Normal	Decreased	Decreased
Pulse pressure	Normal	Decreased	Decreased	Decreased
Respiratory rate (resp/min)	14–20	20–30	30–40	>35
Urine output (mL/h)	>30	20–30	5–15	Negligible
Mental status	Slightly anxious	Mildly anxious	Anxious/confused	Confused/lethargic

vary based on age. In particular, elderly patients have less capacity to increase their heart rate to maintain cardiac output (especially if they are taking beta blockers). Likewise, pediatric patients have an incredible capacity to maintain blood pressure through vasoconstriction. Children can suffer from profound hemorrhagic shock but maintain a normal blood pressure until moments before a cardiac arrest occurs. Sometimes, abnormal vital signs will indicate other types of shock. For instance, patients with blunt cardiac injury may present with arrhythmias, heart block, and bradycardia. Patients with a high spinal cord injury may present with a low heart rate (cardiac accelerator fibers are present from T1 to T4), but may simultaneously suffer from severe neurogenic shock resulting in the vasodilation of peripheral blood vessels.

Signs of poor perfusion include a weak pulse, cool or clammy extremities, dry mucus membranes, pale skin, and confusion. A normal mental status exam confirms the presence of acceptable cerebral perfusion.

In addition to serving as an assessment for the presence of shock, the physical exam can also reveal etiology. A tension pneumothorax or hemothorax, found in a patient with absent unilateral breath sounds, could explain poor perfusion. Abdominal distension, pelvic instability, and long bone deformities can be associated with blood loss. The presence of lacerations and wounds (especially gunshot wounds) should be noted, and if active bleeding is present it should be controlled with direct digital pressure, a proximal tourniquet, stapling, or clips (Raney clips are especially useful for scalp lacerations).

Rapidly diagnosing the source of blood loss in a trauma patient is critical for hemorrhage control and should be done in conjunction with the most skilled member of the trauma team.

Resuscitation of the trauma patient should begin as early as possible and often occurs in the pre-hospital setting. The first priority is to obtain vascular access. The standard of care is the rapid placement of two large bore intravenous (IV) lines in the upper extremities. If this cannot be performed in an expeditious manner, alternate vascular access such as an intraosseous (IO) line or central line placement should be performed. In the past, IO lines were used only in pediatric patients, but new designs and insertion devices have made IO access a viable option in adult patients. IO lines can be comparable to central access in the care of trauma patients [10]. The location of intravascular access should be dictated by injuries and suspected sites of blood loss, and severely traumatized extremities should not be used for IV sites when possible. In general, patients with a suspected injury below the diaphragm such as a liver laceration or pelvic fracture benefit from vascular access above the diaphragm (such as an upper extremity peripheral IV, subclavian/internal jugular central line, or humerus/sternal IO line). Similarly, patients with trauma above the diaphragm such as a slash wound to the neck should be provided access below the diaphragm such as femoral central line or a tibial IO line.

In a patient who may be hypoperfused, resuscitation with crystalloid fluids (or blood products in severe cases) should begin immediately after vascular access is obtained. ATLS recommends starting with an initial bolus of 1–2 L of warmed isotonic IV fluids in adults or 20 mL/kg in pediatric patients [3]. If a patient becomes hemodynamically stable following this bolus and hemorrhage control is obtained, then this may be the only fluid resuscitation that is needed. However, a patient who remains hypotensive after this intervention, or has only a transient response, requires further resuscitation utilizing blood products. Cross-matched and screened blood products are preferred, however, in urgent cases. O negative blood may be used while the team is waiting for type specific blood to arrive.

The goal of resuscitation is to maintain tissue perfusion and homeostasis. Over resuscitation (in particular with isotonic fluids) can lead to complications of volume overload. Aggressive efforts must be made to preserve homeostasis during resuscitation with particular attention paid to the avoidance of hypothermia, acidosis, and coagulopathy, the so-called "triad of death." In particular, coagulopathy can be caused by the simultaneous consumption and dilution (with IV fluids) of platelets and clotting factors. Deliberate attention must be focused on making blood products available in large amounts and ensuring that packed red blood cells, plasma, and platelets are transfused in an appropriate ratio. Most trauma centers employ a massive transfusion protocol (MTP) to be instituted for those trauma patients who require the rapid administration of large amounts of blood products [11]. Recently, substantial literature has supported transfusion of a high ratio of FFP and platelets to packed red blood cells [12, 13], and the components of the MTP have evolved accordingly [14]. While the ideal ratio of plasma and platelets to packed red blood cells, as well as the use of other pro-coagulants is often debated, the mainstay of treatment for hemorrhagic shock continues to be fluid resuscitation with warm crystalloid fluids followed by blood products, and immediate localization and source control of bleeding.

Table 1.3 Glasgow Coma Scale scoring system

Eye opening (E)
• 4 = spontaneous
• 3 = to voice
• 2 = to pain
• 1 = none
Verbal response (V)
• 5 = normal conversation
• 4 = disoriented conversation
• 3 = words, but not coherent
• 2 = no words, only sounds
• 1 = none
Motor response (M)
• 6 = normal
• 5 = localized to pain
• 4 = withdraws to pain
• 3 = decorticate posture
• 2 = decerebrate posture
• 1 = none

The score in each section is added for a cumulative score of 3–15:

- GCS 3–8: severely depressed consciousness
- GCS 9–12: moderately depressed consciousness
- GCS 13–15: normal to mildly depressed consciousness

Disability

Once airway, breathing, and circulation are addressed in the primary survey, the next priority is to assess disability. The primary focus is on rapidly determining a patient's mental status and neurologic function via physical exam.

The Glasgow Coma Scale (GCS) is a rapid and reliable way to quantify a patient's level of consciousness (Table 1.3) [15]. The GCS score allows for quick communication among clinicians about a patient's current mental status and can be important for decision-making.

The neurologic assessment also includes an examination of the cranial nerves, pupils, and sensory and motor function. If there is an obvious extremity deformity or wound, the clinician should document gross neurologic and vascular function distal to the injury prior to any manipulation, wound exploration, or tourniquet application. For severely deformed limbs with obvious underlying fractures, a gross reduction should be performed to approximate more normal alignment (if tolerated by the patient), which will often result in improved perfusion of the limb.

One serious disorder that will be diagnosed and treated during the disability segment of the primary survey is intracranial hypertension. Signs of intracranial hypertension include an abnormal GCS, a unilaterally blown pupil, and Cushing's triad (bradycardia, hypertension, and abnormal respiratory variation) in a patient with a suspected head injury. Mild hyperventilation is a temporary way to control elevated intracranial pressure (ICP), with a goal pCO_2 of 30–35 mmHg. Deep sedation is also helpful, but may obscure the clinician's ability to assess the patient. All patients suspected of having an elevated ICP should be considered for hyperosmolar therapy until neurosurgical assessment and intervention can be performed. Hyperosmolar therapy consists of either a bolus of 23.4 % hypertonic saline (0.5 mL/kg) or the administration of mannitol (1 g/kg). Note that mannitol can precipitate hypotension, so it should be administered carefully, and its use may necessitate subsequent resuscitation with isotonic crystalloid.

Exposure/Environment

Exposure and environment are the final components of the primary survey. While lowest in priority, they are still vital to the successful management of the trauma patient. The patient should be completely exposed (all clothing removed) so that injuries can be fully assessed. Decontamination may also be needed, depending on the nature of the trauma. Protection from hypothermia and continuous temperature monitoring are essential. Warm resuscitation fluids should be given. The patient should be covered with warm blankets or a forced-air warming device (e.g. Bair Hugger), and the temperature in the resuscitation area should be warm. If the patient is wet, he or she should be dried immediately. Critically injured patients with hypothermia may require more aggressive methods of rewarming, such as warm lavage of body cavities (e.g., pleural, peritoneal, and bladder lavage), warming/cooling catheters, and/or extracorporeal blood warming (e.g. venovenous cardiopulmonary bypass) [16].

Reevaluation

Frequent reevaluation should be the rule for trauma patients, even after all five components of the primary survey have been addressed. For some patients the primary survey will need to be completed multiple times. For the critically ill, it is often helpful to repeat the primary survey every time the patient is transferred to a new area of care (e.g., from the emergency department to the intensive care unit). The physiology of the trauma patient is dynamic as injuries may evolve during the assessment. If at any point, the patient begins to respond in a way not consistent with the initial primary survey, then the primary survey should be repeated quickly to assess if a new, immediately life-threatening situation has arisen.

Adjuncts to the Primary Survey

Monitoring

While not explicitly a part of the primary survey, monitors should be placed on the patient to facilitate assessment as soon as possible. Continuous monitoring of cardiac rhythm is helpful to quickly detect changes in heart rate as well as arrhythmias. Continuous O_2 saturation and continuous end-tidal CO_2 monitoring are essential to remain vigilant about changes in the respiratory status of a patient. Automatic noninvasive blood pressure measurements can alert the trauma team to trends or sudden changes in blood pressure. In some patients with hemodynamic variability, a more invasive monitor will be needed such as an arterial line to monitor blood pressure continuously. Monitoring central venous pressure or pulmonary artery pressure can be a useful adjunct to managing complex trauma patients, especially those with known cardiac disease or suspected cardiac injury.

Imaging

In most trauma centers, rapid portable X-rays are available in the emergency department. X-rays are only adjuncts to the primary survey, but can be very helpful in identifying problems that may impact the primary survey. Most commonly, a portable chest radiograph is performed in the resuscitation area of the emergency department. Chest radiography can confirm the position of an advanced airway, as well as diagnose pneumo-thorax, hemothorax, pulmonary contusion, aspiration, and broken ribs, all common diagnoses which are important to identify early. Blunt trauma patients often benefit from a portable pelvic plain film. The presence of a pelvic fracture can explain occult blood loss in a hemodynamically unstable patient. Patients with penetrating trauma, especially from a projectile, also can benefit from a plain film to localize the presence of any foreign bodies and guide interventions.

Ultrasound has an important role as an adjunct to the primary survey in localizing occult hemor-rhage. In particular, the Focused Assessment Sonography in Trauma (FAST) exam is used to rapidly and reliably identify free fluid in the peritoneum or fluid around the heart. The FAST Exam is a bedside sonographic exam that utilizes four views or "windows." Three abdominal views examine the perihepatic space, the perisplenic space, and the pelvis. The fourth view looks for fluid in the pericardium. For example, in a hemodynamically unstable patient, the FAST exam can quickly identify intra-abdominal hemorrhage as the likely source of bleeding and alert the trauma team that the patient should be transferred to the operating room expeditiously for laparotomy and hemor-rhage control [17]. Likewise, a positive

pericardial view (especially in a patient with penetrating trauma to the chest) can alert the surgeon that exploration of the chest may be needed [18]. The FAST exam has become the modality of choice to assess the unstable trauma patient and has supplanted diagnostic peritoneal lavage (DPL) as a noninvasive way to look for intra-abdominal hemorrhage [19]. DPL should be used when ultrasound is unavailable, the FAST is equivocal, or a patient has unexplained profound hypotension despite a negative FAST exam.

Computed tomography (CT) is a useful tool in the management of trauma patients, due to the fact that it is more sensitive and specific for most anatomic injury patterns than plain films or ultrasound. In particular, for head injury, CT scan is the primary modality used to guide intervention. For the unstable patient, however, a CT scan can be unsafe due to the time required for the scan, as well as the relatively uncontrolled environment that occurs during transportation and within the scanner. The barriers to obtaining a CT scan expediently and safely vary greatly between institutions, but the general rule is that only patients with a stable airway, good oxygenation and ventilation (mechanical or spontaneous), and hemodynamic stability should receive a CT scan. If a patient becomes unstable in the CT scanner, the team should reevaluate according to the primary survey paradigm and consider abandoning the study if the patient cannot be stabilized.

Laboratory

While laboratory studies are not considered to be an integral component of the primary survey, they can often serve as useful adjuncts. During resuscitation, an arterial blood gas measurement is performed to assess oxygenation, ventilation, and pH. Often, rapid arterial blood gas results are used for close monitoring and to help establish an end point for resuscitation. Venous blood samples are usually obtained during the primary survey, while IV access is being obtained. Importantly, a "type and screen" must be sent to establish blood type and screen for antibodies to red blood cells. A complete blood count and coagulation studies are especially important in patients who are anemic or anticoagulated. A pregnancy test should be performed in any woman of child-bearing age. Toxicology studies are also helpful in any patient with altered mental status. In patients with abdominal or pelvic trauma, a urinalysis should be checked for hematuria. Blood sugar and other chemistries are also important, especially in patients with unexplained altered mental status.

Tubes

A clinician must be particularly cautious when placing a urinary catheter in a patient with a pelvic fracture (especially in a male patient) or penetrating trauma near the pelvis and perineum. This is particularly true when there is concomitant gross hematuria or blood at the urethral meatus.

Gastric tubes are helpful adjuncts in patients who are mechanically ventilated, to decompress the stomach and decrease the risk of aspiration of stomach contents. After confirmation of correct positioning of the gastric tube, medication and later enteral nutrition can be delivered. In a patient with a complex facial or basilar skull fracture, a nasogastric tube could inadvertently be passed through the fracture site and into the intracranial space. An orogastric tube is a safer alternative until the presence of these types of injuries can be excluded.

Secondary Survey

Next, attention is turned to the secondary survey, whose purpose is to characterize injuries and uncover any occult injuries that did not require immediate attention during the primary survey. In practice, the secondary survey often begins while the primary survey is still being completed. The primary survey, however, should never be interrupted by the secondary survey. Additionally, at any time, a change in the status of the patient may necessitate a return to the primary survey.

History

In the conscious individual, a history can be obtained directly; however, in a severely incapacitated trauma patient, this information must be acquired from pre-hospital personnel, witnesses, and friends or family members. Due to the time-sensitive nature of treatment, a concise history is gathered utilizing the mnemonic AMPLE:
Allergies
Medications
Past medical problems and surgery
Last Meal
Events related to the Injury

In some cases, this information will be obtained from items in the patient's belongings such as medical bracelets, medication bottles, or medical/insurance wallet cards. Pre-hospital personnel may have spoken to witnesses of the traumatic event and can give information about the patient's status in the field and treatment delivered. Taking a trauma history is skill that improves with experience. As a provider sees certain patterns of injury repeatedly, history taking will become tailored for those circumstances. For example, inquiries should be made as to tetanus status in patients with lacerations or abrasions, helmet use in motorcyclists, and weapons and ballistics in patients with gunshot wounds.

Physical Exam

The secondary survey should include a careful "head to toe" physical exam. Remember that the primary survey is focused on an assessment for immediately life-threatening problems, and the secondary survey is used to uncover occult injuries that might have substantial morbidity and mortality if missed. The physical exam will guide the diagnostic and therapeutic approach to be undertaken during the critical hours after the initial resuscitation and assessment, therefore ensuring that the problems with greatest priority are addressed most expeditiously.

Neurologic assessment in the primary survey focuses on the level of consciousness (Glasgow Coma Score and gross neurologic function). The secondary survey goes into greater detail. For instance, in a conscious patient with a GCS of 15, it may be important to assess the level of orientation or confusion. More subtle deficits might be found with a mini-mental exam, for example, when attempting to determine if a patient can safely be discharged after a concussion. Other parts of the neurologic assessment that occur during the secondary survey include cranial nerve assessment, rectal tone, reflexes, and coordination. In addition, obvious injuries should elicit a careful neurologic assessment. For instance, cranial nerve VII will be checked carefully in a patient with a deep facial laceration. Likewise, a complete neurologic and functional examination of the hand should be performed in a patient with a wrist deformity or fracture.

The head, scalp, and face require careful attention on the secondary survey. Ongoing blood loss from a scalp laceration can be hidden in long hair. The skull should be palpated for discontinuities, "step-offs", or other signs of fracture. Rhinorrhea, hemotympanum, raccoon's eyes (bruising around the eyes), or Battle's sign (blood over the mastoid process) are suggestive of basilar skull fracture and should be noted during the secondary survey. Facial lacerations and fractures are common in trauma, can be quite disfiguring, and often impact long-term function. An unstable midfacial area or maxilla are physical exam signs that may help diagnose a LeFort fracture prior to imaging studies. The presence of malocclusion or difficulties in mouth opening should be noted and are especially relevant in cases in which a patient later needs an advanced airway.

The neck receives special attention in trauma patients. Patients usually arrive in the emergency room with a rigid cervical collar in place. For the neck exam, this collar should be removed while the spine is held in an immobilized position. In particular, tracheal deviation, neck hematomas, bruits, subcutaneous emphysema, lacerations, and gunshot wounds should be considered carefully. If the cervical spine collar is interfering with the ability to care for obvious neck injuries, it should not be used, and an individual should hold the spine in alignment until these injuries are stabilized and the collar can be replaced.

The chest, abdominal, back, and genital exams should be performed more carefully during the secondary survey. Chest wall point tenderness, rales, and wheezing may be found. Abdominal tenderness, especially in patients with penetrating trauma, is an indication for urgent surgical exploration. The back exam is performed with the patient's spine in stable alignment using the "log roll" maneuver. The clinician should look for any additional penetrating wounds to the back or axillae. In men, the genitalia are examined to look for gross blood at the urethral meatus, priapism, or degloving injuries. In women, blood at the vaginal introitus and any lacerations to the perineum should be noted.

Extremities should be inspected for deformity and color and palpated for point tenderness, instability, or crepitus. All limbs should be moved throughout their range of motion to assess for mobility or laxity in the joints. A peripheral vascular and neurologic evaluation of the extremity should be carefully performed when an injury is found.

Disposition from the Trauma Resuscitation Area

The amount of time a patient initially spends in the emergency department resuscitation area can vary greatly. Some patients will be whisked away to the operating room for treatment of life-threatening injuries after mere seconds. Others may require more than an hour of resuscitation, reevaluation, and intervention. The care of every patient begins with the primary survey. If life-threatening injuries are encountered that can only be managed elsewhere, such as the operating room or angiography suite, then the primary survey will continue until that life-threatening problem is addressed. The primary survey is not complete until the patient is stabilized. Most trauma patients will receive a complete primary survey and secondary survey before being transferred from the resuscitation area. Commonly, patients will be transferred to one of the following destinations: radiology (CT scan, MRI), intensive care unit, inpatient unit, procedure/treatment room (operating room, angiography, endoscopy), or to a less acute section of the emergency department for observation and possible discharge to home. It is important that patients are monitored appropriately and that the new care team receives adequate information as part of transfer. Oftentimes, a nurse, respiratory therapist, physician, and transport personnel will accompany the patient to the next level of care (e.g., the ICU). Vigilance is key. A suicidal patient may have an unremarkable primary and secondary survey, but will need careful monitoring for elopement or self-injury. Evolution of a trauma patient's condition can be quick and occur in the hours after the patient's initial assessment. For example, a patient with a delayed hemorrhage will deteriorate over the next several hours, even in the presence of initially normal vital signs. The clinician should have a low threshold to return to the primary survey if anything unexpected occurs. Good care of the trauma patient means going "back to the ABCs" as many times as it takes until the patient is truly stable.

References

1. Collicott PE, Hughes I. Training in advanced trauma life support. JAMA. 1980;243(11):1156–9.
2. Collicott PE. Advanced Trauma Life Support (ATLS): past, present, future–16th Stone Lecture, American Trauma Society. J Trauma. 1992;33(5):749–53.
3. Advance trauma life support student course manual. 9th ed. American College of Surgeons Committee on Trauma. 2012.
4. Weiss ES, Cornell III EE, Wang T, et al. Human immunodeficiency virus and hepatitis testing and prevalence among surgical patients in an urban university hospital. Am J Surg. 2007;193(1):55–60.
5. Petrie D, Lane P, Stewart TC. An evaluation of patient outcomes comparing trauma team activated versus trauma team not activated using TRISS analysis. Trauma and Injury Severity Score. J Trauma. 1996;41(5):870–3.
6. Purtill MA, Benedict K, Hernandez-Boussard T, et al. Validatin of a prehospital triage tool: a 10-year perspective. J Trauma. 2008;65(6):1253–7.
7. Driscoll PA, Vincent CA. Organizing an efficient trauma team. Injury. 1992;23(2):107–10.
8. Sinclair A, Jacobs Jr LM. Emergency department autotransfusion for trauma victims. Med Instrum. 1982;16(6):283–6.
9. Broadie TA, Glover JL, Bang N, et al. Clotting competency of intracavitary blood in trauma victims. Ann Emerg Med. 1981;10(3):127–30.
10. Leidel BA, Kirchhoff C, Bogner V, et al. IS the intraosseous access route fast and efficacious compared to conventional central venous catheterization in adult patients under resuscitation in the emergency department? A prospective observational pilot study. Patient Saf Surg. 2009;3(1):24.
11. Fraga GP, Banal V, Coimbra R. Transfusion of blood products in trauma: an update. J Emerg Med. 2010;39:253–60.
12. Borgman MA, Spinella PC, Perkins JG, et al. The ratio of blood products transfused affects mortality in patients receiving massive transfusions at a combat support hospital. J Trauma. 2007;63(4):805–13.
13. Texeira PG, Inaba K, Shulman I, et al. Impact of plasma transfusion in massively transfused trauma patients. J Trauma. 2009;66(3):693–7.
14. Riskin DJ, Tsai TC, Riskin L, et al. Massive transfusion protocols: the role of aggressive resuscitation versus product ratio in mortality reduction. J Am Coll Surg. 2009;209(2):198–205.
15. Teasdale G, Jennett B. Assessment and prognosis of coma after head injury. Acta Neurochir. 1976;34 (1–4):45–55.
16. Gentellio LM, Jurkovich GJ, Stark MS, et al. Is hypothermia in the victim of major trauma protective or harmful? A randomized, prospective study. Ann Surg. 1997;226(4):439–49.
17. Liu M, Lee CH, P'eng FK. Prospective comparison of diagnostic peritoneal lavage, computed tomographic scanning and ultrasonography for the diagnosis of blunt abdominal trauma. J Trauma. 1993;35 (2):267–70.
18. Rozycki GS, Feliciano DV, Ochner MG, et al. The role of ultrasound in patients with possible penetrating cardiac wounds: a prospective multicenter study. J Trauma. 1999;46(4):543–52.
19. Rozycki GS, Shackford SR. Ultrasound, what every trauma surgeon should know. J Trauma. 1996;40(1):1–4.

Levon M. Capan and Sanford M. Miller

Ultimately, the goal of airway management in trauma is to establish and/or maintain adequate oxygenation, ventilation, and airway protection. It is the first priority in the acute phase of care of the trauma patient and consists of evaluation and, when indicated, intervention using various techniques and devices. It involves the recognition of any trauma to the airway or surrounding tissues, anticipation of their respiratory consequences, and planning and application of management, keeping in mind the potential for exacerbation of existing airway or other injuries by the contemplated strategies. It also involves prediction and prevention of progression of airway or surrounding tissue injury with increasing airway compromise.

Although with certain modifications, the American Society of Anesthesiologists (ASA) difficult airway algorithm can be applied to various trauma-induced airway issues [1], it may not be applicable in some clinical scenarios. For example, cancellation of airway management when difficulty arises may not be an option in the acute trauma setting. Likewise, awake rather than asleep intubation or a surgical airway from the outset may be the preferred choice in some situations. Modifications of the ASA difficult airway algorithm are available for various trauma-induced clinical situations [2].

Frequently Encountered Clinical Conditions

Full Stomach

Commonly, the unknown time of the last food intake, the frequent presence of alcohol and/or illicit drugs, and trauma-induced reduction or absence of gastrointestinal motility imply that almost all acute trauma victims have a full stomach and are at risk for pulmonary aspiration. Pharyngeal blood, secretions, and foreign bodies in some maxillofacial and neck injuries are additional factors for aspiration after trauma. It is generally considered, although without much proof, that at least 24 h are needed after injury to decrease the risk of aspiration from a full stomach. In most instances, the urgency of securing the airway does not permit adequate time for pharmacologic measures such as bicarbonate or H_2 blockers to reduce gastric volume and acidity, and indeed these agents may be unreliable. Thus, rather than depending on pharmacology, emphasis should be placed on selection of a safe technique for securing the airway when necessary. Rapid-sequence induction (RSI) is recommended for those patients without serious airway problems. Awake intubation, with sedation and topical anesthesia, if possible, should be performed in

L.M. Capan, M.D. (✉) • S.M. Miller, M.D.
Department of Anesthesiology, NYU School of Medicine, Bellevue Hospital Center, 550 First Avenue, New York, NY 10016, USA
e-mail: levon.capan@nymuc.org;
Sanford.miller@nyumc.org

C.S. Scher (ed.), *Anesthesia for Trauma*, DOI 10.1007/978-1-4939-0909-4_2,
© Springer Science+Business Media New York 2014

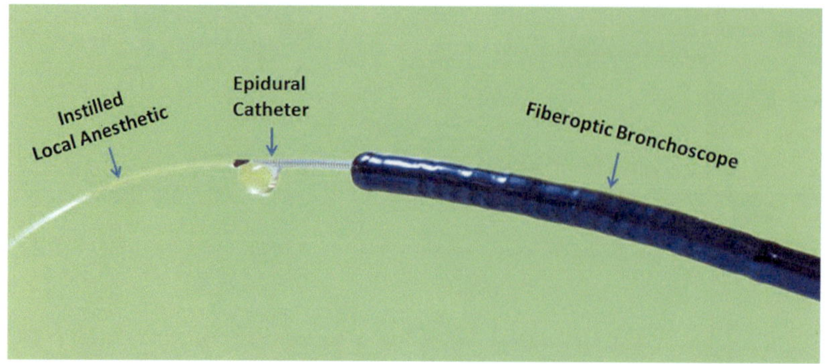

Fig. 2.1 Local anesthetic solution injected via the epidural catheter introduced through the working channel of the fiberoptic bronchoscope provides topical anesthesia of the larynx and trachea under direct vision with minimal stimulation during intubation attempt

those with anticipated serious airway difficulties, in whom taking irretrievable steps such as administering intravenous anesthetics and muscle relaxants may be associated with uncorrectable airway obstruction and severe hypoxia.

Rapid sequence induction should be achieved with the following objectives in mind: (a) adequate sedation and paralysis, (b) adequate oxygenation, (c) optimal hemodynamics and perfusion, (d) avoidance of intracranial hypertension, and (e) prevention of vomiting and aspiration. Any of the intravenous agents including propofol, etomidate, ketamine, or midazolam can be used provided that their doses are adjusted to satisfy the above objectives [3]. Although even a single dose of etomidate has been shown to cause adrenocortical suppression [4], increased likelihood of adult respiratory distress syndrome (ARDS), and multiple organ failure (MOF) [5], it is still used for emergency airway management because of its rapid onset and relatively lower risk of hypotension in comparison to propofol. Succinylcholine is still the preferred agent for muscle relaxation, because it has the shortest time to effect in relation to other agents. Large doses (1.2–1.5 mg/kg) of rocuronium may provide an onset of action comparable to succinylcholine, but its long duration may represent a disadvantage in patients with difficult mask ventilation or tracheal intubation, since return of spontaneous breathing may be excessively delayed. As in any tracheal intubation the use of pulse oximetry, end tidal CO_2 monitoring, and an available experienced operator is essential. Additionally, the neck must be maintained in neutral position and equipment and personnel for invasive airway management must be present.

The use of cricoid pressure for RSI is controversial. Although standard since Sellick's recommendation in 1960s [6], recent findings from 402 trauma patients suggest that its use actually decreases the view of the larynx during direct laryngoscopy and does not seem to prevent regurgitation and aspiration [7, 8]. Although it is difficult to recommend elimination of cricoid pressure during RSI at this time, its removal when the laryngeal view is compromised during direct laryngoscopy or when mask ventilation is hindered appears to be an appropriate maneuver.

Awake intubation with preservation of spontaneous breathing should be performed, if at all, with minimal sedation and topical anesthesia of the tongue, pharynx, epiglottis, and the superior surface of the vocal cords. Topical anesthesia of the trachea can be obtained just before introduction of the tracheal tube during direct laryngoscopy or fiberoptic bronchoscopy (FOB) using a tracheal local anesthetic applicator or the working channel of the FOB. Advancement of an epidural catheter that fits the working channel of the FOB, beyond the tip of the device and into the laryngotracheal opening, decreases laryngeal stimulation, minimizing cough and patient movement (Fig. 2.1).

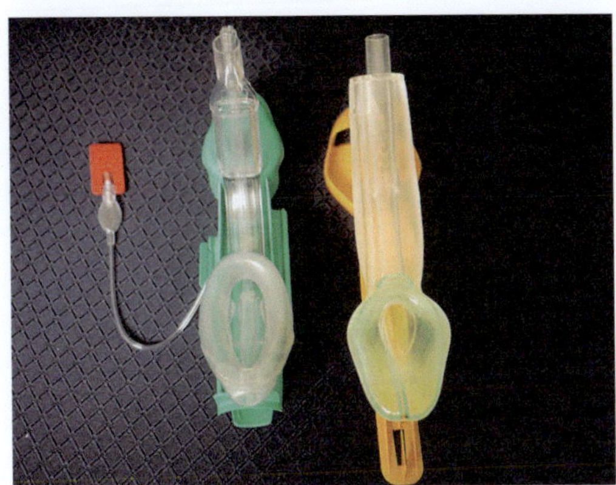

Fig. 2.2 Laryngeal airways. Laryngeal Mask Airway Supreme (LMA Supreme) on the *left*, and I-Gel Airway on the *right*

The high probability of a full stomach precludes the use of any supraglottic device, such as the Laryngeal Mask Airway (LMA) (Fig. 2.2), Combitube (Fig. 2.3), or King's airway (LT, LTS, LTS-D) (Fig. 2.4), which does not protect the trachea from aspiration of gastric or pharyngeal contents, as a definitive airway in trauma patients. However, these devices can serve as a bridge for a brief period to establish airway patency or to facilitate intubation. In patients with maxillofacial injuries, aspiration of pharyngeal blood or secretions is more likely than aspiration of gastric contents. If they can be inserted in these circumstances, supraglottic airways may protect the lungs. Although positive-pressure ventilation may be used with supraglottic airways, patients with pulmonary contusion, edema, or aspiration may be difficult to ventilate with these devices. Supraglottic airways may permit rapid blind or FOB-guided tracheal intubation while temporarily allowing ventilation. An important disadvantage of the original intubating LMA is its metal stem that may exert considerable pressure against the cervical vertebrae, potentially exacerbating an unstable injury in this region [9].

Many trauma victims with abdominal injuries return to the operating room several times after damage control surgery performed during the acute stage of injury. These repeat procedures are performed to debride and wash the abdominal cavity and to close the abdomen when the initial

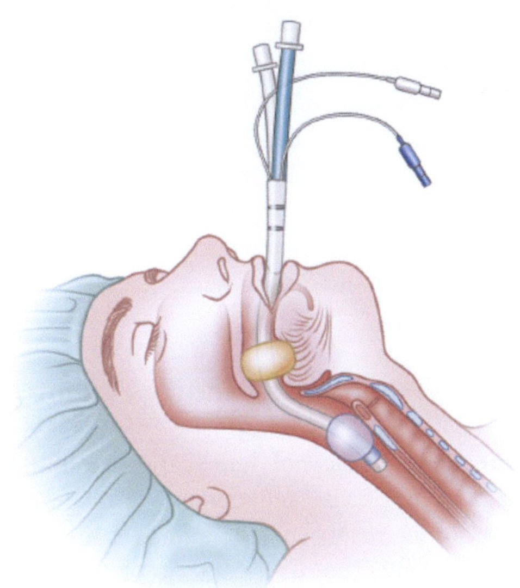

Fig. 2.3 Combitube. In this position of the tube with distal cuff in the esophagus, ventilation takes place by the air delivered through the openings below the proximal cuff

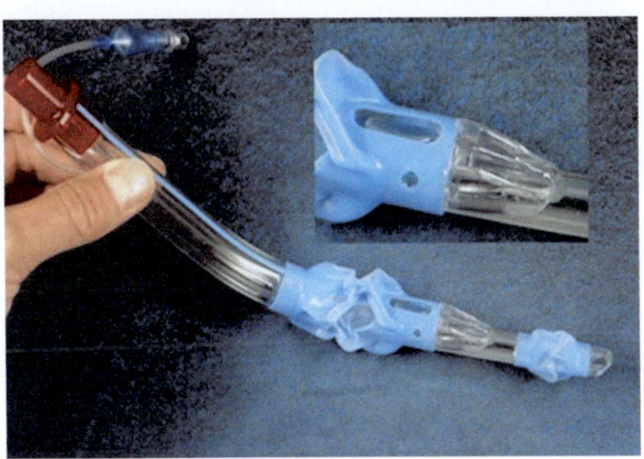

Fig. 2.4 King Airway. The tube with distal cuff enters into the esophagus and permits nasogastric tube introduced from a proximal port to proceed into the stomach. Ventilation takes place by the air exiting through the openings below the proximal cuff. Detailed view of the openings below the proximal cuff is shown in the *inset*

edema subsides. Many of these patients present with a vacuum dressing placed over the open abdomen. They are often extubated and many have been fed with a feeding tube which allows one-way entry of formula into the stomach owing to an internal valve that prevents drainage of gastric contents. These tubes, unlike sump nasogastric tubes, do not decompress the stomach. Even when the feeding tube is removed and the patient is kept NPO for several hours, these patients should be considered to have full stomachs because of hypoactive bowel function, the open abdomen, continuous accumulation of gastroduodenal fluid, and remaining feeding solution in the stomach. Airway management in these patients necessitates using rapid sequence induction with cricoid pressure.

The Agitated Uncooperative Patient

Pain, anxiety, alcohol intoxication, and illicit drug use may cause agitation and uncooperative behavior in many acutely injured patients. In these patients, topical anesthesia of the airway may be impossible, whereas administration of sedative agents may result in apnea or airway obstruction, with an increased risk of aspiration of gastric contents and inadequate conditions for tracheal intubation. These patients are best managed with RSI with direct laryngoscopy, provided that the cricothyroid membrane is located, the lung is denitrogenated, and personnel and material necessary to perform translaryngeal ventilation or cricothyroidotomy are prepared and ready to provide a rapid surgical airway if intubation with RSI fails.

Airway Obstruction

Airway obstruction is probably the most frequent cause of asphyxia; it may result from pharyngeal soft tissue edema, laceration, hematoma, bleeding, secretions, foreign bodies, or displaced bone or cartilage fragments. Bleeding into the cervical region may produce airway obstruction not only because of compression by the hematoma, but also from venous congestion and upper airway edema as a result of neck vein compression. Signs of upper and lower airway obstruction include dyspnea, cyanosis, hoarseness, stridor, dysphonia, subcutaneous emphysema, and hemoptysis. Cervical deformity, edema, crepitation, tracheal tug and/or deviation, or jugular venous distention may be present before these

symptoms appear and may help indicate that specialized techniques are required to secure the airway.

The initial steps in airway management are chin lift, jaw thrust, clearing of the oropharyngeal cavity, placement of an oropharyngeal or nasopharyngeal airway and, in inadequately breathing patients, ventilation with a self-inflating bag/mask assembly. Cervical spine immobilization and administration of oxygen are essential. Blind passage of a nasopharyngeal airway or a nasogastric or nasotracheal tube should be avoided if a basilar skull or maxillary sinus fracture is suspected; it may enter the cranial cavity or the periocular fat pad. Supraglottic airways may permit ventilation with a self-inflating bag, although they do not provide protection against aspiration of gastric contents. They may be used as temporary measures, and if they do not provide adequate ventilation, the trachea must be intubated immediately using either direct laryngoscopy or videolaryngoscopy. Cricothyroidotomy may have to be performed if mask or supraglottic airway ventilation fails to overcome airway obstruction, tracheal intubation is unsuccessful, and hypoxia is severe and cannot be corrected. In all trauma patients airway assessment should include a rapid examination of the anterior neck for feasibility of access to the cricothyroid membrane. Between 0.3 % and 2.7 % of airway management attempts fail in the trauma population, necessitating cricothyroidotomy [10, 11]. Tracheostomy is not desirable during initial management because it takes longer to perform than a cricothyroidotomy and requires neck extension, which may cause or exacerbate cord trauma in patients with cervical spine injuries. Conversion to a tracheostomy should be considered later to prevent laryngeal damage if a cricothyroidotomy will be in place for more than 2–3 days. Possible contraindications to cricothyroidotomy include age younger than 12 years and suspected laryngeal trauma; permanent laryngeal damage may result in the former, and uncorrectable airway obstruction may occur in the latter situation.

Airway Evaluation in the Trauma Patient

As in any patient requiring airway management, airway evaluation in trauma victims is of crucial importance for optimal preparation and thus prevention of undesirable outcomes. Assessment should be made for mask ventilation, tracheal intubation, and a surgical airway. The LEMON score, an airway assessment tool for trauma patients, is included in the current version (8th edition) of the Advanced Trauma Life Support Manual (ATLS) [12, 13]. The components of the score are similar to those used in routine airway assessment, but it is more organized and standardized for trauma patients. Following are the criteria that may indicate difficulty:

L stands for **Look** at the cervicofacial region for evaluation of facial or neck trauma, large incisors, presence of beard, large tongue, or orofacial soft tissue stiffness such as the effect of radiation therapy. One point is assigned for each of four conditions present that can possibly cause difficulty. Thus, this criteria leads to a maximum of four points.

E stands for **Evaluate**. The 3-3-2 rule is used for this purpose to specify an interincisor distance <3 fingers, mentum to hyoid distance <3 fingers, and floor of the mouth to thyroid notch distance <2 fingers. One point is assigned for each abnormal findings yielding a maximum of three points.

M stands for **Mallampati score**, in which inability to visualize the uvula suggests a grade 3 or 4 view during laryngoscopy. One point is assigned for Mallampati Grade 3 and 4 view.

O stands for **Obstruction**. Airway obstruction from any cause, and the signs and symptoms described above are detected with this part of the assessment tool. One point is assigned to the presence of airway obstruction.

N stands for **Neck Mobility**. Apart from preexisting cervical diseases, the trauma patient with a cervical collar may have significant limitation of neck mobility causing reduction of the laryngeal view during direct laryngoscopy. One point is assigned to the presence of neck mobility caused by any reason.

Thus, by addition of points from each item of LEMON a maximum of 10 and a minimum score of 0 is obtained.

High LEMON scores have been shown to be associated with a greater likelihood of difficult intubation [12]. It should be emphasized that as in any airway evaluation method, this method as well provides information only about the likelihood of difficulty and is not a definite marker of difficult airway management.

Airway evaluation in patients requiring emergency tracheal intubation shortly after trauma is solely based on clinical examination. During the later stages of treatment, radiographic evaluation of the craniofacial region may additionally contribute to airway evaluation. Computed tomography (CT) examination and magnetic resonance (MR) imaging have largely replaced conventional radiographic evaluation for this purpose during the past decade. They will be discussed during the review of specific injuries below.

Ultrasound technology has recently emerged as a tool for airway management. It aids in both airway evaluation and intervention, and its potential benefit is especially relevant in the time of critical immediate phase after trauma. The airway can be evaluated with this method all the way from the mouth to the lung (Table 2.1), and airway structures such as the tongue, oropharynx, hypopharynx, hyoid bone, epiglottis, larynx, vocal cords, cricothyroid membrane, cricoid cartilage, trachea, esophagus, lung, and pleura can be imaged. It is also possible to identify the stomach and predict the volume of its contents after placing the patient in right lateral position [14]. Ultrasound imaging for upper airway evaluation is performed by using an 8–15 MHz linear array probe placed in the transverse axis in the submandibular area and moved downward to the level of the suprasternal notch. In this region the focus of evaluation is usually centered in four levels: (a) submandibular region where the muscles in the floor of the mouth (geniohyoid) and the tongue are imaged; (b) over the hyoid bone where the soft tissue thickness of the anterior neck, which appears to correlate with difficulty of laryngoscopy if it exceeds 2.8 cm, can be measured [15]; (c) the

Table 2.1 Possible uses of ultrasonography for airway management

Clinical application	Comment
Predicting difficult airway management [96]	Demonstrated to be useful in small series of obese patients
Diagnosis of head and neck pathology with potential of causing difficulty of airway management [97]	Both intrinsic and extrinsic head and neck pathology can be diagnosed
Measuring gastric content [98]	Best results are obtained if the patient is placed in right lateral decubitus position
Predicting appropriate diameter of endotracheal, endobronchial, and tracheostomy tubes [99]	
Differentiating between tracheal and endobronchial intubation	
Differentiating between tracheal and esophageal intubation [38]	Allows detection of esophageal intubation and it is especially helpful in the presence of no circulation (cardiac arrest)
Diagnosing pneumothorax [100]	Fastest way to rule out a suspicion of intraoperative pneumothorax
Identifying the cricothyroid membrane [101]	For preparation of emergency cricothyroidotomy, transtracheal O_2 insufflation, translaryngeal (retrograde) intubation, administration of local anesthetics when palpation of the cricothyroid membrane is not possible
Identifying trachea and trachea and tracheal ring interspaces for tracheostomy and percutaneous dilatational tracheostomy [102]	Usually needed in the intensive care unit few days after trauma

Modified from Kristensen MS and Teoh WHL. Ultrasound probe in the hands of the anesthesiologist: a powerful new tool for airway management. Anesthesiology News Supplement on Guide to Airway Management. 2013; page 23-30

thyrohyoid membrane between the hyoid bone and the thyroid cartilage where, in addition to measurement of the soft tissue thickness, the preepiglottic space and epiglottis can be identified. At this level, moving the transducer slightly caudad to the level of the thyroid cartilage allows imaging of the larynx at the level of the vocal cords with demonstration of the thyroid and cricoid cartilages, vocal ligaments, and the anterior commissure; and (d) at the level of the thyroid isthmus and suprasternal notch where the posterior air/mucosa interface can be identified (Fig. 2.5) [16]. It should be emphasized that the position of the probe as it is moved distally over the airway is gradually tilted from parallel to the axis of the body at the submandibular area to perpendicular to the axis of the body at the thyroid or cricoid cartilage level. Pneumothorax and endobronchial intubation can be diagnosed in B-mode ultrasound imaging by transverse placement of the ultrasound probe over two adjacent ribs and observing lung sliding [17, 18]. If M-mode imaging is used, the presence of a succession of horizontal lines may be related to endobronchial intubation or pneumothorax. The "lung pulse" observed in M-mode normally results from movement of the visceral over the parietal pleura with every heartbeat and may give the false impression that pneumothorax or endobronchial intubation do not exist. Of course in patients with cardiac arrest the "lung pulse" is absent (Fig. 2.6) [19].

Indications for Emergency Tracheal Intubation

Absolute indications for emergency tracheal intubation for trauma and smoke inhalation victims are provided by the Eastern Association for the Surgery of Trauma (EAST) guidelines. Essentially, as mentioned above, the criteria for these indications are based on the presence of hypoxia, hypoventilation, and inability to protect the airway (Table 2.2) [20].

Several retrospective studies, however, have identified additional indications for emergency

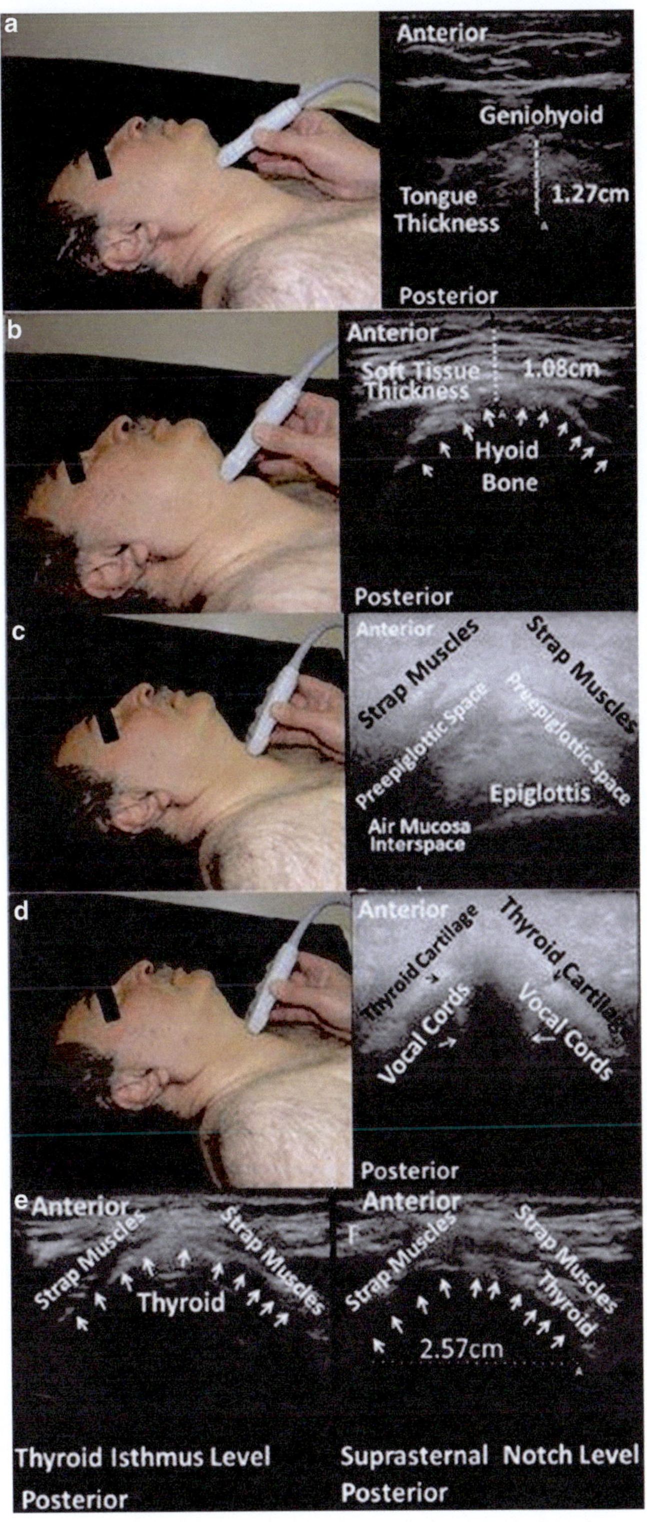

Fig. 2.5 Ultrasonographic evaluation of the upper airway. (**a**) In supine position of the patient the ultrasound probe is placed submentally to image the geniohyoid and the tongue. (**b**) The probe is moved downward over the hyoid bone to measure the soft tissue thickness over the hyoid. Soft tissue thickness exceeding 2.5–3.0 cm may be

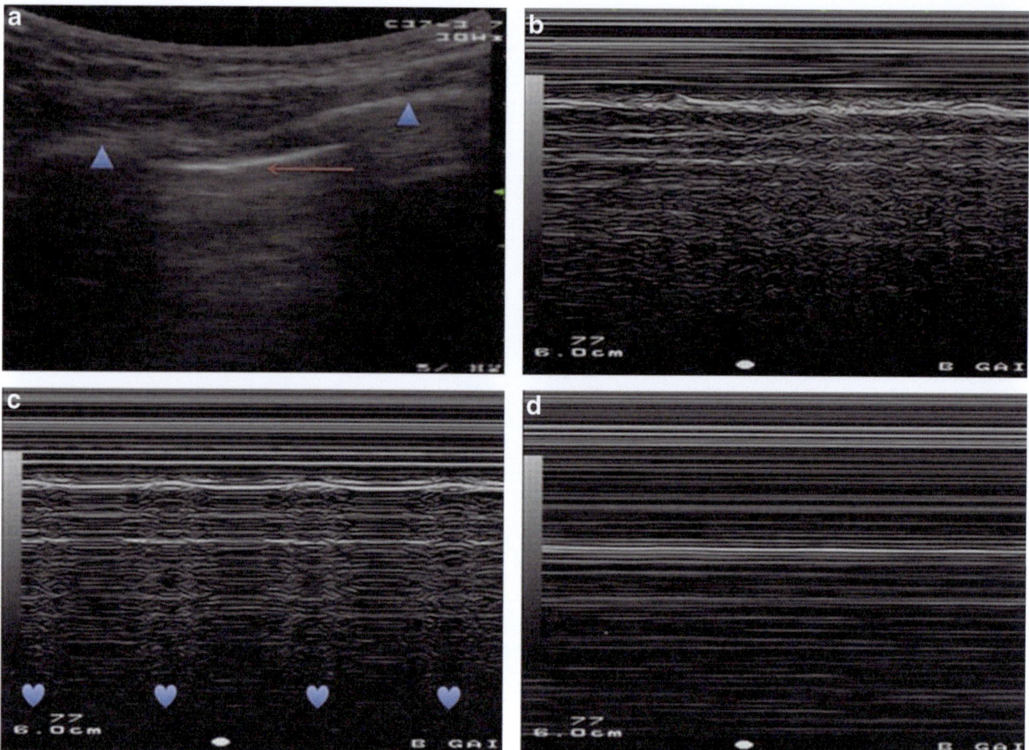

Fig. 2.6 Ultrasonographic views of lung sliding (**a**, **b**) and absence of lung sliding (**c**, **d**). (**a**) Ultrasound probe placed longitudinally over the chest showing 2D image of pleural lines (*arrow*) and successive ribs (*arrowheads*). On a dynamic image sliding of the visceral over parietal pleura suggests absence of pneumothorax. (**b**) With M-mode image lung sliding generated a sandy pattern which is often described as a seashore sign. (**c**) M-mode image obtained in the absence of lung sliding. Succession of *horizontal lines* is interrupted by intermittent fluctuations at points marked by *heart shapes*. These fluctuations are caused by heart beats and are called lung pulse. (**d**) Absence of lung sliding in the absence of heart beat effect is reflected over the M-mode image as uninterrupted horizontal lines termed as the stratosphere sign. Reproduced with permission from Sim S-S, Lien WC, Chou HC et al.: Ultrasonographic lung sliding sign in confirming proper endotracheal intubation during emergency intubation. Resuscitation 2012; 83:307-312

tracheal intubation in other trauma patients [21–24]. These include moderate cognitive impairment (GCS score 9–12), persistent combativeness unresponsive to mild to moderate sedation, respiratory distress without hypoxia or hypoventilation, cervical spinal cord injury (CSCI) with evidence of respiratory insufficiency (complete or incomplete SCI at C5 or above) [20]. Interestingly, these studies show that one of the three patients intubated with these criteria had a head injury.

Techniques of Airway Management

The objective in airway management of trauma patients is to achieve a safe tracheal intubation in the shortest possible time without causing a

Fig. 2.5 (continued) associated with difficult tracheal intubation. (**c**) Ultrasound image at the thyrohyoid membrane demonstrates strap muscles, preepiglottic space, epiglottis, and the air–mucosa interspace. (**d**) Ultrasound probe placed over the thyroid cartilage showing the image of thyroid cartilage and vocal cords. (**e**) Ultrasound image at the level of the thyroid isthmus showing the image of thyroid and the subglottic airway. (**f**) Ultrasound image at the suprasternal notch showing the airway. The diameter of the airway can be measured at each level of the airway

Table 2.2 Absolute indications for emergency tracheal intubations in trauma and smoke inhalation victims

Trauma victims
Airway obstruction
Hypoventilation
Persistent hypoxemia ($SaO_2 < 90$ %) despite supplemental oxygen
Severe cognitive impairment (Glasgow Coma Scale [GCS] score < 8)
Severe hemorrhagic shock
Cardiac arrest
Smoke inhalation victims
Airway obstruction
Severe cognitive impairment (GCS score < 8)
Major cutaneous burn (body surface area > 10 %)
Major burns and/or smoke inhalation with an anticipated prolonged transport time to definitive care
Impending airway obstruction as follows:
Moderate-to-severe facial burn
Moderate-to-severe oropharyngeal burn
Moderate-to-severe airway injury observed during endoscopy

decrease in blood pressure or blood O_2 saturation, or an increase in CO_2 tension. This is especially important in head-injured patients in whom even short periods of hypoxia and/or hypotension are likely to increase the size of secondary injury, worsening the outcome. Based on the EAST airway management guidelines, orotracheal intubation guided by direct laryngoscopy is the technique of choice for emergency tracheal intubation of trauma patients [20].

There are, however, other alternatives which may be used as rescue devices when difficulty arises with classical mask ventilation and tracheal intubation using direct laryngoscopy with conventional blades. Supraglottic airway devices, by bypassing the oropharynx, offer the benefits of rapid blind placement as well as a high success rate in situations of combined difficult mask ventilation, laryngoscopy, and cricothyroidotomy that may be experienced in patients with obesity, obstructive sleep apnea, short neck, limited neck movement, previous radiotherapy to the cervicofacial region, beard, etc. Although extensive information exists about the use of supraglottic devices in the nontrauma in-hospital setting, data for trauma patients in this area are limited mainly to prehospital airway management by nonphysician personnel. The success rate of these devices as a rescue technique after failed tracheal intubation in prehospital trauma varies between 87 % and 100 %. Since there are more than ten supraglottic devices available on the market, it is difficult to recommend a specific one for this purpose; familiarity of the operator with a specific device appears to be the most important factor.

Videolaryngoscopes provide an indirect view of the larynx. Unless there is intrinsic distortion of the airway, these devices enable the operator to visualize the larynx almost every time. However, depending on the oropharyngeal anatomy, direction of the tracheal tube into the larynx may not always be successful. Videolaryngoscopes can be divided into two groups: those guiding the tube toward the laryngeal inlet (Airtraq, Pentax AWS) and those requiring the operator to direct the tube into the larynx (GlideScope, Storz, etc.). Some devices in the second category such as the GlideScope have stylets designed to facilitate manipulation of the tube. Besides improving the Cormack and Lehane grade, videolaryngoscopes may decrease cervical spine motion and the force and pressure applied to the posterior pharynx, features that may be advantageous during management of cervical spine injury [25–28].

Although experience with videolaryngoscopes in nontrauma patients is extensive,

Table 2.3 Performance characteristics of GlideScope in 2,004 patients

Performance criteria tested	Number (%)
Overall success rate	1,944 of 2,004 (97 %)
Success in predicted difficult intubation	1,377 of 1,428 (96 %)
Success after failed conventional laryngoscopy	224 of 239 (94 %)
Complications	21 of 2,004 (1 %)
Major complications[a]	6 of 2,004 (0.3 %)
Predictors of GlideScope failure	Altered neck anatomy[b]

[a]Dental, pharyngeal, tracheal, and laryngeal injury
[b]Surgical scar, radiation changes, neck mass
Reproduced with permission from Aziz MF, Healy D, Kheterpal S et al.: Routine clinical practice effectiveness of the Glidescope in difficult airway management: an analysis of 2004 Glidescope intubations, complications, and failures from two institutions. Anesthesiology 2011; 114:34-41

few studies have evaluated these devices in the trauma setting. In one study, the laryngeal view with the GlideScope was superior to that obtained with the Macintosh blade [29]. In another study involving 822 emergency room patients, of whom more than 60 % had sustained trauma, the first attempt success rate with the GlideScope was higher than that with conventional laryngoscopes; nevertheless the overall success rate was similar between the two techniques [30]. The overall success rate was also found to be similar in another study of trauma patients, although intubation times were longer with the GlideScope [31]. A recent prospective randomized study comparing the Macintosh blade and videolaryngoscope (GlideScope) for intubation of a group of trauma patients ($n = 623$) demonstrated no difference in mortality. Intubation with the GlideScope took longer (median 56 s vs. 40 s). Although the difference in duration of intubation, while statistically significant, may appear relatively small, it was associated with a longer duration of decreased O_2 saturation. In fact, the severe head injury patients in the study, who are expected to be most vulnerable to hypoxia in the early post-trauma phase because of the likelihood of development or expansion of secondary injury, had a higher incidence of hypoxia (O_2 saturation <80 %) during intubation with the videolaryngoscope than with the Macintosh blade (50 % vs. 24 %). The authors suspected that this may have been one of the reasons for a statistically significant higher mortality rate in the head-injured patients intubated with the GlideScope (30 % vs. 14 %) [32]. Inability to demonstrate a difference in success of intubation between direct laryngoscopy and videolaryngoscopy may be related to the use of an unselected population in whom direct laryngoscopy has a high success rate. It is now clear that in the nontrauma population many, but not all, patients in whom tracheal intubation with direct laryngoscopy failed, video laryngoscopic intubation was successful. Likewise in patients known to be difficult, video laryngoscopy was more successful in tracheal intubation than direct laryngoscopy (Tables 2.3, 2.4, and 2.5) [33–37].

Ultrasound can be useful for airway intervention. Apart from identifying esophageal intubation, especially in patients with cardiac arrest or low flow states when the end tidal CO_2 measurement is unreliable [38], and helping to recognize endobronchial intubation, its most valuable use for airway intervention is in identification of the cricoid cartilage and cricothyroid membrane for emergency cricothyrotomy when these structures cannot be identified by palpation [39, 40].

Airway Management in Specific Injuries

Head, Open Eye, and Contained Major Vessel Injuries

In addition to adequate oxygenation and ventilation, patients with these injuries require deep anesthesia and profound muscle relaxation before airway manipulation. This helps prevent

Table 2.4 Comparison of performance characteristics of Macintosh and C-MAC laryngoscopes in 300 patients having at least one predictor of difficult intubation

	Macintosh	C-MAC	
	Number (%)	Number (%)	p
First attempt intubation	124 of 147 (84 %)	138 of 149 (93 %)	0.026
Grade 1 or 2 view	119 of 147 (81 %)	139 of 149 (93 %)	<0.01
Laryngoscopy time	33 s (95 %) (CI 29–36)	46 s (95 %) (CI 40–51)	<0.001
Facilitatory manipulation needed[a]	46 of 124 (37 %)	33 of 138 (24 %)	<0.020
Complications	16 of 124 (13 %)	27 of 138 (20 %)	

[a]External laryngeal pressure or gum elastic bougie
Reproduced with permission from Aziz MF, Healy D, Kheterpal S et al.: Routine clinical practice effectiveness of the Glidescope in difficult airway management: an analysis of 2004 Glidescope intubations, complications, and failures from two institutions. Anesthesiology 2011; 114:34-41

Table 2.5 Comparative intubating characteristics of airway scope (Pentax), C-MAC (Storz), and GlideScope

	Airway scope (Pentax)	C-MAC (Storz)	GlideScope
Intubation time (s)	20.6 ± 11.5	31.9 ± 17.6	31.2 ± 15
Grade 1 view (%)	97	87	78
First attempt intubation rate (%)	95	93	91

Reproduced with permission from Teoh WH, Saxena S, Shah MK, Sia AT: Comparison of three videolaryngoscopes: Pentax airway scope, C-MAC, Glidescope vs Macintosh laryngoscope for tracheal intubation. Anaesthesia 2010; 65:1126-32

hypertension, coughing, and bucking, and thereby minimizes intracranial, intraocular, or intravascular pressure elevation, which can result in herniation of the brain, extrusion of eye contents, or dislodgment of a hemostatic clot from an injured vessel, respectively.

Anesthetic agents selected for management of brain injury should produce the least increase in intracranial pressure (ICP), the least decrease in mean arterial pressure, and the greatest reduction in cerebral metabolic rate ($CMRO_2$). One of the most important factors in the etiology of cerebral ischemia is increased ICP from intracranial hematoma and/or cerebral edema. Prompt decompression of the cranial contents is the most crucial means of ensuring cerebral well-being. Hypotension caused by anesthetics or other factors contributes to the development or progression of cerebral ischemia. Utmost attention should be paid during anesthesia to avoid hypotension and hypoxia. A minimal mean arterial pressure of 60 mmHg is generally accepted as the threshold for brain ischemia or as the lower limit of autoregulation, but depending on the patient, the duration of hypotension, the anesthetic technique, and the state of the cerebral vasculature, this threshold may be as high as 70–80 mmHg. The preferred anesthetic sequence to achieve optimal brain oxygenation includes preoxygenation and opioid loading, followed by an intravenous anesthetic and muscle relaxant. Systemic hypotension, ICP elevation, and decreased cerebral perfusion pressure (CPP = mean arterial pressure − ICP) should be avoided. Intravenous anesthetics are the most common causes of hypotension during induction. This problem can be ameliorated by administering pretreatment doses of opioids (fentanyl, 2–3 µg/kg), which permit reduction of the intravenous anesthetic dose. This may also prevent the myoclonic movements associated with etomidate and occasionally with propofol, and thus reduce the risks of ICP and IOP increase. Nevertheless, myoclonus is best prevented by careful timing of the dose of muscle relaxants. Another measure to preserve CPP during anesthesia is to administer vasopressors, being aware that hypovolemia may be masked by their use. Alpha-1 agonist agents, although considered cerebral vasoconstrictors and thus contraindicated, do not actually produce this effect in the usual doses [41].

Opioid loading, however, may also be responsible for hypotension, as it inhibits the overactive sympathetic activity that is likely to be present in trauma patients with or without head injury. In head-injured patients this may occur whether cerebral autoregulation is present or absent, and if untreated can produce secondary ischemic insults. Thus, hemodynamic responses to the opioid should be carefully monitored and promptly corrected [42].

For many years ketamine was considered to be contraindicated in patients with head and vascular injuries because it may increase both intracranial and systemic vascular pressures; it does not increase intraocular pressure (IOP). Its effect on ICP when used as an induction agent has recently been questioned, and actually some studies have demonstrated decreases in ICP when it is used for sedation [43–46].

Any muscle relaxant, including succinylcholine, may be used as long as the fasciculation produced by this agent is inhibited by prior administration of an adequate dose of a nondepolarizing muscle relaxant. More recently, however, the use of defasciculating doses of nondepolarizing muscle relaxants for head-injured patients has also been questioned, as the evidence that succinylcholine-induced fasciculations produce significant elevation of ICP in this setting is lacking [47]. However, fasciculations do increase IOP, necessitating the use of intravenous anesthetics and defasciculating doses of nondepolarizing agents [48]. Avoiding succinylcholine usually does not alleviate the problem because laryngoscopy and tracheal intubation produce a greater and longer-lasting increase in IOP [49]. Alternatively, rocuronium can provide intubating conditions within 60 s following a dose of 1.6–2.0 mg/kg, although the neuromuscular blockade produced by this dose lasts approximately 2 h [50]. Intravenous lidocaine has an attenuating effect on the pressor response to airway instrumentation, but it is mild and unpredictable. Of course, neither muscle relaxants nor intravenous anesthetics are indicated when initial assessment suggests a difficult airway. Airway management with mild sedation and gentle topical anesthesia of the airway to prevent bucking and coughing may be needed in these patients. As in any other trauma patient, hypotension dictates either reduced or no intravenous anesthetic administration. None of the nondepolarizing muscle relaxants causes elevation of ICP or IOP in the absence of associated tracheal intubation.

Cervical Spine Injury

Overall incidence of cervical spine injury after blunt trauma is estimated to be 2 % [51]. Concomitant craniofacial injury and Glasgow coma scale of 8 or less triples this risk [51]. As in brain injury, secondary injury by factors such as hypoxia and hypotension is also likely in spinal cord injuries; estimated rate of this complication varies between 10 % and 30 % [51], indicating the importance of appropriate airway management. In the cervical spine (C-spine)-injured patient as well, airway management consists of two components: evaluation and intervention. In this instance evaluation includes not only the airway but also the spine itself, as the presence of a C-spine injury greatly affects the strategy for intervention. The definitive method of diagnosis of C-spine injury in the early phase after injury is thin slice (2 or 3 mm) computed tomography (CT). Subjecting every patient with suspected C-spine injury to CT, however, would result in many unnecessary radiographic studies, radiation exposure, high costs, and delays in patient care. In the beginning of the millennium, a prospective observational study performed in 34,000 patients in 21 centers across the United States produced a simple decision instrument, in which a clinical evaluation showing absence of posterior cervical pain and tenderness, no focal neurological deficit, normal alertness, no evidence of intoxication, and no obvious distracting injury indicated a low probability of a C-spine injury and justified ruling it out without the need for radiographic evaluation [52]. This decision rule, the National Emergency X-radiography (NEXUS) criteria, has been embraced by the EAST and is used throughout

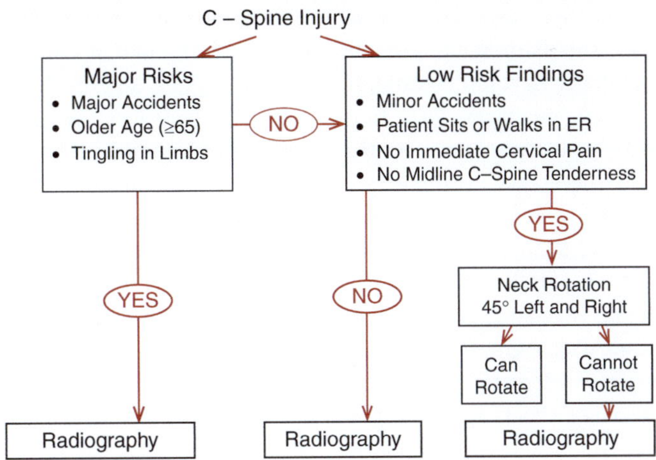

Fig. 2.7 Management algorithm followed by the Canadian C-spine rule for the initial care of cervical spine injuries

the US. There is, however, no definition of a distracting injury, and the decision about its presence and its impact on evaluation is left to the perception and judgment of the clinician. Recently there has been increasing doubt about the effect of a distracting injury on the recognition of a C-spine injury. At least one study demonstrated a similar rate of C-spine injury diagnosis whether there was a presumed distracting injury or not [53]. On the other hand, some trauma surgeons believe that in the major trauma setting, ruling out C-spine injury with the NEXUS criteria alone may be fraught with the danger of missing some clinically important unstable injuries. Thus, they believe that CT evaluation in addition to clinical examination is indicated in all major trauma patients [54].

The relative weakness of the NEXUS criteria compared to the Canadian C-spine rule has also been demonstrated [55, 56]. The latter instrument is based on three high risk and five low risk criteria plus the patient's ability to actively rotate the neck: Age greater than 65 years; dangerous mechanisms of injury such as a fall from an elevation greater than 3 ft or 5 stairs; an axial load to the head, as in diving or in an MVA at a speed greater than 100 km/h with rollover or ejection, bicycle collision, or being hit by a high-speed vehicle; or if the patient reports the development of paresthesias in his extremities,

Table 2.6 Diagnostic performance of NEXUS and Canadian C-spine rule

	Canadian C-spine rule		NEXUS	
Assessment	Injury	No injury	Injury	No injury
Positive	161	3,995	147	3,599
Negative	1	3,281	15	2,677

Data from Stiell JG, Clement CM, McKnight RD et al.: Canadian C-spine rule versus the NEXUS low-risk criteria in patients with trauma. New England Journal of Medicine 2003; 349:2510-8

are high risk factors that mandate radiographic studies. Low risk criteria such as a simple rear-end motor vehicle collision, ability to sit or ambulate in the ER, absence of immediate but not delayed neck pain, or absence of midline C-spine tenderness permit safe assessment of range of motion as the next evaluation step. Finally, the patient's ability to rotate the neck actively 45° in each direction allows clearing the C-spine without radiographic evaluation (Fig. 2.7) [55]. As compared to the NEXUS criteria, the Canadian C-spine rule, which is not used as widely as the NEXUS in the USA, appears to be a safer instrument for evaluating the possibility of a C-spine injury (Table 2.6) [55].

These findings have important implications for the anesthesiologist in that C-spine injury can be ruled out reliably by clinical criteria. However, though with a very small likelihood, patients cleared clinically, especially with NEXUS criteria, may still harbor an unstable injury and could potentially develop neurologic damage during airway management, thus active evaluation and C-spine protection during intubation are generally necessary in all cases.

For those who cannot be cleared clinically and thus require radiographic evaluation, it is now clear that the diagnostic capability of three-view plain films (the previous standard) is inferior to helical (spiral) CT scans with sagittal and coronal reconstruction. Thus, in modern trauma centers radiographic evaluation of the C-spine is now done with thin slice CT, except in pediatric patients who are sensitive to the excessive radiation of the CT scan (six times greater than conventional radiograms), potentially increasing the risk of thyroid cancer later in life [57].

There is, however, a subset of patients who have normal CT results but are either obtunded or have neck pain. Given the fact that CT is not sensitive in diagnosis of soft tissue and ligamentous injury, how can these be ruled out in these patients? The conventional approach used to be to obtain flexion/extension series. However, the efficacy of dynamic fluoroscopy is very limited because of the need for repeated examinations, the difficulty in identifying specific ligamentous injuries, inadequate visualization of lower C-spine, and extremely low yield, combined with the relatively dangerous and cost-ineffective nature of these studies. In the first few days following the injury, active flexion/extension movement of the patient is limited because of pain. Also during this period, the study is fraught with the danger of spinal cord injury and must be done with the participation of a neurosurgeon. Data from two clinical studies demonstrates the low yield of flexion/extension series. In one study only 2 % of the 837 patients with unstable injuries [58], and in another, only 0.7 % of 301 patients were diagnosed [59]. In other patients, the studies were negative, inadequate, or falsely positive or negative [58, 59]. For these reasons many trauma centers no longer perform flexion/extension films.

MRI is currently performed as an adjuvant assessment in cognitively dysfunctional patients with negative CT results. MRI is a reliable tool; when it is normal it can conclusively exclude C-spine injury and is thus established as the gold standard for clearing the C-spine in a clinically suspicious blunt trauma patient [60]. However, it is expensive, requires patient transport and medical supervision during a relatively long study period, and is so sensitive that it can detect subtle stable injuries which are clinically insignificant. Additionally, in the comatose patient with a normal CT and no abnormal neurologic signs, it does not add any information to change clinical management [61]. Also, for several reasons it cannot be done in the first few days of the injury, the time when airway management is most frequently required.

Another possibility is to keep the rigid cervical collar in place until the patient regains cognitive function and can be evaluated. This is the situation encountered in most instances when airway management is needed for the critically injured patient. Immobilization in a rigid cervical collar for more than 48–72 h has its own price, including an increased incidence of pressure sores, intracranial hypertension in the setting of a simultaneous head injury, airway management challenges, compromised central venous access, infection from suboptimal central venous catheter care, and difficult oral hygiene. Thus, every effort must be made to remove the collar as soon as possible.

A more recently proposed approach, practiced by trauma surgeons in Europe, Australia, New Zealand, and Canada, and in many but not all trauma centers in the US, is to rely on the CT study using a modern multidetector device with less than 3 mm cuts. The demonstrated diagnostic ability of this method is excellent, with a 99.99 % sensitivity and specificity and 100 % negative predictive value [62]. In practical terms, this method can miss one unstable C-Spine injury in about 5,000 patients who are not cleared by clinical examination, which in a typical level I trauma center translates into one patient every 10–15 years.

As in any other diagnostic study, there are certain conditions that C-Spine injury theoretically could be missed by CT examination. For example, acute rupture of a transverse atlantal ligament produces significant instability despite the absence of a neurological deficit and normal alignment while the patient is lying supine on a CT scanner. Likewise in a head-injured patient, a mild to moderate central cord syndrome that may occur in situations of spinal cord injury without radiologic findings (SCIWORA) may be difficult to discern with CT scan. Finally, human error is always possible, and misread CT scans by inexperienced clinicians can be a reason for a missed injury.

Although anesthesiologists are not responsible for clearing the C-spine, knowing the process and pitfalls of C-spine clearance may help airway management planning and intervention. Nevertheless, it should be emphasized that many patients present to anesthesiologists for airway management with a C-spine that is not cleared and a hard collar restricting neck flexion and extension; the emergent nature of the injury precludes the use of time-consuming diagnostic measures prior to airway management. The goal is to secure the airway without causing or worsening spinal cord damage. Several studies have reviewed the possibility of new or increasing spinal cord injury resulting from airway management. In 1987, Marshall and colleagues [63] studied the frequency and causes of neurologic deterioration in 154 spinal cord-injured patients after admission to the hospital. The deficits increased in nine patients. None were related to airway management; these complications were caused by placement and adjustment of neck-stabilizing devices. Indeed, although small, some anteroposterior translation and angulation of the unstable spine occurs during application and removal of any one- or two-piece cervical collar [64].

Hindman and colleagues [65] reviewed the closed claims for perioperative cervical cord, root, and spine injury in 48 patients. Interestingly, most cervical cord injuries occurred in the absence of traumatic spine injury, instability, or airway difficulties. Overall, airway management-related neurologic damage represented 11 % (five patients) of the total of 48 claims. Three of these patients had no trauma

but ankylosing spondylitis in two and severe cervical spondylosis with cord compression on the third patient. Cervical spine instability before airway management was present in nine patients. Of these, seven patients had traumatic spinal instability, of whom six underwent cervical cord surgery; neurologic damage was related to the surgery and not to the airway management in these patients. Spinal cord injury attributed to airway management occurred in two of the seven claims with prior trauma-induced unstable C-spines following difficult laryngoscopy and intubation without precautions. McLeod and Calder [66] reviewed nine allegedly intubation-related postoperative spinal cord injuries. Of the nine patients only three in two reports had traumatic C-spine injuries. It is possible that at least two of these cases are the same patients described by Hindman and colleagues [65]. In any case two of the injuries in McLeod and Calder's [66] series were not recognized and laryngoscopy and intubation were performed without precautions. The third patient had an airway obstruction secondary to cervical hematoma. Intubation failed and cricothyroidotomy was performed. Thus, airway management-related spinal cord injury may occur in C-spine-injured patients, but if it does, it is rare. This does not imply, however, that protection of the neck is unnecessary during airway management.

Direct laryngoscopy with manual inline stabilization (MILS) is the standard of care for these patients in the acute stage. In the presence of MILS the glottic view on direct laryngoscopy is restricted because of limitation of neck extension; thus tracheal intubation may be facilitated by the use of adjunctive measures such as bougie, stylet, or external laryngeal pressure. MILS also may require greater anterior pressure on the tongue by the laryngoscope blade. This pressure is transmitted to the spine and can increase the movement of the unstable segment. This has been elegantly demonstrated by Santoni and colleagues [67] who placed multiple pressure transducers on the anterior surface of the Macintosh blade to measure pressures exerted on the tongue (and indirectly to the spine), during various phases of direct

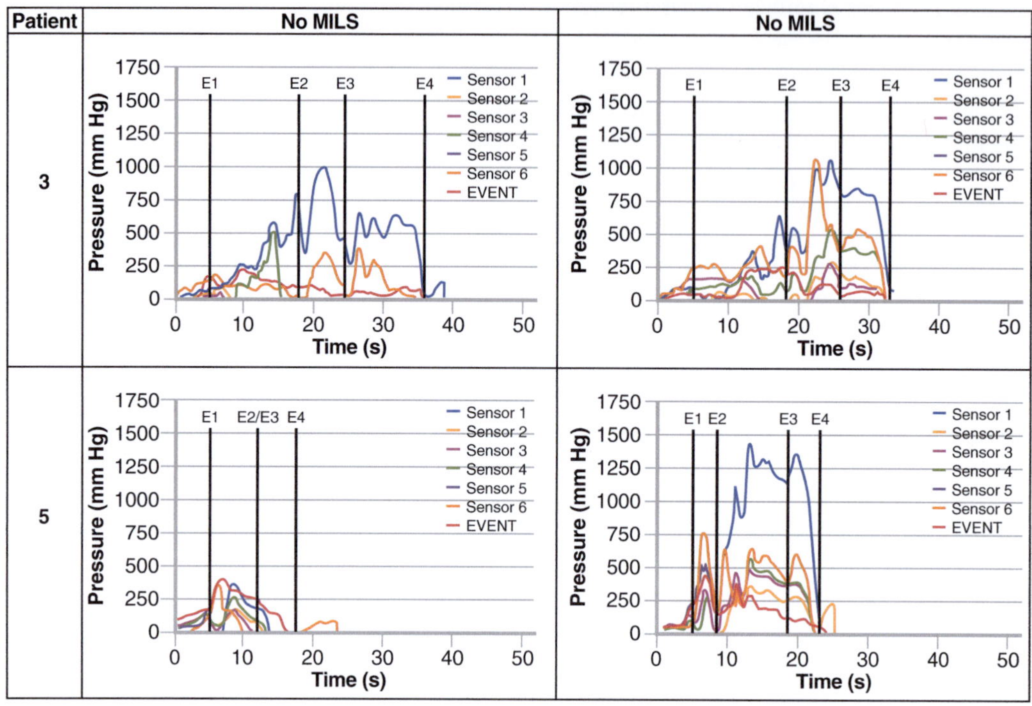

Fig. 2.8 Pressures applied by the MacIntosh laryngoscope blade on the tongue and indirectly on the C-Spine during various phases of direct laryngoscopy and intubation in two patients. Note that applied pressure is greatest from the time of final position of the blade to the completion of intubation, especially with application of manual inline stabilization (MILS) of the head and neck. Reproduced with permission from Santoni BG, Hindman BJ, Puttlitz CM et al.: Manual in-line stabilization increases pressures applied by the laryngoscope blade during direct laryngoscopy and orotracheal intubation. Anesthesiology 2009; 110:24-31

laryngoscopy and intubation. Exerted pressures during the best laryngoscopic view were twice as large with MILS than without (Fig. 2.8). These findings confirm the results of a video fluoroscopic study conducted by Lennarson and colleagues [68] in C4–5 cervical spine destabilized fresh cadavers. They looked at the angular rotation and the anterior/posterior (AP) and axial displacements (change in vertical intervertebral space height) during laryngoscopy with and without MILS. There was no change in angular rotation and axial distraction when the laryngoscopy was done in the presence of MILS. There was, however, significant anteroposterior displacement of as much as 1.9 mm, compared to 1 mm without MILS (Fig. 2.9). The maximum physiologic AP displacement of the C-spine is about 3–3.5 mm [69]. Thus, with or without MILS, movement of the unstable segment during laryngoscopy is still within the physiologic range. However, this change occurred in an experimental C-spine preparation. Under clinical conditions when the extent of injury is unknown, it is difficult to predict the extent of damage even when C-spine movement is within the physiologic range. There are additional reasons for maintaining the practice of applying MILS during airway management of a suspected C-spine-injured patient [70]. First, there is no randomized clinical trial to show conclusively that outcome during airway management is not different with or without MILS. Second,

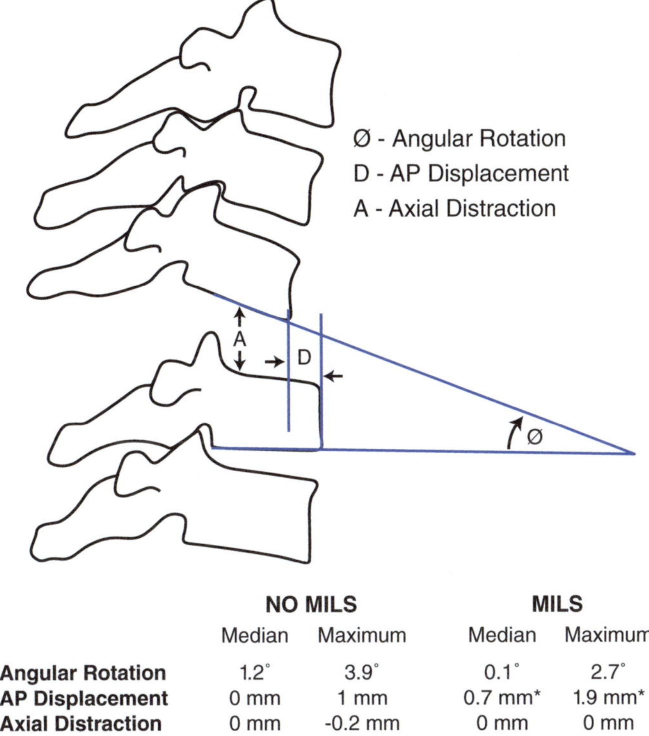

	NO MILS		MILS	
	Median	Maximum	Median	Maximum
Angular Rotation	1.2°	3.9°	0.1°	2.7°
AP Displacement	0 mm	1 mm	0.7 mm*	1.9 mm*
Axial Distraction	0 mm	-0.2 mm	0 mm	0 mm

Fig. 2.9 Effect of manual inline stabilization (MILS) on the cervical spine angular rotation, and the anterior--posterior and axial displacements during laryngoscopy and intubation in C4–C5 destabilized fresh cadavers. *Upper panel* depicts the definitions of angular rotation, and anterior-posterior and axial displacements of the spine. *Lower panel* shows the extent of movement in each of these directions during laryngoscopy and intubation with and without MILS (*Upper panel*, reproduced with permission from Gerling MC, Davis DP, Hamilton RS, Morris GF, Vilke GF, Garfin SR, Hayden SR. Effects of cervical spine immobilization technique and laryngoscope blade selection on an unstable cervical spine in cadaver model of intubation. *Lower panel*, data obtained from Lennarson PJ, Smith DW, Sawin PD et al.: Cervical spinal motion during intubation: efficacy of stabilization maneuvers in the setting of complete segmental instability. Journal of Neurosurgery 2001; 94:265-70)

development or worsening of spinal cord injury after institution of MILS during initial management has been less than that encountered during the prestabilization era, suggesting a protective effect of neck stabilization during airway management. Third, MILS can serve to warn physicians about the possibility of an underlying C-spine injury. It is reasonable, however, to allow some cervical movement by relaxing the MILS to optimize visualization of the larynx when the glottic view is restricted during laryngoscopy. As mentioned Tabove, bougies, stylets, or cricoid pressure in this situation may further facilitate laryngeal view and intubation.

Almost any of the available airway devices cause some C-spine movement [68, 71, 72]. Face mask ventilation with chin lift and jaw thrust results in significant posterior displacement. Supraglottic intubating airways, with or without FOB guidance, can also cause neck motion not much different than that caused by direct laryngoscopy. A wide variety of video laryngoscopes are available and they are evaluated in various conditions that imitate C-spine injury such as simulators, cadavers with destabilized necks, and patients with intact necks. Without doubt video laryngoscopes improve the laryngeal view even in the most difficult airways. They probably reduce neck movement as well, but they do not eliminate it (Table 2.7) [51, 73–75]. As mentioned above video laryngoscopes can be divided into two

Table 2.7 Performance characteristics of four tracheal intubation devices tested in lightly embalmed cadaver model with global ligamentous instability at C5–C6

	Macintosh	ILMA	Lightwand	Airtraq
Time to intubate (s)	22	42	34	27
Failure rate (%)	0	23	0	0
Flexion/ extension (°)	4.7	3	2.4	2.9
Lateral bending (°)	2.7	1.9	1.5	1.9
Axial rotation (°)	4.3	2.9	2.3	2.8
M/L translation (mm)	2.0	1.1	1.1	1.3
AP translation (mm)	5.7	3.6	2.7	3.3
Axial distraction (mm)	2.8	1.9	1.6	2.1

M/L medial/lateral, *AP* anterior/posterior, *ILMA* intubating laryngeal mask airway
Adapted from Prasarn ML, Conrad B, Rubery PT et al.: Comparison of 4 airway devices on cervical spine alignment in a cadaver model with global ligamentous instability at C5-C6. Spine 2012;37: 476-81

categories: those that permit a view of the larynx with a rigid video-furnished blade by which the ET tube can be directed into the larynx by the operator (GlideScope, Storz,), and those which direct the tube into the laryngeal inlet in addition to optimizing the view (Airtraq, Pentax Airway scope, King Vision). Of all these airway techniques FOB-guided nasotracheal intubation causes the least displacement [71, 76], although it may be associated with other problems such as prolonged intubation time, nose bleed, etc. Thus, during the initial phase after trauma when cervical spine injury is suspected, orotracheal intubation by applying MILS and using either a conventional blade or a videolaryngoscope after anesthetic induction is the most appropriate technique of intubation. In the later phases after trauma (24 h or longer), FOB-guided oro- or naso-tracheal intubation after sedation and topicalization of the airway is preferred. This approach allows neurologic testing immediately after securing the airway.

Management of Direct Airway Injuries

Trauma-induced direct damage to the airway or the surrounding tissue can occur anywhere between the nasopharynx and the bronchi. Occasionally injury may involve more than one level of the airway, resulting in persistent dysfunction after one of the problems is corrected.

Maxillofacial Injuries

Both penetrating and blunt mechanisms may be responsible for maxillofacial trauma. The face, head, and neck are vulnerable to missile and explosion injuries. Of the penetrating injuries, high velocity missiles produce severe and unpredictable disfiguring wounds. Battle injuries, which are mostly caused by explosives and ballistics, are more likely to be associated with multiple open and comminuted facial fractures [77]. In the blunt trauma category, injuries caused by altercations are usually less severe than those produced by motor vehicle accidents or falls.

Panfacial fractures involving the lower, middle, and upper face are likely to develop with high impact blunt injuries. This type of trauma is likely to involve more than one of the five regions of the facial skeleton: mandible, maxilla, zygomatic complex, naso-orbito-ethmoid region, and frontal bone [78]. The resistance of individual facial bones to blunt impact varies; the thin nasal bones are least and the thick supraorbital bone is the most resistant. Associated head and/or cervical spine injury should be suspected, especially in the presence of fractures of the more resistant facial bones. Facial fractures may not involve only the anterior bones. The fracture line may extend posteriorly and involve the pterygoid process of the sphenoid bone, the posterior buttress of the facial skeleton, which can cause posterior displacement of the face and obstruction of the nasopharynx. In a LeFort 1 fracture the pterygoid process is damaged at its inferior tip with minimal displacement. LeFort 2 and 3 fractures involve the pterygoid process close to its base, where it is connected to the sphenoid bone, causing significant posterior displacement and giving the face a "dishpan" or "baby face" appearance. These fractures may also involve the cribriform plate causing cerebrospinal fluid leakage with the risk of infection.

Difficulty in airway management may arise from mechanical or functional limitation of mouth opening, soft-tissue edema of the pharynx, peripharyngeal hematoma, and blood or debris in the oropharynx. The result of these is partial or complete airway obstruction which may lead to difficulty in visualizing the larynx in the acute stage of these injuries. Occasionally, teeth or foreign bodies in the pharynx may be aspirated into the airway. If not recognized, these foreign bodies may cause some degree of obstruction in distal airways with subsequent pneumonia. Injured maxillofacial soft tissues are dynamic. Serious airway compromise may develop within a few hours in up to 50 % of patients with major penetrating facial injuries or multiple trauma as a result of an expanding hematoma or progressive inflammation or edema resulting from the trauma itself and/or liberal administration of fluids. Although rare, massive hemorrhage, most frequently from the internal maxillary artery or its branches, may be life threatening, requiring angioembolization. Prophylactic intubation of the trachea may avert airway compromise in these circumstances [79].

As mentioned fracture-induced encroachment on the airway or limitation of mandibular movement, pain, and trismus may limit mouth opening. Fentanyl in titrated doses of up to 2–4 µg/kg over a period of 10–20 min may produce an improvement in the patient's ability to open the mouth if mechanical limitation is not present.

Unless severe airway compromise or bleeding is complicating the clinical picture in panfacial fractures, surgery may be delayed for as long as a week without adverse effect on the repair. Panfacial fractures, most of which are managed after stabilizing hemodynamic and oxygenation status and repair of vital injuries, are usually repaired with the principle of "bottom up and

outside in" in the same session of a prolonged procedure. Thus, the mandible is repaired before the maxilla, and zygomatic fractures before naso-orbito-ethmoid fractures. Some of the reasons for this approach are to maintain the vertical length of the face, repairing the simple mandibular fracture before a complex maxillary fracture, and preventing facial asymmetry [78]. Surgery during the early phase may be limited to intermaxillary fixation, which may be done under local or general anesthesia depending on the type of fracture, patient tolerance, and hemodynamic and respiratory status. Some of these patients may require tracheostomy using either an open or percutaneous technique, preferably over an endotracheal tube [80, 81]. Patients operated for definitive repair a few days after injury will present with a CT scan delineating the skeletal injury. Both two-dimensional spiral CT scanning with axial, coronal, and sagittal projections and three-dimensional CT scans provide adequate evaluation of maxillofacial fractures, aiding in planning of airway management [82].

The selection of an airway management technique in the presence of a maxillofacial fracture is based on the patient's presenting condition. Most patients with isolated facial injuries do not require emergency tracheal intubation. Patients who present with airway compromise may be intubated using direct laryngoscopy; the decision about the use of anesthetics and muscle relaxants is based on the results of airway evaluation. Bleeding into the oropharynx precludes the use of a flexible FOB, and often of a videolaryngoscope, because of obstruction of the view by blood and secretions. A retrograde technique, using a wire or epidural catheter passed through a 14-gauge catheter introduced into the trachea through the cricothyroid membrane, may be used if the patient can open his or her mouth. A surgical airway with either open or percutaneous technique is indicated when there is airway compromise, direct laryngoscopy has failed or is considered impossible, the jaws will be wired, or when a tracheostomy will be performed anyway after definitive repair of the fracture [80,

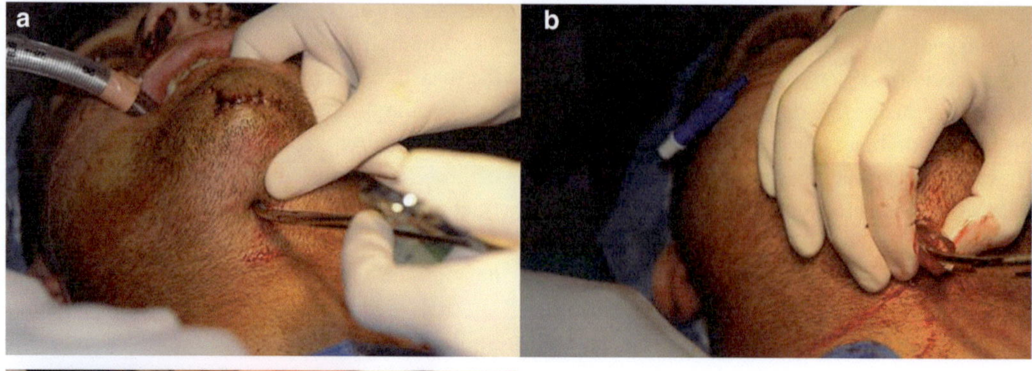

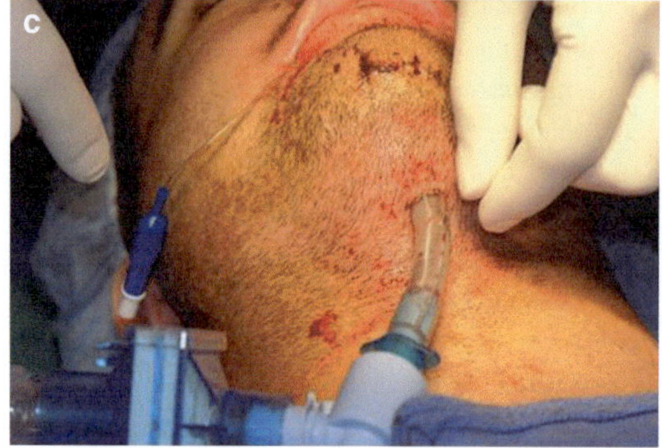

Fig. 2.10 Submental intubation. (**a**) Small submental incision is made and the floor of the mouth is pierced with a clamp introduced through the incision in the patient intubated with a flexible armored tube, (**b**) Proximal end of the endotracheal tube is grabbed with the clamp introduced into the floor of the mouth and pulled through the submental incision, (**c**) The tube is connected to the breathing circuit

81]. Tracheostomy may often be avoided with the use of submental intubation in patients operated electively for definitive repair of injuries [83, 84]. This technique involves making a small submental incision after intubation of the trachea with a flexible armored tube, introducing a clamp through the incision, piercing the floor of the mouth, grabbing the proximal end of the endotracheal tube, and pulling it through the incision (Fig. 2.10). Thus, the oral cavity is free and the tracheal wall remains intact. Postoperatively the tube can be removed or redirected to its original position. Nasogastric or blind nasotracheal intubation should be avoided in the early stage after trauma when a basilar skull or maxillary fracture is suspected: the tube may enter the cranium or the orbital fossa, damaging the brain or the eye. Hemorrhagic shock and life-threatening cranial, cervical, laryngotracheal, thoracic, and cervical spine injuries may accompany major facial fractures; airway management must be tailored accordingly (Fig. 2.11). The likelihood of cranial injury increases in midface fractures involving the frontal sinus, as well as the orbitozygomatic and orbitoethmoid complexes.

Cervical Injuries

Both blunt and penetrating trauma can cause direct laryngotracheal injury. These injuries are relatively rare compared to maxillofacial injuries partly because of protection of the anterior aspect of the neck by the mandible. The incidence of blunt and penetrating laryngotracheal injuries admitted to major trauma centers is 0.34 % and 4 %, respectively [85]. As in maxillofacial injuries, wartime laryngotracheal injuries are more severe and occur more frequently (5 % in United States and 11 % in United Kingdom forces) [86] than peacetime injuries (0.91 %).

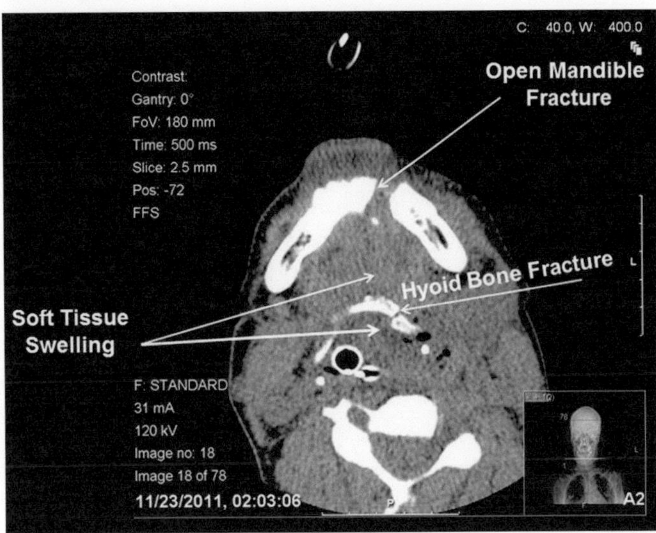

Fig. 2.11 Computed tomography scan of a patient sustaining hyoid bone and open mandibular fracture. Note submandibular edema. Airway obstruction after induction of anesthesia necessitated emergency surgical airway

Interestingly, involvement of the pharynx and esophagus, which are in proximity to the cervical airway, is less likely than airway injuries in peacetime trauma (0.08 % after blunt and 0.9 % after penetrating trauma); [85] they may be more frequent in combat injuries. Although direct injury to the airway is relatively rare, the tightly organized anatomic structures within the neck may result in airway compromise when other cervical structures are injured. For example, vascular injury in this region can cause airway obstruction because of laryngeal edema resulting from shift of the larynx and compression of the veins by the hematoma. Likewise, a retropharyngeal abscess after an unrecognized esophageal injury may result in partial or total airway obstruction. Thus, cervical airway injuries should be considered in conjunction with any neck injury rather than as isolated entities.

Anatomically, the neck is divided into anterior and posterior triangles, and in its anteroposterior direction into three zones (1, 2 and 3, from caudad to cephalad). The boundaries of the anterior triangle are the midline, the lower border of the mandible, and the anterior border of the sternocleidomastoid muscle. A prominent area in this region is the "laryngeal trapezium" which is bounded superiorly by the hyoid bone, inferiorly by the sternal notch, and laterally by the anterior borders of both sternocleidomastoid muscles. The posterior triangle is bounded by the middle third of the clavicle inferiorly, the posterior border of the sternocleidomastoid muscle medially, and the anterior border of the trapezius muscle posteriorly. Wounds in the anterior region compromise the airway more often than posterior injuries because of their proximity to the larynx, trachea, laryngeal nerves, and the important cervical vessels. Zone 1, also called the root of the neck or the thyrocervical region, is the narrow area below the clavicles. Injuries to this area are not only life threatening, but are also difficult to control surgically. On the other hand, this area is protected by the osseous upper anterior chest wall and is injured less often than zone 2. Zone 2 is the region between the clavicle or the cricoid cartilage inferiorly and the angle of the mandible superiorly. It is most likely to be injured by both penetrating and blunt trauma with resulting injuries to the arterial, venous, aerodigestive, and neural structures. Mortality from injuries to this region is relatively low, probably because they are easy to evaluate and treat. Zone 3 comprises the area between the angle of the mandible and the base of the skull.

Fig. 2.12 Management strategy of patients with penetrating neck trauma. Adapted by permission from Inaba K, Branco BC, Menaker J et al.: Evaluation of multidetector computed tomography for penetrating neck injury: a prospective multicenter study. Journal of Trauma 2012; 72:576-84

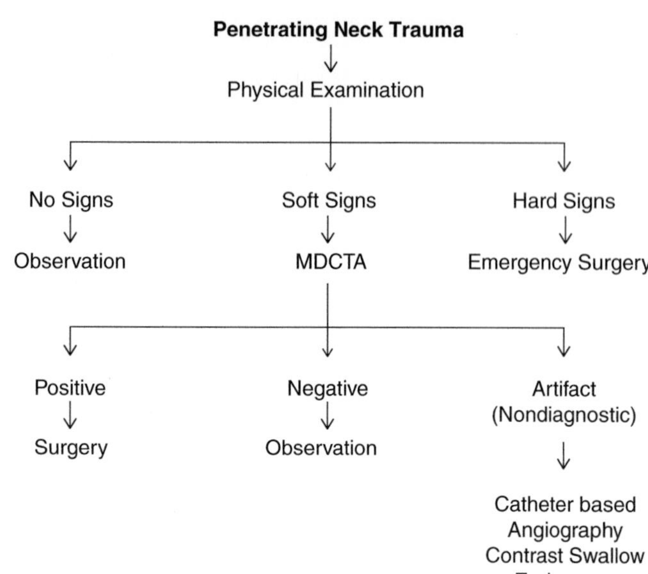

Surgical access is difficult to this area because it is obscured by the ramus of the mandible.

There are several causes of penetrating neck injuries: stab, gunshot, or shotgun wounds, explosions, or occupational hazards. Although explosions can cause injury by several mechanisms, damage is most commonly produced by the energized fragments overlying buried devices [86]. Of the other mechanisms, gunshot wounds usually are the most severe and unpredictable. Penetrating neck wounds are classified not only by their causes, but also by the location of the entry point of the object, the physiologic stability of the patient, and the organs injured. It should be emphasized that entry point may not always correspond to the location of interior damage, especially after high-velocity gunshot wounds [87].

Blunt neck injuries are caused by motor vehicle accidents, falls, and sudden collision with an object at the level of the neck. For example, a chain set between two sides of a dirt road represents a threat of neck injury for a person on a bicycle or motorcycle.

Clinical signs such as air escape, hemoptysis, and coughing spells are present in almost all patients with penetrating injuries, facilitating the diagnosis. In contrast, major blunt laryngotracheal damage may easily be missed, because many patients have mild or no symptoms, which may be missed during the initial evaluation. Hoarseness, muffled voice, dyspnea, stridor, dysphagia, odynophagia, cervical pain and tenderness, ecchymosis, subcutaneous emphysema, and flattening of the thyroid cartilage protuberance (Adam's apple) are the classical signs and symptoms of blunt laryngotracheal injuries. Almost never are all of these symptoms seen in a single patient.

The approach to management of penetrating neck injuries has gone through multiple changes during the last two decades. The current management strategy for penetrating neck injuries is summarized in Fig. 2.12 [88]. It is now clear that physical examination of the neck reliably reveals unstable patients, those with hard signs and soft signs (Table 2.8) and asymptomatic patients. Unstable patients and those with obvious signs (hard signs) (Table 2.8) are candidates for emergency surgical exploration without additional workup. Asymptomatic patients can be observed for 24 h without any radiologic examination. Patients with soft signs and probably those who are asymptomatic but whose injury is

Table 2.8 The list of hard signs that indicate surgery without work-up, and soft signs that indicate evaluation with multidetector computed tomographic angiography (MDCTA) in penetrating cervical injuries

Hard clinical signs after penetrating neck injury	Soft clinical signs after penetrating neck injury
Shock unresponsive to initial fluid resuscitation	Nonexpanding or nonpulsatile hematoma
Active hemorrhage from the neck	Venous oozing
Expanding or pulsatile hematoma	Subcutaneous emphysema
Bruit or thrill in the area of injury	Dysphonia
Massive hemoptysis or hematemesis	Minor hemoptysis
Air bubbling from the injury site	Dysphagia
Neurological signs of cerebral ischemia	Injury proximity to vital organs

Adapted by permission from Inaba K, Branco BC, Menaker J et al.: Evaluation of multidetector computed tomography for penetrating neck injury: a prospective multicenter study. Journal of Trauma 2012; 72:576-84

near vital organs should undergo multidetector computed tomography angiography (MDCTA) scanning with image reconstruction. Surgery may be indicated in those with positive MDCTA findings. Soft signs include non-expanding or non-pulsatile hematoma, venous oozing, subcutaneous emphysema, dysphonia, minor hemoptysis, and dysphagia (Table 2.8). The presence of retained missiles may interfere with the accuracy of the MDCTA image and mask clinically significant injury. These patients may require angiography for the diagnosis of vascular damage, or esophagram or bronchoscopy for diagnosis of esophageal or airway injuries [88]. The insidious and often silent nature of blunt cervical airway injuries requires a high degree of suspicion and often evaluation by computed tomography (CT) and preferably MDCTA, unless the patient is unstable.

Whether the airway injury is blunt or penetrating, attempts at blind tracheal intubation may produce further trauma to the larynx and complete airway obstruction if the endotracheal tube enters a false passage or disrupts the continuity of an already tenuous airway (Fig. 2.13) [89]. Thus, whenever possible, intubation of the trachea should be performed under direct vision using an FOB, or the airway should be secured surgically. The two-man technique, one operator performing laryngoscopy with a conventional blade or a video laryngoscope and directing the second exploring the airway with an FOB, is the preferable technique. A CT scan of the neck provides valuable information and should be viewed, if

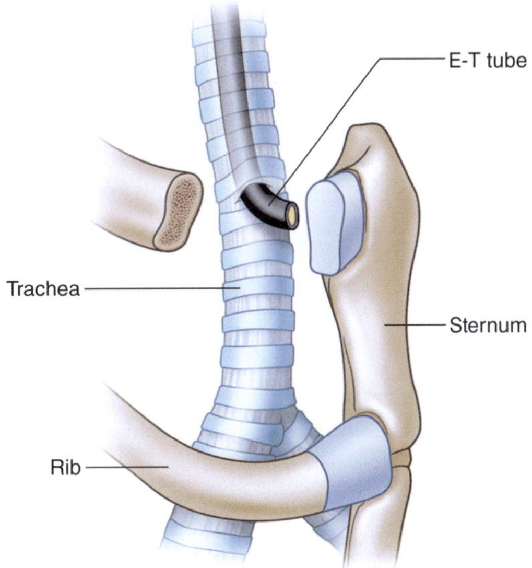

Fig. 2.13 Schematic representation of an endotracheal tube entry into a false passage through the tracheal wall defect caused by the injury

available, before any airway intervention in all stable patients with neck injury and without respiratory and hemodynamic compromise.

Although development of edema and subsequent airway obstruction necessitates securing the airway at the earliest possible time after most cervical airway injuries, the approach to airway management depends on the clinical presentation [89]. Some airway injuries observed on CT scan may be mild with minimal symptoms and without progression. These patients can be managed conservatively without intubation [90]. The tracheas of some patients with penetrating airway injuries may be amenable to intubation through the airway defect in the neck without the need for anesthetics or laryngoscopy. The presence of cartilaginous fractures or mucosal abnormalities necessitates intubation with preservation of spontaneous breathing using an FOB or awake tracheostomy. Laryngeal damage precludes cricothyroidotomy. Tracheostomy should be performed with extreme caution because up to 70 % of patients with blunt laryngeal injuries may have an associated cervical spine injury and neck extension to optimize surgical exposure may jeopardize the integrity of the spinal cord [89]. Uncooperative or confused patients may not tolerate awake airway manipulation. It may be best to transport these patients to the OR, induce anesthesia with inhalational agents, and intubate the trachea without muscle relaxants [89]. Episodes of airway obstruction during spontaneous breathing under an inhalational anesthetic can be managed by positioning the patient upright in addition to the usual maneuvers.

Complete transection of the trachea is rare, but when it occurs it is life-threatening; the distal segment of the trachea retracts into the chest, causing airway obstruction either spontaneously or during airway manipulation. Surgery involves pulling up the distal end and performing an end-to-end anastomosis to the proximal segment or suturing it to the skin as a permanent tracheostomy [91]. In extreme situations, such as complete or near-complete transection of the larynx and trachea, femorofemoral bypass or percutaneous cardiopulmonary support may be considered if time permits [92]. Vascular injuries causing hemorrhagic shock are also an indication for airway management. Bleeding in these patients can be controlled temporarily by the index finger covered with a sterile glove introduced through the cervical wound and compressing the bleeding site. Alternatively, the inflation of the balloon of a Foley catheter introduced through the wound tract can control the bleeding [93]. However, airway management in these patients and in those with cervical hematoma may be challenging because of the shift of the trachea to the contralateral side.

Thoracic Airway Injuries

Although penetrating trauma can cause damage to any segment of the intrathoracic airway, blunt injury usually involves the posterior membranous portion of the trachea and the mainstem bronchi, usually within approximately 3 cm of the carina. A significant number of these injuries results from iatrogenic causes such as tracheal intubation [94]. The usual signs and symptoms include those produced by pneumothorax, pneumomediastinum, pneumopericardium, subcutaneous emphysema, and a continuous air leak from the chest tube; they occur frequently but are not specific for thoracic airway damage. Radiographically, a radiolucent line along the prevertebral fascia due to air tracking up from the mediastinum, peribronchial air or sudden obstruction along an air-filled bronchus, and the "dropped lung" sign that occurs when there is complete intrapleural bronchial transection causing the apex of the collapsed lung to descend to the level of the hilum are important indications of intrathoracic airway injury. Additionally in patients intubated without the suspicion of a tracheal injury, difficulty in obtaining a seal around the endotracheal tube, or the presence on a chest radiograph of a large radiolucent area in the trachea corresponding to the cuff suggests a perforated airway. Airway management is similar to that of cervical airway injury. All airway manipulations must be done under direct vision using an FOB to prevent entry into a false passage. Anesthetics, and especially muscle relaxants, may produce irreversible obstruction, presumably because of relaxation of structures that maintain patency of the airway in the awake patient; however, airway loss may also occur during attempts at awake intubation, often as a result of further distortion of the airway by the endotracheal tube, patient agitation, or bleeding into the airway [95]. After intubation of the trachea, the adequacy of airway intervention is evaluated mainly by auscultation and capnography. Nevertheless, pulmonary contusion, atelectasis, diaphragmatic rupture with thoracic migration of the abdominal contents, and pneumothorax may complicate the interpretation of chest auscultation. Likewise, CO_2 elimination may be decreased or absent in shock and cardiac arrest.

Because the outcome after surgical repair of these injuries is often suboptimal and complicated by stump leak and empyema, suture line stenosis, or the need for tracheostomy or pneumonectomy, many surgeons choose selective conservative management. Patients with lesions larger than 4 cm, cartilaginous rather than membranous injuries, concomitant esophageal trauma, progressive subcutaneous emphysema, severe dyspnea requiring intubation and ventilation, difficulty with mechanical ventilation, pneumothorax with an air leak through the chest drains, and/or mediastinitis are still managed surgically. Those without these problems may be treated nonoperatively with a reasonable outcome [94].

References

1. Apfelbaum JL, Hagberg CA, Caplan RA, Blitt CD, Connis RT, Nickinovich DG, Benumof JL, Berry FA, Bode RH, Cheney FW, Guidry OF, Ovassapian A; Updated by the Committee on Standards and Practice Parameters. Practice guidelines for management of the difficult airway. Anesthesiology. 2013;118:251–70.
2. Wilson W. Trauma: airway management. ASA difficult airway algorithm modified for trauma and five common intubation scenarios. ASA Newsl. 2005;69. 7 p.
3. Fields A, Rosbolt M, Cohn S. Induction agents for intubation of the trauma patient. J Trauma Acute Care Surg. 2009;67. 3 p.
4. Cotton B, Guillamondegui O, Flemin S. Increased risk of adrenal insufficiency following etomidate exposure in critically injured patients. Arch Surg. 2008;143. 5 p.
5. Warner K, Cuschieri J, Jurkovich G. Single-dose etomidate for rapid sequence intubation may impact outcome after severe injury. J Trauma Acute Care Surg. 2009;67. 5 p.
6. Selick B. Cricoid pressure to control regurgitation of stomach contents during induction of anesthesia. Lancet. 1961;2. 2 p.
7. Ellis D, Harris T, Zideman D. Cricoid pressure in emergency department rapid sequence intubations: a risk-benefit analysis. Ann Emerg Med. 2007;50. 12 p.
8. Harris T, Ellis D, Foster L. Cricoid pressure and laryngeal manipulation in 402 pre-hospital emergency anaesthetics: essential safety measure or a hindrance to rapid safe intubation? Resuscitation. 2010;81. 6 p.
9. Keller C, Brimacombe J, Keller K. Pressures exerted against the cervical vertebrae by the standard and intubating laryngeal mask airways: a randomized, controlled, cross-over study in fresh cadavers. Anesth Analg. 1999;89:1296–300.
10. Bair AE, Filbin MR, Kulkarni RG, Walls RM. The failed intubation attempt in the emergency department: analysis of prevalence, rescue techniques, and personnel. J Emerg Med. 2002;23: 131–40.
11. Aarabi B, Simard JM. Traumatic brain injury. Curr Opin Crit Care. 2009;15:548–53.
12. Reed M, Dunn M, McKeown DW. Can an airway assessment score predict difficulty at intubation in the emergency department? Emerg Med J. 2005;22. 3 p.
13. Kortbeek JB, Al Turki SA, Ali J, Antoine JA, Bouillon B, Brasel K, Brenneman F, Brink PR, Brohi K, Burris D, Burton RA, Chapleau W, Cioffi W, Collet e Silva Fde S, Cooper A, Cortes JA, Eskesen V, Fildes J, Gautam S, Gruen RL, Gross R, Hansen KS, Henny W, Hollands MJ, Hunt RC, Jover Navalon JM, Kaufmann CR, Knudson P, Koestner A, Kosir R, Larsen CF, Livaudais W, Luchette F, Mao P, McVicker JH, Meredith JW, Mock C, Mori ND, Morrow C, Parks SN, Pereira PM, Pogetti RS, Ravn J, Rhee P, Salomone JP, Schipper IB, Schoettker P, Schreiber MA, Smith RS, Svendsen LB, Taha W, van Wijngaarden-Stephens M, Varga E, Voiglio EJ, Williams D, Winchell RJ, Winter R. Advanced trauma life support, 8th edition, the evidence for change. J Trauma. 2008;64:1638–50.
14. Perlas A, Mitsakakis N, Liu L, Cino M, Haldipur N, Davis L, Cubillos J, Chan V. Validation of a mathematical model for ultrasound assessment of gastric volume by gastroscopic examination. Anesth Analg. 2013;116:357–63.
15. Adhikari S, Zeger W, Schmier C, Crum T, Craven A, Frrokaj I, Pang H, Shostrom V. Pilot study to determine the utility of point-of-care ultrasound in the assessment of difficult laryngoscopy. Acad Emerg Med. 2011;18:754–8.
16. Kristensen MS. Ultrasonography in the management of the airway. Acta Anaesthesiol Scand. 2011;55: 1155–73.
17. Alrajhi K, Woo M, Villancourt C. Test characteristics of ultrasonography for the detection of pneumothorax: a systematic review and meta-analysis. Chest. 2012;141. 5 p.
18. Lichtenstein D, Meziere G, Lascols N. Ultrasound diagnosis of occult pneumothorax. Crit Care Med. 2005;33. 7 p.
19. Sim SS, Lien WC, Chou HC, Chong KM, Liu SH, Wang CH, Chen SY, Hsu CY, Yen ZS, Chang WT, Huang CH, Ma MH, Chen SC. Ultrasonographic lung sliding sign in confirming proper endotracheal intubation during emergency intubation. Resuscitation. 2012;83:307–12.

20. Mayglothling J, Duane T, Gibbs M, McCunn M, Legome E, Eastman A, Whelan J, Shah K. Emergency tracheal Intubation immediately following traumatic injury: an Eastern Association for the Surgery of Trauma practice management guideline. J Trauma Acute Care Surg. 2012;73. 7 p.

21. Sise MJ, Shackford SR, Sise CB, Sack DI, Paci GM, Yale RS, O'Reilly EB, Norton VC, Huebner BR, Peck KA. Early intubation in the management of trauma patients: indications and outcomes in 1,000 consecutive patients. J Trauma. 2009;66:32–9; discussion 39–40.

22. Hassid V, Schinco M, Tepas J. Definitive establishment of airway control is critical for optimal outcome in lower cervical spinal cord injury. J Trauma Acute Care Surg. 2008;65. 4 pp.

23. Como J, Sutton E, McCunn M. Characterizing the need for mechanical ventilation following cervical spinal cord injury with neurologic deficit. J Trauma Acute Care Surg. 2005;59. 4 p.

24. Velmahos GC, Toutouzas K, Chan L, Tillou A, Rhee P, Murray J, Demetriades D. Intubation after cervical spinal cord injury: to be done selectively or routinely? Am Surg. 2003;69:891–4.

25. Komatsu R, Kamata K, Hoshi I, Sessler DI, Ozaki M. Airway scope and gum elastic bougie with Macintosh laryngoscope for tracheal intubation in patients with simulated restricted neck mobility. Br J Anaesth. 2008;101:863–9.

26. Malik MA, Maharaj CH, Harte BH, Laffey JG. Comparison of Macintosh, Truview EVO2, Glidescope, and Airwayscope laryngoscope use in patients with cervical spine immobilization. Br J Anaesth. 2008;101:723–30.

27. Maruyama K, Yamada T, Kawakami R, Hara K. Randomized cross-over comparison of cervical-spine motion with the AirWay Scope or Macintosh laryngoscope with in-line stabilization: a videofluoroscopic study. Br J Anaesth. 2008;101:563–7.

28. Maruyama K, Yamada T, Kawakami R, Kamata T, Yokochi M, Hara K. Upper cervical spine movement during intubation: fluoroscopic comparison of the AirWay Scope, McCoy laryngoscope, and Macintosh laryngoscope. Br J Anaesth. 2008;100:120–4.

29. Bathory I, Frascarolo P, Kern C, Schoettker P. Evaluation of the GlideScope for tracheal intubation in patients with cervical spine immobilisation by a semi-rigid collar. Anaesthesia. 2009;64:1337–41.

30. Sakles JC, Mosier JM, Chiu S, Keim SM. Tracheal intubation in the emergency department: a comparison of GlideScope(R) video laryngoscopy to direct laryngoscopy in 822 intubations. J Emerg Med. 2012;42:400–5.

31. Platts-Mills TF, Campagne D, Chinnock B, Snowden B, Glickman LT, Hendey GW. A comparison of GlideScope video laryngoscopy versus direct laryngoscopy intubation in the emergency department. Acad Emerg Med. 2009;16:866–71.

32. Yeatts DJ, Dutton RP, Hu PF, Chang YW, Brown CH, Chen H, Grissom TE, Kufera JA, Scalea TM. Effect of video laryngoscopy on trauma patient survival: a randomized controlled trial. J Trauma Acute Care Surg. 2013;75:212–9.

33. Asai T, Liu EH, Matsumoto S, Hirabayashi Y, Seo N, Suzuki A, Toi T, Yasumoto K, Okuda Y. Use of the Pentax-AWS in 293 patients with difficult airways. Anesthesiology. 2009;110:898–904.

34. Lim HC, Goh SH. Utilization of a Glidescope videolaryngoscope for orotracheal intubations in different emergency airway management settings. Eur J Emerg Med. 2009;16:68–73.

35. Aziz MF, Healy D, Kheterpal S, Fu RF, Dillman D, Brambrink AM. Routine clinical practice effectiveness of the Glidescope in difficult airway management: an analysis of 2,004 Glidescope intubations, complications, and failures from two institutions. Anesthesiology. 2011;114:34–41.

36. Aziz MF, Dillman D, Fu R, Brambrink AM. Comparative effectiveness of the C-MAC video laryngoscope versus direct laryngoscopy in the setting of the predicted difficult airway. Anesthesiology. 2012;116:629–36.

37. Teoh WH, Saxena S, Shah MK, Sia AT. Comparison of three videolaryngoscopes: Pentax Airway Scope, C-MAC, Glidescope vs the Macintosh laryngoscope for tracheal intubation. Anaesthesia. 2010;65:1126–32.

38. Pfeiffer P, Bache S, Isbye D, Rudolph S, Rovsing L, Borglum J. Verification of endotracheal intubation in obese patients—temporal comparison of ultrasound vs. ausculatation and capnography. Acta Anaesthesiol Scand. 2012;56. 5 p.

39. Chacko J, Nikahat J, Gagen B, Umesh K, Ramanathan M. Real time ultrasound-guided percutaneous dilatational tracheostomy. Intensive Care Med. 2012;38. 2 p.

40. Kristensen M, Teoh W. The ultrasound probe in the hands of the anesthesiologist: a powerful new tool for airway management. Anesthesiology News. 2013;Supplement Guide to Airway Management:7.

41. Drummond J. Neuroanesthesia: physiology and pharmacology that really matters. ASA Refresher Course Lectures. 2013;Course Number 225:4.

42. de Nadal M, Munar F, Poca MA, et al. Cerebral hemodynamic effects of morphine and fentanyl in patients with severe head injury. Absence of correlation to cerebral autoregulation. Anesthesiology. 2000;92:11–8.

43. Sehdev RS, Symmons DA, Kindl K. Ketamine for rapid sequence induction in patients with head injury in the emergency department. Emerg Med Australas. 2006;18:37–44.

44. Filanovsky Y, Miller P, Kao J. Myth: ketamine should not be used as an induction agent for intubation in patients with head injury. CJEM. 2010;12:154–7.

45. Bar-Joseph G, Guilburd Y, Tamir A, Guilburd JN. Effectiveness of ketamine in decreasing intracranial pressure in children with intracranial hypertension. J Neurosurg Pediatr. 2009;4:40–6.

46. Mayberg TS, Lam AM, Matta BF, Domino KB, Winn HR. Ketamine does not increase cerebral blood flow velocity or intracranial pressure during isoflurane/nitrous oxide anesthesia in patients undergoing craniotomy. Anesth Analg. 1995;81:84–9.

47. Clancy M, Halford S, Walls R, Murphy M. In patients with head injuries who undergo rapid sequence intubation using succinylcholine, does pretreatment with a competitive neuromuscular blocking agent improve outcome? A literature review. Emerg Med J. 2001;18:373–5.

48. Libonati MM, Leahy JJ, Ellison N. The use of succinylcholine in open eye surgery. Anesthesiology. 1985;62:637–40.

49. Zimmerman AA, Funk K, Tidwell JL. Propofol and alfentanil prevent the increase in intraocular pressure caused by succinylcholine and endotracheal intubation during a rapid sequence induction of anesthesia. Anesth Analg. 1996;83:814–7.

50. Heier T, Caldwell JE. Rapid tracheal intubation with large-dose rocuronium: a probability-based approach. Anesth Analg. 2000;90:175–9.

51. Prasarn ML, Conrad B, Rubery PT, Wendling A, Aydog T, Horodyski M, Rechtine GR. Comparison of 4 airway devices on cervical spine alignment in a cadaver model with global ligamentous instability at C5-C6. Spine (Phila Pa 1976). 2012;37:476–81.

52. Hoffman GL, Bock BF, Gallagher EJ, Markovchick VJ, Ham HP, Munger BS. Report of the Task Force on Residency Training Information, American Board of Emergency Medicine. Ann Emerg Med. 1998;31:608–25.

53. Rose MK, Rosal LM, Gonzalez RP, Rostas JW, Baker JA, Simmons JD, Frotan MA, Brevard SB. Clinical clearance of the cervical spine in patients with distracting injuries: it is time to dispel the myth. J Trauma Acute Care Surg. 2012;73:498–502.

54. Duane TM, Mayglothling J, Wilson SP, Wolfe LG, Aboutanos MB, Whelan JF, Malhotra AK, Ivatury RR. National Emergency X-Radiography Utilization Study criteria is inadequate to rule out fracture after significant blunt trauma compared with computed tomography. J Trauma. 2011;70:829–31.

55. Stiell IG, Clement CM, McKnight RD, Brison R, Schull MJ, Rowe BH, Worthington JR, Eisenhauer MA, Cass D, Greenberg G, MacPhail I, Dreyer J, Lee JS, Bandiera G, Reardon M, Holroyd B, Lesiuk H, Wells GA. The Canadian C-spine rule versus the NEXUS low-risk criteria in patients with trauma. N Engl J Med. 2003;349:2510–8.

56. Michaleff ZA, Maher CG, Verhagen AP, Rebbeck T, Lin CW. Accuracy of the Canadian C-spine rule and NEXUS to screen for clinically important cervical spine injury in patients following blunt trauma: a systematic review. CMAJ. 2012;184:E867–76.

57. Booth TN. Cervical spine evaluation in pediatric trauma. AJR Am J Roentgenol. 2012;198:W417–25.

58. Anglen J, Metzler M, Bunn P, Griffiths H. Flexion and extension views are not cost-effective in a cervical spine clearance protocol for obtunded trauma patients. J Trauma. 2002;52:54–9.

59. Davis JW, Kaups KL, Cunningham MA, Parks SN, Nowak TP, Bilello JF, Williams JL. Routine evaluation of the cervical spine in head-injured patients with dynamic fluoroscopy: a reappraisal. J Trauma. 2001;50:1044–7.

60. Muchow RD, Resnick DK, Abdel MP, Munoz A, Anderson PA. Magnetic resonance imaging (MRI) in the clearance of the cervical spine in blunt trauma: a meta-analysis. J Trauma. 2008;64:179–89.

61. Khanna P, Chau C, Dublin A, Kim K, Wisner D. The value of cervical magnetic resonance imaging in the evaluation of the obtunded or comatose patient with cervical trauma, no other abnormal neurological findings, and a normal cervical computed tomography. J Trauma Acute Care Surg. 2012;72:699–702.

62. Panczykowski DM, Tomycz ND, Okonkwo DO. Comparative effectiveness of using computed tomography alone to exclude cervical spine injuries in obtunded or intubated patients: meta-analysis of 14,327 patients with blunt trauma. J Neurosurg. 2011;115:541–9.

63. Marshall LF, Knowlton S, Garfin SR, Klauber MR, Eisenberg HM, Kopaniky D, Miner ME, Tabbador K, Clifton GL. Deterioration following spinal cord injury. A multicenter study. J Neurosurg. 1987;66:400–4.

64. Prasarn ML, Conrad B, Del Rossi G, Horodyski M, Rechtine GR. Motion generated in the unstable cervical spine during the application and removal of cervical immobilization collars. J Trauma Acute Care Surg. 2012;72:1609–13.

65. Hindman BJ, Palecek JP, Posner KL, Traynelis VC, Lee LA, Sawin PD, Tredway TL, Todd MM, Domino KB. Cervical spinal cord, root, and bony spine injuries: a closed claims analysis. Anesthesiology. 2011;114:782–95.

66. McLeod AD, Calder I. Spinal cord injury and direct laryngoscopy—the legend lives on. Br J Anaesth. 2000;84:705–9.

67. Santoni BG, Hindman BJ, Puttlitz CM, Weeks JB, Johnson N, Maktabi MA, Todd MM. Manual in-line stabilization increases pressures applied by the laryngoscope blade during direct laryngoscopy and orotracheal intubation. Anesthesiology. 2009;110:24–31.

68. Lennarson PJ, Smith DW, Sawin PD, Todd MM, Sato Y, Traynelis VC. Cervical spinal motion during intubation: efficacy of stabilization maneuvers in the setting of complete segmental instability. J Neurosurg. 2001;94:265–70.

69. Panjabi MM, Thibodeau LL, Crisco 3rd JJ, White 3rd AA. What constitutes spinal instability? Clin Neurosurg. 1988;34:313–39.

70. Manoach S, Paladino L. Laryngoscopy force, visualization, and intubation failure in acute trauma: should we modify the practice of manual in-line stabilization? Anesthesiology. 2009;110:6–7.

71. Brimacombe J, Keller C, Kunzel KH, Gaber O, Boehler M, Puhringer F. Cervical spine motion during airway management: a cinefluoroscopic study of the posteriorly destabilized third cervical vertebrae in human cadavers. Anesth Analg. 2000;91:1274–8.

72. LeGrand SA, Hindman BJ, Dexter F, Weeks JB, Todd MM. Craniocervical motion during direct laryngoscopy and orotracheal intubation with the Macintosh and Miller blades: an in vivo cinefluoroscopic study. Anesthesiology. 2007;107:884–91.

73. Robitaille A, Williams SR, Tremblay MH, Guilbert F, Theriault M, Drolet P. Cervical spine motion during tracheal intubation with manual in-line stabilization: direct laryngoscopy versus GlideScope videolaryngoscopy. Anesth Analg. 2008;106:935–41, table of contents.

74. Turner CR, Block J, Shanks A, Morris M, Lodhia KR, Gujar SK. Motion of a cadaver model of cervical injury during endotracheal intubation with a Bullard laryngoscope or a Macintosh blade with and without in-line stabilization. J Trauma. 2009;67:61–6.

75. Arslan ZI, Yildiz T, Baykara ZN, Solak M, Toker K. Tracheal intubation in patients with rigid collar immobilisation of the cervical spine: a comparison of Airtraq and LMA CTrach devices. Anaesthesia. 2009;64:1332–6.

76. Houde BJ, Williams SR, Cadrin-Chenevert A, Guilbert F, Drolet P. A comparison of cervical spine motion during orotracheal intubation with the trachlight(r) or the flexible fiberoptic bronchoscope. Anesth Analg. 2009;108:1638–43.

77. Zachar MR, Labella C, Kittle CP, Baer PB, Hale RG, Chan RK. Characterization of mandibular fractures incurred from battle injuries in Iraq and Afghanistan from 2001–2010. J Oral Maxillofac Surg. 2013;71:734–42.

78. Yang R, Zhang C, Liu Y, Li Z, Li Z. Why should we start from mandibular fractures in the treatment of panfacial fractures? J Oral Maxillofac Surg. 2012;70:1386–92.

79. Cogbill TH, Cothren CC, Ahearn MK, Cullinane DC, Kaups KL, Scalea TM, Maggio L, Brasel KJ, Harrison PB, Patel NY, Moore EE, Jurkovich GJ, Ross SE. Management of maxillofacial injuries with severe oronasal hemorrhage: a multicenter perspective. J Trauma. 2008;65:994–9.

80. Susarla SM, Peacock ZS, Alam HB. Percutaneous dilatational tracheostomy: review of technique and evidence for its use. J Oral Maxillofac Surg. 2012;70:74–82.

81. Holmgren EP, Bagheri S, Bell RB, Bobek S, Dierks EJ. Utilization of tracheostomy in craniomaxillofacial trauma at a level-1 trauma center. J Oral Maxillofac Surg. 2007;65:2005–10.

82. Jarrahy R, Vo V, Goenjian HA, Tabit CJ, Katchikian HV, Kumar A, Meals C, Bradley JP. Diagnostic accuracy of maxillofacial trauma two-dimensional and three-dimensional computed tomographic scans: comparison of oral surgeons, head and neck surgeons, plastic surgeons, and neuroradiologists. Plast Reconstr Surg. 2011;127:2432–40.

83. Lima Jr SM, Asprino L, Moreira RW, de Moraes M. A retrospective analysis of submental intubation in maxillofacial trauma patients. J Oral Maxillofac Surg. 2011;69:2001–5.

84. Mohan R, Iyer R, Thaller S. Airway management in patients with facial trauma. J Craniofac Surg. 2009;20:21–3.

85. Demetriades D, Velmahos GG, Asensio JA. Cervical pharyngoesophageal and laryngotracheal injuries. World J Surg. 2001;25:1044–8.

86. Breeze J, Allanson-Bailey LS, Hunt NC, Delaney RS, Hepper AE, Clasper J. Mortality and morbidity from combat neck injury. J Trauma Acute Care Surg. 2012;72:969–74.

87. Danic D, Prgomet D, Sekelj A, Jakovina K, Danic A. External laryngotracheal trauma. Eur Arch Otorhinolaryngol. 2006;263:228–32.

88. Inaba K, Branco BC, Menaker J, Scalea TM, Crane S, DuBose JJ, Tung L, Reddy S, Demetriades D. Evaluation of multidetector computed tomography for penetrating neck injury: a prospective multicenter study. J Trauma Acute Care Surg. 2012;72. 14 p.

89. O'Connor PJ, Russell JD, Moriarty DC. Anesthetic implications of laryngeal trauma. Anesth Analg. 1998;87:1283–4.

90. Kolber MR, Aspler A, Sequeira R. Conservative management of laryngeal perforation in a rural setting: case report and review of the literature on penetrating neck injuries. CJEM. 2011;13:127–32.

91. Bhattacharya P, Mandal MC, Das S, Mukhopadhyay S, Basu SR. Airway management of two patients with penetrating neck trauma. Indian J Anaesth. 2009;53:348–51.

92. Yamazaki M, Sasaki R, Masuda A, Ito Y. Anesthetic management of complete tracheal disruption using percutaneous cardiopulmonary support system. Anesth Analg. 1998;86:998–1000.

93. Van Waes OJ, Cheriex KC, Navsaria PH, van Riet PA, Nicol AJ, Vermeulen J. Management of penetrating neck injuries. Br J Surg. 2012;99 Suppl 1:149–54.

94. Gomez-Caro A, Ausin P, Moradiellos FJ, Diaz-Hellin V, Larru E, Perez JA, de Nicolas JL. Role of conservative medical management of tracheobronchial injuries. J Trauma. 2006;61:1426–34; discussion 1434–5.

95. Martel G, Al-Sabti H, Mulder DS, Sirois C, Evans DC. Acute tracheoesophageal burst injury after blunt chest trauma: case report and review of the literature. J Trauma. 2007;62:236–42.

96. Wojtzak JA. Submandibular sonography. Assessment of hyomental distances and ratio, tongue size, and floor of the mouth musculature using portable sonograph. J Ultrasound Med. 2012;31:523–8.

97. Lixin J, Bing H, Zhigang W, Binghui Z. Sonographic diagnosis features of Zenker diverticulum. Eur J Radiol. 2010;80:e13–9.

98. Perlas A, Mitsakakis N, Liu L, Cino M, Haldipur N, Davis L, Cubillos J, Chan V. Validation of a mathematical model for ultrasound assessment of gastric volume by gastroscopic examination. Anesth Analg. 2013;116:357–63.

99. Shibasaki M, Nakajima Y, Ishii S, Shimizu F, Shime N, Sessler DI. Prediction of pediatric endotracheal tube size by ultrasonography. Anesthesiology. 2010;113:819–24.

100. Alrajhi K, Woo MY, Vaillancourt C. Test characteristics of ultrasonography for the detection of pneumothorax: a systematic review and meta-analysis. Chest. 2012;141:703–8.

101. Kristensen MS. Ultrasonography in the management of the airway. Acta Anaesthesiol Scand. 2011;55:1155–73.

102. Chacko J, Nikahat J, Gagan B, Umesh K, Ramanathan M. Real-time ultrasound-guided percutaneous dilatational tracheostomy. Intensive Care Med. 2012;38:920–21.

Physiological Derangement of the Trauma Patient

3

Henry Liu, Hong Yan, Seth Christian, Santiago Gomez, Frank Rosinia, Mingbing Chen, Juan Tan, Charles J. Fox, and Alan David Kaye

Trauma causes various physiological disturbances dependent upon its nature, location and severity. These physiological derangements can be acute or long-lasting. Some of the derangements are general responses of human body to traumatic injury; some are more specific to a specific organ system. Common responses to trauma in a human body can include stressful reaction [1–3], hemorrhage [4, 5], inflammation [6] and potential sepsis, pain and metabolic alterations. Trauma to specific organ system will have physiological disturbances more specific to the injured organ such as chest trauma may cause pneumothorax which leads to respiratory dysfunctions. This review will discuss all major general responses to trauma and some system-specific injuries.

H. Liu, M.D. (✉) • S. Christian, M.D. • S. Gomez, M.D. • F. Rosinia, M.D.
Department of Anesthesiology, Tulane University Medical Center, 1430 Tulane Avenue, SL-4, New Orleans, LA 70112, USA
e-mail: henryliula@mail.com

H. Yan, M.D.
Department of Anesthesiology, Wuhan Central Hospital, 26 Shengli Street, Wuhan 430014, China

M. Chen, M.D., Ph.D. • J. Tan, M.D., Ph.D.
Department of Anesthesiology, Wuhan Tongji Hospital, 1095 Jiefang Avenue, Wuhan 430030, China

C.J. Fox, M.D.
Department of Anesthesiology, LSUHSC-Shreveport, 1501 Kings Highway, Shreveport, LA 71102, USA

A.D. Kaye, M.D., Ph.D., D.A.B.A., D.A.B.P.M., D.A.B.I.P.P.
Department of Anesthesiology and Department of Pharmacology, Pain Services, LSU School of Medicine T6M5, 1542 Tulane Avenue, Room 656, New Orleans, LA 70112, USA

General Physiological Changes Due to Trauma

Hemorrhage-Related Pathophysiological Changes

Hemorrhagic shock: after a traumatic injury, hemorrhage is responsible for over 35 % of all pre-hospital deaths and over 40 % of deaths within the first 24 h, second only to the rates of death due to severe central nervous system (CNS) injury [7]. Hemorrhagic shock is a severe and life-threatening medical condition. Trauma is one of the most important causes of hemorrhagic shock. Over 21 % of military casualties are in the state of shock upon admission, and over 25 % require a blood transfusion [4]. Sanemia, hyperfibrihock occurs when the blood loss leads to compromised tissue and organ perfusion and oxygen supply, causing a systemic build-up of acidotic substances or metabolites. The patient's body begins to compensate by hyperventilation in an attempt to reverse the acid build-up and release of vasoconstrictors from activated sympathetic system, along with other physiological compensatory changes, to increase blood pressure and diverts blood circulation from the renal system to those more vitally important organs like heart, lungs, and brain. The manifestation of shock symptoms occurs due to the cellular response to

C.S. Scher (ed.), *Anesthesia for Trauma*, DOI 10.1007/978-1-4939-0909-4_3,
© Springer Science+Business Media New York 2014

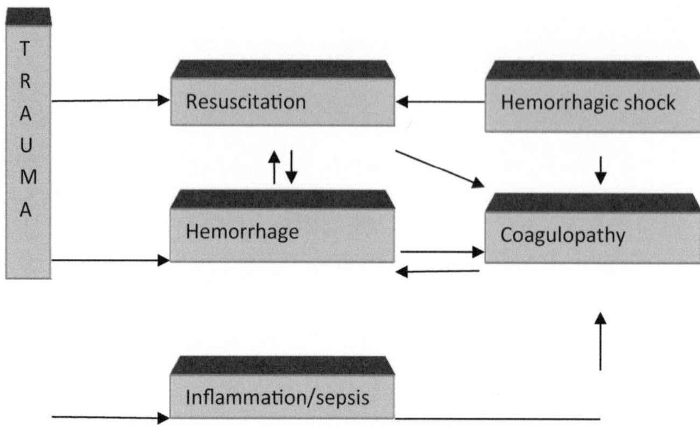

Fig. 3.1 Trauma causes a cascade of conditions: hemorrhage, shock, resuscitation, coagulopathy, and systemic inflammation [8]

the lack of oxygen, and tissue hypoxemia leads to further breakdown and malfunction of cells, prompting various responses in the circulatory system. After a traumatic injury, a cascade of life-threatening medical conditions can begin and many of these occur simultaneously: hemorrhage, impaired tissue perfusion with inadequate resuscitation, shock, systemic inflammation, and coagulopathy, as illustrated in Fig. 3.1 [8]. The severity of each problem condition is commonly associated with the severity and location of the traumatic insult and the extent of overall blood loss. Low blood pressure due to blood loss generally predicts potential immediate complications, including the incidence of multiple organ failure and life-threatening infections [5].

A disease classification generally offers an assessment and summary of a clinical scenario or condition, thus classification helps clinicians to plan more type-specific management. The classification of hemorrhagic shock has puzzlingly gone through enough debates over the last five decades. In 2008, ATLS proposed blood volume loss-based classification of hemorrhagic shock, as shown in Table 3.1 [9], in an attempt to replace the reasonably popular Holcroft Classification of hemorrhagic shock, as shown in Table 3.2.

However, the clinical implementation of ATLS-Blood loss-based classification does not seem to be without difficulty. The main pitfalls are lack of sensitivity and specificity in terms of guiding the timing of clinical management [11].

Table 3.1 ATLS classification of hemorrhagic shock [9]

I <15 % loss of blood volume
II >15 %, <30 % loss of blood volume
III >30 %, <40 % loss of blood volume
IV >40 % loss of blood volume

Table 3.2 Holcroft classification of hemorrhagic shock [10]

Mild	<20 % of blood volume	Skin changes
Moderate	20–40 %	Kidney, bowel, lungs, liver, hypotension
Severe	>40 %	Brain and cardiac dysfunction

Table 3.3 Therapeutic/Physiological classification of hemorrhagic shock [11]

Moderate/mild hemorrhagic shock	Moderate shock is moderate
Severe hemorrhagic shock	Shock with hypotension not responding to blood/volume replacement
Critical hemorrhagic shock	Shock with brain and cardiac involvement or >40 % blood lose; or 40%TBV loss

Thus, a more individual physiology-tailored and therapeutic/decision-making-oriented classification was proposed as illustrated in Table 3.3. This classification is essentially a combination of the above-mentioned two classifications.

The initial response to hemorrhage takes place on the macrocirculatory level and is mediated by

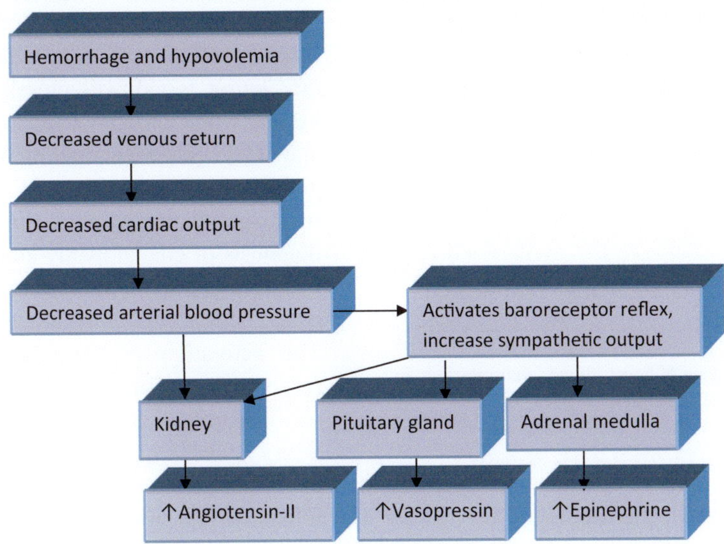

Fig. 3.2 Hemorrhage and endocrine responses

the neuroendocrine system. Trauma causes hemorrhage which consequently induce decreased blood pressure. The hypotension triggers release of catecholamines which lead to vasoconstriction. Heart, liver, and brain blood flow is usually preserved, whereas other regional microvascular beds are constricted. Blood flow to kidneys is initially preserved, but it may decrease as hypovolemia progresses. Pain, hemorrhage, and cortical perception of traumatic injuries lead to the release of hormones and other inflammatory mediators, including renin, angiotensin, vasopressin, antidiuretic hormone, growth hormone, glucagon, cortisol, epinephrine, and norepinephrine, as illustrated in Fig. 3.2. This response sets the stage for the microcirculatory response that follows.

At microcirculatory level, individual tissue cells in ischemia react to hemorrhage by sucking up more interstitial fluid which potentially further compromises intravascular fluid. Moreover, this expansive change in cellular volume and subsequent cellular edema may choke off adjacent capillaries and results in patches of tissues in "no-reflow" status, which will likely eliminate the chance of ischemic reversal, even in the presence of adequate macroperfusion ultimately. Ischemic cells produce lactate and

free radicals, which accumulate in interstitial space if the circulation and perfusion are diminished. These substances may cause direct damage to the cells and form the bulk of the toxic load that washes out to the intravascular circulation when blood flow is reestablished. Ischemic cells also produce and release inflammatory factors: prostacyclin, thromboxane, prostaglandins, leukotrienes, endothelin, complement, interleukins, tumor necrosis factor, and other factors. Most severe trauma patients by the time of admission are in the state of shock, most likely hemorrhagic shock. Hemorrhage remains the major cause of mortality after traumatic injury [12].

Hemorrhage in traumatic patient leads to hypovolemia, acidosis, electrolyte disturbances, hypotension, and coagulopathy. Trauma-induced hemorrhage and coagulopathy may gradually enter a vicious cycle (Fig. 3.3) [13]. Trauma-induced coagulopathy (TIC) is a multi-factorial, global failure of the coagulation system to sustain adequate hemostasis after major trauma. Derangements in coagulation screens are detectable in the acute phase following severe trauma thus supporting the hypothesis of an early endogenous process [14]. This acute traumatic coagulopathy (ATC) is driven by the

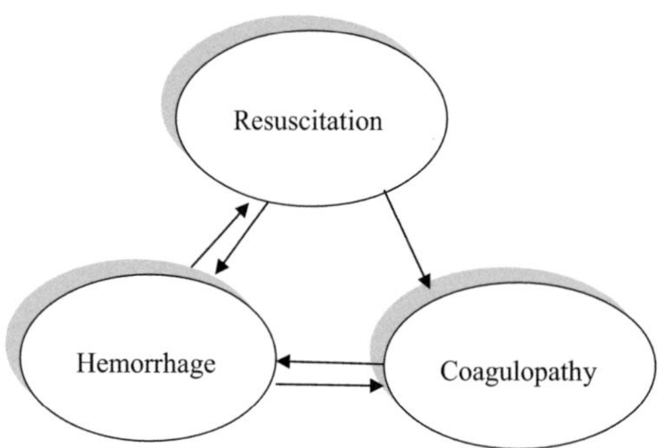

Fig. 3.3 Vicious cycle of hemorrhage, resuscitation, and coagulopathy in trauma patients

combination of tissue trauma and systemic hypoperfusion and characterized by global anticoagulation and hyperfibrinolysis [15]. Coagulation is an integral part component of the innate immune system, and endothelial activation of Protein C (PC) appears to be a central mechanism of ATC [16, 17], possibly as part of the posttraumatic inflammatory response. Further blood loss, hemodilution by intravenous crystalloids or hypocoagulable blood products, e. g., red blood cells (RBCs), acidemia, consumption of clotting factors, and hypothermia occur over time and exacerbate the already deranged coagulation response to give rise to TIC [18].

The main mechanisms involved in ATC are as following:

1. *Excessive activation of coagulation*: About 28 % of patients with severe traumatic injury have dysfunction in the process of coagulation (coagulopathy) when they arrive at the emergency department [19]. This is often caused by dilution of the blood after massive infusion of resuscitation products. Coagulopathy is associated with a 3.5- to 5-fold increase in mortality [14, 19], and especially when combined with hypothermia and acidosis, the scenario entitled "Lethal (or fatal) triad" because of the high likelihood of impending death. Coagulopathy could be prevented or minimized by transfusion of blood products that not only increase fluid/

blood volume but also compensate the diluting effects of resuscitation, thus the circulating blood will closely resemble the normal whole blood with appropriate percentage of all component clotting factors, platelets and auxiliary agents. Detection of early signs of coagulopathy would help establish early diagnosis of coagulopathy and initiate timely management of coagulopathy, thus to limit exacerbation of coagulopathic symptoms. The activation of coagulation cascade in response to traumatic injury and hemorrhage can become excessive due to local tissue injury (thus triggering endothelial injuries and vascular wall injury) and systematic inflammatory reactions. These local and systemic responses are important for the production of tissue factor and factor VII, which can excessively activate coagulation chain reactions. Trauma patients are particularly susceptible to the early development of coagulopathy, and the most severely injured patients are even coagulopathic by the time they are admitted to the hospital [20]. The zenith of the problem seems to be typically seen in patients with head injuries and in those who are massively injured and transfused. The subsequent coagulopathy is characterized by nonsurgical bleeding from mucosal lesions, serosal surfaces, and wound and vascular access sites. Disseminated intravascular coagulopathy (DIC) associated with traumatic injury results from multiple independent but interplaying mechanisms, involving tissue trauma, shock, and systemic inflammation. Therefore, the multi-factorial derangement of hemostasis occurring after massive traumatic injuries is mainly sustained by the release of procoagulants (fats, phospholipids) and constitutive tissue factor from the injured tissue into the circulation, associated with a systemic inflammatory response that also promotes tissue factor hyperexpression on monocytes and the other proinflammatory cells. This hemostatic dysfunction seems to be worse in head trauma patients [20]. The excessive, non-wound-related thrombin generation is insufficiently antagonized by physiological anticoagulant pathways and amplified by impaired endogenous fibrinolysis. The resulting massive systemic thrombin formation, coupled with platelet hyperaggregability, shock, hypothermia, and tissue hypoperfusion, contribute to the development of DIC and microvascular bleeding [20]. Interestingly, Austin et al. observed that psychological stress may also cause changes in coagulation [21].

2. *Hypocalcemia*: Hypocalcemia in traumatic patients is usually caused by hemodilution due to large quantity of fluid resuscitation and/or citrate infusion contained in blood products after massive blood transfusion. Holowaychuk and Monteith et al. investigated the incidence of ionized hypocalcemia with blunt and penetrating traumatic injuries upon presentation to the hospital and the association of ionized hypocalcemia with mortality, duration of hospitalization, and requirement for intensive care management. The incidence of ionized hypocalcemia upon hospital admission with blunt and penetrating trauma is similar to the incidence of ionized hypocalcemia in critically ill group. Subjects with ionized hypocalcemia are more severely injured and subsequently more likely in need of intensive care therapies and have a lower likelihood of survival compared to normocalcemia. Therefore, ionized calcium concentration may be a useful prognostic indicator with blunt and penetrating traumatic injuries [22].

3. *Anemia*: Anemia is almost universal in trauma patients admitted to the intensive care unit (ICU). More than 50 % of patients were anemic on ICU admission, and nearly all were anemic by post-injury day 10. Urinary hepcidin levels were very high. Iron studies confirmed functional iron deficiency. Log hepcidin values were positively correlated with Injury Severity Score (ISS) and negatively correlated with admission Pao_2/FiO_2. Every increase in ISS by 10 was associated with a 40 % increase in hepcidin. Initial hepcidin levels were positively correlated with duration of anemia. The authors believe that hepcidin levels rise to extremely high but variable levels after trauma and are positively correlated with injury severity measured by ISS and duration of anemia and negatively correlated with hypoxia. Hepcidin is likely a key factor in the impaired erythropoiesis seen in critically injured trauma patients [23]. RBC have an important hemostatic role. This seems to be a less well-perceived concept. This is because the flow of RBCs maintains platelets close to the endothelial cells, and they can activate the platelet functions. However, transfusion of packed RBCs (PRBC) can be a double-sided sword, increased hematocrit may help the interaction of platelets and endothelium, but the storage lesion of PRBCs may have untoward effects on coagulation. Aucar and Sheth looked into the effect of storage on the coagulation system by studying how PRBC storage time affects the activated coagulation time (ACT) using an in vitro model. It is well known that storage lesion of PRBCs consists of biochemical changes associated with increased inflammatory mediators and decreased oxygen-carrying capacity. And they found that in an isolated in vitro model, the storage lesion of PRBCs is associated with decreased coagulation function. This may have implications for transfusion practice in coagulation-sensitive circumstances such as trauma [24]. The so-called "Loss-dilution" phenomenon is that bleeding and hemodilution secondary to fluid resuscitation cause a decreased concentration of coagulation factors and platelets.

4. *Fibrinolysis*: The excessive activation of coagulation in trauma patients leads to the transition of fibrinolytic response from its physiological role of controlling coagulation to hyperfibrinolysis and coagulopathy. Hyperfibrinolysis is believed to be a key component of ATC (ATC, it seems that ATC and TIC are used interchangeably in literature)

and present in the majority of severely injured patients [25]. Laboratory markers of fibrinolysis are mostly elevated in the immediate phase after traumatic injury. Unfortunately the detection of this hyperfibrinolysis is limited by the relatively insensitive diagnostic tools available, such as Rotation thromboelastometry (ROTEM), thromboelastography (TEG). Shock, hypoxia, circulating catecholamines, and endothelial damage are potent activators of fibrinolysis, but the precise mechanism by which this hyperfibrinolysis is activated remains unclear. Trauma patients in the state of hemorrhagic shock have been shown to have a reduction in plasminogen activator inhibitor-1 (PAI-1) and elevated tissue plasminogen activity [15]. Excessively activated Protein C (PC) will lead to consumption of large quantity of PAI-1 and results in a "de-repression" of fibrinolytic activity, thus further implicating the PC pathway in the pathogenesis of ATC [15]. Management of this trauma-induced hyperfibrinolysis with antifibrinolytic agents such as tranexamic acid (TXA) has been found to reduce blood loss in elective surgery and more recently improve survival in trauma hemorrhage following the results of the large multicenter CRASH-2 trial in which 20,211 adult trauma patients were studied in 274 hospitals in 40 countries [26]. TXA seems to be especially more effective in shock patients with systolic blood pressure <75 mmHg since this cohort of patients is likely to have maximal activation of fibrinolysis. However, whether early administration of TXA would predict better clinical outcome or not is to be elucidated, though early use of antifibrinolytics should empirically initiate the inhibition of fibrinolysis in the early stages, so to augment clot formation and reduce blood requirements [27].

5. *Hypothermia*: Hypothermia is well known to cause alterations of platelet function, coagulation factors, and fibrinolysis. Trauma patients are prone to develop hypothermia due to multiple factors, such as aggressive fluid resuscitation, potentially hampered heat-generating mechanism, and exposure to ambient temperature.

6. *Trauma-induced platelet dysfunction*: Platelet activation and fibrin generation are mutually dependent and integrated processes. Formation of platelet prothrombinase (FXa/Va) assembly on the phospholipid membrane generates a thrombin burst of sufficient magnitude to polymerize and clot fibrinogen. Platelet dysfunction in ATC is more significant in the severely injured patients. ATC and the combined effects of shock, hypothermia, etc. would likely produce abnormal platelet function through disruption of activation and adhesion pathways, but only very limited mechanistic study has been performed till to date in trauma patients [27]. Massive transfusions of RBCs and Fresh Frozen Plasma (FFP) and other intravenous fluids will empirically cause dilutional thrombocytopenia. But in early stages of trauma hemorrhage, many studies have shown thrombocytes are maintained at reasonable levels not expected to contribute to a clinically significant coagulopathy [28]. Thus, platelet transfusion may not be absolutely necessary for correction of ATC as fibrinogen replacement will reverse the reductions in clot strength evident in thrombocytopenia, especially in earlier stage of trauma. Additionally, in a goal-directed trial utilizing ROTEM and transfusion algorithms for the management of ATC, approximately 1/3 of patients received only fibrinogen and prothrombin complex concentrate with no need for platelet transfusion. An argument to give normally functioning platelets may be their additional benefits such as restoration of the endothelium and modulation of infective and inflammatory sequel. Severe injury results in increased platelet activation and faster rates of adhesion and aggregation. Functional platelet defects as measured by whole blood aggregometry appear minor, but in parallel with platelet count there are significant differences between survivors and nonsurvivors. The most challenging question remains how to study those thrombocytes

actively involved in clot formation at the site of injury. Thus, it remains to be seen if those free, circulating platelets sampled and analyzed are reflective of "active" platelet function [27].

7. *Acidosis*: Metabolic acidosis favors coagulopathy by means of a decrease in the activity of coagulation factors and platelet function and the degradation of fibrinogen [13]. And trauma patients usually have the tendency of accumulation of acidotic substances due to compromised tissue perfusion and oxygen supply.

8. *Increased capillary permeability*: Sawant et al. investigated the effects of inhibiting Fas–Fas ligand interaction on microvascular endothelial barrier integrity. They exposed rat lung microvascular endothelial cells to hemorrhagic shock serum in the presence or absence of the Fas ligand inhibitor, FasFc. The effect of hemorrhagic shock serum on Fas receptor and Fas ligand expression on endothelial cells was determined by flow cytometry. Endothelial cell permeability was determined by monolayer permeability assay and the barrier integrity by β-catenin immunofluorescence. Mitochondrial reactive oxygen species (ROS) formation was determined using dihydrorhodamine 123 probe by fluorescent microscopy. Mitochondrial transmembrane potential was also studied by fluorescent microscopy as well as flow cytometry. Caspase 3 enzyme activity was measured fluorometrically. Rat lung microvascular endothelial cells exposed to hemorrhagic shock serum showed increase in Fas receptor and Fas ligand expression levels. FasFc treatment showed protection against hemorrhagic shock serum-induced disruption of the adherens junctions and monolayer hyperpermeability ($p < 0.05$) in the endothelial cells. Pretreatment with FasFc also decreased hemorrhagic shock serum-induced increase in mitochondrial ROS formation, restored hemorrhagic shock serum-induced drop in mitochondrial transmembrane potential, and reduced hemorrhagic shock serum-induced caspase 3 activity endothelial cells. These investigational findings indicated potential new venues for drug development which manages hemorrhagic shock-induced microvascular hyperpermeability by targeting the Fas–Fas ligand-mediated pathway [29].

Recently, toll-like receptor (TLR)-4 has been found to play an important role in the pathogenesis of multi-organ failure after severe traumatic injury. Hemorrhagic shock and resuscitation following major trauma result in a global ischemia and reperfusion injury that may lead to multiple organ dysfunction syndrome (MODS). Systemic activation of the immune system is fundamental to the development of MODS and shares many features in common with the systemic inflammatory response syndrome (SIRS). An important advancement in the understanding of the innate response to infection might be the identification of mammalian TLRs expressed on cells of the immune system. Ten TLR homologues have been identified in humans and toll-like receptor-4 (TLR4) has been most intensively studied. Initially found able to recognize bacterial lipopolysaccharide (LPS), it has also recently been discovered that TLR4 is capable of activation by endogenous "danger signal" molecules released following cellular injury; this has since implicated TLR4 in several non-infectious pathophysiological processes, including hemorrhagic shock. The exact process leading to multi-organ dysfunction following hemorrhagic shock and resuscitation is not clear yet, although TLR4 is believed to play a central role as both a key mediator and a potential therapeutic target. TLR4 has been shown expressed in vital organs including the liver, lungs, and myocardium following hemorrhagic shock and resuscitation [30]. MODS remains an important cause of morbidity and mortality in trauma patients. Unfortunately almost all current therapy is only based on supportive cares. Better understanding of the pathophysiology of hemorrhagic shock will allow us to develop therapeutic strategies more specifically aimed at minimizing organ dysfunction and improving patient outcomes following traumatic hemorrhage. Xiang et al. found that TLR signaling is related to the pathogenesis of acute lung injury (ALI) which frequently complicates the management of traumatic patients and serves as an important component of SIRS. Hemorrhagic shock that results from major trauma promotes the development of SIRS and ALI by priming the innate immune system for an exaggerated inflammatory response. Recent studies have reported that the mechanism underlying the priming of pulmonary inflammation involves the complicated cross-talk between TLRs and interactions between neutrophils and alveolar macrophages as well as endothelial cells, in which ROS are the key mediator [31].

There are multiple compensatory mechanisms for human body to respond to hemorrhage. These mechanisms include:

1. *Baroreceptor reflexes*: The baroreceptors located in the common carotid bifurcation and aortic arch are sensitive to pressure changes which reach certain magnitude. The baroreceptor reflexes discharge continuously via vagal and glossopharyngeal nerves afferent sensory pathways, to the cardiac and vasomotor centers. The receptors discharge basally and continuously at pressures within a range between 50–60 and 160–180 mmHg and do not respond above or below those values. After 1–2 days the baroreceptors stabilize the pressure to the new values. This is relevant in elderly patients who are hypertensive. Arterioles and venulae are the targets of the sympathetic nervous system vasoconstrictor tone. These reflexes are inhibitory in that more the afferent is stimulated by an increase of pressure more the vasomotor center is inhibited and the vasodilator-bradycardia and other vagal-mediated effects prevail, and vice versa [32].

2. *Vasoconstrictors*: As compensatory effects, patients' body usually releases multiple vasoconstrictors to increase systemic vascular resistance (SVR) in attempt to increase blood pressure. These vasoconstrictors include epinephrine and norepinephrine. Norepinephrine causes predominately vasoconstriction with a mild increase in heart rate, whereas epinephrine predominately causes an increase in heart rate with a small effect on the vascular tone; the combined effect results in an increase in blood pressure.

3. *Chemoreceptor reflexes*: The human chemoreceptor's response to low PaO_2 at decreased MAP increases BP by directly stimulating the vasomotor centers in the medulla oblongata and lower pons. This stimulation causes increased vasoconstriction and increasing arterioles tone via sympathetic nervous system stimulation. When hemoglobin oxygen saturation (HbO_2) reduces to minimal level from the bleeding, and cardiac output (CO) drops from the decreased venous return, and with dissolved PaO_2 unable to sustain CaO_2 at a level to maintain sufficient tissue perfusion, the chemoreceptor reflex gets triggered. By the time the chemoreceptor is triggered, HbO_2 would have reached minimal levels, and so the oxygen delivery (DO_2), and brain and heart are already suffering hypoxia (critical shock). Coronary arteries have a very high oxygen extraction rate (O_2ER) at baseline condition (75 % vs. 25 % of most of the other organs), thus when in hypoxemia, myocardium cannot increase oxygen extraction like other organs do, so myocardium is more prone to ischemic effects in hypoxemic conditions [33]. Adjunctive hyperoxia will paradoxically accelerate the physiological slope, particularly if combined with blood or fluids increasing bleeding rate before source control [11].

4. *Reabsorption of tissue fluids*: In hypovolemic conditions, the body will take up more fluids from interstitial tissue space in attempt to maintain intravascular volume. Capillary pressure will generally fall when MAP and venous pressure decrease, increased precapillary resistance and this will facilitate transcapillary fluid reabsorption (up to 1 l/h autoinfused); capillary plasma oncotic pressure can fall from 25 to 15 mmHg due to autoinfusion, thus limiting capillary fluid reabsorption; hemodilution causes hematocrit to fall which decreases blood viscosity.

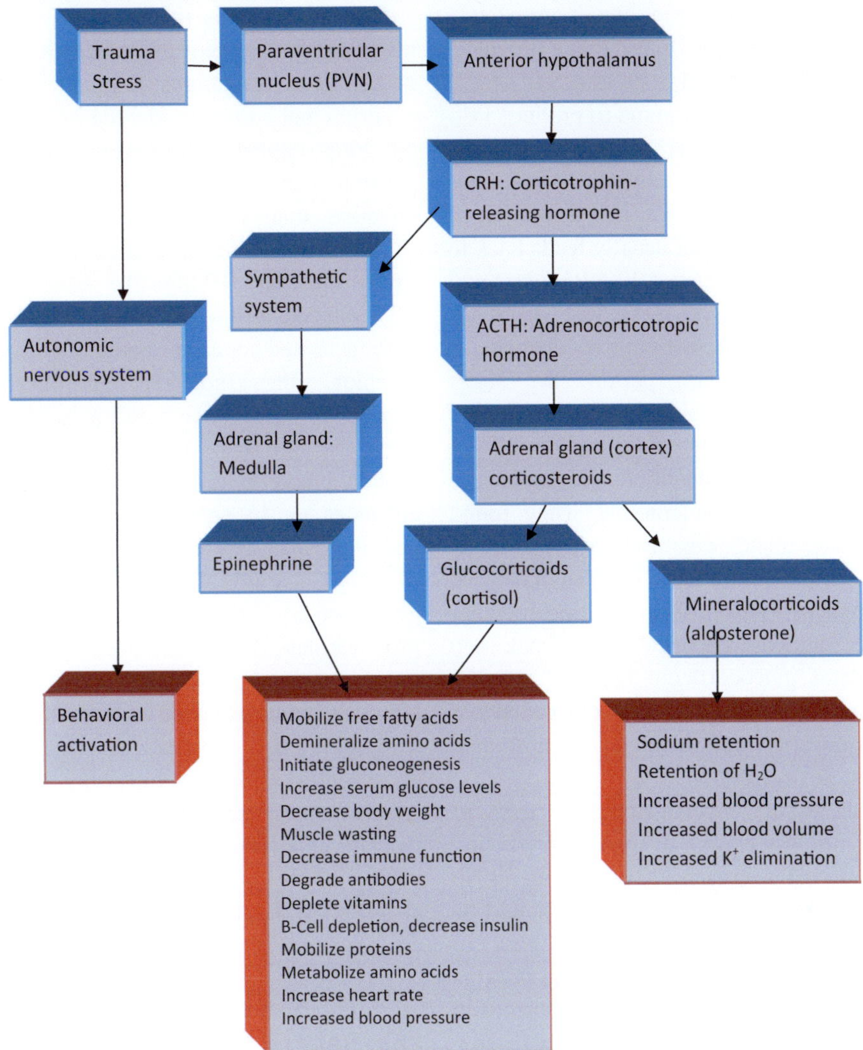

Fig. 3.4 Stress-induced physiological responses

5. *Renal reabsorption of sodium and water*: When intravascular volume is decreased, kidneys will compensate via reabsorbing more water to refill the vascular space by multiple humoral factors: Angiotensin II, aldosterone, and vasopressin.

Stress-Related Physiological Changes

The human autonomic nervous system (ANS) is activated by traumatic injury because autonomic system is responsible for the fight-or-flight responses. As Fig. 3.4 illustrates, trauma can activate ANS to change human behavior, trauma also causes anterior hypothalamus to increase corticotrophin-releasing hormone (CRH) release, which in turn stimulates anterior pituitary gland to produce more adrenocorticotropic hormone (ACTH). Subsequently ACTH works on adrenal gland cortex to release corticosteroids: glucocorticoids (cortisol) and mineralocorticoid (aldosterone) [34].

Trauma can interact with human genotype to increase the risk of conditions as depression or posttraumatic stress disorder (PTSD). The mechanism for the interaction is not completely understood. Klengel et al. found that a polymorphism in the FK506 binding protein 5 (*FKBP5*) gene interacts with early trauma to produce lasting epigenetic changes that increase the risk for such conditions [35]. Glucocorticoids are released in response to stress, and activation of the glucocorticoid receptor usually feeds back to reduce glucocorticoid release. FKBP5 forms part of a negative-feedback loop that regulates glucocorticoid receptor activity, so changes in levels of FKBP5 could perturb the stress response system and make patients vulnerable to conditions like depression and/or PTSD. Klengel et al. also identified the molecular underpinnings of this interaction. They found that the risk allele was associated with an alteration in chromatin structure and increased transcription of *FKBP5*. The resulting increase in FKBP5 "tightens" the negative-feedback loop that regulates glucocorticoid receptor activity, causing relative resistance to glucocorticoid receptor activation and an increased hormonal response to stress [35].

Lindahl et al. investigated the role of chromogranin A in plasma (P-CgA) in predicting mortality in 51 consecutive burn patients in medical intensive care setting. P-CgA could be classified into two types with respect to variability over time. They unveiled that patients with high variability of P-CgA had more deep injuries and were older than those with low variability. All measures of P-CgA correlated with Sequential Organ Failure Assessment (SOFA) score at day 7, but not with total burn size. Univariate regressions showed that age, burn size, and three of four measures of P-CgA predicted organ dysfunction. Multiple regressions showed that age, burn size, and either P-CgA at 24 h, the mean value up to day 7, or the maximum value up to day 7, were all independent predictors for organ dysfunction. Though significant organ dysfunction was best predicted by age, burn area, and the CgA point value at 24 h with an area under curve value of 0.91 in a ROC-analysis. So the investigators concluded that the extent of neuroendocrine activation assessed as P-CgA after a major burn injury is independently related to organ dysfunction [36].

The mechanisms that trauma induces stress reactions have been the research focuses of numerous investigations. Eagle et al. studied in experimental animal model the impacts of stress on hippocampal glucocortical receptor and phosphorylated protein kinase B levels. They unveiled that single prolonged stress (SPS) shows good validity in producing posttraumatic stress disorder (PTSD)-like behavior. While SPS-induced behaviors have been associated with increased gene expression of glucocorticoid receptor, the molecular ramifications of enhanced glucocorticoid receptor gene expression have yet to be identified. Phosphorylated protein kinase B is critical for stress-mediated enhancement in general anxiety and memory and may also be regulated by glucocorticoid receptors. The investigation found that levels of glucocortical receptor and phosphorylated protein kinase B were increased in the hippocampus, but not amygdala. Furthermore, SPS had no effect on unconditioned anxiety-like behavior suggesting that generalized anxiety is not consistently observed following SPS. These results suggest that SPS-enhanced glucocortical receptor expression is associated with phosphorylation of phosphorylated protein kinase B and also suggest that these changes are not related to an anxiogenic phenotype [3].

Pain-Related Physiological Changes

Pain secondary to traumatic injury is very common. Pain induces physiological changes mostly related to stress as discussed in previous paragraphs. However, pain does cause pathophysiological alterations in addition to stress effects.

Pain affects ventilation if chest injury causes rib fractures or other injury in similar nature. This trauma-induced pain will hamper ventilation which subsequently leads to hypoventilation, hypoxemia, and all other complications due to hypoventilation and hypoxemia, such as pneumonia, acute coronary syndrome, stroke, etc. This will be discussed in specific trauma-related physiology changes. Chest trauma has very high mortality rate. The incidence of rib fractures ranges from 10 to 26 % in traumatic thoracic injury and the number of rib fractures independently predicts patients' pulmonary morbidity and mortality. Multiple cardiopulmonary to neurologic causes such as tamponade, hemo- or pneumothorax, and cervical spine injury can be implicated. Severe respiratory distress can also result from breathing-dependent pain where parenteral opioids are often insufficient in addressing the pain and associated respiratory failure. Epidural analgesia is associated with reduction in mortality for all patients with multiple rib fractures; however, this strategy is underused partially due to the potential risks of epidural hematomas. Adequate analgesia will help patient minimize chest injury-related complications [37].

Pain affects mobility: Lower extremity fracture or injury can immobilize patients which may lead to complications due to bed-ridden situation, such as deep vein thrombosis (DVT). Shibata et al. conducted a retrospective analysis of data collected during subject screening following Japan's March 2011 earthquake and tsunami. They did calf ultrasonography for 269 subjects living in 21 shelters during the one-month period immediately following the disaster. They found that lower limb injury, immobility due to pain and/or fracture, dehydration, and reduced frequency of urination are all risk factors of developing DVT [38].

Pain-related cognitive changes and pain-related medication induced mental status changes. Rosenblum et al. reviewed 4,388 studies available in the literature. They found that persistent pain was reported by all studies at variable time points up to 84 months after injury, with wide variation among studies in pain intensity and pain incidence at each time point. The incidence of pain decreased over time within each study. Two studies established significant relationships between injury severity and persistent pain. Frequently cited predictive factors for persistent pain included symptoms of anxiety and depression, patient perception that the injury was attributable to external sources, cognitive avoidance of distressing thoughts, alcohol consumption prior to trauma, lower educational status, being injured at work, eligibility for compensation, pain at initial assessment, and older age [39].

Pain and inflammation: Proinflammatory pathways may be activated under conditions of painful stress, which is hypothesized to worsen the experience of pain and place medically vulnerable populations at high risk for increased morbidity. Griffins evaluated the effects of pain and subjective pain-related stress on proinflammatory activity on 19 healthy control subjects underwent a single standard cold-pressor pain test (CPT) and a no-pain control condition. Indicators of pain and stress were measured and related to inflammatory immune responses [CD8+ cells expressing the integrin molecule CD11a (CD811a), interleukin (IL)-1 receptor agonist (IL-1RA), and IL-6] immediately following the painful stimulus and compared to responses under no-pain conditions. Heart rate and mean arterial pressure were measured as indicators of sympathetic stimulation. The results showed CPT was clearly painful and generated an activation of the sympathetic nervous system. CD811a increased in both conditions, but with no statistically significant greater increase following CPT ($p < 0.06$). IL-1RA demonstrated a non-statistically significant increase following CPT ($p < 0.07$). The change in IL-6 following CPT differed significantly from the response seen in the control condition ($p < 0.02$). Based on these findings the authors concluded that CPT acute pain may affect proinflammatory pathways, possibly through mechanisms related to adrenergic activation [40].

Other pain effects: Xu et al. evaluated the effectiveness of postoperative analgesia on energy metabolism and compare cyclooxygenase-2 selective inhibitor with tramadol in postoperative pain management after major abdominal surgery. They studied 112 patients undergoing major abdominal surgery. The subjects were randomly assigned to one of the four treatment groups before surgery and then scheduled to receive different analgesic drugs after surgery: group parecoxib/control received intravenous parecoxib (40 mg bid) for

3 days; group parecoxib/celecoxib received intravenous parecoxib (40 mg bid) for 3 days and continued oral celecoxib (0.2 mg bid) for 4 days; group tramadol/control received intravenous tramadol (0.1 g tid) for 3 days; and group tramadol/tramadol received intravenous tramadol (0.1 g tid) for 3 days and continued oral tramadol (0.1 g tid) for 4 days. What they found is that Group tramadol/tramadol showed much lower rest energy expenditure 1 week after surgery ($p < 0.05$). The measured rest energy expenditure was significantly lower in patients treated with analgesic drugs administered from day 4–7 after surgery relative to control group ($p < 0.01$). From the fourth day after surgery, groups parecoxib/celecoxib and tramadol/tramadol showed significantly lower pain intensity ratings compared with groups parecoxib/control and tramadol/control during leg raising ($p < 0.05$). The authors thus believe that sufficient postoperative analgesia may be efficacious in reducing some of the stress responses to operative trauma. In addition, intravenous parecoxib (40 mg bid) followed by oral celecoxib (0.2 g bid) is as effective as intravenous tramadol (0.1 g tid) with continued oral tramadol (0.1 g tid) after major abdominal surgery [41].

Systemic Inflammatory Response and Sepsis

Stages of the Immunoinflammatory Response to Traumatic Injury

The immunoinflammatory response to trauma seems to be in two stages: early stage with heightened immune status and delayed responses with depressed immune status in those traumatic patients. The initial response is dominated by excessive activation of innate immune pathways manifested by a pronounced systemic inflammatory response and organ injury. If the trauma patient survives the initial period, a persistent depression in adaptive immunity renders the trauma patient more susceptible to nosocomial infections [42]. This depressed immune status is characterized by a shift toward a TH_2 T-cell phenotype and a depression in T-cell responses.

Unfortunately, the initiator and effector mechanisms involved in driving both innate inflammatory response and the reduced adaptive immune response are unclear, thus multiple investigations aiming at solving this mystery are ongoing. Recent studies indicated that innate immune receptors that detect tissue injury, such as TLR4 [43, 44] and TLR9 [45], are likely associated with the initial proinflammatory response observed in animal models of experimental trauma. Key effector pathways and mediators, such as cytokine/chemokines and complement, are also known to be involved in this initial proinflammatory response [46].

Bacterial Translocation into Blood Circulation and Release of Endotoxin

Patients with trauma and/or hemorrhagic shock are at risk of developing intestinal ischemia associated with decreased bowel integrity and bacterial translocation (BT) that may lead to bacteremia, endotoxinemia, and even multiple organ failure and death. Bowel ischemia is a pathologic status difficult to make a noninvasive diagnosis. Sobhian et al. investigated whether circulating plasma D-lactate is associated with mortality in a clinically relevant two-hit model in baboons. The baboon model of hemorrhagic shock was induced by controlled bleeding to MAP 40 mmHg, base excess (maximum -5 mmol/L), and time (maximum 3 h). All animals underwent a surgical trauma after resuscitation including midshaft osteotomy stabilized with reamed femoral interlocking nailing and were followed up for 7 days. Hemorrhagic shock/surgical trauma resulted in 66 % mortality by day 7. Circulating D-lactate levels were significantly increased (twofold) at 24 h in nonsurvivors compared with survivors, whereas the early increase during hemorrhage and resuscitation declined during the early postresuscitation phase with no difference between survivors and nonsurvivors. Moreover, D-lactate levels remained elevated in the non-survival group until death, whereas the D-lactate levels decreased to baseline value in survivors. It seems that D-lactate levels are accurate in prediction of death in baboon hemorrhagic shock models with an area under curve (days 1–3 after trauma) of 0.85 (95 % confidence interval, 0.72–0.93). The optimal D-lactate cut-off value of 25.34 µg/mL produced sensitivity of 73–99 % and specificity of 50–83 %. These results indicated that elevation of plasma D-lactate after 24 h predicts an increased risk of mortality after hemorrhage and trauma [47]. There is a plethora of animal studies indicating bacterial translocation after trauma, but human studies are relatively scarce. Nieves et al. studied the relationship between trauma and bacterial translocation by removing mesenteric lymph nodes (MLNs) from 36 patients with abdominal trauma during laparotomy and then cultured to detect BT. Postoperative infectious complications in these patients were registered, and both phenotypical and molecular typings (through multilocus sequencing) were investigated for microorganisms isolated from MLN and postoperative infection sites. Associations between clinical variables, BT presence, and postoperative infection development were established. This study found that BT was detected in 33 % of the patients. Postoperative infections were present in 22.2 % of the patients. A statistically significant association was found between postoperative infections in patients with BT evidence (41.6 %), when compared with patients without BT (12.5 %; $p < 0.05$). Bacteria isolated from infection sites were the same as those cultured in MLN in 40 % of the cases. Thus, the authors concluded that there is a higher risk of BT in trauma patients, and trauma is also associated with a significantly increased risk of postoperative infections. An abdominal trauma index ≥ 10 was found to be associated with the development of BT [48].

Cytokine Formation and Release

Inflammatory cytokines are released in trauma patients. These cytokines include tumor necrotizing factor (TNF), multiple interleukins, etc. Sánchez-Aguilar et al. investigated the increased level of inflammatory cytokines after trauma and the beneficial effects of statins. Patients were randomly selected to receive 20 mg of rosuvastatin or placebo for 10 days. The main goal was to determine the effect of rosuvastatin on plasma levels of TNF-α, interleukin (IL)-1β, IL-6, and IL-10 after 72 h of traumatic brain injury (TBI). Amnesia, disorientation, and disability were assessed 3 and 6 months after TBI. The results showed that 36 patients were analyzed according to intention-to-treat analysis; 19 patients received rosuvastatin and 17 received placebo. The best-fit mixed model showed a significant effect of rosuvastatin on the reduction of TNF-α levels ($p = 0.004$). Rosuvastatin treatment did not appear to affect the levels of IL-1β, IL-6, and IL-10. The treatment was associated with a reduction in disability scores ($p = 0.03$), indicating a favorable functional outcome. Life-threatening adverse effects were not observed. This investigation indicated that trauma can induce the release of inflammatory cytokines, such as TNF, IL-1β, IL-6, and IL-10. And therapy with statins may induce an anti-inflammatory effect and may promote recovery after TBI. The role of statins in trauma treatment should be confirmed in larger clinical trials [49].

Bone Marrow Changes

Francis et al. studied the effects of major trauma on bone marrow release of blood cell components. They aspirated bone marrows and blood samples from adult surgical patients with pelvic fractures from major blunt trauma with ISS at least 18, or isolated fractures and control patients undergoing iliac crest bone grafting. ISS, interval to surgery and transfusion in the first 24 h were recorded. Bone marrow aspirate flow cytometry was used to identify hemopoietic progenitor cells (CD34(+)), multipotent cells (CD34(+) CD45(+) CD38(−)), and oligopotent cells (CD34(+) CD45(+) CD38(lo/+) and CD34(+) CD45(+) CD38(BRIGHT(++ +)) subsets). Peripheral plasma levels of inflammatory markers were measured, and the ratio of immature to mature (CD35(−)/CD35(+)) granulocytes was determined. The study found that the median (range) interval between injury and sampling was 7 (1–21) and 5 (1–21) days in the major trauma and isolated fracture groups, respectively. The CD34(+) pool was significantly depleted in the major trauma group ($p = 0.017$), particularly the CD34(+) CD45(+) CD38(BRIGHT(++ +))

oligopotent pool ($p = 0.003$). Immature CD35 (−) granulocytes increased in bone marrow with increasing injury severity ($p = 0.024$) and massive transfusion ($p = 0.019$), and in peripheral blood with increasing interval to surgery ($p = 0.005$). Thus, the investigators concluded that major blunt trauma resulted in changes in the bone marrow CD34(+) progenitor pool. At the point in recovery when these samples were obtained, oligopotent progenitors were lost from the bone marrow with continued release of immature cells [50]. These changes at bone marrow level might be related to the trauma-related infections.

Acute Adrenal Insufficiency After Trauma

Acute adrenal insufficiency (AI) has been increasingly recognized during the past 20 years as a significant contributor to death in the setting of septic shock [51–53]. The mechanism of AI-associated increased mortality might be related to its contribution to cardiovascular collapse in the setting of sepsis, and this process may be mediated by cortisol on essential metabolic, vasoreactive, and immune system functions [51]. Thus, several large randomized trials using steroids to treat patients with sepsis and septic shock have shown efficacy of improving patients' outcome [51]. However, it is not widely accepted yet to utilize steroid for all trauma patients. Stein et al. reported that patients with acute traumatic hemorrhagic shock presenting to a well-known trauma center prospectively had serum cortisol levels collected on admission. The investigators included patients with hypotension and active hemorrhage. Clinicians were blinded to results, and no patient received steroids in the acute phase. They used death from hemorrhage within 24 h of admission as the primary outcome measure. Their results are: mean admission cortisol level was 18.3 ± 8.9 μg/dL in 59 patients. Acute mortality rate from hemorrhage was 27 %. Overall mortality rate was 37 %. Severe hyperacute adrenal insufficiency (HAI) (serum cortisol level <10 μg/dL) was present in 10 patients (17 %). Relative HAI (<25 μg/dL) was present in 51 patients (86 %). Those who died of acute hemorrhage had significantly lower mean cortisol levels (11.4 ± 6.2 μg/dL vs. 20.9 ± 8.4 μg/dL, $p < 0.001$) as did patients who ultimately died in the hospital (12.8 ± 7.6 μg/dL vs. 21.6 ± 8.1 μg/dL, $p < 0.001$). In multivariate analysis, lower cortisol levels were found to be associated with mortality from acute hemorrhage, with an odds ratio of 1.17. Adjusted receiver operating characteristic analysis showed that serum cortisol has a 91 % accuracy in differentiating survivors of acute hemorrhage from non-survivors. Thus, the investigators concluded that AI occurs immediately after acute injury during hemorrhagic shock and is strongly associated with mortality. HAI may be a marker of shock severity, but is potentially rapidly modifiable as opposed to other markers, such as lactate or base deficit. They also stated that it is unclear that steroid administration can change outcome in selected patients or not [54]. Interestingly this adrenal insufficiency has also been reported in cardiogenic shock patients. This may indicate that AI is more from the shock-related hypoperfusion than trauma-related stress. And relative adrenal insufficiency in post-cardiac arrest shock is believed to be under-recognized [55].

Enhanced Nitric Oxide Formation

Trauma induces immune depression as described previously. This state of immune dysfunction following trauma seems to be mediated by cell-mediated immunity, specifically a depression in T-cell function and a shift toward TH$_2$ T-cell phenotype. Studies in both animal models and humans have shown that hemorrhagic shock and severe trauma lead to an early upregulation of inducible nitric oxide synthase (iNOS) in multiple organs like liver, lung, spleen, and vascular system [5, 56]. Investigations in hemorrhagic shock models using knockout mice and selective iNOS inhibitors have revealed that iNOS contributes to the propagation of the inflammatory response and to organ damage that manifests within the first few hours [57]. Upregulation of iNOS is well recognized after injury and contributes to the inflammatory response and organ damage early after trauma.

However, it is unknown whether iNOS plays a role in adaptive immune dysfunction after trauma until Darwiche et al. established this link between iNOS upregulation and trauma-induced immune dysfunction by studying in a murine model of severe peripheral tissue injury and finding that iNOS is rapidly upregulated in macrophages and a myeloid-derived suppressor cell subpopulation in the spleen. Through the use of iNOS knockout mice, a specific iNOS inhibitor, and a nitric oxide (NO) scavenger, this study demonstrated that iNOS-derived NO is required for the depression in T-lymphocyte proliferation, interferon, and interleukin-2- production within the spleen at 48 h after trauma. These findings support the concept that iNOS regulates immune suppression following trauma and suggest that targeting the sustained production of NO by iNOS may attenuate posttraumatic immune depression [58].

Endocrine and Metabolism Changes

Hyperglycemia and insulin resistance are common findings in critical illness. Patients in the surgical ICU are frequently treated for this "critical illness diabetes" with intensive insulin therapy, resulting in a substantial reduction in morbidity and mortality. Adipose tissue is an important insulin target tissue, but it is not known whether adipose tissue is affected by critical illness diabetes. Williams et al. used a rodent model of critical illness diabetes to determine whether adipose tissue becomes acutely insulin-resistant and how insulin signaling pathways are being affected. There was a reduction in insulin-induced phosphorylation of IR, IRS-1, Akt, and GSK-3β. Since insulin resistance occurs rapidly in adipose tissue, but before the insulin resistance develops in skeletal muscle, adipose tissue may play a role in the initial development of critical illness diabetes [59].

Burn injury (BI) is associated with insulin resistance and hyperglycemia which complicate clinical management. Xu et al. investigated the impact of BI on glucose metabolism in a rabbit model of BI using a combination of positron emission tomography (PET) and stable isotope studies under euglycemic insulin clamp conditions. They studied male rabbits which were subjected to either full-thickness BI or sham burn. A euglycemic insulin clamp condition was established by constant infusion of insulin, concomitantly with a variable rate of dextrose infusion 3 days after treatment. PET imaging of the hind limbs was conducted to determine the rates of peripheral O_2 and glucose utilization. Each animal also received a primed constant infusion of glucose to determine endogenous glucose production. What they found are: the fasting blood glucose in the burned rabbits was higher than that in the sham group. Under euglycemic insulin clamp conditions, the sham burn group required more exogenous dextrose than the BI group to maintain blood glucose at physiological levels (22.2 ± 2.6 vs. 13.3 ± 2.9 mg/min, $p < 0.05$), indicating a state of IR. PET imaging demonstrated that the rates of O_2 consumption and (18)F 2-fluoro-2-deoxy-D-glucose utilization by skeletal muscle remained at similar levels in both groups. Hepatic gluconeogenesis determined by the stable isotope tracer study was found significantly increased in the BI group. So they concluded that hyperglycemia and IR develop during the early "flow phase" after BI. Unsuppressed hepatic gluconeogenesis, but not peripheral skeletal muscular utilization of glucose, contributes to hyperglycemia at this stage [60].

System-Specific Physiological Changes Due to Trauma

Head Injury

CNS trauma accounts for almost half of all trauma deaths examined postmortem in population-based analyzes. TBI is usually caused by transfer of mechanical energy into the brain from traumatic events such as rapid acceleration/deceleration, a direct impact to the head, or an explosive blast. Although mild TBI can cause neurological symptoms in the absence of positive neuroimaging findings, the transfer of the extrinsic energy into the brain can cause structural, physiological, and/or functional changes in the brain that may lead to neurological, cognitive, and behavioral symptoms which can be long-lasting [61]. The physiological changes can increase intracranial pressure, which will cause increased blood pressure, decreased heart rate, nausea and vomiting, headache, etc. They can also cause altered mental status due to injury to brain parenchyma or vascular system, induce brain herniation due to asymmetric cerebral spinal fluid pressure, and cause altered ventilation pattern due to compensatory hyperventilation. The primary head injuries inflicted by the traumatic event include skull fracture, subdural hematoma, epidural hematoma, cerebral hematoma, and contusion, diffuse head injury. The secondary head injury occurs after initial injury due to multiple insults and secondary injury may or may not be preventable. The pathophysiology of secondary injury includes metabolic failure, oxidative stress, and a cascade of biochemical and molecular events leading to both delayed necrotic and apoptotic cell death. Secondary injury is often exacerbated by tissue hypoxia/ischemia and by inflammatory responses. The risk factors for secondary injury can be cerebral factors: increased intracranial pressure, expanding mass lesion, hypercarbia, venous obstruction, hypoxemia, excessive hyperventilation, seizures; or systemic factors: hypoxemia, hypotension, anemia, hypovolemia, hyperglycemia, coagulopathy [62].

Chest Injury

The major medical concerns of chest trauma are (1) hypoventilation due to pneumothorax, pleural effusion, rib fracture-related pain, etc; (2) negative impact on hemodynamics due to intrathoracic hemorrhage, pulmonary contusion, cardiac injury, major vascular perforation, etc; (3) cardiac dysrhythmia due to traumatic injury to the myocardium; (4) hypoxemia due to changes causing hypoventilation or affecting oxygen exchange, etc. Injuries to the lung parenchyma or bronchial trees that produce pneumothorax can generally be managed by tube thoracostomy to relieve tension, drain accumulated blood, and apply suction to the pleural space until the air leak spontaneously resolves. Bleeding from the low-pressure pulmonary circulation can usually be self-limiting. Thoracostomy is utilized only when there is evidence of mediastinal injury, chest tube drainage output exceeds 1,500 mL in the first hours after injury, tracheal or bronchial injury and massive air leak are apparent. Or the patient is hemodynamically unstable with apparent thoracic pathology. Blood collected from the pleural space is generally non-clotting and can be directly reinfused after washing and filtering with any FDA-approved commercial system. Hemorrhage necessitating surgery may be from injured intracostal or internal mammary arteries, as well as from the lung parenchyma. Wedge resection of injured lung or even anatomic lobectomy is not uncommon, particularly after penetrating chest trauma. Historically chest trauma necessitating pneumonectomy resulted in very high mortality, almost approaching 100 %. According to a recent multicenter retrospective review reports, intraoperative deaths are often the result of uncontrollable hemorrhage, acute right ventricular failure, and air embolism. Patients who survive the initial procedure are at risk for early postoperative morbidity and mortality. Fluid management may be complicated by the need to weigh on ongoing resuscitation against the treatment of right ventricular failure. Blunt thoracic trauma requiring pneumonectomy is often associated with abdominal and pelvic coexisting injuries. Volume replacement must be judicious, and the use of a pulmonary artery catheter (placed with care in a postpneumonectomy patient) or TEE may be beneficial. Echocardiography will also play an important role in assessing right ventricular function and pulmonary hypertension. Treatment of right ventricular failure after traumatic pneumonectomy is often very difficult.

Without doubt, double-lumen endotracheal tube (DLT) intubation is desirable during urgent thoracotomy, particularly in trauma patients with one-sided penetrating injury; DLT intubation may not be the initial approach for most patients, especially in situations with limited resources and inexperienced personnel. Reliable rapid endotracheal intubation with a large-caliber (at least 8.0 mm in internal diameter) conventional endotracheal tube will allow anesthesia provider to secure airway faster and more reliably, so to protect the patient from aspiration during intubation before passage of a gastric tube for the suction of the stomach contents. Additionally large-caliber single lumen tube will accommodate future diagnostic bronchoscopy, pulmonary lavage, or other endobronchial procedures. Switch to DLT can then be attempted under controlled conditions in the presence of adequate oxygenation, anesthesia, muscle relaxation, and especially a suctioned stomach. Tolerability of single-lung ventilation is variable in the trauma population and depends largely on the nature of the traumatic injury and absence of significant pathology in the ventilated lung. Many patients with blunt thoracic injury have bilateral pulmonary contusions and will require increased FiO_2 and high levels of PEEP to maintain adequate oxygenation, even when both lungs are ventilated. During hypovolemic shock there is a disproportionate increase in pulmonary vascular resistance with respect to SVR, as well as high mortality with combined hemorrhagic shock and pneumonectomy.

Tracheal-bronchial injury can be caused by either blunt force or penetrating trauma. Usually penetrating injuries are more promptly diagnosed and treated. Blunt trauma most commonly results in an injury to the tracheobronchial tree within 2.5 cm of the carina and may initially be unrecognized. Physicians should be alert to possible tracheobronchial injury in the presence of subcutaneous emphysema, pneumomediastinum, pneumopericardium, or pneumoperitoneum but without apparent cause. If the traumatic injury is just an incomplete tear, it may heal with stenosis, subsequent atelectasis, pneumonia, pulmonary destruction, and sepsis. When surgery is required for a delayed, incomplete tracheobronchial injury, pulmonary resection may be

required if there is significant tissue destruction, whereas complete transection may be amenable to reconstruction with preservation of pulmonary tissue. The level of injury dictates the surgical approach.

Van Wessem et al. investigated the effect of high-volume ventilation on the inflammatory response in blunt chest trauma in rat model, because patients with lung contusion often need ventilatory support after incurring trauma. Lung contusion usually induces an inflammatory response manifested by primed polymorph neutrophil granulocytes (PMNs) in blood and tissue. Mechanical ventilation (MV) can also cause an inflammatory response. Twenty-three male Sprague–Dawley rats were assigned to undergo either MV or bilateral lung contusion followed by MV. Lung contusion was induced by a blast generator. The tissue and systemic inflammation were measured by absolute PMN numbers in blood and bronchoalveolar lavage fluid (BALF), myeloperoxidase, interleukin (IL)-6, IL 1β, growth-related oncogene-KC, and IL-10 in both plasma and BALF. The results were both MV and blast plus MV rats showed increased systemic and pulmonary inflammation, expressed by higher PMNs, myeloperoxidase levels, and cytokine levels in both blood and BALF. Blast plus MV rats showed a significantly higher systemic and pulmonary inflammatory response than MV only rats. These results indicated that mechanical ventilation after lung contusion induced a larger overall inflammatory response than MV alone, which indicates that local damage contributes not only to local inflammation, but also to systemic inflammation. This emphasizes the importance of lung protective ventilation strategies after pulmonary contusion [63].

Rib fractures are the most common injury resulting from blunt chest trauma. The fracture itself generally requires no specific treatment and will heal spontaneously over a period of several weeks. But multiple rib fractures can be associated with significant morbidity and mortality. Fracture of multiple neighboring ribs will result in the "flail chest" syndrome, characterized by paradoxical chest wall motion during spontaneous ventilation. Common complications of multiple rib fractures include hypoventilation leading to atelectasis, pneumonia, and respiratory failure. Pain management was thus recognized as a very important factor in preventing complications in these patients. And management of the respiratory system became more widely recognized as a major factor in patients' medical care. It is now known that patients with multiple rib fractures benefit most from adequate pain control, rapid mobilization, and meticulous respiratory care to prevent complications [64].

Cardiac Injury

Blunt cardiac injury is rare but it must be ruled out in any patient who has sustained a frontal impact to the chest. Functional differentiation between bruising or edema of the myocardium will be very difficult. The pathophysiology of cardiac contusion may involve forcible dislodgement of unstable atherosclerotic plaque in the coronary arteries. If the patient is hemodynamically stable and the ECG does not demonstrate conduction disturbances or tachyarrhythmia, blunt cardiac injury can generally be excluded safely. However, if a new dysrrhythmia subsequently develops or the patient has unexplained hypotension, other causes (hypovolemia, electrolyte disturbances, renal failure) should be ruled out first. Echocardiography (transthoracic or/and transesophageal) can help determine the pathological nature and physiological status.

Abdominal Trauma and Digestive System Changes

Abdominal cavity holds many different organs. Traumatic injury to abdominal organs is relatively common in clinical practice. Abdominal injury can be blunt or penetrating. Traditionally blunt trauma causes more mortality than penetrating trauma, but this has been changing as more accurate diagnostic modalities becoming more readily available. The injury can be inflicted to hollow organs like gastrointestinal system, bladder, causing peritonitis; or solid organs like liver, spleen, or kidneys causing major hemorrhage and shock. The several main concerns after abdominal trauma are: hemorrhage and hemorrhagic shock due to injury to liver, spleen, kidney, or major abdominal vessels; Peritonitis due to introduction of exterior bacteria from trauma, or from the perforation of visceral organs in the abdomen; Electrolytes disturbances due to loss of gastrointestinal fluids, hypovolemia, inflammation; Systemic infection, bacteremia, and sepsis due to exposure of abdominal cavity, gastrointestinal leakage into peritoneal cavity, and bacterial translocation; Abdominal pain and abdominal rigidity can cause hypoventilations, thus lead to hypoxemia and pertinent complications as stroke, myocardial infarction; And malnutrition due to bowel resection or functional decline.

Summary

Trauma causes remarkable physiological derangements if it reaches certain severity. These derangements can pose significant impact on patient's life. The response of patient's body to trauma can be general which is more common to all kinds of trauma, or more specific to certain organ system involved in the traumatic injury. The general responses include hemorrhage-related changes, stress, pain, sepsis, and metabolic alterations. Hemorrhage can initially have macrocirculatory effects mediated by neuroendocrine system leading to release of epinephrine, vasopressin, and angiotensin-II. Hypovolemia, hypotension, and compromised tissue perfusion will cause ischemia at cellular level, leading to the release of inflammatory factors as prostacyclin, thromboxane, prostaglandin, leukotrienes, endothelin, complement, TNF, and interleukins. TIC, resuscitation, and hemorrhage can form a vicious cycle. The mechanisms for TIC can be excessive activation of coagulation, hypocalcemia, anemia, hyperfibrinolysis, hypothermia, and trauma-induced platelet dysfunction. Multiple compensatory reactions can develop during hemorrhage, including baroreceptor reflexes, release of vasoconstrictors, chemoreceptor reflexes, reabsorption of tissue fluid, and increased fluid uptake by kidneys. TLRs have been recognized in recent years as important players in the pathogenesis of multiorgan dysfunction. Pain and stress are also patient's physiological exposures in traumatic injury. Adequate analgesia has been associated with better outcome in trauma patients. Infection and sepsis are the important factors causing morbidity and mortality in trauma patients. Multiple mechanisms are involved in the sepsis, cytokine releases (TNF, interleukins), bacterial translocation, bone marrow's change causes release of immature immune cells, increased nitric oxide formation, and acute adrenal insufficiency. Better understanding of these physiological alterations after trauma will help anesthesia providers better care the injured patients in perioperative settings.

References

1. Jones R. Neurogenetics: trauma and stress, from child to adult. Nat Rev Neurosci. 2013;14(2):77. doi:10.1038/nrn3425.
2. An LN, Yue Y, Guo WZ, Miao YL, Mi WD, Zhang H, Lei ZL, Han SJ, Dong L. Surgical trauma induces iron accumulation and oxidative stress in a rodent model of postoperative cognitive dysfunction. Biol Trace Elem Res. 2013;151(2):277–83. doi:10.1007/s12011-012-9564-9.
3. Eagle AL, Knox D, Roberts MM, Mulo K, Liberzon I, Galloway MP, Perrine SA. Single prolonged stress enhances hippocampal glucocorticoid receptor and phosphorylated protein kinase B levels. Neurosci Res. 2013;75(2):130–7. pii: S0168-0102(12)00205-2. DOI:10.1016/j.neures.2012.11.001.
4. Eastridge B. Joint Theater Trauma Registry Data. (June 2006–November 2008) 2009.
5. Franklin GA, Boaz PW, Spain DA, Lukan JK, Carrillo EH, Richardson JD. Prehospital hypotension as a valid indicator of trauma team activation. J Trauma. 2000;48:1034–7. discussion 1037-1039.
6. Venereau E, Schiraldi M, Uguccioni M, Bianchi ME. HMGB1 and leukocyte migration during trauma and sterile inflammation. Mol Immunol. 2013;55(1):76–82. pii: S0161-5890(12)00451-8. DOI:10.1016/j.molimm.2012.10.037.
7. Kauvar DS, Lefering R, Wade CE. Impact of hemorrhage on trauma outcome: an overview of epidemiology, clinical presentations, and therapeutic considerations. J Trauma. 2006;60:S3–S11.
8. http://www.nationaltraumainstitute.org/home/hemorrhage.html
9. Kortbeek JB, Al Turki SA, Ali J, Antoine JA, Bouiloon B, Brasel K, et al. Advanced trauma life support, 8th edition, the evidence for change. J Trauma. 2008;64:1638–50.
10. Holcroft JW. Shock. In: Dunphy JE, Way DL, editors. Current surgical diagnosis and treatment. 5th ed. Los Altos, CA: Lange Medical Publication; 1981. p. 172–81.
11. Bonanno FG. Hemorrhagic shock: the "physiology approach". J Emerg Trauma Shock. 2012;5 (4):285–95. doi:10.4103/0974-2700.102357.
12. Kauvar DS, Wade CE. The epidemiology and modern management of traumatic hemorrhage: US and international perspectives. Crit Care. 2005;9 Suppl 5:S1–9.
13. Bouglé A, Harrois A, Duranteau J. Resuscitative strategies in traumatic hemorrhagic shock. Ann Intensive Care. 2013;3(1):1.
14. Brohi K, Cohen MJ, Davenport RA. Acute coagulopathy of trauma: mechanism, identification and effect. Curr Opin Crit Care. 2007;13:680–5.
15. Brohi K, Cohen MJ, Ganter MT, Schultz MJ, Levi M, Mackersie RC, Pittet JF. Acute coagulopathy of trauma: hypoperfusion induces systemic anticoagulation and hyperfibrinolysis. J Trauma. 2008;64:1211–7. discussion 1217.
16. Floccard B, Rugeri L, Faure A, Denis MS, Boyle EM, Peguet O, Levrat A, Guillaume C, Marcotte G, Vulliez A, Hautin E, David JS, Negrier C, Allaouchiche B. Early coagulopathy in trauma patients: an on-scene and hospital admission study. Injury. 2012;43:26–32.
17. Cohen MJ, Call M, Nelson M, Calfee CS, Esmon CT, Brohi K, Pittet JF. Critical role of activated protein C in early coagulopathy and later organ failure, infection and death in trauma patients. Ann Surg. 2012;255:379–85.
18. Hess JR, Brohi K, Dutton RP, Hauser CJ, Holcomb JB, Kluger Y, Mackway-Jones K, Parr MJ, Rizoli SB, Yukioka T, Hoyt DB, Bouillon B. The coagulopathy of trauma: a review of mechanisms. J Trauma. 2008;65:748–54.
19. MacLeod JB, Lynn M, McKenney MG, Cohn SM, Murtha M. Early coagulopathy predicts mortality in trauma. J Trauma. 2003;55:39–44.
20. Lippi G, Cervellin G. Disseminated intravascular coagulation in trauma injuries. Semin Thromb Hemost. 2010;36(4):378–87. doi:10.1055/s-0030-1254047.
21. Austin AW, Wirtz PH, Patterson SM, Stutz M, von Känel R. Stress-induced alterations in coagulation: assessment of a new hemoconcentration correction technique. Psychosom Med. 2012;74(3):288–95. doi:10.1097/PSY.0b013e318245d950.
22. Holowaychuk MK, Monteith G. Ionized hypocalcemia as a prognostic indicator in dogs following trauma. J Vet Emerg Crit Care (San Antonio). 2011;21(5):521–30. doi:10.1111/j.1476-4431.2011.00675.x.

23. Sihler KC, Raghavendran K, Westerman M, Ye W, Napolitano LM. Hepcidin in trauma: linking injury, inflammation, and anemia. J Trauma. 2010;69 (4):831–7. doi:10.1097/TA.0b013e3181f066d5.

24. Aucar JA, Sheth M. The storage lesion of packed red blood cells affects coagulation. Surgery. 2012;152 (4):697–702. doi:10.1016/j.surg.2012.07.011. discussion 702-3.

25. Raza I, Davenport R, Rourke C, Platton S, Manson J, Spoors C, Khan S, De'Ath HD, Allard S, Hart DP, Pasi KJ, Hunt BJ, Stanworth S, MacCallum PK, Brohi K. The incidence and magnitude of fibrinolytic activation in trauma patients. J Thromb Haemost. 2013 Feb;11(2):307-14. doi: 10.1111/jth.12078.

26. Shakur H, Roberts I, Bautista R, Caballero J, Coats T, Dewan Y, El-Sayed H, Gogichaishvili T, Gupta S, Herrera J, Hunt B, Iribhogbe P, Izurieta M, Khamis H, Komolafe E, Marrero MA, Mejia-Mantilla J, Miranda J, Morales C, Olaomi O, Olldashi F, Perel P, Peto R, Ramana PV, Yutthakasemsunt S, et al. Effects of tranexamic acid on death, vascular occlusive events, and blood transfusion in trauma patients with significant hemorrhage (CRASH-2): a randomized, placebo-controlled trial. Lancet. 2010;376:23–32.

27. Davenport R. Pathogenesis of acute traumatic coagulopathy. Transfusion. 2013;53 Suppl 1:23S–7S. doi:10.1111/trf.12032. PMID: 23301969.

28. Frith D, Davenport R, Brohi K. Acute traumatic coagulopathy. Curr Opin Anaesthesiol. 2012;25:229–34.

29. Sawant DA, Tharakan B, Tobin RP, Stagg HW, Hunter FA, Newell MK, Smythe WR, Childs EW. Inhibition of fas-fas ligand interaction attenuates microvascular hyperpermeability following hemorrhagic shock. Shock. 2013;39(2):161–7. doi:10.1097/SHK.0b013e31827bba73.

30. McGhan LJ, Jaroszewski DE. The role of toll-like receptor-4 in the development of multi-organ failure following traumatichaemorrhagic shock and resuscitation. Injury. 2012;43(2):129–36. doi:10.1016/j.injury.2011.05.032.

31. Xiang M, Fan J, Fan J. Association of Toll-like receptor signaling and reactive oxygen species: a potential therapeutic target for posttrauma acute lung injury. Mediators Inflamm. 2010. pii: 916425. DOI: 10.1155/2010/916425

32. Bonanno FG. Physiopathology of shock. J Emerg Trauma Shock. 2011;4(2):222–32.

33. Schumacker PT, Samsel RW. Oxygen delivery and uptake by peripheral tissues: physiology and pathophysiology. Crit Care Clin. 1989;5:255–69.

34. http://www.jblearning.com/samples/0763740411/Ch %202_Seaward_Managing%20Stress_5e.pdf

35. Klengel T, et al. Allele-specific FKBP5 DNA demethylation mediates gene–childhood trauma interactions. Nature Neurosci. 2013;16:33–41. doi:10.1038/nn.3275.

36. Lindahl AE, Low A, Stridsberg M, Sjöberg F, Ekselius L, Gerdin B. Plasma chromogranin A after severe burn trauma. Neuropeptides. 2013;47 (3):207–12. pii: S0143-4179(12)00109-6. DOI: 10.1016/j.npep.2012.10.004.

37. Ahn Y, Görlinger K, Alam HB, Eikermann M. Pain-associated respiratory failure in chest trauma. Anesthesiology. 2013;118(3):701–8.

38. Shibata M, Hanzawa K, Ueda S, Yambe T. Deep venous thrombosis among disaster shelter inhabitants following the March 2011 earthquake and tsunami in Japan: a descriptive study. Phlebology. 2014;29 (4):257–66.

39. Rosenbloom BN, Khan S, McCartney C, Katz J. Systematic review of persistent pain and psychological outcomes following traumatic musculoskeletal injury. J Pain Res. 2013;6:39–51. doi:10.2147/JPR. S38878.

40. Griffis CA, Crabb Breen E, Compton P, Goldberg A, Witarama T, Kotlerman J, Irwin MR. Acute painful stress and inflammatory mediator production. Neuroimmunomodulation. 2013;20(3):127–33.

41. Xu Z, Li Y, Wang J, Li J. Effect of postoperative analgesia on energy metabolism and role of cyclooxygenase-2 inhibitors for postoperative pain management after abdominal surgery in adults. Clin J Pain. 2013;29(7):570–6.

42. Chaudry IH, Ayala A. Mechanism of increased susceptibility to infection following hemorrhage. Am J Surg. 1993;165(2A Suppl):59SY67S.

43. Mollen KP, Anand RJ, Tsung A, Prince JM, Levy RM, Billiar TR. Emerging paradigm: toll-like receptor 4 sentinel for the detection of tissue damage. Shock. 2006;26(5):430Y437.

44. Kobbe P, Kaczorowski DJ, Vodovotz Y, Tzioupis CH, Mollen KP, Billiar TR, Pape HC. Local exposure of bone components to injured soft tissue induces toll-like receptor 4Ydependent systemic inflammation with acute lung injury. Shock. 2008;30(6):686Y691.

45. Zhang Q, Raoof M, Chen Y, Sumi Y, Sursal T, Junger W, Brohi K, Itagaki K, Hauser CJ. Circulating mitochondrial DAMPs cause inflammatory responses to injury. Nature. 2010;464:104Y107.

46. Cai C, Gill R, Eum HA, Cao Z, Loughran PA, Darwiche S, Edmonds RD, Menzel CL, Billiar TR. Complement factor 3 deficiency attenuates hemorrhagic shock related hepatic injury and systemic inflammatory response syndrome. Am J Physiol Regul Integr Comp Physiol. 2010;299(5):R1175YR1182.

47. Sobhian B, Kröpfl A, Hölzenbein T, Khadem A, Redl H, Bahrami S. Increased circulating D-lactate levels predict risk of mortality after hemorrhage and surgical trauma in baboons. Shock. 2012;37(5):473–7. doi:10. 1097/SHK.0b013e318249cb96.

48. Nieves E, Tobón LF, Ríos DI, Isaza A, Ramírez M, Beltrán JA, Garzón-Ospina D, Patarroyo MA, Gómez A. Bacterial translocation in abdominal trauma and postoperative infections. J Trauma. 2011;71(5):1258–61.

49. Sánchez-Aguilar M, Tapia-Pérez JH, Sánchez-Rodríguez JJ, Viñas-Ríos JM, Martínez-Pérez P,

de la Cruz-Mendoza E, Sánchez-Reyna M, Torres-Corzo JG, Gordillo-Moscoso A. Effect of rosuvastatin on cytokines after traumatic head injury. J Neurosurg. 2013;118(3):669–75.

50. Francis WR, Bodger OG, Pallister I. Altered leucocyte progenitor profile in human bone marrow from patients with major trauma during the recovery phase. Br J Surg. 2012;99(11):1591–9. doi:10.1002/bjs.8919.

51. Marik PE, Pastores SM, Annane D, Meduri U, Sprung CL, Arlt W, Keh D, Briegel J, Beishuizen A, Dimopoulou I, et al. Recommendations for the diagnosis and management of corticosteroid insufficiency in critically ill adult patients: consensus statements from an international task force by the American College of Critical Care Medicine. Crit Care Med. 2008;36:1937–49.

52. Annane D, Maxime V, Ibrahim F, Alvarez JC, Abe E, Boudou P. Diagnosis of adrenal insufficiency in severe sepsis and septic shock. Am J Respir Crit Care Med. 2006;174:1319–26.

53. Maxime V, Lesur O, Annane D. Adrenal insufficiency in septic shock. Clin Chest Med. 2009;30:17–27.

54. Stein DM, Jessie EM, Crane S, Kufera JA, Timmons T, Rodriguez CJ, Menaker J, Scalea TM. Hyperacute adrenal insufficiency after hemorrhagic shock exists and is associated with poor outcomes. J Trauma Acute Care Surg. 2013;74(2):363–70. doi:10.1097/TA. 0b013e31827e2aaf.

55. Miller JB, Donnino MW, Rogan M, Goyal N. Relative adrenal insufficiency in post-cardiac arrest shock is under-recognized. Resuscitation. 2008;76(2):221–5.

56. Thiemermann C, Szabo C, Mitchell JA, Vane JR. Vascular hyporeactivity to vasoconstrictor agents and hemodynamic decompensation in hemorrhagic shock is mediated by nitric oxide. Proc Natl Acad Sci U S A. 1993;90:267Y271.

57. Hierholzer C, Harbrecht B, Menezes JM, Kane J, MacMicking J, Nathan CF, Peitzman AH, Billiar TR, Tweardy DJ. Essential role of induced nitric oxide I the initiation of the inflammatory response after hemorrhagic shock. J Exp Med. 1998;187 (6):917Y928.

58. Darwiche SS, Pfeifer R, Menzel C, Ruan X, Hoffman M, Cai C, Chanthaphavong RS, Loughran P, Pitt BR, Hoffman R, Pape HC, Billiar TR. Inducible nitric oxide synthase contributes to immune dysfunction following trauma. Shock. 2012;38(5):499–507. doi:10.1097/SHK.0b013e31826c5afe.

59. Williams VL, Martin RE, Franklin JL, Hardy RW, Messina JL. Injury-induced insulin resistance in adipose tissue. Biochem Biophys Res Commun. 2012;421 (3):442–8. doi:10.1016/j.bbrc.2012.03.146.

60. Xu H, Yu YM, Ma H, Carter EA, Fagan S, Tompkins RG, Fischman AJ. Glucose metabolism during the early "flow phase" after burn injury. J Surg Res. 2013;179(1):e83–90. doi:10.1016/j.jss. 2012.02.037.

61. Jeter CB, Hergenroeder GW, Hylin MJ, Redell JB, Moore AN, Dash PK. Biomarkers for the diagnosis and prognosis of mild traumatic brain injury/concussion. J Neurotrauma. 2013;30(8):657–70.

62. Tenenbein P, Kincaid MS, Lam AM. Head trauma-anesthetic considerations and management. In: Smith C, editor. Trauma anesthesia. Cambridge: Cambridge University Press; 2008. Chapter 11.

63. van Wessem KJ, Hennus MP, van Wagenberg L, Koenderman L, Leenen LP. Mechanical ventilation increases the inflammatory response induced by lung contusion. J Surg Res. 2013;183(1):377–84. pii: S0022-4804(12)01986-5. DOI:10.1016/j.jss.2012. 12.042.

64. Easter A. Management of patients with multiple rib fractures. Am J Crit Care. 2001;10(5):320–7.

Blood Transfusion and Coagulation Disorders

4

L. Yvette Fouché-Weber and Richard P. Dutton

Introduction

One-third to one-half of all mortality due to trauma is attributable to bleeding. Most deaths occur in the first hours after injury, as the result of uncontrolled hemorrhage from major vessels or organs. A smaller proportion occurs in the days or weeks that follow, as a long-term complication of shock and resuscitation. Tissue ischemia leads to an inflammatory response that creates the conditions for organ system failure and recurrent sepsis. Hours of mechanical ventilation become days, days of intensive care become weeks, and patients who are no longer bleeding can nonetheless die from the long-term consequences of shock and resuscitation months following the original injury.

Resuscitation is the restoration of normal physiology and tissue oxygen delivery following injury or illness. Optimizing resuscitation after trauma reduces the risk for both short-term death from uncontrolled hemorrhage and late death in the intensive care unit from inflammation and organ system failure [1, 2]. Optimal resuscitation prioritizes control of bleeding, followed by restoration of tissue oxygen delivery and complete return to normal physiology. Clinical care of the patient in hemorrhagic shock must weigh early priorities (control of bleeding and preservation of clotting function) vs. late considerations, such as the negative inflammatory effects of blood transfusion. The basic principles of early resuscitation are shown in Table 4.1 and will be the topics addressed in the remainder of this chapter, with an emphasis on transfusion and coagulation.

Control of Hemorrhage

Following trauma, hemorrhage is diagnosed by the symptoms of shock. Diminished tissue perfusion is evident in skin pallor, diaphoresis, altered mental status, and change in vital signs. While the traditional stages of hemorrhagic shock are defined by heart rate and blood pressure, there is enormous variation in response across individual patients. Age, physical fitness, medical comorbidities, genetic predisposition, and the effects of systemic toxins (e.g., alcohol, cocaine) all contribute to the change in vital signs associated with blood loss. Hypotension associated with tachycardia is the most common response. However, the amount of blood loss that causes a measurable decrease in pressure may vary from 5 to 50 % of normal blood volume, while an increase in heart rate is seen

L.Y. Fouché-Weber, M.D.
Department of Anesthesiology, University of Maryland Shock Trauma Center, 22 S. Greene Street, Baltimore, MD 21201, USA

R.P. Dutton, M.D., M.B.A. (✉)
Department of Anesthesia and Critical Care, University of Chicago, 5841 South Maryland Avenue, Chicago, IL 60637, USA
e-mail: r.dutton@asahq.org

C.S. Scher (ed.), *Anesthesia for Trauma*, DOI 10.1007/978-1-4939-0909-4_4, © Springer Science+Business Media New York 2014

Table 4.1 Principles of early resuscitation (before definitive control of hemorrhage)

Follow ABCs: control of airway and breathing; manual pressure on external bleeding sites
Expedite diagnostic and therapeutic maneuvers to control anatomic source of bleeding
Activate massive transfusion protocol as soon as uncontrolled hemorrhage is recognized
Maintain lower-than-normal blood pressure (systolic 80–100 mmHg)
Administer tranexemic acid: 1 g bolus, 1 g by infusion
Avoid excessive infusion of crystalloid or colloid solutions
Replace blood loss with blood products (red blood cells, plasma, and platelets)
Closely monitor critical laboratory values: arterial pH, lactate, ionized calcium, coagulation function; consider guiding transfusion therapy by viscoelastic testing
Achieve and maintain deep anesthesia

in only two-thirds of patients that become hypotensive [3].

Under most circumstances, loss of circulating blood volume causes a sympathetic nervous system response that vasoconstricts peripheral and low-priority vascular beds, while increasing blood flow to the heart. This compensatory response preserves blood pressure and central organ perfusion, and may be subtly indicated by narrowing pulse pressure within the normal range. Changes at the cellular level may include increased procoagulant tendency, with mobilization of clotting factor and platelet reserves, increased blood sugar, and increased cellular oxygen extraction [4–6]. Pain from tissue injury and conscious awareness of trauma enhance these responses. Circulating analgesic or anesthetic agents (e.g., alcohol, narcotics, sedatives) may blunt the sympathetic response to trauma, leading to earlier hypotension (without tachycardia). This may paradoxically allow earlier recognition and diagnosis of bleeding. Age, underlying cardiac disease, and the use of medications such as beta-adrenergic antagonists may also alter the normal physiologic response to hemorrhage [7, 8].

The degree of shock associated with a given injury is roughly proportional to the amount of blood lost. One of the key clinical distinctions which must be made early in the diagnosis of any trauma patient is the amount of blood already lost and the presence and rate of ongoing hemorrhage [9]. Certain injuries—isolated femur fracture for example—are associated with substantial blood loss (20–30 % of normal blood volume) but are less likely to cause ongoing bleeding. Otherwise healthy patients will be hypotensive early after such an injury (typically during initial assessment in the field), but will compensate rapidly as vasoconstriction and coagulation end ongoing blood loss and extravascular fluid is mobilized to preserve perfusion. These patients will often be normotensive at the time of trauma center presentation, and will generally do well with gentle isotonic fluid replacement [10, 11].

Other common injuries—splenic laceration, for example—may be associated with less immediate blood loss but more sustained bleeding. There is less opportunity for tamponade in the peritoneum than in the muscular compartments of the leg, and less effective vasoconstrictive control of splenic vessels. These patients may become hypotensive later than the first group. When treated with fluids, the blood pressure will typically respond immediately, but then drift down again as ongoing hemorrhage occurs. Identifying these "transient responders" is critical, because the ongoing cycle of hypotension and fluid therapy will lead to progressive coagulopathy, increased inflammatory perturbation, and protracted resuscitation [12, 13]. Life-threatening ongoing hemorrhage can occur into one of five compartments, as noted in Table 4.2. Investigation of each is required for any patient suffering high-energy trauma, or exhibiting early hemodynamic instability.

Individual trauma patients may have multiple combinations of bleeding and non-bleeding injuries, superimposed on the full human spectrum of genetics and comorbidities. Early laboratory assessment can assist the clinician in recognizing the seriousness of shock and hemorrhage. Base deficit and pH, assessed by arterial blood gas, indicate the instantaneous degree of hypoperfusion. Arterial or serum lactate approximates the cumulated "dose" of shock, or the integer over time of hypoperfusion. Providing adequate hemodynamic support to stabilize base

Table 4.2 Location of life-threatening hemorrhage

Location	Revealed by
Thorax	Chest radiograph or computed tomography (CT); tube thoracostomy output
Abdomen	Focused abdominal sonography for trauma (FAST); diagnostic peritoneal lavage
Retroperitoneum	Physical examination (unstable pelvic ring); CT scan
Thighs	Physical examination (obvious femur fracture)
Street	Visible bleeding outside the body; common with head and neck lacerations

deficit deterioration (or improve it to normal) should be the first target of fluid resuscitation during active hemorrhage. Once bleeding is controlled, the rate at which serum lactate is returned to normal is an excellent proxy for the quality of resuscitation. Rapid normalization of lactate after major trauma is associated with improved patient outcome [14].

More sophisticated assessments of tissue perfusion are increasingly available. Continuous monitoring of mixed-venous oxygenation via central line provides an accurate and dynamic guide to resuscitation. Transesophageal echocardiography can provide an immediate view of heart filling and contractility, and can rule out nonhemorrhagic causes of hypotension such as pericardial tamponade or valve disruption. Noninvasive monitors of tissue oxygenation, using near-infrared spectroscopy, are good indicators of perfusion in the intensive care unit and during elective surgery; their value during the highly dynamic moments of early resuscitation, during active hemorrhage, has yet to be definitively established [15, 16].

Early measurement of hemoglobin or hematocrit is not an accurate guide to the degree of hemorrhage. Rapid bleeding consumes whole blood and will thus not change the percent of red cells in a serum sample, while the rate of fluid mobilization from the extravascular space (and thus the degree of decrease in hematocrit) is unpredictable. Coagulation function, on the other hand, is an important secondary indicator of the

degree of shock [17]. A review of more than 30,000 admissions to a single trauma center documented abnormality in prothrombin time on initial blood draw as a highly precise predictor of mortality (Fig. 4.1). Other studies have confirmed the dire prognosis associated with early coagulation abnormalities. The observation that severe tissue ischemia, associated with trauma, produces a systemic increase in fibrinolysis is a key concept in resuscitation [18]. This has led in recent years to a number of studies examining the potential benefit of antifibrinolytic therapy and more aggressive support of clotting mechanisms.

Once hemorrhage has been identified, it must be controlled and the patient resuscitated. If physical examination and serial vital signs indicate that the patient is not actively bleeding, then further interventional care can be planned after a careful secondary assessment. Resuscitation can be completed with gentle administration of isotonic crystalloid to restore total-body fluids, guided by normalization of lactate. The patient with spontaneous resolution of hemorrhage is unlikely to need transfusion on an urgent basis but may require red blood cell (RBC) administration following restoration of adequate blood volume, especially if starting with a lower-than-normal hematocrit. Care should be taken with the rate of fluid administration in patients who have achieved spontaneous hemostasis. Too rapid infusion will increase cardiac output and blood pressure abruptly in the vasoconstricted patient with elevated sympathetic tone and may lead to rebleeding if fragile early clots are washed away [13, 19]. On the other hand, restoration of adequate circulating blood volume is highly recommended before pursuing any surgical or angiographic interventions. Many non-actively bleeding trauma patients will require early surgery for orthopedic, neurologic or soft-tissue injuries. A pause to assess the adequacy of resuscitation before proceeding to the OR can improve patient management and long-term outcomes in this population [1].

In the patient with active hemorrhage there are few activities that take priority over rapid transfer to the interventional radiology suite or operating room. This short list consists of airway

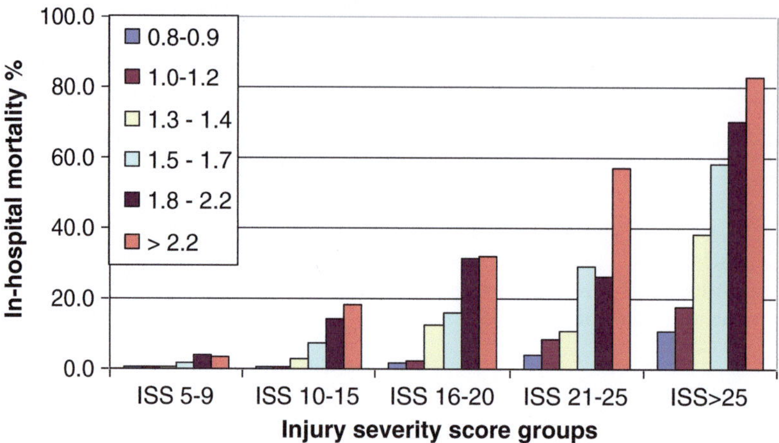

Fig. 4.1 Association of admission prothrombin time and injury severity on survival to hospital discharge. Reprinted with permission from Hess JR, Lindell AL, Stansbury LG, Dutton RP, Scalea TM. The prevalence of abnormal results of conventional coagulation tests on admission to a trauma center. Transfusion. 2009;49 (1):34–9

management and support of ventilation, relief of tension pneumothorax or pericardial tamponade, and application of direct pressure to any site of active external bleeding. Rapid anatomic control of hemorrhage limits the overall quantity of blood lost and directly improves outcomes [20]. While transfusion therapy and support of coagulation have advanced rapidly in the past two decades there is still no resuscitative fluid better than the patient's own blood. Keeping as much of that in circulation as possible is beneficial in both the short and the long term.

Anesthesiologists play a critical role in the rapid control of traumatic hemorrhage. Facilitating rapid physical transfer of the patient to the OR or angiography suite is one component. Other components include judging the desired degree of preoperative resuscitation, the adequacy of intravascular access, the appropriate depth of analgesia and sedation, and the need for advanced monitoring. In general, however, speed wins. Better outcomes will usually be achieved by getting the unstable patient to the OR and initiating surgery, while simultaneously adding vascular access, establishing arterial pressure monitoring and monitoring laboratory results [12].

Support of Intravascular Volume

While surgical intervention is underway in the patient with active hemorrhage, the anesthesiologist must manage the patient's hemodynamic status. This consists of balancing administration of resuscitative fluids (which will improve blood pressure) against administration of anesthetic and analgesic agents (which will lower it). Optimal fluid administration can be thought of in two dimensions: what fluid or fluids to give, and how to titrate the quantity of fluid to the patient's response.

Beginning with the latter point: the quantity of fluid to administer during active resuscitation has been debated for almost a century. In one of the first descriptions of intravenous fluid therapy, in 1919, Cannon noted about his practice in casualty care during World War I: "Injection of a fluid that will increase blood pressure has dangers in itself … If the pressure is raised before the surgeon is ready to check any bleeding that might take place, blood that is sorely needed may be lost." This principle was lost and then rediscovered by military physicians several times during the twentieth century. In the 1950s, however, development of the "Wiggers Model" of controlled resuscitation in laboratory animals emphasized the importance of generous volume replacement to preserving post-hemorrhage organ system function. This concept was embodied in the principles of Advanced Trauma Life Support in the 1970s and 1980s. In management of operative hemorrhage during elective surgical procedures, the recommendation was to replace blood loss with isotonic crystalloid infusion on a 3:1 basis (to allow for extravascular redistribution) up until the "allowable blood loss" was reached. The goal was to restore normal blood pressure as rapidly as possible, on the theory that this would lead to the best tissue and organ perfusion.

Dr. Cannon's observation that rapid fluid infusion could lead to further bleeding was not quantified in the laboratory until the 1960s, when Shaftan noted that femoral artery bleeding in the dog was perpetuated by volume administration and/or the use of vasopressors. Bleeding resolved most rapidly when the dog was allowed to become hypotensive, and no fluids were given. The use of vasodilating agents also decreased the duration and volume of hemorrhage. Sophisticated animal models of uncontrolled hemorrhage appeared in the late 1980s, and allowed for the study of resuscitation strategy in models of abdominal hemorrhage that approximated large-vessel traumatic injury. Total blood loss was reduced, and survival improved, when resuscitation was titrated to a lower-than-normal blood pressure. This finding has been confirmed in active-bleeding models in swine, rats, mice, dogs, and sheep, leading to the following summary conclusion reached by a panel of clinicians and researchers and published in 1996: "[during active traumatic hemorrhage] attempting to normalize blood pressure seems to be counterproductive."

Consistent findings in animal models led to clinical trials of "deliberate hypotensive resuscitation' in the 1990s. The first and most important of these was the landmark work of Bickell et al., published in the New England Journal of Medicine in 1994. Hypotensive victims of penetrating torso trauma in the city of Houston were randomized (based on the day of the month) to either conventional care or deliberate fluid restriction from the moment of first contact with the emergency medical system until reaching the OR in the trauma center. More than 600 patients were randomized, with an average 2 L difference in crystalloid infusion between groups observed at the time of surgery. Of note, mean systolic blood pressure (SBP) was identical on OR arrival between groups, although the fluid-restricted group experienced more hypotension during the study period. The hypotensive resuscitation group had improved survival (10 % vs. 62 %, $p=0.04$).

While controversial, this study prompted clinical interest in controlled hypotension as a technique to control traumatic hemorrhage, as well as further and more elaborate studies. One such was a trial in Baltimore which randomized patients arriving at the trauma center to management of fluids targeted at SBP of >80 vs. >100 mmHg. Hypotensive patients had shorter OR times and similar survival to normotensive patients [21]. By the turn of the millennium, deliberate hypotensive management was the norm at most large trauma centers. Hypotension is typically sustained by limitation of infused fluids, especially non-sanguineous crystalloids, which makes this approach a trade-off between the short-term risks of exacerbating coagulopathy and bleeding to death vs. the long-term risks of decreased organ perfusion. A new large clinical trial of deliberate hypotensive management is underway at this time; a preliminary report suggests that the results will again favor hypotension during active hemorrhage.

While the value of sustained hypotension in limiting blood loss seems clear, and is supported by the use of deliberate hypotension to limit blood loss in major elective surgery, the way in which hypotension is achieved and sustained may strongly influence outcomes. In trauma patients hypotension is achieved by loss of circulating blood volume, and is associated with tissue hypoperfusion: shock. Hypotension is then sustained by restricting fluid administration,

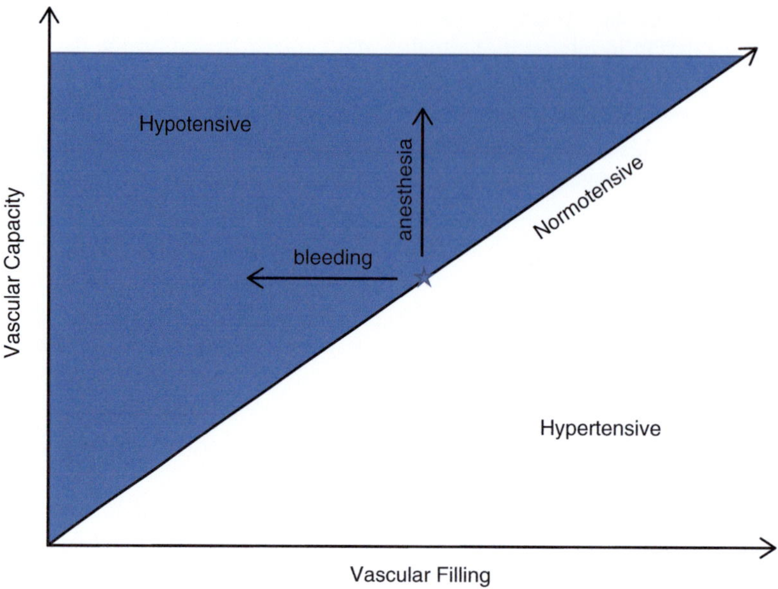

Fig. 4.2 Hemorrhagic shock followed by deliberate hypotension vs. deep anesthesia followed by bleeding. The patient is hypotensive, but the physiologic state is different

allowing the vasoconstricted, hypoperfused physiology to persist. During early resuscitation this typically occurs in the setting of minimal analgesia and sedation. Although counterintuitive, this approach can improve outcomes if it results in earlier hemostasis and reduced overall blood loss [21]. By comparison, deliberate hypotension in elective surgery is achieved with administration of vasodilating agents (usually anesthetics) in the setting of normovolemia. Figure 4.2 shows this distinction graphically, and illustrates the critical difference in physiology. It is possible that outcomes of deliberate hypotension in trauma could be improved by following a similar approach: restore fluid volume aggressively, but simultaneously increase anesthetic depth to sustain hypotension. The desired physiologic state would be one of controlled hypotension (limiting blood loss) but sympathetic relaxation (allowing the maximum possible tissue perfusion for a given pressure). The authors' anecdotal experience with this approach has been positive, but it has yet to be experimentally validated; animal models of acute hemorrhage using minimal anesthesia are difficult to construct in an ethical fashion.

Choice of Fluids

While the volume of fluid administered to a hemorrhaging trauma patient has an impact on the rate and volume of bleeding, and on associated long-term outcome, the types of fluid administered are likely at least as significant. Specific products are summarized in Table 4.3. Options fall into four basic categories:
- Isotonic crystalloids
- Non-blood colloids such as 5 % albumin solution and the various hetastarches
- RBCs
- Non-RBC blood products (plasma, platelets, cryoprecipitate)

The latter two categories are forms of transfusion—or blood transplantation—and are associated with the greatest controversy. Support of oxygen carrying capacity (RBC) and coagulation (plasma, platelets, cryoprecipitate) is a lifesaving necessity in patients with severe, active hemorrhage [22]. Yet numerous retrospective studies have documented the increased risk for organ system failure and long-term mortality associated with transfusion [23–25]. The immune

Table 4.3 Products for fluid resuscitation

Product	Comment
Isotonic crystalloids	Lactated Ringers solution; Plasmalyte A. Normal saline should be avoided due to hyperchloremic metabolic acidosis
Colloids	Albumin 5 % is only one available in the US Hetastarch solutions still available in Europe but falling out of favor due to concern with renal impairment
Fresh whole blood	Only available in military medicine. Viral testing of donated whole blood requires 3 days to complete, at which point platelet count is negligible
Red blood cells	Normal hematocrit of component unit is 55–60 %. Must be blood type specific (or type-O). Carries oxygen, but does not include clotting factors
Plasma	May be thawed from frozen units or kept liquid. Includes all serum clotting factors in relatively dilute solution. Requires blood typing (or type-AB)
Platelets	Usually obtained from plasmapheresis (equivalent to a pool of 4–6 random donor units). Relatively concentrated product; includes a significant amount of plasma
Plasma concentrates	Assembled from donor plasma units; specific concentrations of selected clotting factors
Factor concentrates	Purified or recombinant single factor products: Fibrinogen, Factor VIII, Factor VII available in the USA. Typically only used for addressing known defects due to genetic disorders

modulation associated with transfusion increases the risk for perfusion-related syndromes (e.g., acute tubular necrosis), pulmonary dysfunction (acute lung injury), and infectious complications. Interpreting this evidence is challenging, because of the numerous confounding variables seen in retrospective studies. Patients who receive transfusion are sicker or more badly injured than those who do not, and no amount of propensity matching and logistic regression can compensate for this reality. Prospective studies of transfusion thresholds have generally confirmed a higher risk for complications associated with one or two unit transfusions, but cannot be extended to include patients with rapid hemorrhage and more massive transfusions [26]. On the other hand, studies of severe bleeding have shown that earlier and more

aggressive use of blood products can reduce the risk of hemorrhagic death [25, 27]. The clinician must therefore practice schizophrenically, doing everything possible to avoid transfusion in marginal situations, but being aggressive with blood products when there is a real risk of exsanguination or irreversible coagulopathy.

The trauma patient with active, ongoing hemorrhage presents unique challenges to the clinician. First, resuscitation must start at a time when the anatomic source of injury is not clearly defined. Second, the amount of blood the patient has already lost is unknown. Third, the duration and severity of future bleeding can only be estimated. And fourth, the patient is in a severely vasoconstricted state very different from the vasodilated hypotension more common in elective anesthesia practice.

The impact of shock and injury on the coagulation system has been better defined in the past decade. Patients who reach medical care but subsequently die of acute hemorrhagic shock are universally acidotic, hypothermic, and coagulopathic at the time of exsanguination [18]. Coagulopathy was formerly thought to trigger from consumption of clotting factors and dilution of blood by administered fluids, and be exacerbated by acidosis and hypothermia. While these mechanisms remain important and relevant, another contributor has been discovered: the body's innate response to tissue injury and ischemia. Observational studies in patients with high injury severity score (ISS) have documented the onset of coagulopathy very early after injury, *prior to* administration of resuscitative fluids [28]. This concept was illustrated in Fig. 4.1, above; the large majority of patients had received less than 1 L of crystalloid fluid prior to the time of first laboratory assessment. While multiple mediators are likely contributing to early coagulopathy, one identified change is increased release of Protein C leading to enhanced fibrinolysis [29]. While maladaptive in trauma patients this reaction at the tissue level may reflect an evolutionary response to ischemia caused by thrombosis and embolism, which is a more common threat than hemorrhage.

Further understanding of the complex interplay between the vascular endothelium and

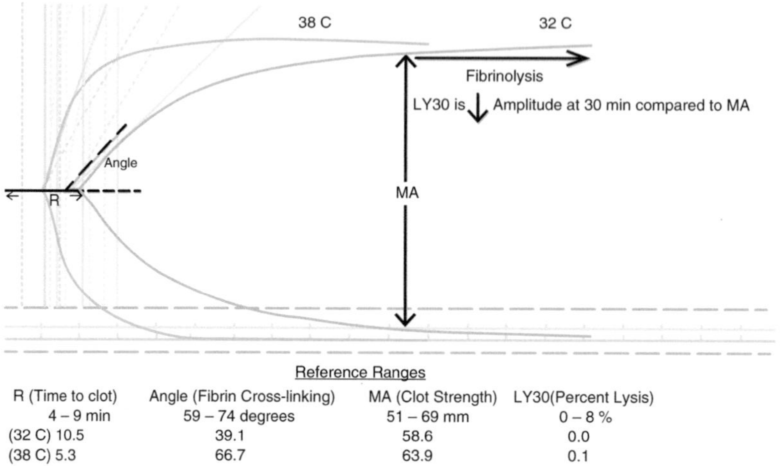

Reference Ranges			
R (Time to clot)	Angle (Fibrin Cross-linking)	MA (Clot Strength)	LY30(Percent Lysis)
4 – 9 min	59 – 74 degrees	51 – 69 mm	0 – 8 %
(32 C) 10.5	39.1	58.6	0.0
(38 C) 5.3	66.7	63.9	0.1

Fig. 4.3 Normal and abnormal thromboelastograph tests

humoral components of clotting (e.g., RBC, platelets, and circulating factors) is slowly emerging, fueled by increased diagnostic capability. At the University of Texas in Houston traditional coagulation assessment by prothrombin time, partial thromboplastin time and platelet count has been replaced by early whole blood viscoelastic testing. While the thromboelastograph (TEG) and rotational thromboelastometer (ROTEM) have been available for some years, their use in the management of acute traumatic hemorrhage is just beginning. TEG and ROTEM use slightly different technology to produce similar "pictures" of clot formation in the patient's whole blood. The onset, rate, and strength of clot formation can be visualized in real time, as well as the rate and severity of fibrinolysis and clot destruction. Figure 4.3 shows normal and abnormal TEG patterns. Viscoelastic testing provides a more precise assessment of which clotting element is most likely lacking in the coagulopathic patient: platelets, soluble factors or fibrinogen, and what the contribution of fibrinolysis may be. Resuscitation guided by TEG or ROTEM has been reported to improve outcomes and reduce transfusion in several small series, but a definitive prospective, randomized trial is still lacking [30].

Absent the availability of rapid bedside testing, and confronted with a hemodynamically unstable patient, the clinician must make empiric decisions about what products to transfuse. RBC, plasma, and platelets, administered in a 1:1:1 ratio, have been proposed as a simple and obvious approach. While this recipe is intended to replicate the whole blood that the patient is losing, the reality of modern component therapy preparation is that the resulting solution still falls substantially short. This concept is illustrated in Fig. 4.4. The ratio of plasma to RBC units for empiric resuscitation that produces the greatest survival has been hotly debated in recent years, with proposals ranging from 1:1 to as low as 1:2, but in any case the early support of the coagulation system in severe trauma patients has become much more common.

Observational data in both military and civilian trauma centers has been used to support the theory that earlier administration of plasma improves outcomes. Any unadjusted large series of hemorrhaging patients will show improved outcomes in those that receive a higher ratio of plasma to RBC but this data is strongly confounded by the logistics of most trauma centers, which cause RBC to reach the bedside in advance of plasma. Patients with the most rapid bleeding may receive RBC prior to dying, but never have the chance to receive plasma. This "survivor bias" is present in many observational studies of resuscitation ratio; when the effect is controlled for the results are more equivocal. DiBiasi and colleagues examined this problem

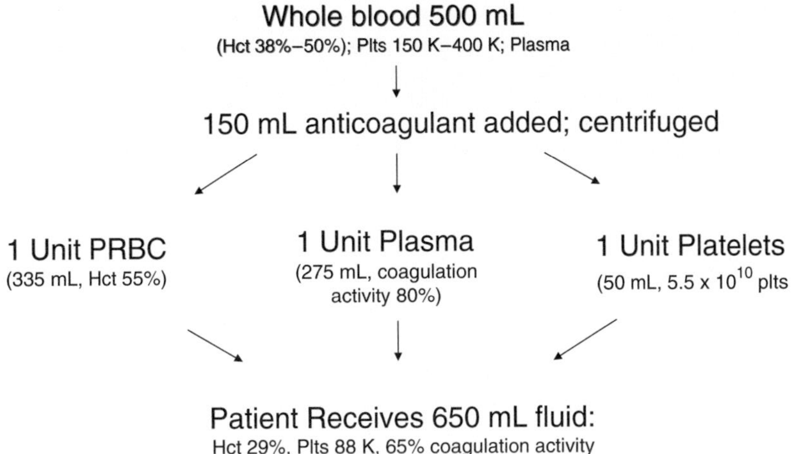

Fig. 4.4 Donated whole blood vs. component therapy

using the idea of instantaneous plasma deficit (RBC units minus plasma units at any point in time), and discovered that a higher deficit was associated with greater mortality, but only in the first three hours after trauma center admission. Beyond that time anatomic control of hemorrhage has typically occurred, and administration of blood products is less likely to be empiric and more likely to be driven by specific laboratory assessment.

Adjuvant Therapies

Successful resuscitation from traumatic hemorrhage is dependent on rapid anatomic control of the source of bleeding, careful management of blood pressure, and precise transfusion therapy. Other adjuvant therapies are worthy of consideration, driven by an improved understanding of the pathophysiology of shock, advancing pharmaceutical and monitoring technology, and empiric data.

Transfusion of large quantities of banked blood necessarily includes infusion of citrate-based anticoagulants. Citrate works by binding free calcium in the stored units, thus preventing activation of clotting. When administered in a rapid transfusion, citrate will reduce the patient's ionized calcium level. While this will have a mild adverse effect on coagulation it may have

a marked effect on myocardial contractility, which is another calcium-dependent process. The result is hypotension unresponsive to further fluid therapy. Close monitoring of ionized calcium is important during ongoing resuscitation, and the need for administration of calcium is likely whenever more than 4 units of blood products per hour are infused. (Slower rates of transfusion are less likely to cause citrate intoxication, as the body has time to mobilize calcium reserves.) During massive transfusion, hypotension unresponsive to a fluid volume bolus should be empirically treated with administration of 1 g of calcium, while awaiting the return of laboratory results. This dose, in and of itself, is unlikely to cause adverse effects, whereas observation of a positive response in blood pressure indicates ongoing citrate poisoning and the potential need for further therapy.

Because fibrinolysis may be activated early after trauma, and may contribute to coagulopathy, some investigators have focused on the potential benefits of antifibrinolytic therapy. The CRASH-2 trial enrolled some 20,000 trauma patients with ongoing hemorrhage and randomized them to receive either tranexemic acid (TXA) or placebo. This international trial was conducted in more than 100 countries around the world (although not in the USA), and may be the largest prospective trial ever published in trauma. CRASH-2 demonstrated a substantial improvement in survival in the patients who received TXA within 3 h of injury, making this a near-instantaneous recommendation for early therapy [31]. Patients who received TXA later than 3 h from injury did not benefit [31]. Also noteworthy was the absence of a difference in transfusion requirements between the patient groups. This has raised the possibility that some other anti-inflammatory effect of TXA is truly beneficial, rather than antifibrinolysis. A smaller observational study conducted in US military casualties in Afghanistan confirmed an association between TXA and improved survival [32]. Administration of TXA as earlier as possible after injury has become routine in most major trauma centers around the world, although controversy remains as to which patient populations should be included. The results of CRASH-2 have led to renewed interest in antifibrinolytics in other conditions, including total joint replacement and postpartum hemorrhage, and studies are ongoing in these and other models.

Other efforts to treat the coagulopathy of traumatic shock with specific, concentrated clotting factors have not been as universally successful. Recombinant human Factor VIIa (FVIIa) has been available for more than a decade as an off-label rescue therapy for patients with acute hemorrhage and coagulopathy. Initial enthusiasm for FVIIa, and widespread use, has been replaced by a conservative and highly selective approach. FVIIa will rapidly normalize PT in almost any patient, and early use of FVIIa has been shown to reduce transfusion requirement in seriously injured trauma patients. However, this benefit has not been associated with improved survival, and off-label use of FVIIa may be a risk factor for thromboembolic complications. The best prospective data available comes from the CONTROL trial, which enrolled nearly 600 patients with acute, ongoing traumatic hemorrhage, and randomized them to receive either a large dose of FVIIa or placebo. Transfusion requirement was reduced, but survival was unchanged [33]. The rate of thromboembolic complications did not vary between groups. Of note, the overall survival of all patients in CONTROL was about half what was predicted by the pre-study power analysis. The investigators attributed this finding to other improvements in trauma care, including evidence-based protocols for operative management, transfusion, and post-injury ventilator weaning. This observation mirrors clinical experience with FVIIa in the US and British military and in major civilian trauma centers: the need to "rescue" patients with FVIIa declined sharply as the speed and precision of resuscitation improved.

Prothrombin complex concentrates, which may include FVIIa, have improved in purity and consistency in recent years, and have been advocated by some for trauma resuscitation. At present there is insufficient data to know whether they represent a viable alternative to plasma therapy in a 1:1:1 model of early resuscitation. Recombinant fibrinogen concentrate is another blood-derived product that may also be of use in actively bleeding patients. Positive small studies in single centers await multicenter confirmation.

A final potential adjuvant therapy for management of uncontrolled hemorrhage is the administration of deep general anesthesia. Patients who require massive transfusion during elective surgical procedures have approximately 10 times better survival than trauma patients receiving similar volumes of blood products [34]. While there are many potential explanations for this finding, one important observation is that elective surgery patients are anesthetized at the time when hemorrhage occurs, and are therefore in a low-catecholamine state and relatively vasodilated. Trauma patients, on the other hand, are in pain and shock when bleeding is diagnosed, and may be profoundly vasoconstricted. This difference may contribute to a difference in outcomes, and begs the question of whether provision of deep anesthesia can improve tissue perfusion and reduce the risk of organ system failure and death. Literature from animal studies is of relatively little benefit in assessing this issue, because laboratory study of acute hemorrhagic shock (such as the models presented above) typically requires general anesthesia. In real clinical practice in trauma patients with unstable vital signs there is a strong tendency to provide minimal anesthesia, or to manage the patient with amnestics such as scopolamine and midazolam but limited analgesic or sedative therapy. This preserves the patient's high sympathetic tone and certainly improves measured blood pressure in the short term, but at the expense of perpetuating tissue hypoperfusion. It may be that better results would be achieved with titration toward deep anesthesia, balanced by more aggressive administration of fluids. This approach allows for continued hypotension to preserve hemostasis, while hopefully improving perfusion over time. A technique of early deep anesthesia is used in some trauma centers now, but awaits evidence-based assessment.

Late Resuscitation

The anesthesiologist is often the first to know when bleeding has been definitively controlled. As shown in Fig. 4.5, patients with active bleeding will have very labile blood pressure due to dynamic changes in blood volume and catecholamine level. Constriction of the normal 5 L vascular volume leads to an exaggerated response to fluid boluses or further hemorrhage, especially when a hypotensive pressure is targeted by the anesthesiologist. Once further bleeding is removed from this equation, due to ligation of a bleeding vessel, excision of an injured organ or angiographic embolization, the patient's vital signs will rapidly stabilize. Even absent the administration of any further exogenous fluids intravascular volume will be recruited from the interstitium. Blood pressure will normalize spontaneously as the patient "auto-resuscitates." This effect can be seen in those patients who bleed but then coagulate (e.g., the patient with an isolated femur fracture described above), and explains why they are hypotensive in the field but often normotensive at the time of trauma center arrival. Recovery of hemodynamic stability is also seen in the OR when a given fluid bolus produces a sustained increase in blood pressure, or when administration of additional anesthetics is tolerated without a change in vital signs.

When this happy moment occurs, the anesthesiologist should take the opportunity to pause any active transfusions and reassess the situation. First is a consideration of the patient's anatomy. Is hemorrhage really over? Are unrecognized injuries a possibility? What is the risk for rebleeding? When hemostasis is associated with an arterial ligature or completion of splenectomy, for example, rebleeding is less likely than if bleeding was originally from the liver, pelvis, or any other organ where complete anatomic resolution may not be possible. The next step should be a return to evidence-based (rather than empiric) resuscitation. Laboratory variables should be assessed, and further fluid and transfusion therapy guided by the results. Electrolytes should be normalized, especially ionized calcium. Fluid therapy should be continuing, recognizing that normovolemia must still be achieved. The need for replacement of total-body fluid volume after hemorrhage, to enable improved clinical outcomes, was first made more than 50 years ago. The adequacy of volume restoration in late resuscitation can be judged in several ways. Serial measurement of cardiac output, with fluid titration titrated to the highest achievable value, is one approach. Titration to maximal mixed-venous oxygen saturation is another. Normalization of serum lactate indicates restoration of adequate systemic perfusion; the more rapidly this is achieved post-hemorrhage, the better the associated clinical outcome [14]. Note, however, that simple restoration of a normal blood pressure is an inadequate indicator of perfusion; the phenomenon of "occult hypoperfusion" occurs in ICU patients with normal systolic pressure but persistent vasoconstriction and hypoperfusion [10]. This condition, indicated by persistent metabolic acidosis or elevated serum lactate, is associated with increased organ system dysfunction and late mortality.

As in early resuscitation, consideration should be given to what kind of fluid is administered. In general, isotonic crystalloid solutions will be the least expensive and most effective. The role of colloid solutions, including both albumin and hetastarches, has been hotly debated. While

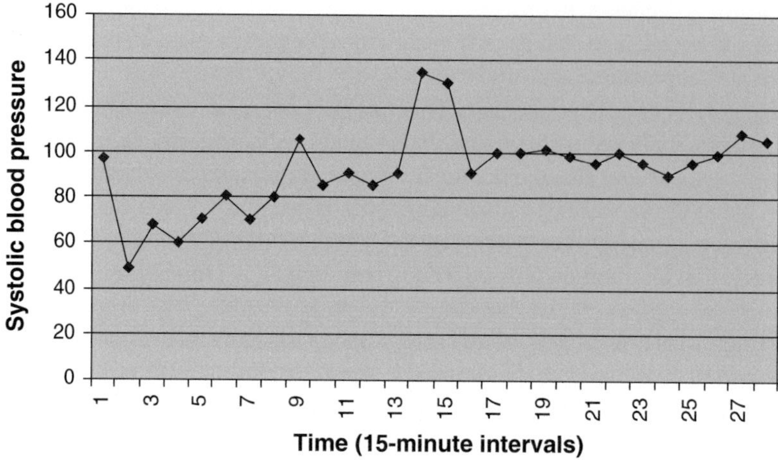

Fig. 4.5 Blood pressure lability during uncontrolled hemorrhage with deliberate hypotensive resuscitation. Reprinted with permission from Dutton RP, Mackenzie CF, Scalea TM. Hypotensive Resuscitation during Active Hemorrhage: Impact on In-Hospital Mortality. J Trauma. 2002;52:1141–6

numerous publications have taken up this topic, the global consensus is that colloids offer no particular benefit and may be associated with adverse outcomes under some conditions (i.e., renal failure associated with starch solutions) [24, 35]. Further transfusion of blood products should be limited, because of the known adverse inflammatory effects and association with adverse outcomes. An acceptable hematocrit in the non-bleeding patient may be as low as 20 %, but should take into account the patient's age and comorbidities. Transfusion of plasma or platelets is unlikely to benefit a non-bleeding patient, but may have prophylactic value in selected cases (e.g., traumatic brain injury with abnormal coagulation studies; liver injuries with potential for rebleeding; the need for early orthopedic surgery). Any transfusion during late resuscitation should be guided by laboratory assessment, including viscoelastic testing if available.

Future Research

The field of resuscitation has made enormous strides in the past 20 years, driven by evolution of laboratory science, a series of large prospective human trials and the ability to translate between the two.

References

1. Bickell WH, et al. Immediate versus delayed fluid resuscitation for hypotensive patients with penetrating torso injuries. N Engl J Med. 1994;331(17):1105–9.
2. Douzinas EE. Hemorrhagic shock resuscitation: a critical issue on the development of posttraumatic multiple organ failure. Crit Care Med. 2012;40(4):1348–9.
3. Davis JW, et al. Are automated blood pressure measurements accurate in trauma patients? J Trauma. 2003;55(5):860–3.
4. Bogner V, et al. Very early posttraumatic serum alterations are significantly associated to initial massive RBC substitution, injury severity, multiple organ failure and adverse clinical outcome in multiple injured patients. Eur J Med Res. 2009;14(7):284–91.
5. Collins JA. The pathophysiology of hemorrhagic shock. Prog Clin Biol Res. 1982;108:5–29.
6. Sung J, et al. Admission hyperglycemia is predictive of outcome in critically ill trauma patients. J Trauma. 2005;59(1):80–3.
7. Amr YM, Amin SM. Effects of preoperative beta-blocker on blood loss and blood transfusion during spinal surgeries with sodium nitroprusside-controlled hypotension. Saudi J Anaesth. 2012;6(3):263–7.
8. Dark PM, et al. Monitoring the circulatory responses of shocked patients during fluid resuscitation in the emergency department. Intensive Care Med. 2000;26(2):173–9.
9. Tarnoky K, Nagy S. Effect of the rate of blood loss on the plasma catecholamine response. Acta Physiol Hung. 1985;66(2):143–53.
10. Martin JT, et al. 'Normal' vital signs belie occult hypoperfusion in geriatric trauma patients. Am Surg. 2010;76(1):65–9.

11. Hirshberg A, Hoyt DB, Mattox KL. Timing of fluid resuscitation shapes the hemodynamic response to uncontrolled hemorrhage: analysis using dynamic modeling. J Trauma. 2006;60(6):1221–7.

12. Carlino W. Damage control resuscitation from major haemorrhage in polytrauma. Eur J Orthop Surg Traumatol. 2014;24(2):137–41.

13. Hahn RG. Fluid therapy in uncontrolled hemorrhage—what experimental models have taught us. Acta Anaesthesiol Scand. 2013;57(1):16–28.

14. Reynolds PS, Barbee RW, Ward KR. Lactate profiles as a resuscitation assessment tool in a rat model of battlefield hemorrhage resuscitation. Shock. 2008;30(1):48–54.

15. Jorge MA, Irrazabal CL. Assessing shock resuscitation strategies by oxygen debt repayment. Shock. 2011;35(1):100. author reply 100-2.

16. Ba ZF, et al. Alterations in tissue oxygen consumption and extraction after trauma and hemorrhagic shock. Crit Care Med. 2000;28(8):2837–42.

17. Fries D, et al. Management of coagulation after multiple trauma. Anaesthesist. 2005;54(2):137–44.

18. Schlag G, Redl H. Current findings in the pathogenesis of the shock process in traumatology. Unfallchirurgie. 1988;14(1):3–11.

19. Sondeen JL, Coppes VG, Holcomb JB. Blood pressure at which rebleeding occurs after resuscitation in swine with aortic injury. J Trauma. 2003;54(5 Suppl):S110–7.

20. Baron BJ, Scalea TM. Acute blood loss. Emerg Med Clin North Am. 1996;14(1):35–55.

21. Dutton RP, Mackenzie CF, Scalea TM. Hypotensive resuscitation during active hemorrhage: impact on in-hospital mortality. J Trauma. 2002;52(6):1141–6.

22. Cabrales P, Intaglietta M, Tsai AG. Transfusion restores blood viscosity and reinstates microvascular conditions from hemorrhagic shock independent of oxygen carrying capacity. Resuscitation. 2007;75(1):124–34.

23. Atzil S, et al. Blood transfusion promotes cancer progression: a critical role for aged erythrocytes. Anesthesiology. 2008;109(6):989–97.

24. Brakenridge SC, et al. Early blood product and crystalloid volume resuscitation: risk association with multiple organ dysfunction after severe blunt traumatic injury. J Trauma. 2011;71(2):299–305.

25. Maetani S, et al. Role of blood transfusion in organ system failure following major abdominal surgery. Ann Surg. 1986;203(3):275–81.

26. Al-Faris L, et al. Blood transfusion practice in critically ill patients: a single institutional experience. Med Princ Pract. 2012;21(6):560–5.

27. de Biasi AR, et al. Blood product use in trauma resuscitation: plasma deficit versus plasma ratio as predictors of mortality in trauma (CME). Transfusion. 2011;51(9):1925–32.

28. Engels PT, et al. The natural history of trauma-related coagulopathy: implications for treatment. J Trauma. 2011;71(5 Suppl 1):S448–55.

29. Ely EW, Bernard GR, Vincent JL. Activated protein C for severe sepsis. N Engl J Med. 2002;347(13):1035–6.

30. Tauber H, et al. Prevalence and impact of abnormal ROTEM(R) assays in severe blunt trauma: results of the 'Diagnosis and Treatment of Trauma-Induced Coagulopathy (DIA-TRE-TIC) study'. Br J Anaesth. 2011;107(3):378–87.

31. Perel P, et al. CRASH-2 (Clinical Randomisation of an Antifibrinolytic in Significant Haemorrhage) intracranial bleeding study: the effect of tranexamic acid in traumatic brain injury—a nested randomised, placebo-controlled trial. Health Technol Assess. 2012;16(13):iii–xii. 1–54.

32. Morrison JJ, et al. Military application of tranexamic acid in trauma emergency resuscitation (MATTERs) study. Arch Surg. 2012;147(2):113–9.

33. Hauser CJ, et al. Results of the CONTROL trial: efficacy and safety of recombinant activated Factor VII in the management of refractory traumatic hemorrhage. J Trauma. 2010;69(3):489–500.

34. Dutton RP. Haemostatic resuscitation. Br J Anaesth. 2012;109 Suppl 1:i39–46.

35. Phillips DP, et al. Crystalloids vs. colloids: KO at the twelfth round? Crit Care. 2013;17(3):319.

General Principles of Intraoperative Management of the Severe Blunt or Polytrauma Patient: The Resuscitative Phase

Corey S. Scher, Inca Chui, and Sanford M. Miller

Case Entry Point

A 57-year-old mailman made a delivery in a high rise office building in the financial district in New York City. As he left the building, a car going 60 miles per hour hit him and pinned him against a wall of the building. He immediately lost consciousness. Witnesses at the scene called 911 and tried to help. With a concerted effort, they tried to remove the driver as well as the mailman from the scene. The New York City Fire Department and emergency medical services arrived within 5 min. One witness was able to feel pulses in both patients, and said that both driver and mailman were breathing.

The fire department personnel towed the car backwards, enabling the rescue team to place a rigid cervical collar on the mailman and remove him from the scene on a spine board. Two large bore IV's were started and oxygen was given via facemask. The first set of vital signs was BP 66/42, pulse 110, and respirations 17. Tympanic temperature was 35.4 °C. The driver received similar treatment in a separate ambulance. All of her vital signs were stable. There was a strong smell of alcohol and vomit on her body. EMS

C.S. Scher, M.D. (✉) • S.M. Miller, M.D.
Department of Anesthesiology, NYU/Bellevue Hospital Center, 462 First Avenue, New York, NY 10016, USA
e-mail: coreyscher@gmail.com

I. Chui, M.D.
Department of Anesthesiology, New York University Langone Medical Center, 550 First Avenue, New York, NY 10016, USA

called ahead to the nearest Level I trauma center. Two designated trauma beepers went off: one for the attending anesthesiologist on call, the second for the senior anesthesia resident on trauma.

Both patients were transported to the trauma bay, an area in the emergency department designated for a total trauma assessment by the emergency room and trauma attending physicians. It is imperative that all members of the anesthesia trauma team also attend this assessment in order to prepare for a resuscitation strategy that yields the best outcome.

The initial strategy for handling trauma has been called "damage control resuscitation" by the military. This needs to be initiated in the first or "golden" hour [1]. Damage control in the United States Navy consists of (1) control of bleeding, (2) control of contamination, and (3) restoring a survivable physiological state. The growth of trauma medicine as a unique discipline is rooted in numerous trauma specialists advocating for the development of a standardized treatment format.

The term "golden hour" has been used in several arenas of critical care, described by Tobin and Varon, and applied by R. Adams Cowley [2]. The philosophy of the "golden hour" is that the outcome of the patient resuscitated in the first hour following injury will be better than one resuscitated hours later. The evidence supporting this may not be strong, since trauma remains a difficult subject to study. Many victims of trauma have poor outcomes whether or not they are resuscitated within the

C.S. Scher (ed.), *Anesthesia for Trauma*, DOI 10.1007/978-1-4939-0909-4_5,
© Springer Science+Business Media New York 2014

"golden hour." Additionally, there is so much variation among severe trauma patients that it is very difficult to attain data that would yield therapeutic strategies with a high level of evidence.

In the trauma bay, a rapid assessment of the mailman was made based on his unstable condition, and the trauma attending and anesthesiologist agreed that the rapid transfusion protocol should be initiated. The focused assessment with sonography for trauma (FAST) revealed a significant amount of blood in the peritoneal and retroperitoneal spaces. There were no obvious facial fractures noted that might make intubation difficult. For intubation, a Macintosh 4 laryngoscope blade was gently placed in the patient's mouth for airway assessment. The patient bit down mildly on the blade and gagged. This "awake look" revealed that a rapid sequence intubation could be done. The cervical collar was removed and an assistant provided inline stabilization of the cervical spine. Ketamine and succinylcholine were administered and an endotracheal tube was placed atraumatically. Vital signs after intubation were essentially unchanged, with a systolic pressure in the low 70s and a pulse of 120. Rapid ultrasound of the abdomen was positive in addition for blood. Both legs had open fractures. The most outstanding finding was an open pelvic fracture, which was considered by the trauma team as a lethal injury by itself because of iliac vein bleeding.

Due to the ongoing circulatory instability and severe bleeding, a "damage control" laparotomy was chosen over any further imaging, including CT scan of the head and neck. A vasopressin bolus followed by an infusion was initiated to both increase the blood pressure and decrease the rate of bleeding. A triple lumen central line was placed into the right femoral vein and an arterial line was placed in the right radial artery. The patient was rushed to the operating room with an abdominal binder and cervical collar. This step towards the operating room is part of "overlapping care," as the patient will receive critical care after surgery and probably return later to the operating room, where he will get a hybrid of care based on both anesthesia and critical care principles.

Etomidate is often chosen for rapid sequence induction in unstable patients. However, the incidence of the complications of adrenal suppression appears to be much higher than originally thought. This may be a serious issue in the severe polytrauma patient. In trauma patients, a single dose of etomidate increased the incidence of pneumonia (56.7 vs. 25.9), prolonged ICU stay (6.3 vs. 25.9), and prolonged hospital stay (11.6 vs.6.4). Etomidate causes inhibition of 11β-hydroxylase, leading to adrenal inhibition, and results in a relative risk of death of 1.22 in 3,715 septic patients reported by de la Grandville et al. [3]. In our patient, there was a distinct possibility of a closed head injury, and the increase in intracranial pressure caused by ketamine must thus be weighed against the adrenal suppression caused by etomidate. There is a significant body of literature showing that ketamine does not elevate an already increased intracranial [4] pressure, making it a reasonable selection in the trauma patient with a possible intracranial injury. Of note, carboetomidate: an analog of etomidate that interacts weakly with 11β-hydroxylase, is in final trials and appears to have little impact on the synthesis of steroids [5]. This should make it an excellent replacement for etomidate.

There is a growing opinion among trauma experts that bypassing the operating room and going immediately to interventional radiology may be the best first step in the massively bleeding patient. The goals of the "golden hour" may be appreciated and met by measuring the time from diagnostic angiogram and embolization of essential bleeding vessels as compared to exploration and surgical control of the hemorrhage leading to control of acidosis and hypothermia. In our case, the interventional radiology suite was several floors away, and mobilizing the interventional radiology team would have taken more than 30 min.

Upon arrival in the trauma bay the driver was awake and cooperative. Rapid ultrasound assessment of her abdomen was negative. She underwent a full CT evaluation of her head and neck, and a toxicology screen was positive for alcohol and cocaine. With no definitive injury, she was sent to the surgical ICU with a cervical collar for observation.

This chapter will discuss the possible approaches to operating room management according to a slowly developing consensus of practice. The clinical bar of excellence met in this chapter has not been attempted by all. We believe that some of these new concepts will become part of the standard of care in the severe trauma patient.

Goals and Objectives of Anesthesia Care for the Severe Trauma Patient in the Operating Room

1. Determine the clinical path that leads to damage control of bleeding, coagulopathy, acidosis, and hypothermia [6].
2. Start resuscitation by diminishing the size of the circulation with vasopressin.
3. Have a plan for increasing the blood volume if blood is not available, such as hypertonic saline solution (HSS), albumin, hemoglobin-based oxygen carriers, and standard crystalloids.
4. Have a goal for each vital sign, and determine whether the patient is a candidate for hypotensive resuscitation.
5. Use point-of-care tests to drive the resuscitation while understanding their deficiencies.
6. Determine if immunotherapy is an option.

Preparation

What is predictable about the severe trauma patient is that very little is predictable. Unlike neurosurgical or orthopedic trauma, details of blunt abdominal trauma are discovered during surgery. Level I trauma centers have a dedicated operating room always ready for the severely injured patient. A standard setup includes three pressure transducers, fluid and body warmers, and a minimum of two vasopressors ready to be administered on pumps. While there is great variability of vasopressor use from institution to institution, we usually have norepinephrine and vasopressin readily available. We tend to start norepinephrine at 0.1 µg/kg/min and vasopressin

at 5 units/h after a 5 unit bolus. It is essential that the room be kept warm and fully stocked with the medications and medical devices normally used in a polytrauma case. The interventional radiology suite should be set up for trauma in the same way as the operating room.

In our institution the trauma room setup is as follows.

Rapid Infuser

We use the "Belmont" (www.belmontinstrument. com), and have had great success with his device. There are several rapid infusers on the market that differ only slightly from the Belmont. This device has a feature that we would call essential. It has a large reservoir that accommodates several liters of blood products at once. The faster blood products are infused, the greater the warming capability. The device has a line pressure monitor which stops flow and indicates an obstruction when the line pressure exceeds 300 mmHg, Internal jugular or subclavian lines provide relatively little resistance to flow and the infusion pressure is usually less than 70 mmHg. Large bore peripheral IVs (14 gauge or lower) may infiltrate when attached to the rapid infuser at high infusion rates. Air entrainment is also detected by the infuser. When air is detected, it will stop the infusion and allow the air to be removed. Blood products, with the exception of platelets, can be placed in the rapid transfuser reservoir in the ratio of the institution's rapid transfusion protocol. Since the flow is fast, warm, and turbulent, platelets cannot be poured into the reservoir without destroying them. Blood may be infused or bolused. We recommend not using the continuous infusion mode as the clinician may become distracted by another aspect of the case and only later realize that an excessive amount of blood products had been given. In bolus mode, the pump must be restarted after each unit is complete, allowing the clinician to determine if more blood products are needed. A fresh cassette is easily placed and can be primed in under a minute. Bolus rates can reach up to 500 mL/min with the Belmont and may be higher with other rapid infusers. Ideally; two rapid infusers should be kept in the dedicated trauma room. With the advent of rapid infusers, it is rare that mortality is related to exsanguination, unless blood becomes unavailable. We do not hang fluid bags and prime lines until we are sure a trauma is coming to the operating room. Another distinct advantage of a rapid infuser is that it can be operated by one user, with an assistant to check blood products.

Ultrasound Machine

Most clinicians have been using ultrasound for central line placement, since it has been shown in several reports to aid in avoiding arterial cannulation. Our policy for placement of central lines includes the anesthesiologist scrubbing, gowning, and gloving. An assistant sterilely preps both sides of the neck and places a drape covering the body from head to toe. For our patient with an unstable cervical spine, the C-collar was removed without movement of the head. With the neck in the neutral position, the ultrasound (Sonosite, Inc.) will still show excellent anatomy [7]. We recommend the "double stick" approach to venous access. An ultrasound guide wire placed in the internal jugular is followed by a second ultrasound-guided placement of a wire next to the first wire. The longer wire accommodates a triple lumen catheter and the shorter is used to place for a 9.0 French introducer. The two wires should be almost touching at the level of the skin, as placing both catheters will otherwise require two incisions. If the two catheters are touching, they will tamponade any bleeding that may occur during dilation prior to placement of the catheters. Once the catheters are placed, their position should be reconfirmed by ultrasound. Placing a pulmonary artery (PA) catheter through the introducer may give important diagnostic information, but the utility of this information must be weighed against the use of the introducer for rapid infusion. A (PA) catheter will decrease flow and increase line pressure. If a pulmonary artery catheter is desired, we suggest preparing the other side of the neck as described above, and placing an 8.5 or 9 French introducer to accommodate the catheter.

In non-trauma patients who require central venous access, strict protocols for aseptic technique have become the standard of care. If the decision is made to take the trauma patient to the operating room as soon as possible, it is impractical to follow this standard as the surgeons are rushing to control the bleeding in an unstable patient. The goal is "clean" central venous access. Classically defined anatomic landmarks cannot be relied upon in a trauma patient, therefore ultrasound is extremely useful. While safety is always dependent on the operator, the "straight neck" or neutral position should not impair central line placement [8]. The volume status of the patient may create difficulty in identifying the internal jugulars. An "empty" patient may have an intermittently identifiable internal jugular vein, which may disappear depending on the mode of ventilation. There are three steps one can perform to assure cannulation of a vein and not an artery. The first is ultrasound visualization of the needle or plastic catheter in the vein. The second involves attaching a length of pressure tubing to the catheter. Once attached, the open end of the tubing is raised above the patient. If the catheter is in a vein, the level of blood in the tubing will fluctuate with ventilation and may empty into the patient. If the catheter is in an artery, the blood in the tubing will pulse continually and not return to the patient. The third is performed by attaching an angiocatheter to a pressure transducer and viewing a distinct venous pressure tracing as opposed to the arterial line tracing consistent with carotid artery placement.

Underbody Forced Air Warmer

Hypothermia a significant factor in morbidity and mortality [9]. In many polytrauma cases the abdomen, chest, and extremities are exposed for the surgical procedure. Heat loss is inevitable; therefore every effort should be made to create a neutral thermal environment. Underbody forced air devices tend to work well. In addition, the room temperature should be kept above 70 °F at all times, as warming the room, when the patient arrives in the OR rarely, achieves the goal of preventing further cooling. All fluids should be warmed. The rapid infuser works well to warm fluids at high flow rates.

Additional Essential Equipment

Three transducers are set up for arterial and any other necessary pressure measurements, including intracranial pressure and tissue pressures for compartment syndromes. In addition, a BIS monitor, cerebral co-oximetry, pulse pressure variation monitor, HSS, multiple infusion pumps, blood filters, large bore introducer kits, single and triple lumen central line kits, ACT monitor, and defibrillation pads are essential. The "crash cart" must be brought into the room at the inception of the case.

Goal-Directed Tests and Therapy for the Trauma Patient

Thromboelastography

Conventional tests for coagulation are generally of little value in trauma, particularly in the severely injured patient, since their results may be normal in the face of coagulopathy. Fibrinolysis, clot instability and breakdown, which may commonly occur in liver transplantation and open cardiac operations, are not detected by conventional testing. TEG, and more recently thromboelastometry, are goal-directed point-of-care tests that indicate clot stability [10]. While thromboelastography was first described in 1948 by Hartert, there remains some resistance in many institutions to make it part of point-of-care testing. TEG and thromboelastometry are not routinely taught to most medical students or residents, and even many of our trauma surgeons are unfamiliar with these tests. However, the concepts of TEG and examples of TEG printouts are now part of the American Board of Anesthesiology Certification exam. Thromboelastography (2012 Haemonetics Corporation) measures the life of a clot, including clot retraction or fibrinolysis, from 0.36 mL of blood. Thromboelastography is performed by taking a sample of blood and placing it in a small cup called a cuvette. Moving the cuvette back and forth in a $4°$ arc mimics sluggish venous flow, which is a main extrinsic component of clot formation (Fig. 5.1a). A sensor (torsion wire) attached to a computer is placed in the cuvette. When fibrinogen and platelets interact, a clot begins to form, and the computer senses the ongoing forces that develop from the bonds forming in the clot, and thus creates a trace of clot formation and dissolution (Fig. 5.1b).

Figure 5.2 is a computer generated diagram of the TEG. The "torsion wire" is the sensor. The top of the image "R" is the beginning of clot formation and the bottom is the end of the computer trace. In general, the time from top to bottom in a normal patient is about 45 min.

If R exceeds the limits of normal, the patient needs clotting factors. The management of clotting factor deficiency is evolving, with the production of procoagulants like recombinant factor VII. For the most part, a prolonged R time is treated with fresh frozen plasma. There is no exact correlation of the R time with how many units of FFP are needed. While a full TEG takes 45 min, evaluating the R time takes only a few minutes after the trace begins (Fig. 5.3).

MA stands for maximum amplitude. If the MA exceeds normal reference values, the patient is hypercoaguable. If the MA is narrow, the patient is deficient in platelets, platelet function, and/or fibrinogen. To sort out a narrow MA, monoclonal antibodies targeted at platelets can be administered prior to running the TEG. The MA would then be representative of only fibrinogen. This trial can also be done by adding heparinase in the cuvette in the heparnized cardiac patient. The image in Fig. 5.1 is a computerized generated TEG with the reference points added.

K is the time from beginning of clot formation until the amplitude of the thromboelastogram is 20 mm. A prolonged k-time is ominous and therapy should be initiated before complete TEG results are available.

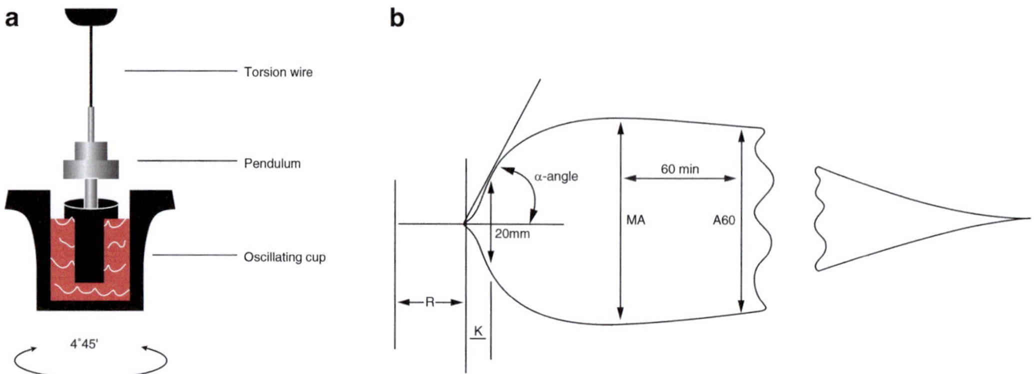

Fig. 5.1 The technology of thromboelastography. (**a**) The thromboelastograph cup (cuvette) rotates through an arc. Blood is placed in an oscillating cuvette. As the blood begins to clot, the cup slows down and transmits a force to the torsion wire that generates an image drawn by a computer. Different rates of slowing lead to different forces on the torsion wire and different images (With permission from Hemologix.) (**b**) R represents clotting factors. If the R is very long and exceeds the limits of a normal R time, the patient needs clotting factors. MA stands for maximum amplitude. If the MA exceeds the normal reference values, the patient is hypercoaguable. If the MA is narrow, the patient is deficient in platelets, platelet function, and/or fibrinogen. K is the time from beginning of clot formation until the amplitude of the thromboelastogram is 20 mm. A prolonged k is very ominous and is a sign that therapy should be initiated while waiting for complete TEG results. Alpha angle is the angle between the line in the middle of the TEG(r) tracing and the line tangential to the evolving "body" of the TEG(r). The angle represents the speeding up process of fibrin build-up and cross-linking (TEG® tracing and parameters are used by permission of Haemonetics. TEG® and Thromboelastograph® are registered trademarks of Haemonetics Corporation in the USA, other countries, or both.)

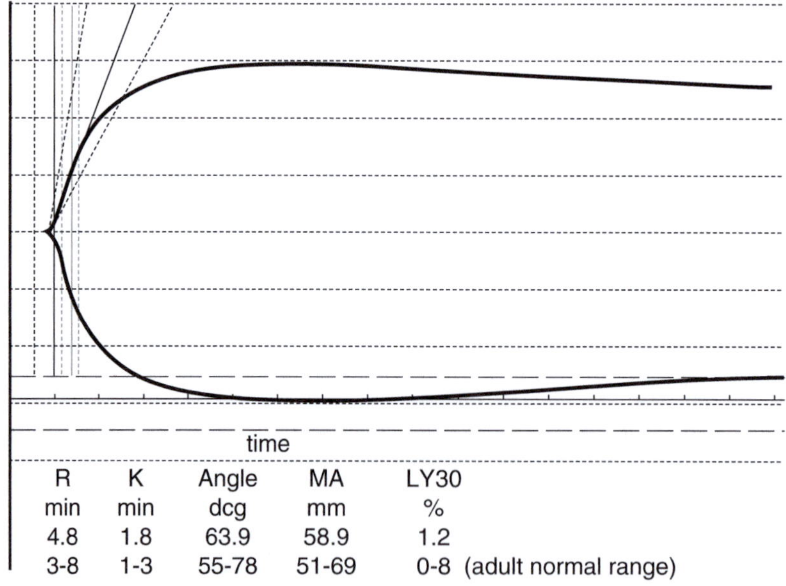

Fig. 5.2 The final computerized generated thromboelastogram. The top set of numbers represents normal values and the bottom number represents the patient. All of this patient's numbers are normal and the image looks perfectly normal (With kind permission from Springer Science + Business Media: Pediatr Cardiol, Thromboelastography of patients after fontan compared with healthy children, 2009;30(6):771–6, Raffini L, Schwed A, Zheng XL, Tanzer M, Nicolson S, Gaynor JW, Jobes D.)

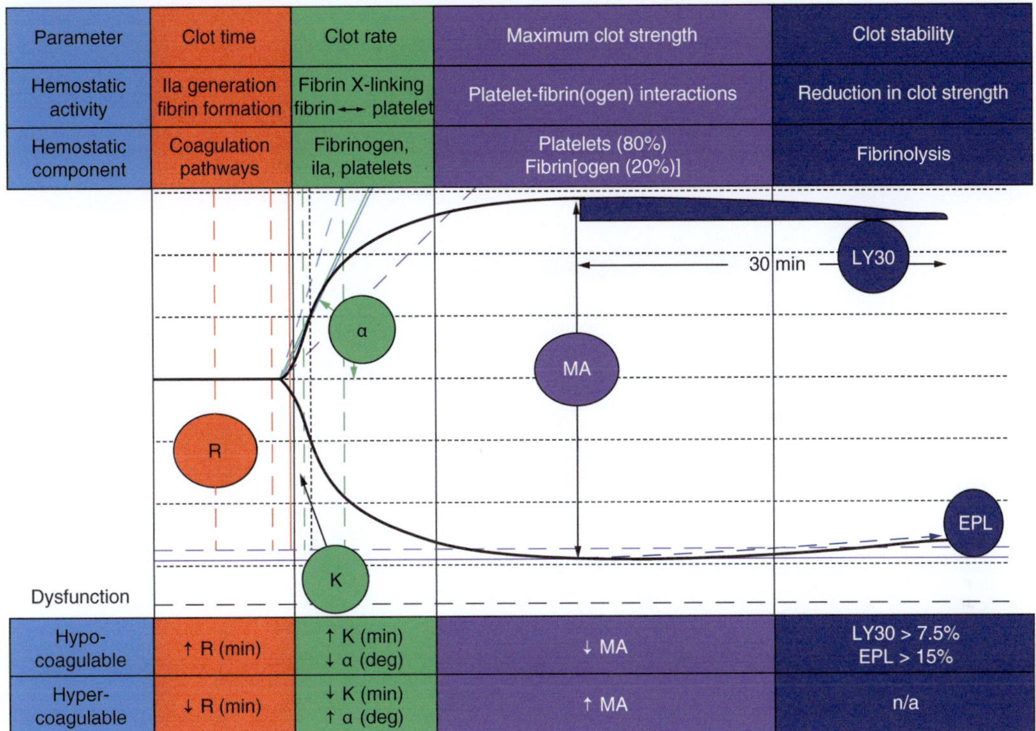

Fig. 5.3 The integration of the TEG and the components of the coagulation cascade (With permission from TEM Systems, Inc.)

The α-angle is the angle between the middle line of the TEG(r) tracing and the line tangential to the evolving "body" of the TEG(r). It represents the acceleration of fibrin build-up and cross-linking. Like the k-time, a narrow angle represents poor acceleration and is likely that the patient has become coagulopathic.

Figure 5.4 demonstrates what standard coagulation tests do not show. The patient is bleeding and the R-time is normal. We can deduce that we do not need factors. The TEG starts out looking normal, but then the MA narrows.

This demonstrates loss of clot stability and the onset of fibrinolysis, which is very difficult to treat. [11]. There are currently two antifibrinolytic agents available to the clinician: ε-aminocaproic acid and tranxemic acid. Much of what we know about them comes from the cardiac literature where they are used prophylactically from the start of each procedure. The efficacy of these drugs is highest when administered before fibrinolyis occurs. There is growing evidence for

the use of these medications in trauma. It is common that patients become hypercoaguable during major surgery. There is an argument against aiming for a normal coagulation state during many operations as hypercoagulation and the threat of pulmonary emboli may develop with an overzealous attempt at perfection. We give antifibrinolytics prophylactically when the rapid transfusion protocol is activated. Our team cannot state at this time if this fairly benign treatment is actually effective. Figure 5.4 demonstrates the TEG changes in other pathologic states. Treatments are suggested for each illustration.

The TEG permits goal-directed transfusion of blood products. While manufactured procoagulants and synthetic blood are in development, thromboelastography and thromboelastometry are essential for guiding the resuscitation of the hemorrhaging patient in the operating room. Recently the sensitivity of TEG and TEM has been disputed in the literature. In Raza et al. [11], blood was drawn on arrival for TEM and

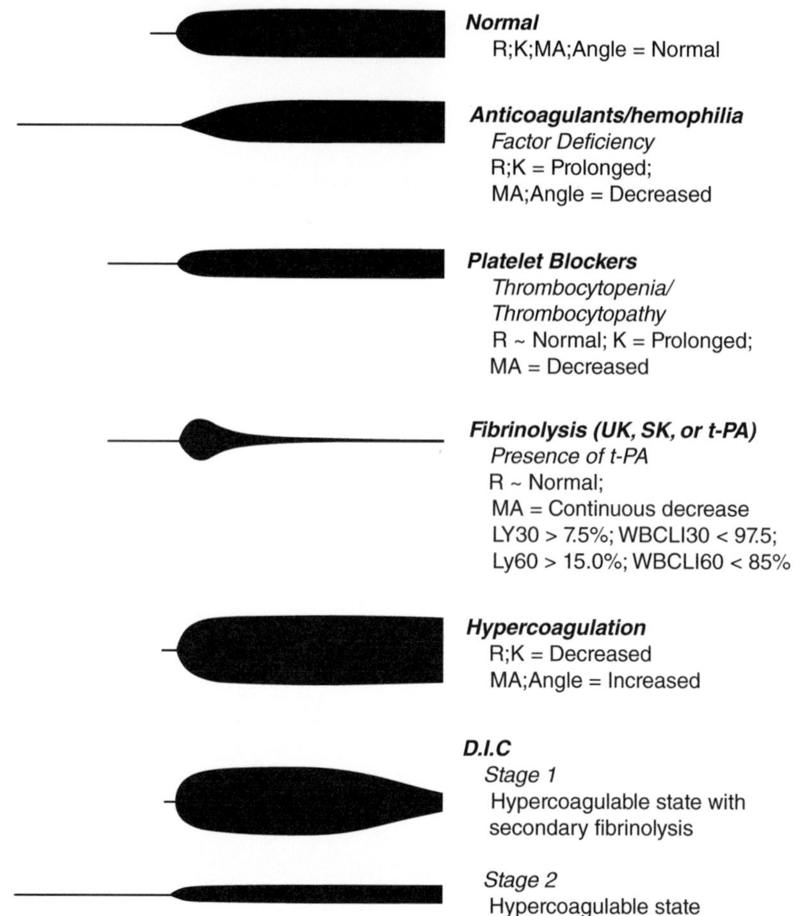

Fig. 5.4 Examples of goal-directed TEGs. These TEGs are typical for the disorders that are shown here

coagulation assays. TEM hyperfibrinolysis was defined as maximum clot lysis of >15 %. Fibrinolytic activation (FA) was determined according to plasmin–antiplasmin (PAP) complex and d-dimer levels. Only 5 % of patients had severe fibrinolysis on TEM, but 57 % showed evidence of "moderate" fibrinolysis, with PAP complex levels elevated to over twice normal (>1,500 µg/L) while no lysis was seen on TEM. TEM detected clot lysis only when PAP complex levels were increased to 30 times normal ($p < 0.001$) and antiplasmin levels were <75 % of normal. This one study has led investigators to determine actual procoagulant factors and inhibitors, and to compare them to TEG/TEM and clinical events. Many clinicians do not follow the thromboelastogram, since many trauma thromboelastograms appear the same as each other and institutional standard treatment is given irrespective of the TEG.

Thromboelastometry

Rotational thromboelastometry is another technique that determines clot stability [12]. As in TEG, the test is performed by placing blood in a cuvette. A sensor fixed on the tip of a rotating axis is placed in the cuvette. It is important to note that in the TEG, the cuvette is moving and in thromboelastometry the sensor is moving (Rotem.de). The shaft of the sensor is rotated back and forth over an arc of 4.75°, mimicking low venous flow. As a clot begins to form, the

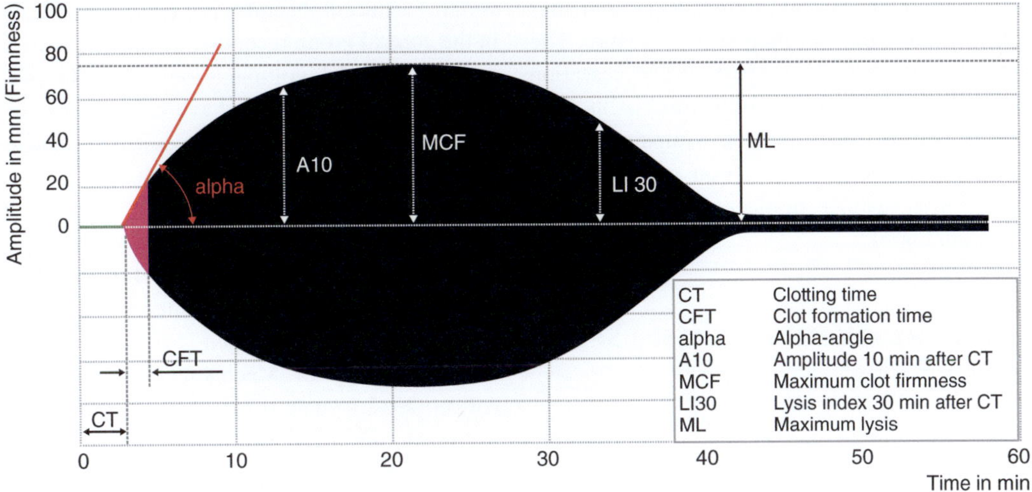

Fig. 5.5 Terms and explanations of Rotem components (With permission from TEM Systems, Inc.)

shaft movement slows. The shaft is connected to a spring that measures elasticity. The exact position of the shaft is determined by light reflection from a small mirror on the shaft. Data from the detected light is processed by computer that generates a graph similar to the one created by the TEG, with related parameters including clotting time (CT) and maximum clot firmness (MCF) (Fig. 5.5). Similar to TEG, there are specific reagents that can be added to the blood sample to help define the exact etiology of a clotting disorder.

The ROTEM permits several tests at different points in the coagulation cascade that cannot be done with the TEG (Fig 5.6a–e). Essentially, thromboelastometry indicates more specific disorders. The following are some of the tests offered by ROTEM:

INTEM	Contains phospholipid and ellagic acid as activators and provides information similar to that of the APTT
EXTEM	Contains Tissue Factor as an activator and provides information similar to that of the PT
HEPTEM	Contains lyophilised heparinase for neutralizing heparin
APTEM	Contains aprotinin for inhibiting fibrinolysis
IBTEM	Utilizes cytochalasin D, a platelet inhibitor which blocks the platelet contribution to clot formation, allowing qualitative analysis of the functional fibrinogen component.

There are cases when TEG results are different from those obtained by the TEM, even when samples are taken concurrently [13]. It is believed the mismatch is related to the differences in the technologies that generate the clot. Until this variance is better understood, we recommend developing different treatment algorithms based on specific results [14].

PFA-Platelet Function Analyzer

PFA-platelet function analyzer determines the total platelet count and the percentage of platelets that are actually functioning [15]. A system for the detection of platelet dysfunction, the PFA-100 is widely used in centers that perform cardiac, liver transplantation, and trauma surgery. There is rarely a major trauma case in which platelet function does not come into question. The PFA-100 (Siemens Healthcare Diagnostics) measures platelet function in citrated whole blood in a few minutes. The instrument aspirates blood from a reservoir through a capillary and a microscopic aperture in a membrane which is coated with collagen and epinephrine, or collagen and adenosine 5′-diphosphate. The presence of these coatings combined with high shear rates, results in platelet activation, adhesion, and aggregation, and thus builds a stable platelet plug at the aperture. The time to occlusion of the aperture and cessation of blood flow is called closure time. Abnormal closure times may indicate impairment of platelet enhancers like Von Willebrand's factor, low platelet numbers, or medications like clopidogrel.

Goal-Directed Ventilation of the Severe Trauma Patient

Other than during exceptional circumstances, when jet ventilation or oscillators are needed, modern anesthesia machines do an acceptable job of ventilating patients. Trauma patients are at high risk for developing acute respiratory distress syndrome [16]. In a pig model, Roy et al. [16] determined that early airway pressure release ventilation stabilized alveoli, reduced pulmonary edema, and prevented ARDS. This "pig model" has interesting significance for the human trauma patient, as ARDS carries significant mortality. Simply stated, early treatment of the patient who is at high risk for ARDS with ARDS paradigm for ventilation, may prevent the development of the syndrome. Low tidal volumes and fluid-conservative management comprise the essentials of management of the ARDS patient [17]. Arguments against low tidal volume ventilation include the risk of bilateral atelectasis that might occur if tidal volumes fall below 6 cm^3/kg/breath. Without recruitment maneuvers, atelectasis may lead to ARDS and pneumonia in the postoperative period. This can be avoided with manual distention of the lungs every 30 min.

The evidence that clinicians should change from high volume to low volume ventilation first appeared in the ARMA clinical trial, which was followed by numerous papers praising the non-volutrauma approach to ARDS patients [18]. While the science in many of these studies may be flawed, the conclusions of these studies have been proven by a high number of good clinical outcomes. Trials suggest that a strategy of low tidal volume ventilation (6–8 mL/kg ideal body weight) reduced absolute mortality from 42.5 % in the control group receiving 10 cm^3/kg to 34 % in the low tidal volume group. On the other hand, high tidal volumes have historically been recommended for mechanically ventilated patients during general anesthesia [19]. As a result, a protective ventilation strategy is underutilized, even in patients with ARDS. However, recent data support LTVV for almost all mechanically ventilated patients beginning immediately after intubation [17].

The Strategy of Mechanical Ventilation in ARDS: 2012 Update (From ARDSNet.org).

1. Start in any ventilator mode with initial tidal volumes of 8 mL/kg predicted body weight in kg, calculated by: [2.3 (height in inches—60) +45.5 for women or +50 for men].
2. Set the respiratory rate to 35 breaths/min to deliver the expected minute ventilation requirement (generally, 7–9 L/min).
3. Set positive end-expiratory pressure (PEEP) to at least 5 cm H_2O (higher is better), and FiO_2 to maintain an arterial oxygen saturation (SaO_2) of 88–95 % (paO_2 55–80 mmHg). Maintain FiO_2 below 70 % when feasible.
4. Over a period of less than 4 h, reduce tidal volumes to 7 mL/kg, and then 6 mL/kg. Ventilator settings are adjusted to keep the plateau pressure (measured during an inspiratory hold of 0.5 s) less than 30 cmH_2O (preferably as low as possible), while maintaining reasonable blood gas parameters. Hypercapnea is usually well tolerated. An elevated pCO_2 should be accepted, as elevated plateau pressures may worsen alveolar damage and contribute to mortality. If the plateau pressure remains elevated, one can employ several techniques to reduce it. Tidal volume may be reduced to as low as 4 mL/kg in 1 mL/kg steps. Heavy sedation to minimize fighting the ventilator should be considered. Other factors unrelated to the lungs that can increase plateau pressures, such as a pneumoperitoneum from a laparoscopic procedure, or lack of muscle relaxation should also be considered.

Using this strategy, arterial blood gases will demonstrate respiratory acidosis. Treatment of respiratory acidosis with sodium bicarbonate or

THAM is often employed by clinicians with minimal evidence of positive outcome. There are scenarios in trauma when prophylactic ARDS ventilation is not acceptable, such as traumatic brain injury, when there is evidence of elevated intracranial pressure. Permitting a pCO_2 greater than 50 may further increase ICP. In this scenario, the brain takes preference over the lungs. The same holds true in cases of severe hypovolemia and coronary artery disease.

Intraoperative Fluid Monitoring and Treatment with Pulse Pressure Variation

Whether administering crystalloids or colloids, the formulas normally used to calculate fluid administration are inaccurate and potentially dangerous in the severely injured patient. Even in the non-trauma patient the standard formula for maintenance fluids often leads to over-resuscitation. Giving crystalloids to increase hemodynamic stability often results in transfer of 2/3 of the administered fluid into the extravascular space within minutes. Thus each liter of crystalloid contributes only one-third of a liter to increasing the blood pressure and should not be counted on to correct hypotension.

The goal of fluid management in the trauma patient is to optimize stroke volume. Monitoring pulse pressure variation has been proven effective in guiding fluid resuscitation [20]. Pulse pressure is the difference between the systolic and diastolic pressures.

Low or narrow pulse pressure: Pulse pressure is considered low if it is less than 25 % of the systolic value. The most common cause of a low pulse pressure is a decrease in ventricular stroke volume. In trauma, a narrow pulse pressure suggests significant blood loss. By increasing pleural pressure, mechanical ventilation induces cyclic variations in cardiac preload that result in cyclic changes in left ventricular stroke volume and arterial pulse pressure. The variation in arterial pulse pressure (ΔPP) induced by mechanical ventilation is an accurate predictor of fluid responsiveness during resuscitation. Simply stated, if the height of arterial systole varies with each positive pressure breath, the patient does not have an optimal stroke volume. When patients are hypovolemic, they are on the steep portion of the Frank-Starling curve in terms of the preload/stroke volume relationship. Patients who are on the flat portion of the curve are insensitive to cyclic changes in preload induced by mechanical ventilation, and thus ΔPP is low: increasing circulating volume will not cause a significant increase in stroke volume (GE Healthcare).

By increasing cardiac preload, volume loading induces a rightward shift on the preload/stroke volume relationship and causes a decrease in ΔPP. The goal of maximizing stroke volume can therefore be achieved simply by minimizing ΔPP [20].

Positive pressure ventilation causes vascular pressure changes in the thoracic cavity. Inspiration increases and expiration decreases pressures. Systolic pressure variation (SPV) and pulse pressure variation (dPP) reflect these respiratory changes. The magnitude of change depends on the fluid status of the patient. In our hypovolemic trauma patient, the degree of pressure change was greater than in those who are normovolemic or hypervolemic [21] (Fig. 5.6a,b).

SPV and dPP are calculated from the invasive arterial blood pressure using the following equations:

$$SPV\,[mmHg] = SBP_{max} - SBP_{min}$$

$$dPP\,[\%] = \frac{(PP_{max} - PP_{min})}{[(PP_{max} + PP_{min})/2]} \times 100$$

SBP_{max} and SBP_{min} represent the highest and lowest values of the systolic blood pressure over the measurement period. We measure SPV/dPP to determine fluid responsiveness. Will the patient's stroke volume and cardiac output improve with fluid resuscitation? It is important to note that dPP is given as a percentage and SPV as mmHg (Fig. 5.7).

Monitoring arterial pressure variation, i.e., SPV/dPP, helps to answer the question of fluid responsiveness and can be used to guide fluid

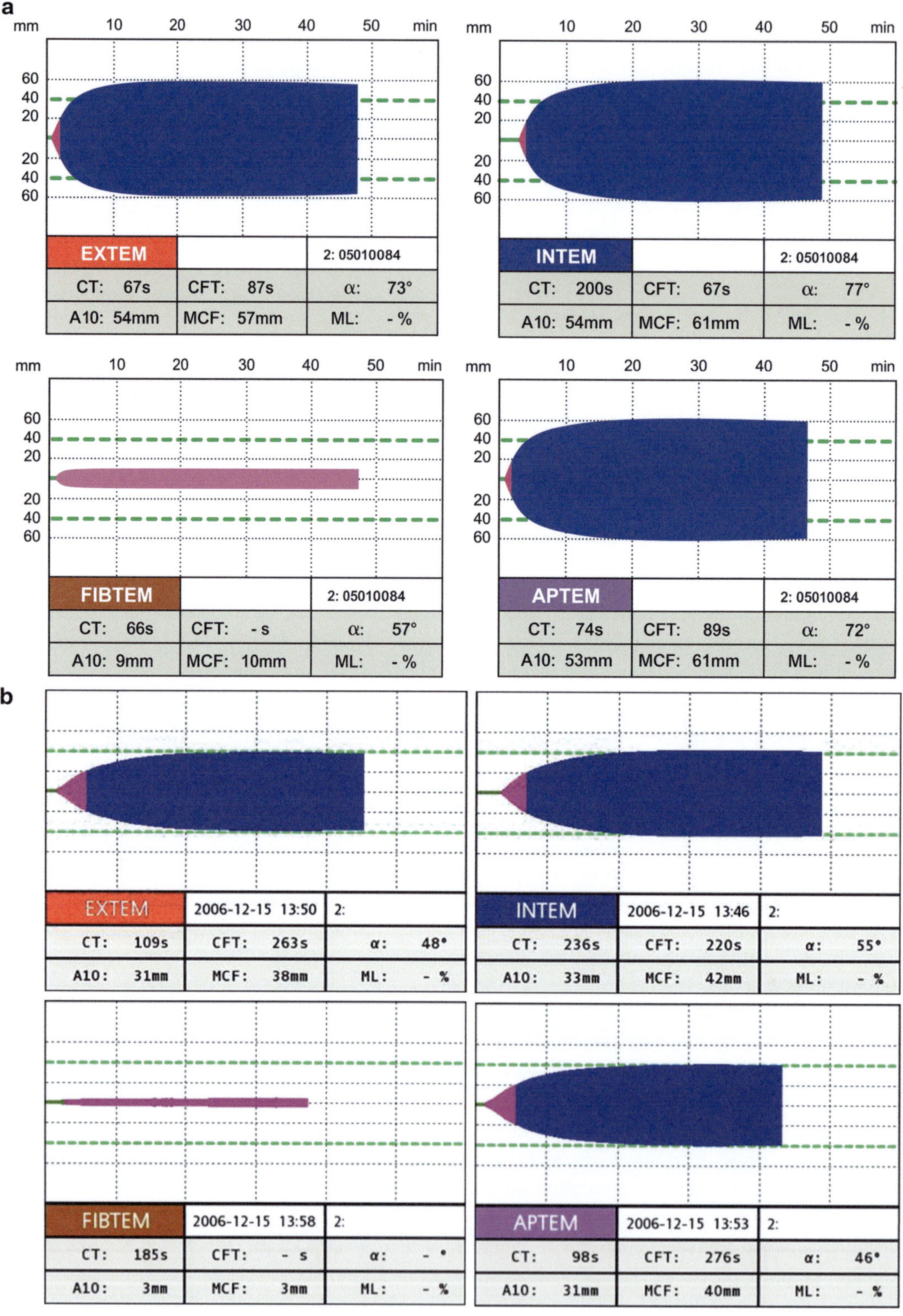

Fig. 5.6 (Continued)

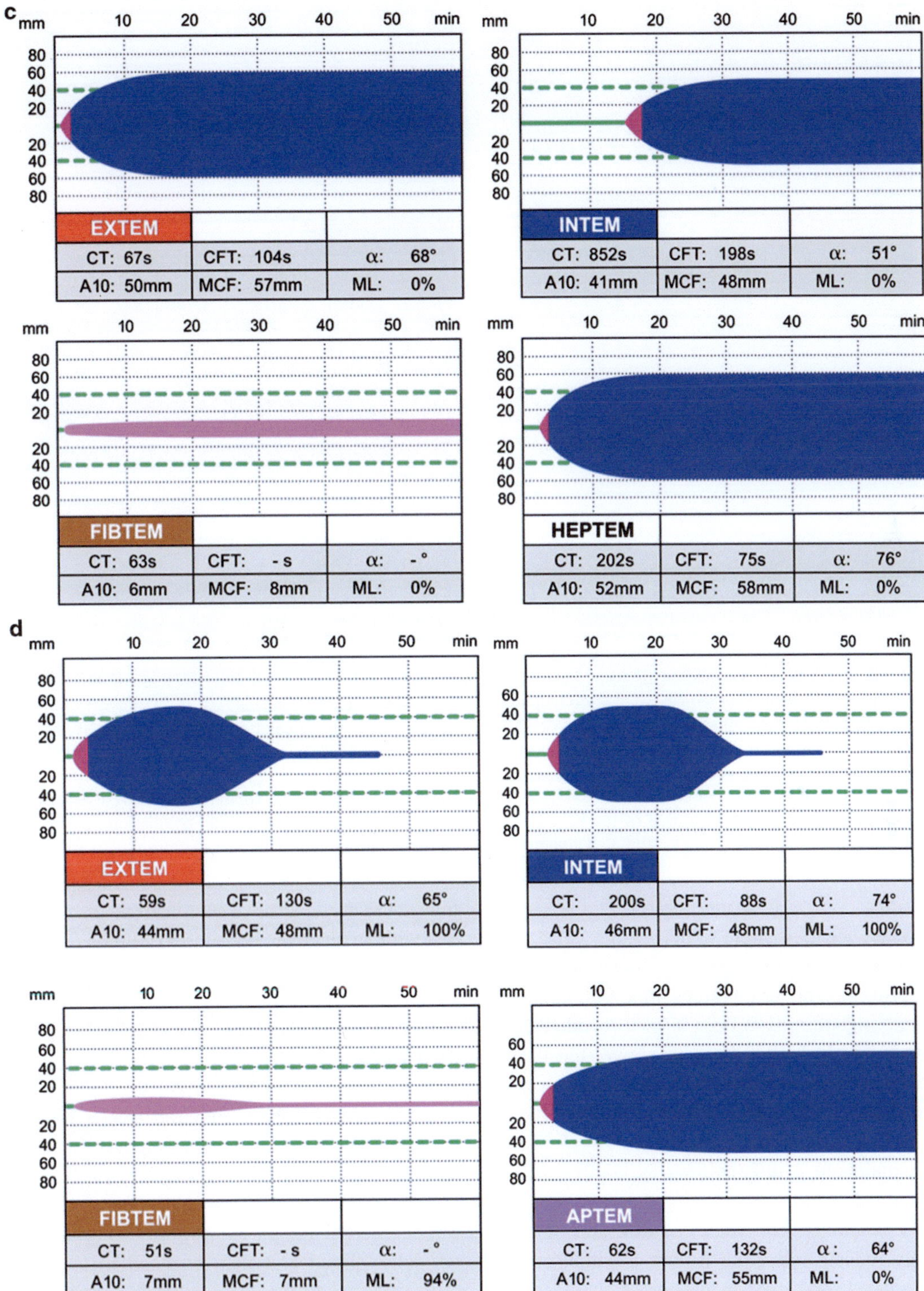

Fig. 5.6 (Continued)

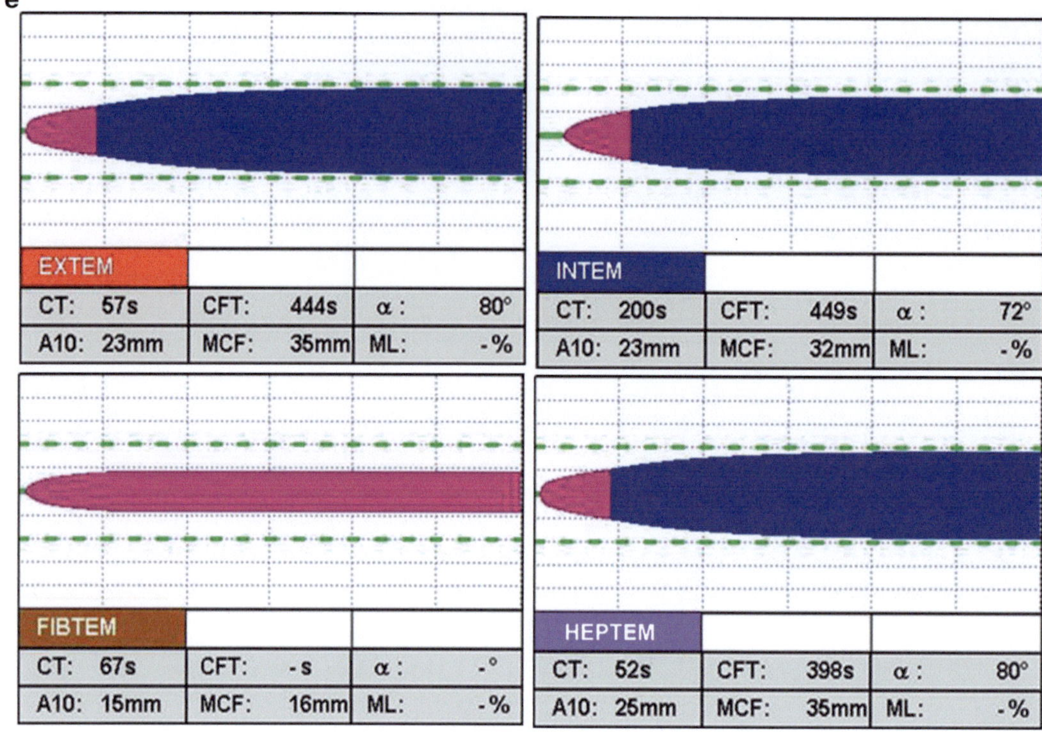

Fig. 5.6 ROTEM and coagulation disorders from Rotem. de with permission, mixing various reagents to help make a coagulation disorder diagnosis (**a**) Normal ROTEM images, (**b**) Fibrinogen deficiency (**c**) Heparin influence (**d**) Hyperfibrinolysis, and (**e**) Platelet deficiency. EXTEM, contains tissue factor as an activator and provides information similar to that of the PT; INTEM, contains phospholipid and ellagic acid as activators and provides information similar to that of the APTT; FIBTEM, utilizes cytochalasin D, a platelet inhibitor which blocks the platelet contribution to clot formation, allowing qualitative analysis of the functional fibrinogen component; APTEM, contains aprotinin for inhibiting fibrinolysis; HEPTEM, contains lyophilized heparinase for neutralizing heparin (With permission from TEM Systems, Inc.)

therapy. While it seems logical that a colloid would contribute more to decreasing pulse pressure variation, this remains controversial and unproven. The dPP values that indicate fluid responsiveness have been shown to range from 10 to 15 %. In the diagram above, the dPP is 27 %, which suggests that the patient may be extremely responsive to fluid. Fluids would be given until the value decreases to 10–15 % [20] Hydrating to a dPP below this could result in overhydration.

Limitations: The values of dPP and SPV are only reliable when the patient is intubated and ventilated, and only in patients without cardiac arrhythmias. Since SPV and dPP values are calculated from an invasive arterial blood pressure waveform, they are reliable only if the readings of the arterial line are reliable. The pressure transducer needs to be at mid-heart level, zeroed, and without air in the transducer or in the catheter line.

Monitors

Placing standard ASA monitors on a trauma patient can be a significant challenge. If the chest and back are sites of injury, standard EKG leads will not work. Eighteen or nineteen gauge needles can be inserted into the skin where EKG leads are normally placed and then attached to alligator clips that fit into the ECG cable to monitor the EKG. Two sets of these vital substitutes should be available. They are particularly useful for the burn patient. Some injuries may also preclude proper placement of a noninvasive blood pressure cuff;

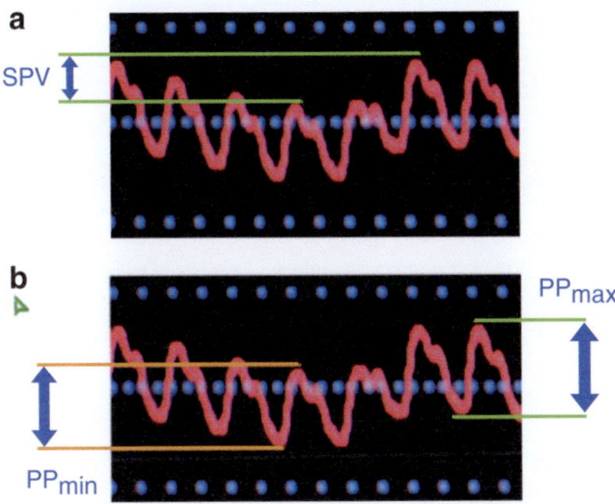

Fig. 5.7 (**a**) Systolic pressure variation; (**b**) pulse pressure variation (Used with permission of GE Healthcare.)

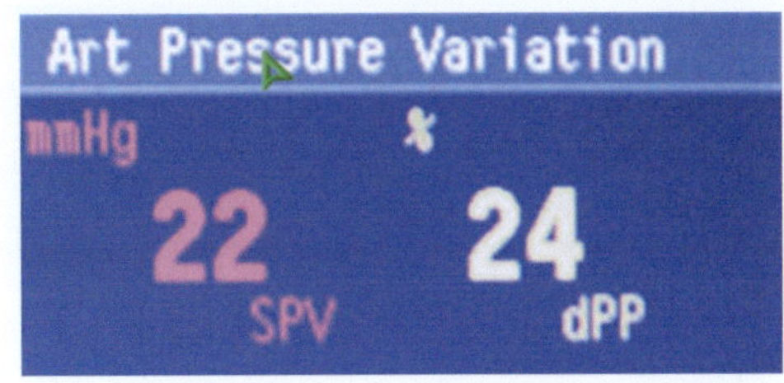

Fig. 5.8 Pulse pressure variation monitor. The dPP represents the difference in pulse pressure on the Arterial line tracing before and after a positive pressure is given by mechanical ventilation. It is recommended that volume is administered to a dPP of 15 %. At 15 %, patients will have an optimal stroke volume (Used with permission of GE Healthcare.)

an arterial line should be used instead. In severe trauma cases at least two anesthesiologists should be placing lines. Femoral and axillary catheters may be considered, but they must be inserted with caution. Arterial lines that require repeated manual flushing are suboptimal. The dorsalis pedis artery is not optimal for blood pressure monitoring, as it typically does not represent central arterial pressure. A small gauge brachial arterial catheter with vigilant monitoring of the insertion site and the hand (for perfusion), may have to be an alternative.

In addition to standard ASA monitors, there is growing evidence that cerebral oximetry may be useful in the prevention of neurologic injury. If hypotensive technique is chosen, they may be essential in preventing brain injury. A low pressure may result in a low saturation.

Transcranial Doppler differs from cerebral oximetry in that it looks at larger arteries (middle cerebral) and is helpful for major embolic phenomena. It has lost popularity since data from this monitor are difficult to interpret. Perioperative neurologic injury may often be related to an imbalance in regional cerebral microcirculation, which may be monitored by the cerebral oximeter. In a prospective study of over 11,000 patients, Likosky and colleagues [22] found that 75 % of strokes occur among the 90 % of patients with low to intermediate risk undergoing coronary artery bypass grafting (CABG) surgery. These neurologic insults often occur despite well-maintained blood pressure and cardiac output. The leads of the cerebral oximeter are placed symmetrically on the forehead (Fig. 5.8) and estimate regional tissue oxygenation by transcutaneous measurement of areas most vulnerable to changes in oxygen supply and demand (frontal cerebral cortex). Light from the oximeter penetrates the skull and is used to determine hemoglobin oxygenation according to the amount of infrared light absorbed by hemoglobin. Cerebral oximetry differs from pulse oximetry by utilizing two photodetectors with each light source, allowing sampling of tissue within a specified depth. Near-field (scalp and skull) detection is subtracted from the far-field (scalp, skull, and brain) reading to provide a measurement of brain oxygenation beyond a predefined depth (Fig. 5.9a).

Cerebral oximetry also differs from pulse oximetry in that the results represent primarily (70–75 %) venous, rather than (20–25 %) arterial blood. Monitoring is not dependent upon pulsatile flow. Normal saturations are ~70 % (Fig. 5.9b). A saturation below 50 % is a call for clinical action either by increasing cerebral circulation or by increasing oxygen carrying capacity. The target mean arterial pressure for the young trauma patient is 50–60 mmHg. This MAP is associated with a more rapid improvement of trauma-induced coagulopathy and significantly less blood product administration (Fig. 5.7). To treat patients with the goal of a systemic MAP of 50 compels the clinician to use the cerebral oximeter. A mean pressure of 50

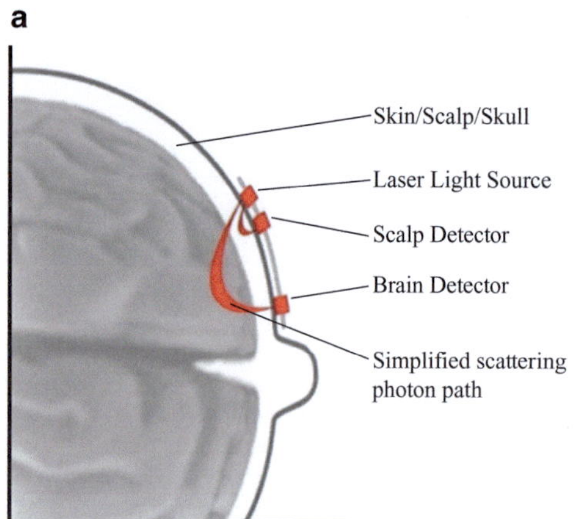

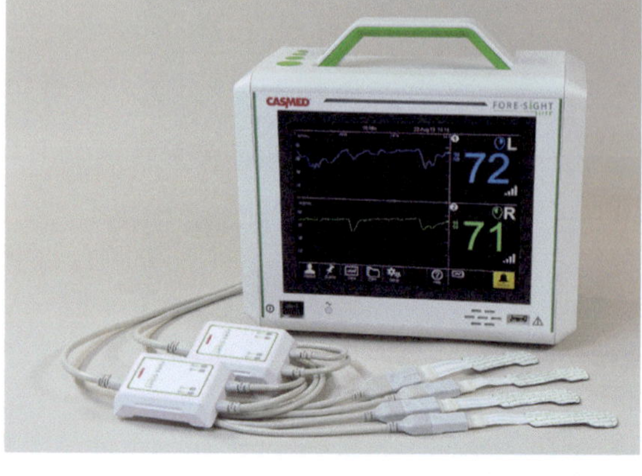

Fig. 5.9 Cerebral oximetry. (**a**) Cerebral oximetry differs from pulse oximetry by utilizing two photodetectors with each light source, thereby allowing sampling of tissue beyond a specified depth beneath the skin. Near-field photodetection is subtracted from far-field photodetection to provide tissue oxygenation measurement beyond a predefined depth. (**b**) A state-of-the-art oximeter with the two numbers representing the oxygen saturation of the right and left side of the brains (FORE-SIGHT Elite™ Absolute Tissue Oximeter. Courtesy of CASMED, Inc.)

with a low cerebral O_2 saturation, necessitates raising the pressure despite the possible clinical disadvantages of doing so. The frontal cortex is most common region of neurologic damage in a trauma patient. While cerebral oximetry has been used in cardiac surgery for years, evidence to support its use in other settings has grown. Several recent articles have demonstrated an association between decreased cerebral oximetric values and neurocognitive decline, increased major organ morbidity, and increased hospital length of stay (LOS) after major surgery [23]. Monitoring cerebral oxygenation has helped guide clinicians in the operating room, although its utility has yet to be determined fully in severe trauma. It may be of great value during surgery, especially in patients with multiple comorbidities. There are many possible therapeutic interventions for a fall in cerebral saturation, including increasing blood pressure, cardiac output and/or FiO_2; increasing $PaCO_2$ to >40 mmHg by decreasing minute ventilation; administering anesthesia and/or muscle relaxants as indicated; and finally, red blood cell transfusion if the patient's hematocrit is <20 %. Patients with cerebral desaturation during non-cardiac surgery have been shown to demonstrate decreases in their Mini Mental State Examination (MMSE) scores.

Casati and colleagues [23] studied 122 patients older than 65 years scheduled for major abdominal, nonvascular surgery under general anesthesia, with an expected duration of surgery greater than two hours. Patients were randomly assigned to an intervention group (the monitor was visible and rSO_2 maintained at >75 % of preinduction values) or a control group (the monitor was blinded and anesthesia was managed routinely). There was a significant correlation between the area under the curve of $rSO_2 < 75 \%$ of baseline and postoperative decrease in MMSE score from preoperative values. Control group patients with intraoperative cerebral desaturation also experienced a longer time to post-anesthesia care unit (PACU) discharge compared with patients in the treatment group.

Another useful area for the cerebral co-oximeter is in patients positioned in the sitting or "beach chair" position, for instance in shoulder surgery. Cerebral co-oximetry has identified cerebral hypoperfusion when blood pressure is measured in the nonoperated arm positioned well below the level of the brain. The physiologic and anatomic changes that occur with the beach chair position may include decreased venous return, vasodilation, and head flexion, which may impede jugular venous flow and thus decrease cerebral perfusion. Providing deliberate hypotension along with these physiologic changes requires enhanced vigilance. The use of a cerebral oximeter in this setting provides a tool to assess adequate oxygen delivery to vulnerable cerebral tissue.

The clinical studies described above demonstrate the potential benefits of cerebral oximetric monitoring in a variety of clinical situations. Although the majority of studies have been conducted during cardiac surgery, the application of cerebral oximetry to non-cardiac patients is compelling in certain clinical situations. The previously described work by Casati demonstrated the benefits of using cerebral oximetry among elderly patients undergoing major abdominal surgery. In our trauma patient, intubated and brought to the OR without any brain imaging, the cerebral oximeter could be a vital monitor for ICP management.

Temperature monitors: Trentsch et al. [24] determined that hypothermia is a powerful independent predictor of death in the severely injured blunt trauma patient, based on data from the Trauma Registry of the German Society for Trauma Surgery (TR-DGU). The investigators utilized the Revised Injury Classification Score (RISC score). Data from 5,197 severe trauma patients were reviewed. Hypothermia was defined as a temperature of 35 °C or less. Statistical analysis revealed that hypothermic patients were more severely injured and had higher rates of shock, organ failure, and sepsis. Hypothermia was also shown to correlate with hemorrhage and coagulopathy.

While Foley catheters with temperature probes are ideal for measuring temperature in trauma patients, not all centers have them. For patients with facial fractures or significant neck or chest trauma, often an esophageal temperature probe cannot be used. Temperature reading from the axilla or skin using esophageal temperature probes is often inaccurate. Recent advances in NASA's telemetry and miniaturizing technologies have led to the development of a CorTemp [25].

Ingestible Temperature Sensor, or "pill" (HQ, Inc.). If the pill cannot be ingested by the patient, it can be placed inside a surgically exposed body cavity. The pill is a small electronic device that senses the body's temperature and transmits it via a radio signal to an external receiver. The advantage of the pill over other temperature measurement devices is that it enables core temperature measurement for many hours without the need for wired connections. This is an ideal tool for temperature measurement in or out of the hospital location, or for continuous monitoring of ambulatory patients over long periods. The pill temperature values usually fall between the (higher) rectal and the (lower) esophageal values, considered the gold standard for core temperature measurement. Core body temperature is normally tightly regulated. All general anesthetics produce a profound dose-dependent reduction in the core temperature, triggering responses including arteriovenous shunt, vasoconstriction, and shivering. The primary cause of hypothermia in most patients in the operating room is anesthetic-induced impairment of normal thermoregulatory control, and the resulting core-to-peripheral redistribution of body heat.

Key Management Concerns in Our Patient

In the operating room for "damage control laparotomy," our patient presented dilemmas inherent to many major trauma cases. He had a penetrating abdominal wound, bilateral pelvic fractures, disruption of both iliac arteries, and lacerations of the spleen, liver, and stomach. His abdominal and vascular injuries, combined with dilutional coagulopathy, hypothermia, and acidosis precluded completion of the laparotomy. "Damage control" (DC), defined as initial control of hemorrhage and contamination followed by intraperitoneal packing and rapid closure, allows resuscitation to normal physiology in the intensive care unit and subsequent definitive reexploration and repair.

Although the Massive Transfusion Protocol was activated for our patient, no blood was available in the operating room on arrival. The patient was receiving normal saline. There has been an ongoing debate among anesthesiologists and surgeons about fluid administration in hemorrhagic shock when blood is not available. Hemoglobin-based oxygen carriers and hypertonic saline, although not ideal, have advantages over other fluids in this circumstance. Hemoglobin-based oxygen carriers have been approved for use in Russia and South Africa, while phase III trials are ongoing in the USA.

A Cochrane database review in 2003 [26] explored the "continuing uncertainty" about the timing of fluid resuscitation in the bleeding patient. Large volume fluid infusions (blood products, colloids, crystalloids) have been linked to multiorgan failure (MOF), coagulopathy, acute lung injury, compartment syndrome, edema, immune suppression, promotion of further blood loss, and hypothermia. In addition, the 1:1:1 ratio of FFP, PRBCs, and platelets in the massive transfusion protocol supplies a mean hematocrit of 29 %, a hematocrit upon equilibration may be too low.

Volume Replacement While Waiting for Blood

The goals of the early resuscitative stage are: (1) to restore an effective blood volume, (2) to optimize tissue perfusion (early initiation of vasopressin infusion), and (3) to limit ischemic and reperfusion injury (antioxidants, complement inactivators). By establishing adequate blood pressure through appropriate volume resuscitation, it is possible to lessen reperfusion injury. Although the colloid vs. crystalloid debate may never be resolved, there is increasing evidence suggesting that lactated ringers is proinflammatory and contributes to end organ damage [27]. Resuscitation with large volumes of crystalloids has also been linked to abdominal compartment syndrome [28]. These findings have led to the use of hypertonic saline 7.5 % in initial volume resuscitation.

In 1980, a critically ill, hypotensive Brazilian man inadvertently received 100 cm^3 of 7.5 % hypertonic saline. His rapid and remarkable recovery stimulated much interest in hypertonic solutions for resuscitation. Many investigators have established a recommended dose of 4 cm^3/kg of 7.5 % saline [29], which correlates to large volume resuscitation with respect to cardiac

output and organ perfusion. Theoretical, practical, and physiological advantages of HSS over all other crystalloids for hemorrhagic shock have been reported in the literature. HSS promotes rapid mobilization of fluids from intracellular to extracellular space by creating an osmotic gradient [30]. The increased oncotic pressure expands the vascular space and increases mean arterial blood pressure. Transcapillary refill is restored or increased, with fluid movement into the vascular space, resulting in increased blood flow to the tissues. Dextran 70, a high molecular weight colloid, can be given with HSS. Dextran helps to maintain the oncotic gradient and thus the intravascular volume for a longer period of time than HSS alone [31]. Other attributes of HSS include reduction of pulmonary and systemic vascular resistance, expansion of the interstitial and plasma volumes, increased cardiac output, natriuresis, restoration of membrane potentials, prevention of cellular edema, improved microcirculation, and a smaller overall volume of solution needed for resuscitation. Animal models have shown that HSS has several immune and inflammation modulating effects. Additionally, HSS has been shown to impede oxidative stress, apoptosis, and degranulation of neutrophils, and to lower the rate of bacterial translocation.

However, HSS has not been shown to have any survival advantage over other crystalloids. In traumatic or hemorrhagic shock, the nature of the injury is usually the most important factor determining survival. In clinical trials, boluses of 250 mL of 5, 6, or 7.5 % HSS with dextran 70 have been studied. The most commonly used formulation studied in humans has been 7.5 % with 6 % dextran 70. When HSS is used alone, 3–5 % HSS in a dose of 4–6 cm^3/kg is infused, and repeated as needed. When administering HSS, serum sodium, potassium, and creatinine should be measured at least every 6–8 h. HSS should not be infused through a peripheral IV, as it has been associated with regional vascular complications.

The main concerning side effect of HSS is theoretical: osmotic demyelination syndrome (ODS). There has been only one reported case of ODS when HSS was used for resuscitation. Repeated doses of HSS more commonly may lead to hypernatremia, hypokalemia, and metabolic acidosis. Dextran may cause anaphylaxis and dextran-induced renal failure.

Hemoglobin-Based Oxygen Carriers

The oxygen carrying solutions are blood, cell free hemoglobin-based oxygen carriers (HEBOC), cell free hemoglobin encapsulated in artificial cells, and perfluorocarbon solutions. Only the HEBOC solutions are devoid of antigenicity issues and can carry a high concentration of oxygen. HEBOC fluids do not have cellular rheology, making them ideal in the massively bleeding patient. They have a shelf life of 3 months, which permits stockpiling in areas of shortage. HEBOC carries universal donor status due to its lack of red blood cell antigens. It appears to be an ideal resuscitation fluid [31]. Clinicians have been waiting for decades for these products to be released in the USA, but lingering issues remain before FDA approval.

There are currently two HEBOCs that have undergone phase three clinical trials. Hemopure (HBOC-21) (Bio-Pure Products, Inc.) has been approved for human use in South Africa and Russia. It has been used in over 800 humans in clinical trials, and in over 70 people for compassionate use. It has not received FDA approval and has been given the status of available under the Code of Federal Regulations, Title 21, Parts 312 and 316. (Expanded access to investigational drugs for treatment use.) The FDA noted several deficiencies when HEBOC-21 was used in humans. In compromised elderly patients with multiple comorbidities, clinical mismanagement occurred, ranging from congestive heart failure to failure to maintain adequate hemoglobin levels because of its brief (19 h) half-life compared to the 22–33 day half-life of PRBCs. It also has vasoconstrictive properties; therefore patients must be closely monitored for hypertension during infusion of the agent. When infusing HEBOC, the total hemoglobin includes the patient's hemoglobin plus that from HEBOC. As HEBOCs are acellular, the hematocrit level is not useful. The dosing schedule of HEBOC is targeted at keeping the hemoglobin level above 5 g/dL by a continuous infusion over 2–6 h. The infusion should be repeated in 12–18 h.

HBOC is not a substitute for blood. The hemoglobin content of PRBCs is 32–36 g/dL while HBOC-201 has a hemoglobin level of 13 g/dL. The significant difference in hemoglobin content between HEBOC and blood is another reason why HEBOC has not yet been FDA approved.

Blood Pressure Management in Our Patient

Our patient entered the operating room hypotensive and bleeding. There are several studies that suggest that permissive hypotension during initial resuscitation may improve trauma outcomes [32]. This strategy, while long standing, remains controversial. It should never be used for a patient with traumatic brain injury, as poor neurologic outcomes have been reported after hypotension in those patients.

Morrison, et al. reported that hypotensive resuscitation reduces transfusion requirements and severe postoperative coagulopathy in trauma patients with hemorrhagic shock [32]. In their randomized controlled trial, once a patient had a systolic pressure of 90 mmhg, they were randomized to a target mean pressure of 50 or 65. The mean arterial pressures were kept at 50 or 65 by means at the discretion of the anesthesiologists. If the patient's pressure responded to treatment, their pressures were allowed to drift up to a level that the patient could sustain without support.

Patients in the lower mean arterial pressure group received significantly less blood products and intravenous fluids than those patients targeted to a mean of 65. The most important outcomes of the study were that postoperative coagulopathy was decreased in the low pressure group, and early postoperative mortality was significantly lower. However, there was no difference between the two groups in late mortality (>24 h), duration of mechanical ventilator support, organ failure, infection, or LOS in the ICU or hospital.

With high volume resuscitation, the lethal triad of acidemia, coagulopathy, and hypothermia are almost always exacerbated. While the INR was elevated in both groups, the average INR was drastically higher in the higher MAP group. Of note, more patients died from bleeding and coagulopathy within the first 24 h in the higher MAP group than in the lower MAP group, despite the fact that patients with higher MAP received more FFP. The smaller doses of FFP did not result in increased coagulopathy in the lower MAP group, and mortality from coagulopathy was significantly reduced.

Both groups had nearly equal hemoglobin levels in the early postoperative period, as well as similar platelet counts. The fact that significantly less blood products are used with the hypotensive resuscitation strategy has great implications for cost and blood use.

It is important to note that the study randomized more blunt trauma patients to the higher MAP group, and thus it is possible that the results may have been confounded by the severity of the injuries in that group. In summary, the evidence supports maintaining a MAP of 50 for trauma patients in hemorrhagic shock, without the use of hypotensive agents. Control of blood pressure during resuscitation for hemorrhagic shock affects morbidity and mortality, and permissive hypotension may be beneficial. Among the likely reasons, lower MAP was tolerated, was that trauma patients tend to be young and healthy, with a mean age of 29.

This study provides evidence to modify the current standard of care for trauma patients, which includes massive transfusion of blood and fluids [33]. The massive transfusion protocol, with an equal ratio of factors and red cells, suffers from a lack of strong evidence of improved survival [33, 34]. In many severe trauma cases, the nature of the injury is the greatest predictor of survival.

The design of Morison's study of hypotensive resuscitation is worthy of discussion as it brings out many issues related to trauma care and research. When a new approach to a clinical situation arises, it is customary that multiple clinical trials revealing strong evidence for the new approach are done before it becomes acceptable, if not the standard of care. In the trauma arena, investigators try to obtain a waiver of consent for research, as trauma patients are not usually capable of understanding the research study, nor are they able to sign consent.

According to federal law, trauma or emergency medicine researchers seeking a waiver of consent must first consult with "representatives of the communities in which the research will be conducted" who are willing to move forward with the trial. The community in Morrison's trial was defined as patients who used the emergency room at the study institution for their own care. The community gave consent before the initiation of the trial. In addition, the institutional IRB and the Center for Medical Ethics and Health Policy at Baylor College of Medicine approved the study, which was also registered with the National Institutes of Health. This approach was successful in obtaining a waiver of consent from trauma patients. The study was accomplished by including the community, ethical board, IRB, and the United States government. This trial serves as an excellent model for others who would like to study new strategies for trauma treatment.

Vasopressors in Our Patient

Arginine vasopressin (AVP), also known as vasopressin or antidiuretic hormone (ADH), is a neural hormone derived from a precursor made in the hypothalamus and secreted by the posterior pituitary gland. Its two primary functions are to constrict blood vessels and to regulate the body's water by increasing water absorption from the collecting ducts of the kidney [34]. It also increases peripheral vascular resistance, which in turn increases arterial blood pressure. It plays a key role in homeostasis by regulation of water, glucose, and electrolyte concentrations in the blood.

During hemorrhagic stress, blood levels of AVP fall. An infusion of vasopressin can restore blood pressure. In both animal and limited human investigations, the use of AVP for circulatory support has been linked to improved outcomes. Part of AVP's efficacy lies in its ability to increase the sensitivity of vascular smooth muscle to calcium in an acidotic environment. Vasopressin is also associated with a "steal" phenomenon in which blood is shunted from the periphery to the vital organs.

In the massively hemorrhaging patient, administration of vasopressin is essential as an early, if not first-line, treatment [35]. Vasopressin supports vascular tone by binding to the V1 receptors responsible for vascular smooth muscle constriction, and modulates nitric oxide and ATP sensitive K-channels, as well as potentiating adrenergic agents [36]. Vasopressin also binds to V2 (renal) receptors which are located in the distal renal tubules to increase free water absorption. By binding to both V1 and V2 receptors, vasopressin increases volume retention and increases blood pressure, commonly producing an adequate perfusion pressure. Endogenous vasopressin blood levels increase dramatically in the bleeding patient, stimulated by increased osmolarity and decreased circulating volume. Volume loss is a greater stimulus to increased output of vasopressin than is osmolarity. These levels decline in 24 h, coinciding with the refractory hypotension seen in some patients [36].

In hemorrhagic shock, 10–20 % of AVP stores are released from the pituitary, and as the shock state continues, the supply of endogenous vasopressin becomes exhausted, resulting in worsening of the shock state. In a low perfusion state, lactic acidosis develops, resulting in an acidic environment. Acidosis hyperpolarizes calcium-sensitive potassium channels. This decreased sensitivity to calcium leads to poor vascular tone, decreased perfusion pressure and persistence of shock. Therefore, exogenous vasopressin should be started early when hemorrhage is present. There is strong evidence that in hemorrhagic shock vasopressin works more physiologically than catacholamines, since epinephrine and norepinephrine are not as effective as vasopressin for increasing blood pressure in the severely hemorrhaging patient.

The usual starting dose of AVP is a bolus of 2–4 units followed by an infusion of 0.04 units/ min, which is then titrated to effect. As with all vasopressors, there may be adverse effects depending on the dose and the physiological state of the patient. Doses of vasopressin that elevate liver enzymes also decrease blood flow to abdominal organs. At therapeutic doses, perfusion to abdominal organs is usually not dangerously impaired.

The delivery of oxygen to the liver is carried out by the hepatic artery and portal vein. Fifty percent of oxygen is carried by the portal vein and 50 % by the hepatic artery. When the flow is decreased in one vessel, a hepatic flow buffering mechanism takes over and increases flow in the other vessel. Vasopressin is unique in that its effect on the portal vein is temporary, while the hepatic artery flow remains high. With vasopressin, the microcirculation of the liver usually remains unchanged. Elevated bilirubin and liver enzymes associated with vasopressin administration have not been shown to be related to patient mortality [36].

In summary, by increasing the circulatory volume, vasopressin enables the clinician to decrease the amount of blood products and fluids given. Although the adverse effects of a unit of blood are extremely low, morbidity quickly becomes an issue when multiple and various blood products are administered.

Antimicrobial Therapy in Our Patient

Broad spectrum antibiotics are initially administered to blunt trauma patients. If a single area is contaminated, more specific antibiotic coverage is used. Facial fractures involving the sinuses often contain different microbes from a fractured hip. The bacterial contamination in polytrauma cases can be extensive, with multiple large lacerations, open fractures, and violation of the abdominal or thoracic cavity. Anesthesiologists play a significant role in both selection and administration of antimicrobial therapy. In a large meta-analysis by Shiu et al. comparing intermittent vs. continuous infusion of antibiotics [37], no difference was found in mortality, infection recurrence, clinical cure, superinfection post therapy, and safety outcomes between the two methods.

The Surgical Care Improvement Project (SCIP) established antibiotic prophylaxis guidelines for surgical patients. These guidelines did not include trauma patients. The guidelines include (1) prophylactic antibiotic administration, (2) antibiotic received within one hour of incision, (3) correct antibiotic selection, and (4) discontinuation of antibiotics 24 h after surgery. In a sentinel retrospective review of severe trauma patients, those who received antibiotics according to the four SCIP guidelines did not have a higher infection rate than normal surgical patients irrespective of severity or location of trauma. Trauma patients treated by SCIP guidelines had less than half the infections than those not treated by the guidelines [38].

The Anesthesiologist and the Immune System: The New Frontier

The trauma literature refers to the initial immunological response in the injured patient the "first hit." Until recently there was poor understanding of the "second hit," which consists of the subsequent immunological reactions that make the victim vulnerable to further injury. The activation of the immune system within the first hours after the traumatic event is the early phase of hyperinflammation, which may occur locally in isolated injuries, or may manifest as massive systemic immune activation in the polytrauma patient [39]. The endogenous triggers of trauma-associated inflammation have been recently elucidated. The very early stage of trauma is characterized by activation of complement [40] and neutrophils. The complement system is the critical effector of immune responses; it functions in the elimination of invading pathogens by opsonization for phagocytosis, chemotaxis of leukocytes, and by direct lysis of pathogens through the membrane attack complex. The complement system "complements" the ability of antibodies and phagocytic cells to clear pathogens. The complement system consists of small proteins in the blood, synthesized by the liver. They normally circulate as inactive pro-proteins. When triggered, proteases in the system cleave specific proteins to release cytokines and start an amplifying cascade of further cleavages. The end result of this activation cascade is massive augmentation of the response and activation of the cell-killing membrane attack complex. Three biochemical pathways activate the complement system: the classical complement pathway, the alternative complement pathway, and the lectin pathway [41].

Anaphylatoxins C3a and C5a are chemoattractants for phagocytes and neutrophils and recruit immune cells to a site of injury. In addition degranulation occurs in mast cells, basophils, and eosinophils. Many studies have demonstrated that trauma activates complement locally at the site of injury as well as systemically. The complement cascade is activated at the level of C3, and the extent of activation correlates with the severity of injury.

As the complement system is the humoral response to injury, neutrophil activation is the cellular response. Within minutes of injury and up to several days, neutrophils mount an immunologic response, and are essential to the debridement of injured or devitalized tissue. Neutrophils release cytokines, chemokines, reactive oxygen species, and tissue-toxic enzymes such as myeloperoxidase and elastase, all of which contribute to the massive inflammatory response [42]. which involves not only the site of injury but also healthy tissues. This reaction is not completely understood. Shortly after the inflammatory response is initiated, a significant failure of components of the innate immune system follows, including reduced proliferation of T lymphocytes [43]. Simply stated, all patients suffer from an impairment of lymphocytes and monocytes.

The majority of polytrauma patients receive blood; a therapy that ignites the immune system. Other than issues related to blood storage injury, transfusion has a negative impact on the patient's immune system and hyperinflammatory response. Proinflammatory cytokines (Interleukins) IL-8, IL-6, and counterregulatory cytokines (IL-10) are markedly elevated in patients resuscitated with PRBCs [44]. It is unlikely that such high levels came from the donated cells. More likely, the elevated cytokines are the host's response to the transfusion. These isolated cytokines are now being evaluated to determine if they are involved in MOF [44].

Over the years, a large body of scientific evidence has accumulated from evaluating over 100 monoclonal antibodies, antiendotoxins, and antioxidants. Testing of these agents on severely injured patients has become infrequent, since attempts to control the immune response have not been successful [45]. Timing and treatment of inflammatory changes is essential in preventing MOF. IL-1 and TNF were the first to be elucidated in the inflammatory response; however, antibodies to them worked well in animal models but not at all in humans. In the 1980s, antibodies to endotoxin component lipid and HA-1 proved to be both neuro- and hepatotoxic. Protein C and corticosteroids did not give meaningful results. Clearly, full understanding of the proinflammatory response and immunomodulation needs further research.

The most significant trials to halt the massive immunological response to trauma are targeted at the complement system, in attempts to moderate or avoid the multiorgan failure associated with severe trauma. Recombinant C1 inhibitor concentrates (C1-INH) and the anti-C5 Ab eculizumab (Alexion pharmaceuticals) are the first anticomplement drugs to be approved and utilized [46]. These agents prevent complement initiation at the classical and lecithin pathways. Clinical trials have begun for the attenuation of thromboinflammatory responses in trauma (ClinicalTrials.gov identifier NCT01275976). In contrast to C1-INH, eculizumab is complement-specific. It works at the C5 level, preventing the generation of C5a which attacks cell membranes [46]. Countless other substances that attack various levels of the complement system are under investigation and are likely to be available to anesthesiologists for trauma cases as well as for a host of other areas like transplants and medical diseases.

This brief introduction to proinflammatory/immunosuppression and catabolism (PICS)

reactions is important for the anesthesiologist, as these responses are the basis of multiorgan failure. This complex inflammatory response is likely responsible for the dysphoria and exhaustion those patients feel after surgery. Prevention of MOF by controlling the immune system and the hyperinflammatory response will be a new challenge for clinicians.

Case Summary

The patient arrived in the operating room at 8:00 PM, with a blood pressure of 55/35. 100 cm^3 of HSS were administered while the anesthesia team was waiting for blood. A total bolus of 10 units of vasopressin was given followed by an infusion of 10 units/h. The blood pressure responded to both therapies. Two radial arterial lines were placed and the pulse pressure showed a 35 % variation with respiration. Packed red blood cells were alternated with fresh frozen plasma and platelets until the pulse pressure variation was 12 %. The hematocrit at that time was 27. The infusion of vasopressin was decreased until a mean pressure of 50 mmHg was sustained. A bolus of 5 g of ε-aminocaproic acid was administered upon arrival and an infusion was maintained at 1 g/h. The TEG demonstrated a significant decrease in the MA, which proved to be related to low fibrinogen as the platelet function analyzer showed 90,000 platelets with 80 % function. Cryoprecipitate was administered to address the fibrinogen deficit.

During the damage control laparotomy, the left iliac vein was traumatized and could not be repaired, and therefore had to be ligated. The abdomen was packed and the patient was sent to the ICU. The patient was stable for only a short period of time as both coagulopathy and overt bleeding were worse. The patient was transferred to the interventional radiology suite and the anesthesiologists resumed their resuscitation plan while the interventional radiologists coiled every bleeding vessel they could find. It was discovered that the other iliac had become aneurysmal and after much discussion among the surgeons, anesthesiologists, and radiologists, it was embolized. With both iliacs "down," the patient's legs, rectum, bladder, and perineum began to "die." The patient was not eligible for a hemicorpectomy both because of his medical condition as well as the wishes of the family. When he arrived back in the ICU, "comfort" care was started. The patient was extubated and morphine sulfate was administered each time the patient had a respiratory rate greater than 20 and when he appeared to be uncomfortable. Death was pronounced 5 h after extubation.

Many of the concepts presented here are not "mainstream" clinical practice. It is essential to note that the consensus of practice for the severe trauma patient is evolving. There is an ongoing explosion in investigations related to blood transfusion, immunology, oxidative stress, and MOF. Of equal importance, there is evolution in the ethics of dealing with these complex cases. In all of these areas, anesthesiologists will be playing a vital role.

References

1. Wye H, Lefering R, Maegele M, Brockamp T, Wafaisade A, Wutzler S, Walcher F, Marzi I. The golden hour of shock; how time is running out: prehospital time intervals in Germany—a multivariat analysis of 15,103 patients from the TraumaRegister DGU(R). Emerg Med J. 2013;30(12):1048–5.
2. Tobin JM, Varon AK. Update in trauma anesthesiology: perioperative resuscitation management. Anesth Analg. 2012;115(6):1326–33.
3. de la Grandville B, Arroyo D, Walder B. Etomidate for critically ill patients. Con: do you really want to weaken the frail? Eur J Anaesthesiol. 2012;29 (11):511–4.
4. Bar-Joseph G, Guilburd Y, et al. Effectiveness of ketamine in decreasing intracranial pressure in children with intracranial hypertension. J Neurosurg Pediatr. 2009;4(1):40–6.
5. Shanmugasundararaj S, Zhou X, Neunzig J, Bernhardt R, Cotten JF, Ge R, Miller KW, Raines DE. Carboetomidate: an analog of etomidate that interacts weakly with 11β-hydroxylase. Anesth Analg. 2013;116 (6):1249–56. doi:10.1213/ANE.0b013e31828b3637. Epub 2013 Mar 14. PMID:23492967.
6. Waibel BH, Rotondo M. Damage control surgery: its evolution over the last 20 years. Rev Col Bras Cir. 2012;39(4):314–21.
7. Bruzoni M, Slater BJ, Wall J, St Peter SD, Dutta S. A prospective randomized trial of ultrasound- vs landmark-guided central venous access in the pediatric population. J Am Coll Surg. 2013;216(5):939–43. doi:10.1016/j.jamcollsurg.2013.01.054. Epub 2013 Mar 7.
8. Lamperti M, Subert M, Cortellazzi P, Vailati D, Borrelli P, Montomoli C, D'Onofrio G, Caldiroli D. Is a neutral head position safer than 45-degree neck rotation during ultrasound-guided internal jugular vein cannulation? Results of a randomized controlled clinical trial. Anesth Analg. 2012;114(4):777–84. doi:10.1213/ANE.0b013e3182459917. Epub 2012 Jan 17.
9. Moffatt SE. Hypothermia in trauma. Emerg Med J. 2013;30(12):989–96. Dec 14 PMID:23243045.
10. Walsh M, Thomas SG, Howard JC, Evans E, Guyer K, Medvecz A, Swearingen A, Navari RM, Ploplis V, Castellino FJ. Blood component therapy in trauma guided with the utilization of the perfusionist and thromboelastography. J Extra Corpor Technol. 2011;43(3):162–7.
11. Raza I, Davenport R, Rourke C, Platton S, Manson J, Spoors C, Khan S, De'Ath HD, Allard S, Hart DP, Pasi KJ, Hunt BJ, Stanworth S, MacCallum PK, Brohi K. The incidence and magnitude of fibrinolytic activation in trauma patients. J Thromb Haemost. 2013;11:307–14.
12. The ROTEM website ROTEM.de 2013.
13. Sankarankutty A, Nascimento B, Teodoro da Luz L, Rizoli S. TEG® and ROTEM® in trauma: similar test but different results? World J Emerg Surg. 2012;7 Suppl 1:S3. 10.1186/1749-7922-7-S1-S32. Epub 2012 Aug 22.
14. Hagemo JS, Næss PA, Johansson P, et al. Evaluation of TEG(®) and RoTEM(®) inter-changeability in trauma patients. Injury. 2013;44(5):600–5.
15. Vucelić D, Golubović M, Bjelović M. PFA-100 test in the detection of platelet dysfunction and monitoring DDAVP in a patient with liver cirrhosis undergoing inguinal hernia repair. Srp Arh Celok Lek. 2012;140 (11–12):782–5.
16. Matthay MA, Ware LB, Zimmerman GA. The acute respiratory distress syndrome. J Clin Invest. 2012;122 (8):2731–40.
17. Roy S, Sadowitz B, Andrews P, Gatto LA, Marx W, Ge L, Wang G, Lin X, Dean DA, Kuhn M, Ghosh A, Satalin J, Snyder K, Vodovotz Y, Nieman G, Habashi N. Early stabilizing alveolar ventilation prevents acute respiratory distress syndrome: a novel timing-based ventilatory intervention to avert lung injury. J Trauma Acute Care Surg. 2012;73(2):391–400.
18. Lellouche F, Lipes J. Prophylactic protective ventilation: lower tidal volumes for all critically ill patients? Intensive Care Med. 2013;39(1):6–15.
19. Freitas FG, Bafi AT, Nascente AP, Assunção M, Mazza B, Azevedo LC, Machado FR. Predictive value of pulse pressure variation for fluid responsiveness in septic patients using lung-protective ventilation strategies. Br J Anaesth. 2013;110 (3):402–8. 10.1093/bja/aes398. Epub 2012 Nov 15.

20. Auler Jr JO, Galas FR, Sundin MR, Hajjar LA. Arterial pulse pressure variation predicting fluid responsiveness in critically ill patients. Shock. 2008;30 Suppl 1:18–22.

21. Santos L, Thiago C, Michard F. Online monitoring of pulse pressure variation to guide fluid therapy after cardiac surgery. Anesth Analg. 2008;106 (4):1201–6.

22. Goodney PP, Likosky DS, Cronenwett JL. Factors associated with stroke or death after carotid endarterectomy in Northern New England; Vascular Study Group of Northern New England. J Vasc Surg. 2008;48(5):1139–45.

23. Casati A, Fanelli G, Pietropaoli P, Proietti R, Tufano R, Danelli G, Fierro G, De Cosmo G, Servillo G. Continuous monitoring of cerebral oxygen saturation in elderly patients undergoing major abdominal surgery minimizes brain exposure to potential hypoxia. Anesth Analg. 2005;101(3):740–7. table of contents. Erratum in: Anesth Analg. 2006 Jun; 102(6):1645.

24. Trentzsch H, Huber-Wagner S, Hildebrand F, Kanz KG, Faist E, Piltz S, Lefering R. Trauma registry DGU hypothermia for prediction of death in severely injured blunt trauma patients. Shock. 2012;37 (2):131–9.

25. Hoffmann ME, Rodriguez SM, Zeiss DM, Wachsberg KN, Kushner RF, Landsberg L. Linsenmeier RA 24-h core temperature in obese and lean men and women. Obesity (Silver Spring). 2012;20(8):1585–90.

26. Kwan I, Bunn F, Roberts I. Timing and volume of fluid administration for patients with bleeding. Cochrane Database of Systemic Reviews 2003; CD002245.

27. Rhee P, Burris D, Kaufman C, et al. Lactated Ringers solution resuscitation causes neutrophil activation after hemorrhagic shock. J Trauma. 1998;44:313–9.

28. Balogh Z, McKineley BA, Cocanour CS, et al. Supranormal trauma resuscitation causes more cases of abdominal compartment syndrome. Arch Surg. 2013;138:637–43.

29. Patanwala A, Amini A, Erstad B. Use of hypertonic saline injection in trauma. Am J Syst Pharm. 2010;67:1920–8.

30. Kramer G. Hypertonic resuscitation: physiological mechanisms and recommendations for trauma care. J Trauma. 2003;54:S89–99.

31. Galvagno SM, Mackenzie CF. Trauma new and future resuscitation fluids for trauma patients using hemoglobin and hypertonic saline. Anesthesiol Clin. 2013;31(1):1–19.

32. Morrison AC, Carrick MM, Norman MA, et al. Hypotensive resuscitation strategy reduces transfusion requirements and severe postoperative coagulopathy in trauma patients with hemorrhagic shock: preliminary results of a randomized controlled trial. J Trauma. 2011;70(3):652–63.

33. Riskin DJ, Tsai TC, et al. Massive transfusion protocols: the role of aggressive resuscitation versus product ratio in mortality reduction. J Am Coll Surg. 2009;209:198.

34. Anand T, Skinner R. Arginine vasopressin: the future of pressure-support resuscitation in hemorrhagic shock. J Surg Res. 2012;178(1):321–9.

35. Holmes CL, Landry DW, Granton JT. Science review: vasopressin and the cardiovascular system Part 1-receptor physiology. Crit Care. 2003;7:427.

36. Nemenoff RA. Vasopressin signaling pathways in vascular smooth muscle. Front Biosci. 1998;3:194–207.

37. Shiu J, Wang E, Tejani AM, Wasdell M. Continuous versus intermittent infusions of antibiotics for the treatment of severe acute infections. Cochrane Database Syst Rev. 2013; Mar 28;3:CD008481. doi: 10.1002/14651858.CD008481.pub2.

38. Smith BP, Fox N, Fakhro A, Lachant M, et al. "Scip"ing antibiotic prophylaxis guidelines in trauma: The consequences of noncompliance. J Trauma Acute Care Surg. 2012;73(2):452–6.

39. Neher MD, Weckbach S, Huber-Lang MS, Stahel PF. New insights into the role of peroxisome proliferator-activated receptors in regulating the inflammatory response after tissue injury. PPAR Res. 2012;2012:728461.

40. Janeway Jr CA, Travers P, Walport M, et al. The complement system and innate immunity. Immunobiology: the immune system in health and disease. New York: Garland Science; 2001. Retrieved 25 February 2013.

41. Gentile LF, Cuenca AG, et al. Persistent inflammation and immunosuppression: a common syndrome and new horizon for surgical intensive care. J Trauma Acute Care Surg. 2023;72(6):1491–501.

42. Rivers EP, Jaehne AK, Nguyen HB, Papamatheakis DG, Singer D, Yang JJ, Brown S, Klausner H. Early biomarker activity in severe sepsis and septic shock and a contemporary review of immunotherapy trials: not a time to give up, but to give it earlier. Shock. 2013;39 (2):127–37. doi:10.1097/SHK.0b013e31827dafa7.

43. Menges P, Kessler W, Kloecker C, Feuerherd M, Gaubert S, Diedrich S, van der Linde J, Hegenbart A, Busemann A, Traeger T, Cziupka K, Heidecke CD, Maier S. Surgical trauma and postoperative immune dysfunction. Eur Surg Res. 2012;48(4):180–6. doi:10.1159/000338196. Epub 2012 May 25.

44. Johnson JL, Moore EE, Gonzalez RJ, Fedel N, Partrick DA, Silliman CC. Alteration of the postinjury hyperinflammatory response by means of resuscitation with a red cell substitute. J Trauma. 2003;54 (1):133–40.

45. Groeneveld K, Leenan L, et al. Immunotherapy after trauma: timing is essential. Curr Opin Anesthesiol. 2011;24(2):219–23.

46. Woodruff TM, Nandakumar KS, Tedesco F. Inhibiting the C5-C5a receptor axis. Mol Immunol. 2011;48(14):1631–42. doi:10.1016/j.molimm.2011.04.014. Epub 2011 May 6.

Pain Control in Acute Trauma

Christopher K. Merritt, Orlando J. Salinas, and Alan David Kaye

The management of pain is one of the primary and most noble goals of medicine. Pain is a complex phenomenon involving physical stimuli, physiologic and pathologic responses, all shadowed by personal experience and psychology. Although pain in acute trauma can have diverse causes and characteristics, inadequately treated results in a common set of negative physiological and psychological consequences.

Physiological and Psychological Consequences of Acute Pain

Undermanaged acute pain presents not only psychological but also multifactorial physiological stress on the cardiopulmonary, renal, immunologic, and gastrointestinal systems [1]. Acute pain results in the increased secretion of catecholamines and stress hormones. Ultimately this has effects on nearly every organ system and may impair recovery. Pain can result in increase in heart rate, blood pressure, and myocardial contraction [1, 2]. Together these increase myocardial oxygen consumption and could contribute to ischemia. Uncontrolled pain in the thorax or upper abdomen can result in impaired ventilation and increased atelectasis resulting in decreased vital capacity, hypoventilation, increased shunting, and increased risk of pneumonia [1, 3]. In the gastrointestinal tract, pain decreases intestinal motility and contributes to nausea and vomiting, though unfortunately so do opioids that form the cornerstone of pain management [1, 4]. Pain stimulates the secretion of antidiuretic hormone that can result in oliguria and urinary retention, and it potentiates the prothrombotic state of the postoperative period with increase in platelet aggregation and the risk of venous thrombosis or myocardial infarction [1, 5].

In addition to these deleterious physiologic consequences of pain, acute pain can also contribute to the development of chronic pain syndromes after surgery and trauma as well as having long-term psychological consequences beyond the suffering of discomfort [1, 6–10]. Pain is associated with the development of acute and chronic anxiety, and this in turn may increase the fear and perception of future pain. In burn and trauma patients, higher pain scores are associated with the development of clinical depression and post-traumatic stress disorder (PTSD) [11]. More recent evidence suggests that improving the treatment of acute pain may decrease the risk of subsequent PTSD [12–16].

C.K. Merritt, M.D. • O.J. Salinas, M.D.
Department of Anesthesiology, LSU Health Sciences Center, 1542 Tulane Avenue Suite 659, New Orleans, LA 70115, USA

A.D. Kaye, M.D., Ph.D., D.A.B.A., D.A.B.P.M. (✉)
Departments of Anesthesiology and Pharmacology, LSU School of Medicine T6M5, 1542 Tulane Avenue, Room 656, New Orleans, LA 70112, USA
e-mail: alankaye44@hotmail.com

C.S. Scher (ed.), *Anesthesia for Trauma*, DOI 10.1007/978-1-4939-0909-4_6,
© Springer Science+Business Media New York 2014

The suffering of pain, anxiety, and PTSD are more than reason enough to strive for aggressive pain control in trauma, but these psychological consequences can further result in societal costs and worse physiologic patient outcome. Specifically, the development of PTSD is associated with increased risks of subsequent hypertension, hypercholesterolemia, coronary artery disease, substance abuse, suicide, and overall mortality in addition to societal costs such as lost productivity and increased health care costs [17–22].

Thankfully, the aggressive management of acute pain may prevent some of these physiologic and psychological consequences, particularly in the setting of thoracic and abdominal surgery [2, 3, 7, 12, 13, 15, 23–31]. In the trauma specifically, Buckenmaier et al. have published extensively on the application and benefits of regional anesthesia and aggressive acute pain management in the wounded soldier [10, 24, 28, 32–36]. The work of their group has clearly demonstrated outcomes benefit of regional anesthesia as a component of multimodal analgesia in improving the pain control of wounded soldiers [28]. In addition to improved pain control, the early and successful control of pain may be associated with improvement in the psychological consequences of trauma such as anxiety, chronic pain, and potentially long-term psychological distress [2, 3, 7, 12, 13, 15, 23–31, 34].

Management of Acute Pain in Trauma

Strategies of Pain Management and Guidelines from the WHO

The World Health Organization has developed recommendations for the treatment of cancer pain, though its principals are broadly applicable to the treatment of acute pain in trauma as well [37]. The foundation of the WHO management plan is a three-step "ladder" for the management of cancer pain. The structure of the ladder encourages the use of non-opioid analgesics and adjuvant medications followed by the addition of mild and then strong opioids. In addition to this

escalation of treatment based on pain severity, "by the ladder," the WHO also emphasizes delivering pain medications "by mouth" when possible, "by the clock," and "with attention to detail." These principals apply to pain in trauma as well, i.e., dosing on a scheduled basis when pain is constant allows for better baseline control of pain and avoids peaks and valleys in management. In addition, tailoring regimens "for the individual," and always with "attention to detail," e.g., timing administration, match a patient's sleep cycle [37]. These considerations may be as important as choosing appropriate medications.

Within the WHO ladder, the first rung consists of non-opioid medications such as acetaminophen and non-steroidal anti-inflammatories with or without adjuvant agents such as antidepressants or anticonvulsants. Higher rungs of the ladder are based on the use of opioids with or without those non-opioid agents and adjuvants. The ideal pain management regimen should incorporate this strategy of both escalating and multimodal analgesia. Agents that act through different mechanisms should be combined to maximize their benefits and minimize their side effects. Regional anesthesia should be considered as a key component of multimodal analgesia in combination with non-opioid and opioid pain medications. Often the efficacy of non-opioid analgesics in patients with severe acute pain is discounted. Non-opioid analgesics are dismissed as "not strong enough" for the trauma patient. Unfortunately, this belief denies patients both the significant analgesic benefit of these agents and their opioid-sparing effect. Decreasing patients' opioid requirement through multimodal analgesia may allow for superior pain control with decreased opioid-induced respiratory depression, delirium, sedation, constipation, urinary retention, etc.

Non-opioid Analgesics

Acetaminophen/Paracetamol

Acetaminophen is non-opioid analgesic with mild-moderate analgesic potency. It lacks peripheral anti-inflammatory properties and has a likely primarily central mechanism of analgesic and antipyretic properties. Despite the lack of anti-inflammatory effects, evidence suggests that acetaminophen exerts its effects through neuraxial inhibition of cyclo-oxygenase-II (COX-II) enzyme system [38, 39]. Despite its reputation as a mild pain reliever, acetaminophen can have profound analgesic benefit. Alone, acetaminophen has an analgesic equivalent of 10–20 mg of ketorolac, though without NSAID-associated risks of platelet inhibition, gastritis, or acute nephrotoxicity [40]. The primary risk of acetaminophen is hepatotoxicity. Overdose of acetaminophen can cause fulminant hepatic failure and is in fact the leading cause of acute liver failure in the USA [41]. Doses exceeding 3 g per day should be avoided, and care should be taken in those with pre-existing hepatic disease. In addition, the physician should consider all medications in which a patient may receive acetaminophen, as combination formulations of acetaminophen with opioids are common. When possible, it is best to prescribe these agents individually to decrease the risk of acetaminophen overdose.

Few trauma patients have pain that can be adequately controlled by acetaminophen alone. Nevertheless, acetaminophen remains a useful agent even in patients with moderate or severe pain and can be given in enteral or intravenous formulations. A Cochrane review evaluating oxycodone versus oxycodone with acetaminophen for postoperative pain found that acetaminophen 650 mg combined with oxycodone 10 mg is nearly two times as effective as 15 mg of oxycodone alone [42]. The net result of the addition of acetaminophen is not only superior pain relief but also a decrease in opioid requirements and therefore side effects. Intravenous acetaminophen given every 6 h for the first 24 h after major orthopedic surgery not only improved pain scores but resulted in reduced morphine PCA consumption by 33 % [43, 44]. Similar analgesic- and opioid-sparing benefits have been noted after abdominal surgery and orthopedic trauma [45, 46]. In the emergency room, 1 g of intravenous acetaminophen was found to provide equivalent analgesia to 10 mg of intravenous morphine, though with significantly fewer side effects [47]. Unless contraindicated, scheduled acetaminophen should be strongly considered as part of a multimodal analgesic regimen for all trauma patients.

Non-steroidal Anti-inflammatory Drugs

NSAIDs include a wide variety of analgesic, anti-inflammatory, and antipyretic medications with benefits primarily via COX-II inhibition. Serious adverse effects associated with NSAIDs may limit their use in trauma patients. COX-I blockade results in inhibition of platelet binding that may result in unacceptable risk of bleeding in patients requiring surgery or those with CNS trauma. In addition, NSAIDs are nephrotoxic and increase the risk of gastroenteritis that can result in gastrointestinal ulceration or perforation, and may result in bronchospasm in patients with asthma [48]. Furthermore, evidence suggests increased risk of cardiovascular thrombotic events including myocardial infarction and stroke in patients who use long-term or potent NSAIDs [49]. This is thought to be a result of a relative increase in thromboxane levels from potent COX-II inhibition resulting in a prothrombotic state that offsets the platelet inhibiting effects of COX-I blockade [50].

COX-II Selective Inhibitors

A newer generation of COX-II selective inhibitors, e.g., celecoxib and rofecoxib, provided superior pain relief with decreased gastrointestinal side effects and platelet inhibition. However, subsequent studies revealed evidence of increased cardiovascular risk associated with these agents and resulted in the removal of rofecoxib from the US market [49]. Subsequent studies have demonstrated that this is a common risk even with nonselective NSAIDs [51]. Celecoxib remains available, and can be considered for pain management in trauma. Celecoxib provides potent analgesia and decreases opioid consumption without risks of platelet inhibition or gastrointestinal damage. Clearly these are desirable effects in the trauma patient. Care with celecoxib should be taken in patients at risk for cardiovascular disease and those with sulfa allergies. In addition, concerns exist regarding potential impairment of bone healing with NSAIDs, particularly after fractures and spinal fusion [52–54]. This impairment may be more pronounced with COX-II inhibitors, and does not appear to occur with acetaminophen [52, 53].

Use of NSAIDs

A wide variety of NSAIDs are available in oral, enteral, and parenteral formulations. Among the most commonly prescribed agents for postoperative pain include ketorolac, ibuprofen, diclofenac, naproxen, and celecoxib. Each of these agents represents a different balance of COX-I and COX-II inhibition and they share the risks and side effects discussed above though in varying degrees. Ketorolac remains one of the most potent NSAIDs used in the perioperative setting, and it is available in oral, intramuscular, and intravenous formulations. Ketorolac is a very useful drug for a variety of acute pain conditions. 10 mg of ketorolac results in the analgesic equivalence of 1,000 mg of acetaminophen [40, 55]. At doses greater than 10 mg, the duration of pain relief may be extended though not the peak analgesic effect. This may be important as side effects including the risks of gastritis, platelet inhibition, and renal damage continue to increase with higher doses though with no significant additional benefit.

Ketamine

Ketamine is an antagonist of the N-methyl-D-aspartate (NMDA) glutamate receptor within the phencyclidine family of medications. The effects of ketamine vary greatly with the dose administered, producing analgesia at low doses and general dissociative anesthesia at high doses. Notable side effects of ketamine include the possibility of dysphoric or psychotic reactions, indirect sympathetic stimulation that can increase blood pressure and heart rate, bronchodilation, increased salivation, and it can impair airway protective reflexes or act as a direct cardiac depressant at high doses. Among the primary benefits of ketamine are its lack of respiratory depressant effects and its profound

and persistent analgesic properties. Multiple studies have demonstrated the analgesic- and opioid-sparing effects of ketamine in forms ranging from a single intraoperative dose, to postoperative bolus or infusions, to ketamine as a component of patient-controlled analgesia (PCA) systems. Bolus intravenous administration of ketamine results in peak plasma concentrations within 1 min, allowing for rapid pain control with subanesthetic doses 0.1–0.4 mg/kg IV or induction of general anesthesia with doses of 1–2 mg/kg IV.

In the trauma patient, ketamine is often considered as an induction agent due to the benefits of its relative hemodynamic stability. It remains underutilized, however, as an analgesic and may be particularly useful in opioid tolerant patients, those with a history of chronic pain, or those on opioid agonist/antagonists or partial agonists such as buprenorphine. Even a single perioperative sub-anesthetic dose, e.g., 0.5 mg iv, decreases postoperative pain, nausea, and morphine consumption for 24 h or longer [56]. As a postoperative analgesic, ketamine can be administered as small IV boluses of 5–20 mg to achieve rapid pain control, typically in the post-anesthesia care unit or intensive care unit. As part of a multimodal analgesic regimen in the trauma patient, ketamine can be initiated as an infusion at ~0.1–0.4 mg/kg/h or ketamine may be added as part of a PCA with a demand dose of 0.01–0.02 mg/kg with a 5–10 min lockout interval. Ketamine may also be administered by oral, sublingual, subcutaneous, or intranasal routes, though these are less commonly performed.

Dysphoric reactions to sub-anesthetic doses are uncommon, but may occur [56]. Any patient receiving ketamine should be monitored for hallucinations or alterations in mood; undesirable reactions can usually be controlled with coadministration of a benzodiazepine. Infrequently, even low dose ketamine may need to be discontinued. Often practitioners are uneasy prescribing ketamine to patients with a history of psychiatric illness, though emerging research suggests that ketamine may benefit patients with depression or those at risk for PTSD [15, 16, 57–59].

Analgesic Adjuncts

In addition to the analgesics above, multiple adjunct medications may contribute to pain relief and can be considered as part of an analgesic regimen in the trauma patient. These include anticonvulsants such as gabapentin or pregabalin, antidepressants such as tricyclics, selective serotonin reuptake inhibitors or selective norepinephrine reuptake inhibitors, and alpha-2 agonists such as clonidine or dexmedetomidine. Evidence of analgesic benefit for each of these exists but does not yet place them in the category of routine pain medications. Although adjuvant medications are listed among the first rung of the WHO ladder, they are not frequently included in the routine management of pain in the trauma population. They may be useful, however, for patients with pain that is difficult to manage despite the first-line treatment with opioids, non-opioid analgesics, or regional techniques. Limiting side effects for anticonvulsants typically include sedation, and for alpha-2 agonists include hypotension, bradycardia, and sedation.

Opioids

Opioid pain medications are the cornerstone of management of moderate to severe pain. Opioids include a diverse collection of endogenous, naturally occurring, and synthetic agents who exert their action through opioid receptor. These receptors include mu, kappa, delta, and sigma receptors as well as multiple subtypes. Their primary sites of action include the dorsal horn of the spinal cord, brainstem, cortex, and some portions of the peripheral nervous system. The therapeutic and side effect profile of specific opioids is determined by the balance of receptor activity. Desired clinical effects such as analgesia, antitussive, and anti-shivering effects must be balanced with undesirable effects such as respiratory depression, nausea, urinary retention, decreased gastrointestinal motility, and constipation. Analgesia, euphoria, and sedation are primarily mediated via mu receptor agonism, where kappa and delta receptor activation results in sedation and weak analgesia.

The category of opioid medications is extremely broad and beyond the scope of this chapter to discuss in full detail, instead, the following section will focus on the guiding principles in the administration of opioids in trauma patients. Opioids possess no anti-inflammatory properties, but instead it increases the pain threshold and modifies the perception of pain. Dull, continuous pain is relieved by opioids more effectively than sharp, intermittent pain, and opioid analgesia is superior when administered prior to the painful stimulus.

The most commonly used opioids in the management of acute pain after trauma include morphine (the prototypical opioid), hydromorphone, and fentanyl through intravenous administration, or the oral administration of morphine, oxycodone, or hydrocodone. Alternative delivery methods are also available including intramuscular (e.g., morphine, hydromorphone), transdermal (fentanyl), and transmucosal (fentanyl, sufentanil). Moderate to severe pain after acute trauma is typically best controlled initially with intravenous agents due to their reliable and rapid action and their utility in those who are unable to take oral agents due to thoracoabdominal trauma. PCA should be considered for any patient requiring intravenous opioids who is alert enough to participate with the PCA. PCA results in improved patient pain control and satisfaction, and although PCA is associated with higher total dose of opioid, it is not associated with increased risks of dangerous side effects such as respiratory depression [60].

PCA systems use a programmable pump to deliver a physician-determined demand dose of opioid, lockout interval, hourly or four-hour maximum dose, and an optional basal infusion rate. Morphine, hydromorphone, and fentanyl remain the most common agents for PCA administration with typical doses of 1 mg, 0.2 mg, and 12.5 mcg q6–10 min for those agents, respectively. The inherent safety mechanism of PCA lies in the fact that a patient who is comfortable or becomes sedated will not push the button to deliver another dose of medication. Family members and visitors must have a clear understanding that the PCA is only to be administered by the patient, as additional PCA demand dosing given to a sedated patient may result in serious respiratory depression. A basal infusion rate or the administration of other oral or intravenous opioids while on PCA is generally not advisable due to this increased risk of unintentional overdose and respiratory depression. A basal infusion can, however, be used to replace a patient's baseline opioid requirement, e.g., in those patients who are on chronic long-term opioids. If it is used, the basal dose should be calculated based on the opioid equivalence of the patient's total daily chronic opioid and then reduced by 30–50 %. For example, a patient on oxycontin 20 mg TID prior to trauma has a total daily dose of 60 mg of oxycodone. This is equivalent to 20 mg of intravenous morphine. A basal rate of 0.5 mg per hour of intravenous morphine would deliver 12 mg/day and replace 60 % of the patient's chronic opioid amount. A similar strategy can be used in reverse when converting a patient from a high dose PCA to oral agents. For example, a patient receiving a cumulative daily dose of 60 mg of intravenous morphine through a PCA has an oral equivalence of 180 mg of oxycodone. 30–50 % of this can be given orally to the patient via extended release opioids, e.g., oxycontin, and the patient can receive as needed dosing for breakthrough.

Among the common IV opioids prescribed for PCA, hydromorphone may have the best pharmacologic profile. It has a similar onset and duration as morphine, though with decreased itching and nausea, and the absence of any significantly active metabolites. Similarly, fentanyl does not have active metabolites and induces less nausea and itching than morphine. However, the rapid redistribution half-life of fentanyl results in a short duration of effect that can make it a frustrating choice for patients as an agent for PCA. Newer PCA systems may allow the delivery of rapid titratable PCA through routes other than intravenous. For example, the Ionsys™ iontophoretic PCA system delivers patient-controlled transdermal demand doses of fentanyl with efficacy and safety similar to that of morphine PCA [61]. The sufentanil NanoTab™ represents another alternative PCA system based on the buccal delivery of the potent opioid sufentanil and shows promise for the control of postoperative pain [62].

Regional Anesthesia in the Trauma Patient

Regional anesthesia represents a potentially invaluable tool for pain management in the trauma patient. Regional or neuraxial techniques can be used as the primary anesthetic for patients with trauma limited the extremities, and it can supplement the anesthetic and postoperative pain control of patients with more extensive injuries including thoracoabdominal trauma. Strong evidence exists for the benefit of regional and neuraxial anesthesia in pain control, patient satisfaction, decreased physiologic stress response to surgery, improved return of bowel function after laparotomy, decreased opioid-related side effects, and possibly improved pulmonary mechanics, and decreased development of chronic pain [9, 63–68].

Nevertheless, there are multiple common concerns that prevent the widespread use of regional and neuraxial anesthesia in trauma patients. Neuraxial techniques may be contraindicated in trauma patients due to factors such as hypovolemia, hemodynamic instability, the presence of increased intracranial pressure, patient refusal or inability to obtain consent, coagulopathy, thrombocytopenia or pharmacologic anticoagulation, patient inability to cooperate with the procedure (e.g., the anesthetized, disoriented, or intubated/sedated patient), spinal trauma, and patients at risk of compartment syndrome, e.g., crush injuries or tibial plateau fractures. Many of these concerns are lessened in consideration of peripheral nerve blockade compared to neuraxial. For example, many peripheral nerve blocks can be safely performed in hypovolemic patients or those patients receiving low-molecular-weight heparin where neuraxial techniques may not be suitable.

The possibility of compartment syndrome remains a common relative contraindication to both neuraxial and regional anesthesia. Nerve blocks could mask the symptoms of compartment syndrome including pain, paresthesia, or paralysis, and a delay in diagnosis could contribute to limb-threatening ischemia and tissue damage. Patients at risk for compartment syndrome including those with tibial plateau fractures, certain fractures of the forearm such as distal radius and combined radius and ulnar fractures, patients with crush injuries or following reperfusion in patients after significant limb ischemia. In these patients, the option of regional anesthesia should be thoroughly discussed with the surgical team. Despite the concern of regional anesthesia masking compartment syndrome, there are actually very few reported cases of this occurring [69, 70]. Llewellyn et al. reported a series of over 10,000 pediatric patients with epidural analgesia. In the series four patients developed compartment syndrome, and in none of those four was the diagnosis masked or delayed by the neuraxial block [69]. Other reports of compartment syndrome in the presence of regional block describe cases in which diagnosis may or may not have been delayed [71–73]. One report blamed the delayed diagnosis of an anterior lower leg compartment syndrome on the presence of a femoral nerve block even though a femoral block would not at all affect sensation in the affected area [70]. It is likely that the paucity of reports of regional anesthesia masking compartment syndrome is primarily due to the avoidance of regional anesthesia in patients with predisposing injuries. This seems advisable, even though the actual risk may be low. Most compartment syndromes develop over the course of multiple hours by which point a single-shot block or catheter technique should provide analgesia but would no longer be functioning at the density of a surgical anesthetic. In patients with analgesic blocks there is often neither complete motor block nor complete anesthesia; therefore, symptoms of pain, worsening motor block, or changes in the sensation of paresthesia may still be detectable if a compartment syndrome were to develop.

Regional Anesthesia in Thoracic Trauma

Regional anesthesia for thoracic trauma typically consists of thoracic epidural anesthesia (TEA), paravertebral blockade (PVB), or intercostal nerve blocks. Patients with acute thoracic or abdominal trauma are often not candidates for neuraxial or regional techniques preoperatively due to surgical urgency, concerns about coagulopathy, hypovolemia, and hemodynamic instability. Therefore, neuraxial techniques are more frequently performed postoperatively or for non-operative thoracic trauma such as rib fractures. Logistical challenges are common in this population; patients may not be able to achieve optimal positioning for block placement. Thoracic trauma frequently requires admission to the intensive care unit, and patients may be sedated or even intubated. This can impair the patient's ability to communicate if they experience pain or paresthesia during placement. Furthermore, the use of low-molecular-weight heparins is common in these patients and may prevent the use of neuraxial techniques.

Regional Anesthesia for Rib Fractures

Rib fractures are a common occurrence in major trauma with an estimated incidence as high as 10–16 % [74, 75]. Pain following multiple rib fractures can be severe and furthermore may contribute to increased morbidity. Pain may impair patients' ability to breathe resulting in atelectasis, pneumonia, ICU care, and respiratory failure. Patients of advanced age, those with concomitant pulmonary contusions, and those with multiple and bilateral rib fractures are at increased risk of needing ICU care, mechanical ventilation, and having prolonged ICU and hospital length of stay, pneumonia, pulmonary embolism, and mortality [74, 75].

A variety of analgesic techniques have been used for the management of rib fractures including NSAIDs, opioids, and regional anesthesia including intercostal nerve blocks, PVB, and TEA. Regional techniques tend to provide superior pain relief with fewer side effects, though by their nature they are invasive and carry certain risk. Any regional technique requires careful placement by a skilled provider.

TEA utilizing local anesthetic with opioid is thought to provide the best pain relief for multiple rib fractures. Patients of advanced age, those with multiple fractures or pulmonary contusion may demonstrate the most benefit from thoracic regional anesthesia, and TEA may reduce morbidity or even mortality [74, 76, 77]. TEA provides bilateral segmental analgesia, and TEA catheters can be maintained for days. This can spare the use of opioids and NSAIDs and minimizing their associated side effects of respiratory depression, constipation, gastritis, nephrotoxicity, etc. For best results, the epidural should be placed at a level that corresponds to approximately the middle of multiple fractures. Potential complications of TEA include hypotension due to sympathetic blockade, bradycardia from blockade of cardiac accelerator fibers, dural puncture, headache, systemic local anesthetic toxicity, epidural abscess, meningitis, epidural hematoma, and direct spinal cord injury.

Paravertebral and intercostal nerve blocks may be an alternative to TEA in patients who refuse TEA or in whom TEA is contraindicated. Both techniques provide dermatomal–segmental, unilateral analgesia. PVB may achieve some degree of cepahalocaudal spread to cover more than one rib, where intercostal nerve block is limited to a single rib or dermatomal segment. Because of this limited or absent spread, multiple injections are typically required for multiple rib fracture. Paravertebral or intercostal catheters may be inserted to provide continuous analgesia, though the success of these catheters is lower than TEA and multiple catheters may be required for bilateral or multilevel fractures. Single-shot PVB or intercostal nerve blocks have a duration of effect of up to 12–16 h depending on the local anesthetic utilized. Risks of these techniques include pneumothorax, infection, neuraxial spread of local anesthetic resulting in unintentional epidural or intrathecal blockade, and local anesthetic toxicity. Local anesthetic absorption is high for PVB and intercostal injection, and the risks may be compounded by the need for multiple injections at different levels and serial injections if catheters are unused or ineffective.

Regional Anesthesia for Thoracic Surgery in Trauma

Thoracotomy and video-assisted thoracoscopic surgery (VATS) are associated with significant postoperative pain that can impede recovery. Pain after thoracic surgery may prevent adequate respiration leading to prolonged intubation, atelectasis, infection, and delayed ambulation, and unmanaged pain may impair recovery. In addition, both thoracotomy and VATS present a high risk of the development of chronic pain in approximately 20–60 % of patients [9].

Regional anesthesia and particularly TEA has long been considered the "gold standard" for analgesia after thoracotomy. Benefits are purported to include not only improved analgesia and decreased side effects compared to systemic opioids and non-opioid analgesics but also improved postoperative pulmonary function, oxygen saturation, FVC, FEV1, and shorter duration of intubation. In addition, the use of TEA may decrease the risk of chronic post-thoracotomy or post-VATS pain [9]. These benefits have not been specifically studied in the trauma patient, where the majority of TEA and PVB would be performed postoperatively. Nevertheless, it is likely that regional anesthesia confers benefit in that scenario as well.

The technique of performing a thoracic epidural should be within the skillset of every anesthesiologist. As such the details of placing a thoracic epidural will not be exhaustively discussed in this chapter. Placement of a thoracic epidural catheter is often easier via a paramedian approach compared to midline due to the steep angulation and long overlap of the thoracic spinous processes. Infusion of local anesthetic in combination with an epidural opioid, such as fentanyl or hydromorphone, results in superior analgesia than either alone. The addition of neuraxial opioids is typically well tolerated, though they can cause significant respiratory depression. This requires close monitoring and careful consideration of whether the patient should receive other respiratory depressants such as parenteral or oral narcotics. For the patient whose pain is incompletely controlled with epidural local anesthetic and opioids, a wise strategy may be to continue the epidural with local anesthetic alone and provide the patient with alternative opioids as necessary, e.g., i.v. PCA.

Recent systematic reviews have suggested that continuous PVB may be equivalent to TEA with respect to pain control and pulmonary function, though with decreased risk of adverse effects such as hypotension [30, 31, 77]. In addition, although anticoagulation and coagulopathy are still relative contraindications for PVB, the risk is less than for TEA. There have been multiple case series of PVB performed in anticoagulated patients without report of major complications [78, 79]. In comparison with rib fractures, which often occur at multiple levels and bilaterally, a unilateral thoracotomy typically involves only a few adjacent dermatomal segments. Therefore a single PVB catheter can provide successful analgesia post-thoracotomy. In addition, a PVB catheter can be inserted in an anesthetized patient more safely than TEA. In trauma patients, where preoperative insertion may not be feasible, intraoperative insertion under general anesthesia may be considered at the conclusion of surgery prior to emergence. The insertion site should be approximately 1–2 levels below the thoracotomy incision. The placement of PVB injections and catheters requires significant experience and technical skill. PVB is not inherently difficult to perform, but it requires a tactile sense to perform that is typically gained only through practice. For that reason, it is thought to be an easy block once mastered but difficult to teach and difficult to initially learn.

Anatomically the paravertebral space is a triangular space through which the spinal nerves travel at each dermatomal segment. It is bounded anteriorly by the parietal pleura in the thoracic region or iliopsoas in lumbar region, medially by the vertebral body or disc, and posteriorly by the transverse process. PVB results in unilateral, segmental–dermatomal anesthesia of a similar quality to epidural blockade though there may be cephalocaudal spread of the block 1–2 dermatomal segments. PVB is most frequently performed based on anatomic landmarks though ultrasound-guided techniques have been described. Classically, the patient is positioned sitting with the chin to the chest and spine as rounded as possible. The spinous processes of the chosen levels are carefully identified by palpation, and a point is measured lateral to the midline of the spinous process at the superior border. This point is measured 2.5 cm lateral in the high to mid thoracic region or 2 cm lateral in the low thoracic or lumbar region. A 20–22 g Tuohy needle for single-shot PVB or 18 g Tuohy for catheter PVB is then advanced at this point perpendicular in all planes with the goal of contacting transverse process (TP). The depth of the TP will vary based on patient habitus and level along the spine; typically it ranges from 3 to 5 cm, deepest in the cervical, high thoracic, and lumbar regions and shallowest in the mid thoracic region. If the TP is not contacted at 4 cm, the needle should be redirected cephalad or caudad to seek the TP at the same depth. If it is still not contacted the needle may be advanced to 0.5 cm increments, fanning cephalad and caudad, with each advancement until the TP is found. The goal is very careful advancement to find the transverse process as insertion of the needle too deep may result in pneumothorax. Care must be taken as well to avoid directing the needle medially as this may result in unintentional epidural or intrathecal injection with a high neuraxial block.

Once the TP is contacted the needle is redirected either cephalad or caudad to walk-off the TP and inserted 1 cm further. A subtle fascial pop may be appreciated as the needle pierces the costotransverse ligament. Aspiration should be performed to assess the presence of blood, CSF, or air, and then local anesthetic is slowly injected. Injection in the paravertebral space offers little resistance, similar to the sensation of injection into the epidural space. Loss of resistance techniques have been described for PVB; however, this loss is not as reliable as with epidural placement as the costotransverse does not provide the same resistance as the ligamentum flavum. 3–6 mL of a long-acting local anesthetic with epinephrine is injected at each level blocked, e.g., ropivacaine 0.5 % with epinephrine 2.5 mcg/mL. For continuous blocks, a catheter is threaded through the 18 g Tuohy and inserted 2–5 cm into the paravertebral space. Aspiration through the catheter and a test dose should be administered prior to use, and then an infusion may be started at 4–10 mL/h for postoperative pain relief typically with a low dose local anesthetic such as ropivacaine 0.2 %.

Thoracolumbar Epidurals for Abdominal Surgery in Trauma

The benefits of low thoracic epidural (LTEA) or high lumbar epidurals for abdominal surgery have been well documented. Their use has been associated with superior pain control, improvements in pulmonary outcome, and when utilized in a multimodal enhanced recovery program including early nutrition and ambulation, LTEA is associated with decreased earlier return of bowel function and shorter hospital stay [23, 26, 27, 29, 65, 67, 68, 80]. In addition, the neurohumoral response to pain is suppressed with the use of epidural analgesia, and this may have favorable physiologic effects on inflammation and decreased hypertension and tachycardia postoperatively.

Similar to thoracic trauma, the nature of those patients with trauma that require laparotomy typically precludes the preoperative placement of an epidural in those patients. Postoperative placement in a patient with a fresh laparotomy incision is challenging, and placement in a lateral position may be more successful than upright. LTEA at a T10 level can provide analgesia to nearly the whole abdomen and should not result in any significant lower extremity motor block. Ambulation with assistance should be possible after confirmation of normal lower extremity sensorimotor function.

Peripheral Nerve Blocks to the Abdomen

PVB for Abdominal Surgery

PVB as discussed previously provides unilateral segmental–dermatomal anesthesia of a comparable quality to epidural anesthesia. It is most commonly performed at the high to mid thoracic level thoracotomy or rib fractures in the trauma population or breast surgery in the general population. However, PVB can also be utilized to provide anesthesia or analgesia to the abdomen through low thoracic and lumbar PVB. As with neuraxial anesthesia, in the trauma patient this technique would most likely be performed for postoperative analgesia. In the lumbar region there is less cephalocaudal spread between adjacent dermatomal segments. Therefore blockade must be performed at each individual level. In addition, there may be less benefit from a single continuous PVB due to limitation of its effect to a single dermatome. PVB in abdominal surgery is most beneficial for lateral incisions, as a midline incision requires bilateral multilevel PVB. If lumbar PVBs are performed one should confirm normal quadriceps motor function prior to ambulation. PVB at L2 or lower will affect the lumbar plexus result in lower extremity block.

Transversus Abdominis Plane and Rectus Sheath Blocks

The somatic innervation of the anterior abdomen is derived from the termination of the T7–T11 intercostal nerves, the T12 subcostal nerve, and the L1 ilioinguinal/iliohypogastric nerves. These nerves travel in the fascial plane just deep to the internal oblique muscles and superficial to the transversus abdominis. The most anterior continuation of the T7–T12 nerve roots pierce the peritoneal side of the rectus sheath and provide innervation to the midline of the abdomen both superior and inferior to the umbilicus

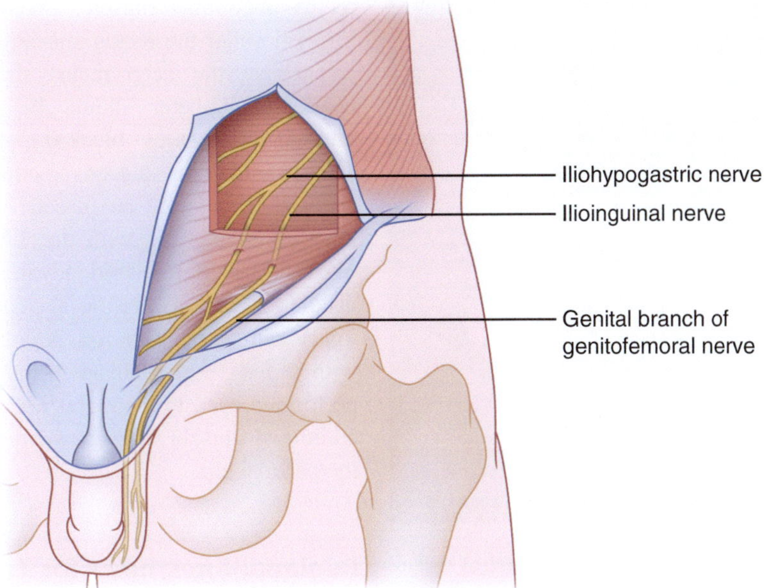

Fig. 6.1 Muscle layers and nerves of the anterior abdomen. *EOM* the external oblique muscle, *IOM* the internal oblique muscle, *TAM* the transverse abdominal muscle, *IH* the iliohypogastric nerve, *IL* the ilioinguinal nerve. Reprinted from [81]. With kind permission from Springer Science and Business Media

(Fig. 6.1). Blockade of these nerves can be performed either in the transversus abdominis plane or within the rectus sheath in order to achieve analgesia to the lower and lateral abdomen or the midline, respectively.

In contrast to neuraxial techniques, TAP and rectus sheath blocks do not provide the same quality of analgesia, nor visceral analgesia, and they provide only unilateral blockade. Nevertheless, these blocks have characteristics that may be very appealing in the trauma patient. They do not result in any significant sympathetic blockade or hypotension and they may be more easily performed postoperatively than LTEA or PVB in patients with abdominal incisions. TAP and rectus sheath blocks are performed with the patient in a supine position compared with the lateral or sitting position for PVB or LTEA. In addition, TAP and rectus sheath blocks can be considered in many patients in whom neuraxial analgesia may be contraindicated, such as those systemic infections, patients with spinal trauma, hypovolemia, or those on prophylactic low-molecular-weight heparins.

The TAP block is typically performed to provide unilateral analgesia to the anterior abdomen below the umbilicus, and it is commonly used for analgesia for lower abdominal incisions. TAP blocks should be performed bilaterally to provide analgesia for either a midline incision or a horizontal incision that crosses midline. This block can be performed with ultrasound by identification of the external oblique, internal oblique, and transversus abdominis muscles (Fig. 6.2). Local anesthetic is injected just deep to the internal oblique within the transversus abdominis plane. Catheters may be placed for continuous blockade. Care must be taken with this block to confidently identify the muscle layers, as advancing the needle too deep may result in peritoneal puncture or bowel injury. For the most reliable result, the block should be performed as posteriorly as possible, i.e., along the lateral abdominal wall between the iliac crest and 12th rib. This allows local to reach the nerves before they form the lateral cutaneous nerves that ascend through the oblique muscles and to the abdominal wall.

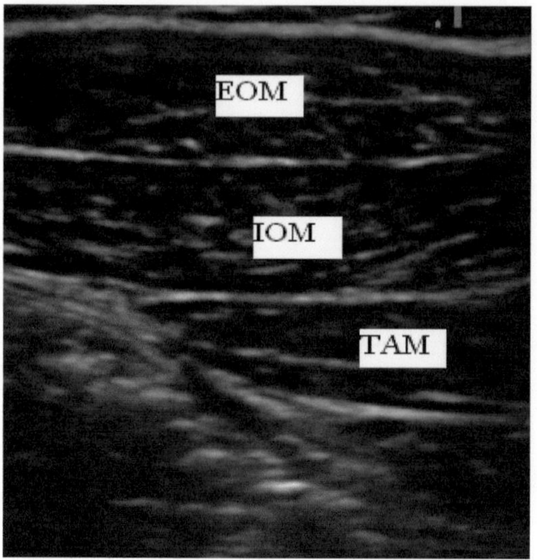

Fig. 6.2 Ultrasound image showing the layers of abdominal muscles. *EOM* the external oblique muscle, *IOM* the internal oblique muscle, *TAM* the transverse abdominal muscle. Reprinted from [81]. With kind permission from Springer Science and Business Media

The TAP block will not provide analgesia to midline of the abdomen above the umbilicus. The T7–T11 intercostal nerves will not be blocked in the transversus abdominis plane below the T12 level as with the above-discussed TAP block. However the midline of the abdomen and the area above the rectus muscles is innervated when the termination of those nerves ascends through the rectus sheath and through the rectus muscles. The midline of the abdomen can therefore be anesthetized by instilling local anesthetic into the deep portion of the rectus sheath.

Rectus sheath block has great potential for use in patients with midline laparotomy incisions and can provide analgesia to the midline above and below the umbilicus. As mentioned it can be utilized in many patients for whom epidural analgesia is contraindicated or not feasible. The block can be most safely performed with ultrasound or under direct vision placed by the surgeon intraoperatively. Bilateral rectus sheath blocks must be performed to cover a midline incision. On ultrasound, the rectus muscles are identified and needle is passed through the superficial aspect of the rectus sheath and the

rectus abdominis muscle. Local anesthetic is injected under the rectus muscle but within and just above the deep rectus sheath. For best results, a catheter should be considered to provide continuous blockade. Rectus sheath catheters may be placed postoperatively with ultrasound, or may be placed by the surgeon intraoperatively. As with the TAP block, care must be taken to avoid advancing the block needle too deep as peritoneal puncture or bowel injury can occur. This risk is potentially higher with rectus sheath blockade because the block is performed deep to the rectus abdominis with no additional muscle layer between the needle and the peritoneum.

Regional Anesthesia for Trauma to the Extremities

Regional anesthesia for trauma to the extremities can provide significant patient benefit through improved pain control, decreased opioid requirements, and in many cases allowing the avoidance of general anesthesia for the treatment of extremity trauma. The use of regional anesthesia in extremity trauma may be limited by some common concerns such as the possibility of it masking a compartment syndrome, the desire for the surgeon to monitor postoperative nerve function, or the presence of associated injuries which make peripheral blockade impractical.

Ultrasound-Guided Versus Nerve Stimulator-Guided Regional Anesthesia

The utilization of ultrasound guidance for the performance of peripheral nerve blocks has dramatically expanded over the last decade and may soon become the standard of care. Ultrasound guidance in experienced hands has the potential benefit of decreasing the risks of regional anesthesia such as intravascular or intraneural injection or needle damage to adjacent structures. In addition it has the potential to improve the efficacy of peripheral nerve blocks by allowing for direct visualization of complete perineural local anesthetic spread.

In addition to these general advantages, ultrasound allows peripheral nerve blockade without nerve stimulation and therefore muscle stimulation. This is a key advantage in the use of ultrasound in trauma and postoperative blocks. Nerve stimulation caused the painful movement of the injured extremity, and avoiding this improves patient satisfaction and often ease of placement. As with any tool however, the use of ultrasound is only as good as the operator, and requires skill, practice, and anatomic knowledge to be used safely and successfully.

Neuraxial Anesthesia for Lower Extremity Trauma

Spinal and lumbar epidural anesthesia and analgesia can be valuable tools in the management of patients with lower extremity trauma patient. However, as with LTEA for coverage of the abdomen, neuraxial anesthesia is underutilized in patients with lower extremity trauma. The most common neuraxial technique performed for lower extremity trauma is a single-shot spinal anesthetic for surgical stabilization of acute hip fractures. Neuraxial anesthesia for hip fracture repair has previously been associated with decreased intraoperative bleeding and postoperative deep venous thrombosis, though the latter benefit may be less significant in the age of aggressive prophylaxis with low-molecular-weight heparins. Regional anesthesia is associated with less postoperative delirium though long-term benefits remain unproven [64].

A neuraxial technique may be appropriate for the primary anesthetic for other simple fracture repairs. With more complicated trauma however, surgical duration, difficulty in patient positioning, risk of significant bleeding or instability, or the need for aggressive DVT prophylaxis can make neuraxial techniques impractical.

Single-Shot Peripheral Nerve Blocks Versus Peripheral Nerve Catheters

Single-shot peripheral nerve blocks provide rapid analgesia but only up to 24 h in duration with long-acting local anesthetics. In order to provide more enduring analgesia, continuous peripheral nerve catheters can be placed near the target nerve to deliver a continuous infusion of local anesthetic and extend the duration of analgesia for days. Initial use of continuous peripheral nerve blockade was limited to the inpatient population, but increasingly patients are being sent home with peripheral nerve catheters. Case series have demonstrated that patients are able to manage and remove their catheters at home with the need to return to care. With adequate instruction and telephone access to health care providers, patients can safely manage and remove continuous peripheral nerve catheters at home [82].

The duration of continuous peripheral nerve blocks is limited primarily by the risk of infection, and the tendency of catheters to dislodge and become ineffective. Both of these are more common as the duration of catheter increases. Most clinicians remove catheters after approximately 3–7 days, though case series have been published with duration greater than 2 weeks [83]. Additional challenges with peripheral nerve catheters include more difficult placement, possibility of malpositioning resulting in failure or complication, and the larger needle used for placement may increase the severity of injury to collateral structures if it were to occur. There may be circumstances where a prolonged block may not be desirable, for example, if prolonged motor block would impair physical therapy. When any nerve block is to be performed in trauma, consideration should be made whether a continuous catheter may be superior. The longer duration of analgesia may improve pain control and allow the decrease in opioid and other pain medications.

Regional Anesthesia for the Upper Extremity

Regional anesthesia for the upper extremity typically involves blockade of the brachial plexus or occasionally blockade of individual terminal nerves. Brachial plexis blockade can be accomplished through the interscalene approach for shoulder and proximal humerus, the supraclavicular or infraclavicular approaches for the mid-humerus to the hand, or the axillary approach for the distal humerus through the hand. In addition, individual nerves can be blocked at the elbow forearm or wrist. Only key upper extremity blocks will be reviewed.

Interscalene Brachial Plexus Block

Background and Indications

The interscalene block targets the brachial plexus at the level of the roots and trunks providing anesthesia to the shoulder and proximal humerus. The distal clavicle may be variably covered as well, and the interscalene block can be supplemented with a superficial cervical plexus block to improve coverage of that area. The interscalene block will not reliably cover the distal arm, specifically the medial distal arm or ulnar distribution and those areas whose innervation is derived from the C8 or T1 nerve roots. In addition the interscalene block and all brachial plexus blocks will not cover the axilla or the proximal/medial upper arm. This area is innervated by the intercostobrachial nerve, which is derived from the T2 nerve root and not the brachial plexus.

Risks and Contraindications

Risks of the interscalene block include neuraxial spread, vascular injection or injury to the vertebral and carotid arteries or the internal or external jugular veins, phrenic blockade or damage, and pneumothorax. Some anesthesiologists have reported that a targeted, small volume (less than 10 mL) interscalene block can be successfully performed without resulting in phrenic blockade.

However, larger volume injections result in nearly universal unilateral phrenic blockade. Therefore, the interscalene block is contraindicated in patients with contralateral phrenic palsy, contralateral pneumonectomy, or those with significant baseline respiratory insufficiency. From a practical standpoint, interscalene block may not be feasible in many trauma patients due to the frequent presence of a rigid cervical collar preventing adequate access to the neck.

Performing the Block

The roots/trunks of the brachial plexus can be reliably identified on ultrasound by scanning proximally with a 25–50 mm linear probe from a supraclavicular view or scanning posteriorly from a view of the carotid and internal jugular vein at the level of the cricoid cartilage. The roots/trunks typically appear as hypoechoic circles resembling a "stoplight" between the anterior and middle scalene muscles and deep/posterior to the posterior border of sternocleidomastoid (Fig. 6.3). Single-shot block or placement of a catheter can be accomplished from an in-plane posterior approach or out-of-plane superior approach. The needle entry site for the out-of-plane superior approach often passes through or near the external jugular vessel.

Supraclavicular Brachial Plexus Block

Background and Indications

The supraclavicular brachial plexus block has gained in popularity with the advent of ultrasound guidance as possibly the most reliable and broadly applicable upper extremity block. Previously nerve stimulator and landmark approaches to the supraclavicular brachial plexus had unacceptably high rates of pneumothorax and arterial puncture in all but the most experienced hands. The skilled use of ultrasound, however, can drastically reduce those risks. Supraclavicular brachial plexus blockade results in anesthesia to the entire upper extremity from approximately mid-humerus down. In contrast to the interscalene block it will cover the hand and

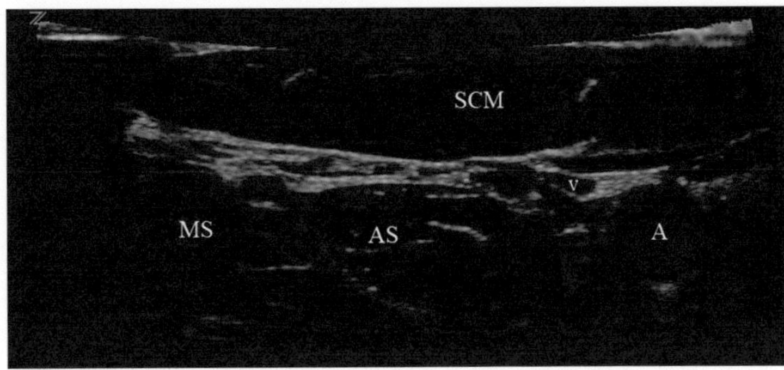

Fig. 6.3 Ultrasonographic appearance of the interscalene and cervical paravertebral brachial plexus (*A* carotid artery, *AS* anterior scalene muscle, *MS* middle scalene muscle, *SCM* sternocleidomastoid muscle, *V* internal jugular vein). Reprinted from [81]. With kind permission from Springer Science and Business Media

medial/ulnar aspects of the upper extremity, though it will not cover the shoulder. As with all brachial plexus blocks, the supraclavicular block will not cover the axilla or proximal medial upper arm in the intercostobrachial distribution. The intercostobrachial nerve should be separately blocked if necessary and is discussed below.

Risks and Contraindications

The most common risks of the supraclavicular block include, not surprisingly, pneumothorax and intravascular injection into the subclavian artery. In addition, the risk of phrenic nerve block is less than with interscalene block but may still be as high as 20–40 %. In addition to the subclavian artery, the path of the needle to the plexus should be examined carefully for the presence of intervening vascular structures. For example, the suprascapular or dorsal scapular arteries may crossover the brachial plexus at this level and may be in the needle path to the plexus. The hypoechoic inferior belly of omohyoid is frequently in view and may be confused as a vessel, though it can be distinguished by the fact that it is neither pulsatile nor compressible. Color Doppler can help identify the presence of intervening vessels. Similar to the interscalene block, the use of the supraclavicular block in trauma is often limited by the presence of a cervical collar.

Performing the Block

The supraclavicular block targets the brachial plexus at the level of the anterior and posterior

divisions, though this distinction is difficult to identify on ultrasound. To find the plexus on ultrasound, a 25–50 mm linear probe is placed along and just posterior to the clavicle at approximately its middle third (Fig. 6.4). Here the subclavian artery can be identified and the plexus will appear as a mix of hyper- and hypoechoic "cluster of grapes" along the posterolateral border of the artery. Deep to the plexus and the artery are the pleura and the first rib. These structures must be confidently identified as both may appear as hyperechoic lines with acoustic shadow behind them. Typically the first rib will appear as a brighter line with a darker shadow behind where the pleura will appear slightly less distinct with a hazy shadow behind it that slides with respiration (lung). The block should be performed from a posterolateral in-plane approach with a view where first rib is deep to the plexus and artery. This adds an additional level of safety that if the needle is inadvertently advanced too deep, it will contact rib instead of piercing pleura. Single-shot or catheter techniques can be used. The "corner pocket" of the plexus, i.e., the portion deep to the artery should be targeted first. Missing this portion of the plexus may result in ulnar sparing or inadequate blockade of the distal/medial hand and forearm. If a catheter is to be placed, its placement should be targeted based on the patients' needs. For example, a patient with injury to the medial side of the forearm or hand should have the catheter placed in the "corner pocket" for the best continuous block result.

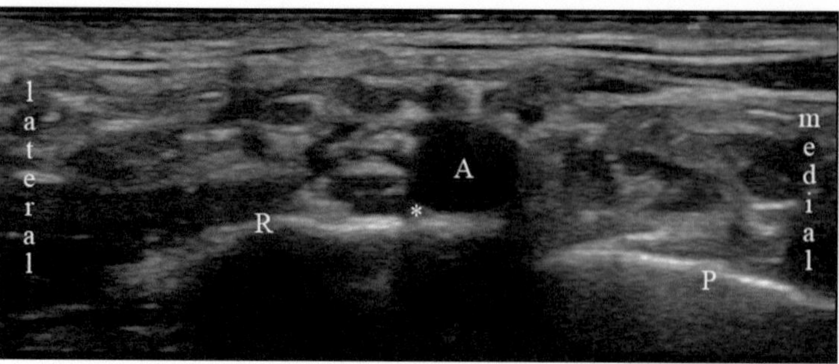

Fig. 6.4 Ultrasonographic appearance of the supraclavicular brachial plexus (*A* subclavian artery, *P* pleura, *R* first rib, *asterisk* indicates target for "corner pocket"). Reprinted from [81]. With kind permission from Springer Science and Business Media

Infraclavicular Brachial Plexus Block

Background and Indications

The infraclavicular block provides a very similar distribution of analgesia as the supraclavicular block, though targeting the plexus at the level of the posterior, medial, and lateral cords. It is more difficult to perform with ultrasound than with supraclavicular block and perhaps slightly less reliable in the blockade of the entire arm. The infraclavicular block possesses two distinct advantages when compared to the supraclavicular block, however. The risk of phrenic block is minimal with an infraclavicular approach, extending its use to those with significant respiratory insufficiency or contralateral phrenic or pulmonary pathology. In addition, the infraclavicular block can be performed in patients with a cervical collar in place. This last fact greatly extends the utility of the infraclavicular block in patients with acute trauma. Furthermore, the risk or pneumothorax is lower with an infraclavicular approach, though vascular puncture and intravascular injection remain concerns.

Risks and Contraindications

The primary risks with infraclavicular block include intravascular injection and pneumothorax. Both of these can be minimized by careful needle visualization. In addition, performing the block more laterally can decrease the risk of pneumothorax. As mentioned, there is no significant risk of phrenic nerve block with the infraclavicular approach.

Performing the Block

With ultrasound a small curvilinear probe or a 25 mm linear probe is placed inferior to the clavicle at approximately its lateral third and oriented in a parasagittal plane. The pectoralis major and minor muscles will be identified, with the subclavian/axillary artery deep to them. Superficial and inferior to the artery will be subclavian/axillary vein (Fig. 6.5). This vein may be compressed by the ultrasound probe and if not visualized one should release pressure on the probe to allow the vein to fill and become apparent. The lateral, posterior, and medial cords of the plexus can be seen surrounding the artery. The lateral cord will be superolateral to the artery, the posterior cord will be deep to the artery, and the medial cord will be inferomedial to the artery often between the vein and artery.

The nerve block needle should be inserted in plane from the superior side of the probe just below the clavicle and advanced with the goal of placing the tip along the posterior border of the artery from the superior side. The steep angle of approach of the needle that is required for this block can make visualization of the needle and tip challenging. To aid in visualization, sterile saline may be connected to the nerve block needle. Small injections of saline as the needle is being advanced can be used to identify a "puff" of tissue movement that indicates the location of the needle tip. Injection at the point immediately behind the deep side of the artery will allow for a "crescent" of local anesthetic to spread around from the posterior aspect of the artery to the medial and lateral aspects covering those cords. Additional local can be injected around the lateral

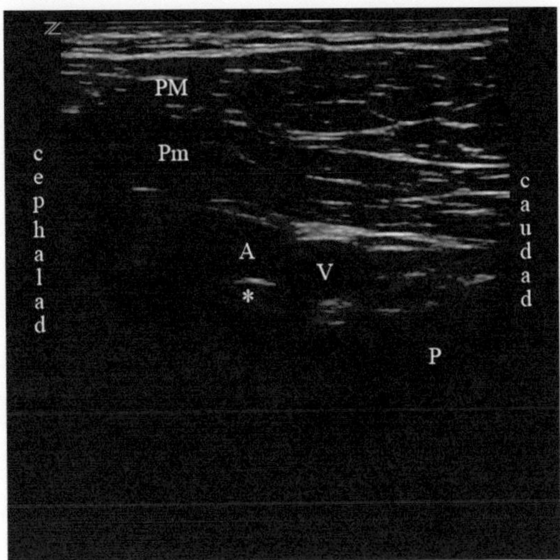

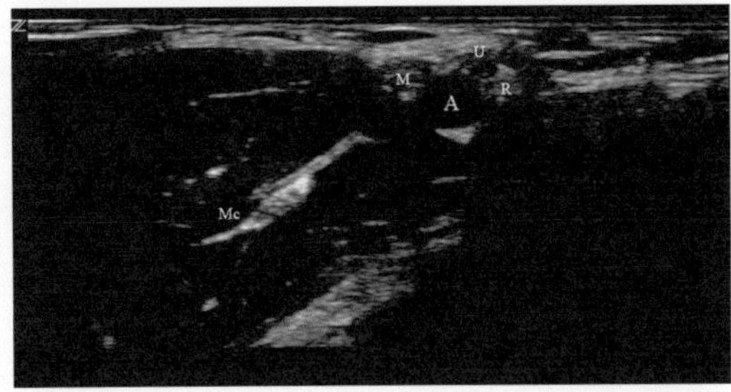

Fig. 6.6 Ultrasonographic appearance of the axillary brachial plexus (*A* axillary artery, *M* median nerve, *Mc* musculocutaneous nerve, *R* radial nerve, *U* ulnar nerve). Reprinted from [81]. With kind permission from Springer Science and Business Media

Fig. 6.5 Ultrasonographic appearance of the infraclavicular brachial plexus (*A* axillary artery, *P* pleura, *PM* pectoralis major muscle, *Pm* pectoralis minor muscle, *V* axillary vein, *asterisk* indicates target). Reprinted from [81]. With kind permission from Springer Science and Business Media

cord as the needle is being withdrawn. If the "crescent" does not appear to adequately cover the medial cord, the needle can be advanced to the medial side alone the superficial/anterior border of the artery to the medial side. Care must be taken with this approach, however, due to the frequent presence of intervening veins. If a catheter is to be placed, it is typically best situated with the tip near the posterior cord behind the deep portion of the artery.

Axillary Block

It is the opinion of this author that the clinical utility of the axillary block has been diminished to near irrelevance in the era of ultrasound-guided brachial plexus blocks at the supraclavicular or infraclavicular level. The axillary block targets the radial, ulnar, and median nerves as they surround the axillary artery, and it must be supplemented with a separate block of the musculocutaneous nerve to provide sensory anesthesia of the ventral forearm. The axillary block does have the advantages compared to

supraclavicular and infraclavicular blocks of having no risk of pneumothorax or phrenic blockade. However, it is an unsuitable location for the placement of a catheter due to axillary hair, increased risk of infection, and the frequent dislodgment of axillary nerve block catheters from movement of the arm. To perform the axillary block with ultrasound, the axillary artery can be identified with the radial, median, and ulnar nerves surrounding the artery (Fig. 6.6). Local anesthetic is injected perivascularly with best results obtained when the individual nerves can also be identified and targeted or when perivascular injection is as proximal along the as. The musculocutaneous nerve can be identified in the fascial plane between biceps and coracobrachialis.

Intercostobrachial and Medial Brachial Cutaneous Nerve Blocks

Background and Indications
The entire sensory and motor innervation of the upper extremity is derived from the brachial plexus with the exception of the axilla and medial upper arm. The intercostobrachial and medial brachial cutaneous nerves supply the sensory innervation of this area. The former of these is derived primarily from the T2 nerve root and the latter has contributions from T1 and T2. The T2 nerve root is not a component of the brachial plexus and therefore the axilla and

medial upper arm are not anesthetized with any of the brachial plexus blocks. The intercosto-brachial and medial brachial cutaneous nerves should be blocked in combination with the brachial plexus whenever a surgical incision may extend into the region of the medial upper arm. In addition, for any circumstance where a brachial plexus block will be utilized as the primary anesthetic for a procedure and an upper arm tourniquet will be used, these nerves should be blocked to cover tourniquet pain.

Risks and Contraindications

The intercostobrachial and medial brachial cutaneous field blocks carry no specific risks other than standard risks of any field block such as infection, inadvertent intravascular injection, and local anesthetic toxicity.

Performing the Block

The intercostobrachial and medial brachial cutaneous nerves can be covered with two sub-cutaneous field blocks. The intercostobrachial nerve is covered by a subcutaneous field block across the proximal axilla and is typically sufficient to cover upper arm tourniquet pain. The medial brachial cutaneous nerve can be blocked by an additional subcutaneous field block across the medial upper arm at the level of the mid-humerus.

Regional Anesthesia for the Lower Extremity

Peripheral regional anesthesia for the lower extremity can be performed via lumbar plexus block, femoral nerve block, saphenous nerve block, proximal sciatic nerve block, distal, i.e., popliteal sciatic nerve block, and ankle block. Unfortunately, the innervation of the lower extremity does not provide as convenient a distribution of anesthesia as the upper extremity. That is, no single peripheral block will provide anesthesia to the entire lower extremity. Only key lower extremity blocks will be reviewed.

Lumbar Plexus Block

Background and Indications

The lumbar plexus is formed from the nerve roots of L2–4 as they exit the foramina of the lumbar vertebrae and enter the fascial plane of the iliopsoas muscle. The terminal nerves derived from the lumbar plexus include the lateral femoral cutaneous, femoral, genitofemoral, and obturator nerves. Together these provide innervation to the lateral, anterior, and medial upper leg as well as the skin of the medial lower leg. The lumbar plexus block can be useful for trauma involving the upper leg though must be combined with a sciatic nerve block to provide complete anesthesia to the leg. Lumbar plexus block can provide reliable postoperative analgesia for surgery on the hip or femur, but it is typically insufficient as a sole anesthetic.

Risks and Contraindications

Lumbar plexus block carries additional utility compared to the more commonly performed femoral block in that it additionally covers the lateral femoral cutaneous, genitofemoral, and obturator nerves. However, it carries additional risk as well. Needle trauma can result in significant retroperitoneal bleeding, and therefore lumbar plexus blockade is contraindicated in patients on anticoagulation, or those with coagulopathy or thrombocytopenia. In addition there are risks of epidural spread, or damage to abdominal viscera including bowel, kidneys, and major vessels. Patients should be warned to expect quadriceps weakness after the block and should not attempt ambulation without assistance until full recovery of motor function.

Performing the Block

Although ultrasound-guided techniques for lumbar plexus blockade have been described, it remains a technique largely based on anatomic landmarks and nerve stimulation. The patient is placed in a lateral decubitus position with the hip and knees partially flexed. The iliac crest is identified as a landmark for the L4 vertebra. The spinous processes are carefully palpated to

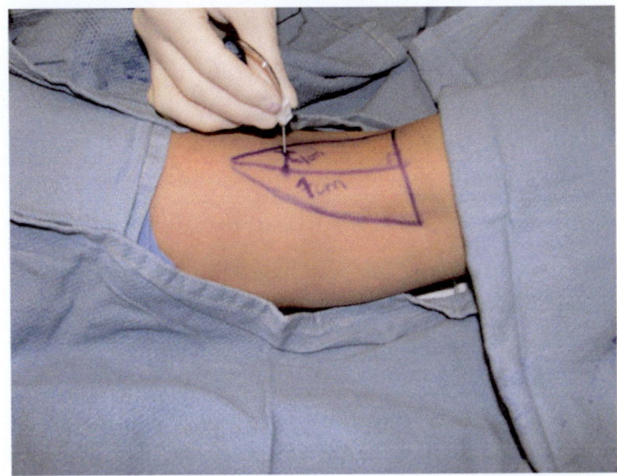

Fig. 6.7 Lumbar plexus nerve block. The intercristal line (*dashed line*) is identified using the posterior iliac crest. The needle insertion site is 4–5 cm from midline and is approximately as lateral as the patient's posterior superior iliac spine (PSIS). Reprinted from [81]. With kind permission from Springer Science and Business Media

identify midline, and a mark is made at the level of L4 4 cm lateral to midline at the level of the iliac crests. This mark should correspond to the intersection of the transverse line that connects the iliac crests, and a line parallel to the midline at the level of the posterior superior iliac spine (Fig. 6.7). After sterile prep a 10 cm insulated needle is inserted perpendicular in all planes with a nerve stimulator attached. At 1–4 cm, stimulation of the paraspinous muscles may be seen, at approximately 4 cm transverse process may be contacted and may need to be redirected to pass the transverse process either cephalad or caudad. Deep to the transverse process at approximately 5–7 cm extension of the quadriceps is sought with nerve stimulation at 0.5–1 mA and local anesthetic is injected. A catheter may also be placed for continuous lumbar plexus block. If extension of the quadriceps is not initially found, stimulation of other muscle groups may provide clues for redirecting the needle. Contraction of the hamstrings results from stimulation of the sciatic nerve via the sacral plexus, and the needle should be redirected cephalad or the insertion site should be moved one level cephalad. Flexion at the hip indicates contraction of iliopsoas from direct muscle stimulation and typically results from needle placement too deep. If the needle is inserted beyond 8 cm with no

twitch response, care must be taken to reassess landmarks and the insertion site and trajectory. Further advancement may result in injury to abdominal viscera.

Femoral Nerve Block and "3-in-1 Block"

Background and Indications

The femoral nerve block is one of the most commonly performed blocks and provides anesthesia to the anterior upper leg including the anterior two-thirds of the knee and the medial lower leg via the saphenous nerve. The femoral nerve block is most commonly utilized for in the non-trauma patient for total knee arthroplasty, though in the trauma population it can be useful for any procedure involving the anterior upper leg. This can include patellar fractures, and it can be a component of analgesia for above or below the knee amputations. A femoral nerve block will not cover the lateral (lateral femoral cutaneous nerve) or medial (obturator nerve) upper leg. The "3-in-1" block is a modified femoral nerve block that attempts to cover those as well by using a large volume of local anesthetic-directed cephalad underneath the fascia iliaca to spread retrograde to the lumbar plexus. This approach has variable success [84].

Risks and Contraindications

The primary risk of the femoral block is intravascular injection. In addition, femoral nerve catheters may be at increased risk for infection based on their location near the groin. Femoral nerve block will result in quadriceps weakness and patients and providers should be warned against ambulation due to falls risk. The presence of prior surgery in the groin or vascular conduit is a relative contraindication to femoral nerve block and favors ultrasound-guided approach.

Procedure

With the patient supine, a 50 mm linear ultrasound probe is used to find the femoral artery below the inguinal ligament. The artery should be followed cephald and caudad to identify the common femoral artery which will be cephalad to its division into the superficial and deep

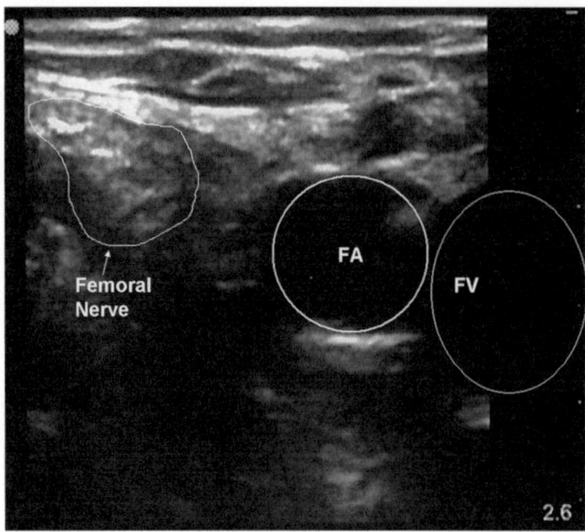

Fig. 6.8 Ultrasound-guided femoral nerve block. Lateral to medial, the femoral nerve (FN), artery (FA), and vein (FV) are identified (*left* is lateral and *right* is medial). Reprinted from [81]. With kind permission from Springer Science and Business Media

femoral arteries. Medial to the common femoral artery will be femoral vein, and lateral to the artery will be femoral nerve (Fig. 6.8). The nerve often appears as a tilted oval underneath two fascial planes, fascia lata and fascia iliaca. A more lateral needle approach may be superior as this helps insure that local anesthetic is delivered deep to fascia iliaca where the nerve resides. Also, the shallow angle of approach improves the needle image, and for catheter placement, a lateral approach keeps the insertion site more distant from the groin.

Sciatic and Popliteal Nerve Blocks

Background and Indications

The sciatic nerve is the longest and largest in the human body and is derived from the lumbosacral plexus with contributions from L4–S3. The sciatic nerve provides sensory innervation to the posterior upper leg and the entire lower leg except the medial saphenous distribution. In addition it provides motor innervation to the hamstrings and entire lower leg. The sciatic nerve contains the tibial component medially and peroneal component laterally, and these

split just above the knee. Sciatic nerve block can be achieved at multiple levels from its most proximal formation down to the split at the popliteal level. Proximal sciatic blocks are typically used to cover the posterior upper leg, for example, in conjunction with femoral blockade to provide analgesia after trauma to the knee or for lower extremity amputation. Distal sciatic nerve block (e.g., popliteal block) is often used to provide analgesia to the lower leg, for example, for foot, ankle, or distal tibial fractures or below knee amputations. Complete anesthesia of the lower leg is achieved by blocking the saphenous (or femoral nerve) as well.

Risks and Contraindications

Risks common to all sciatic blocks include the possibility of foot drop. Any block of the sciatic nerve will result in a temporary foot drop, but damage to the nerve could cause permanent foot drop. Some surgical procedures are associated with surgical risk of foot drop. In those cases, postoperative block may be preferred to allow for neurological exam prior to block placement. Specific sciatic approaches also carry specific risks. For example, parasacral sciatic block risks epidural spread, where popliteal sciatic block risks vascular injury or injection. As mentioned previously, tibial plateau fractures are at high risk for development of compartment syndrome, and therefore sciatic blockade is contraindicated in those situations.

Procedure

Many approaches to block the sciatic nerve have been described. We will discuss one proximal approach, gluteal, and one distal approach, popliteal. The gluteal sciatic block is performed just above the gluteal crease. A large curvilinear ultrasound probe is used to identify the greater trochanter and the ischial tuberosity. The sciatic nerve appears as a flat structure "laying in the hammock" between these two, superficial to quadratus lumborum (Fig. 6.9). The nerve is approached from the lateral side, though local anesthetic should be deposited from both the medial and later sides of the nerve to achieve

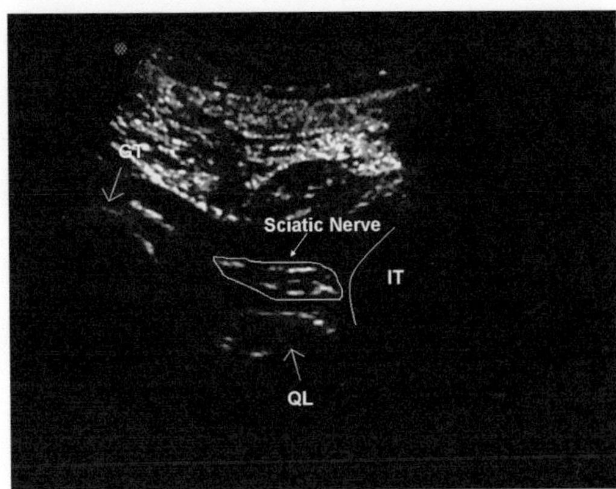

Fig. 6.9 Ultrasound-guided gluteal approach. The *arrow* on the left identifies the greater trochanter. The *arrow* at the bottom identifies the quadratus lumborum. The *curve line* on the right identifies the ischial tuberosity. The sciatic nerve is outlined by a *white line* and lies in the middle of the other structures. Reprinted from [81]. With kind permission from Springer Science and Business Media

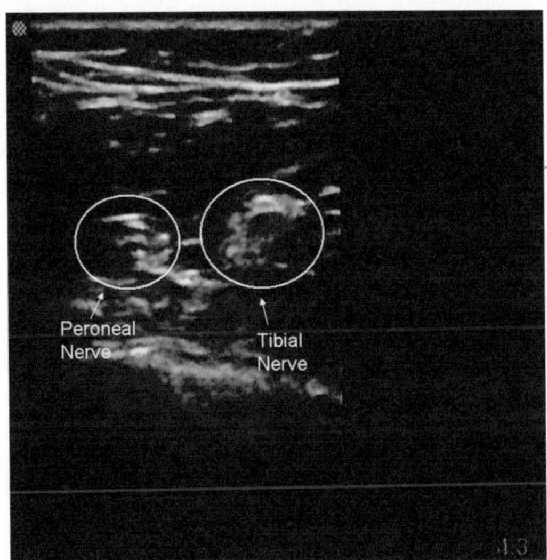

Fig. 6.10 Ultrasound-guided popliteal approach. The common peroneal nerve (lateral) and tibial nerve (medial) are identified in close approximation (*left* is lateral and *right* is medial). The popliteal artery can be seen deep and medial to the tibial nerve. Reprinted from [81]. With kind permission from Springer Science and Business Media

optimal blockade of the tibial and peroneal components.

To identify the sciatic nerve at the popliteal level, a linear ultrasound probe is placed at the popliteal crease to identify the popliteal artery. Superficial to the popliteal artery is the tibial

nerve (Fig. 6.10). These structures are then traced cephalad until the common peroneal nerve is seen coming in from superficial and lateral to join the tibial nerve. This is the level where the sciatic nerve splits into the tibial and common peroneal nerves, and often there will be a characteristic "snowman" on ultrasound consisting of the sciatic nerve superficially, then the popliteal vein and artery deep to the nerve. A 50–100 mm needle is advanced from the lateral side. The popliteal sciatic nerve block can take longer than other peripheral blocks to reach maximum effect. With ropivacaine, 20 min may be required for analgesic effect and up to 40 min to reach surgical anesthesia.

In summary, the ability of the clinical anesthesiologist to manage acute pain in a trauma patient directly provides both short- and long-term benefits. Development of newer drugs with improved side effect profiles and pain management techniques, including ultrasound, offer more promise than ever before to patients involved with trauma.

References

1. Joshi GP, Ogunnaike BO. Consequences of inadequate postoperative pain relief and chronic persistent postoperative pain. Anesthesiol Clin North America. 2005;23(1):21–36.
2. Liu SS, Block BM, Wu CL. Effects of perioperative central neuraxial analgesia on outcome after coronary artery bypass surgery: a meta-analysis. Anesthesiology. 2004;101(1):153–61.
3. Desai PM. Pain management and pulmonary dysfunction. Crit Care Clin. 1999;15(1):151–66. vii.
4. Chia YY, et al. Does postoperative pain induce emesis? Clin J Pain. 2002;18(5):317–23.
5. Rosenfeld BA, et al. Hemostatic effects of stress hormone infusion. Anesthesiology. 1994;81(5):1116–26.
6. Macrae WA. Chronic pain after surgery. Br J Anaesth. 2001;87(1):88–98.
7. Perkins FM, Kehlet H. Chronic pain as an outcome of surgery. A review of predictive factors. Anesthesiology. 2000;93(4):1123–33.
8. Ilfeld BM. Continuous peripheral nerve blocks: a review of the published evidence. Anesth Analg. 2011;113(4):904–25.
9. Andreae MH, Andreae DA. Local anaesthetics and regional anaesthesia for preventing chronic pain after surgery. Cochrane Database Syst Rev. 2012; 10: p. CD007105.

10. Buckenmaier III CC. The role of pain management in recovery following trauma and orthopaedic surgery. J Am Acad Orthop Surg. 2012;20 Suppl 1:S35–8.

11. Norman SB, et al. Pain in the aftermath of trauma is a risk factor for post-traumatic stress disorder. Psychol Med. 2008;38(4):533–42.

12. Saxe G, et al. Relationship between acute morphine and the course of PTSD in children with burns. J Am Acad Child Adolesc Psychiatry. 2001;40(8):915–21.

13. Bryant RA, et al. A study of the protective function of acute morphine administration on subsequent post-traumatic stress disorder. Biol Psychiatry. 2009;65 (5):438–40.

14. Holbrook TL, et al. Morphine use after combat injury in Iraq and post-traumatic stress disorder. N Engl J Med. 2010;362(2):110–7.

15. McGhee LL, et al. The correlation between ketamine and posttraumatic stress disorder in burned service members. J Trauma. 2008;64(2 Suppl):S195–8. Discussion S197-8.

16. Schonenberg M, et al. Effects of peritraumatic ketamine medication on early and sustained posttraumatic stress symptoms in moderately injured accident victims. Psychopharmacology (Berl). 2005;182(3):420–5.

17. O'Donnell ML, et al. The role of post-traumatic stress disorder and depression in predicting disability after injury. Med J Aust. 2009;190(7 Suppl):S71–4.

18. Dedert EA, et al. Posttraumatic stress disorder, cardiovascular, and metabolic disease: a review of the evidence. Ann Behav Med. 2010;39(1):61–78.

19. Ahmadi N, et al. Post-traumatic stress disorder, coronary atherosclerosis, and mortality. Am J Cardiol. 2011;108(1):29–33.

20. Kessler RC, et al. Posttraumatic stress disorder in the National Comorbidity Survey. Arch Gen Psychiatry. 1995;52(12):1048–60.

21. Kessler RC. Posttraumatic stress disorder: the burden to the individual and to society. J Clin Psychiatry. 2000;61 Suppl 5:4–12. discussion 13-4.

22. Schlenger WE, et al. The psychological risks of Vietnam: the NVVRS perspective. J Trauma Stress. 2007;20(4):467–79.

23. Ballantyne JC, et al. The comparative effects of post-operative analgesic therapies on pulmonary outcome: cumulative meta-analyses of randomized, controlled trials. Anesth Analg. 1998;86(3):598–612.

24. Buckenmaier CC, et al. Continuous peripheral nerve block for battlefield anesthesia and evacuation. Reg Anesth Pain Med. 2005;30(2):202–5.

25. Wu CL, et al. The effect of pain on health-related quality of life in the immediate postoperative period. Anesth Analg. 2003;97(4):1078–85.

26. Rigg JR, et al. Epidural anaesthesia and analgesia and outcome of major surgery: a randomised trial. Lancet. 2002;359(9314):1276–82.

27. Fotiadis RJ, et al. Epidural analgesia in gastrointestinal surgery. Br J Surg. 2004;91(7):828–41.

28. Buckenmaier III C, et al. Impact of an acute pain service on pain outcomes with combat-injured soldiers at Camp Bastion. Afghanistan Pain Med. 2012;13(7):919–26.

29. Marret E, et al. Meta-analysis of epidural analgesia versus parenteral opioid analgesia after colorectal surgery. Br J Surg. 2007;94(6):665–73.

30. Wenk M, Schug SA. Perioperative pain management after thoracotomy. Curr Opin Anaesthesiol. 2011;24 (1):8–12.

31. Joshi GP, et al. A systematic review of randomized trials evaluating regional techniques for postthoracotomy analgesia. Anesth Analg. 2008;107 (3):1026–40.

32. Baker BC, et al. Battlefield anesthesia: advances in patient care and pain management. Anesthesiol Clin. 2007;25(1):131–45. x.

33. Buckenmaier III C. Battlefield trauma and pain. J R Nav Med Serv. 2006;92(2):57–63.

34. Buckenmaier III CC, et al. Pain following battlefield injury and evacuation: a survey of 110 casualties from the wars in Iraq and Afghanistan. Pain Med. 2009;10 (8):1487–96.

35. De Buck F, et al. Regional anesthesia outside the operating room: indications and techniques. Curr Opin Anaesthesiol. 2012;25(4):501–7.

36. Kent ML, Upp JJ, Buckenmaier III CC. Acute pain on and off the battlefield: what we do, what we know, and future directions. Int Anesthesiol Clin. 2011;49 (3):10–32.

37. WHO. Cancer pain relief. With a guide to opioid availability. 2nd ed. Geneva: WHO; 1996.

38. Hinz B, Cheremina O, Brune K. Acetaminophen (paracetamol) is a selective cyclooxygenase-2-inhibitor in man. FASEB J. 2008;22(2):383–90.

39. Piletta P, Porchet HC, Dayer P. Central analgesic effect of acetaminophen but not of aspirin. Clin Pharmacol Ther. 1991;49(4):350–4.

40. McQuay HJ, et al. Ketorolac and acetaminophen for orthopedic postoperative pain. Clin Pharmacol Ther. 1986;39(1):89–93.

41. Larson AM, et al. Acetaminophen-induced acute liver failure: results of a United States multicenter, prospective study. Hepatology. 2005;42(6):1364–72.

42. Gaskell H, et al. Single dose oral oxycodone and oxycodone plus paracetamol (acetaminophen) for acute postoperative pain in adults. Cochrane Database Syst Rev. 2009(3): p. CD002763.

43. Sinatra RS, et al. Intravenous acetaminophen for pain after major orthopedic surgery: an expanded analysis. Pain Pract. 2012;12(5):357–65.

44. Sinatra RS, et al. Efficacy and safety of single and repeated administration of 1 gram intravenous acetaminophen injection (paracetamol) for pain management after major orthopedic surgery. Anesthesiology. 2005;102(4):822–31.

45. Tsang KS, Page J, Mackenney P. Can intravenous paracetamol reduce opioid use in preoperative hip fracture patients? Orthopedics. 2013;36(2):20–4.

46. Wininger SJ, et al. A randomized, double-blind, placebo-controlled, multicenter, repeat-dose study of

two intravenous acetaminophen dosing regimens for the treatment of pain after abdominal laparoscopic surgery. Clin Ther. 2010;32(14):2348–69.

47. Craig M, et al. Randomised comparison of intravenous paracetamol and intravenous morphine for acute traumatic limb pain in the emergency department. Emerg Med J. 2012;29(1):37–9.

48. Davies NM, et al. Minimizing risks of NSAIDs: cardiovascular, gastrointestinal and renal. Expert Rev Neurother. 2006;6(11):1643–55.

49. Mukherjee D, Nissen SE, Topol EJ. Risk of cardiovascular events associated with selective COX-2-inhibitors. JAMA. 2001;286(8):954–9.

50. Bing RJ, Lomnicka M. Why do cyclo-oxygenase-2 inhibitors cause cardiovascular events? J Am Coll Cardiol. 2002;39(3):521–2.

51. Gislason GH, et al. Increased mortality and cardiovascular morbidity associated with use of nonsteroidal anti-inflammatory drugs in chronic heart failure. Arch Intern Med. 2009;169(2):141–9.

52. Bergenstock M, et al. A comparison between the effects of acetaminophen and celecoxib on bone fracture healing in rats. J Orthop Trauma. 2005;19(10):717–23.

53. Simon AM, Manigrasso MB, O'Connor JP. Cyclooxygenase 2 function is essential for bone fracture healing. J Bone Miner Res. 2002;17(6):963–76.

54. Long J, et al. The effect of cyclooxygenase-2 inhibitors on spinal fusion. J Bone Joint Surg Am. 2002;84-A(10):1763–8.

55. Forbes JA, et al. Evaluation of ketorolac, ibuprofen, acetaminophen, and an acetaminophen-codeine combination in postoperative oral surgery pain. Pharmacotherapy. 1990;10(6 Pt 2):94S–105S.

56. Bell RF, et al. Perioperative ketamine for acute postoperative pain. Cochrane Database Syst Rev. 2006(1): p. CD004603.

57. Bloch MH, et al. Effects of ketamine in treatment-refractory obsessive-compulsive disorder. Biol Psychiatry. 2012;72(11):964–70.

58. Rao TS, Andrade C. Innovative approaches to treatment—refractory depression: the ketamine story. Indian J Psychiatry. 2010;52(2):97–9.

59. Stefanczyk-Sapieha L, Oneschuk D, Demas M. Intravenous ketamine "burst" for refractory depression in a patient with advanced cancer. J Palliat Med. 2008;11(9):1268–71.

60. Hudcova J, et al. Patient controlled opioid analgesia versus conventional opioid analgesia for postoperative pain. Cochrane Database Syst Rev. 2006(4): p. CD003348.

61. Mattia C, et al. Efficacy and safety of fentanyl HCl iontophoretic transdermal system compared with morphine intravenous patient-controlled analgesia for postoperative pain management for patient subgroups. Eur J Anaesthesiol. 2010;27(5):433–40.

62. Griffin DW, Skowronski RJ, Dasu BN, Palmer PP. A phase 2 open-label functionality, safety, and efficacy study of the sufentanil NanoTabTM PCA system in patients following elective unilateral knee replacement surgery, 2010: American Society of Regional Anesthesia and Pain Medicine: Poster Presentation, 35th annual spring meeting and workshops.

63. Charlton S, et al. Perioperative transversus abdominis plane (TAP) blocks for analgesia after abdominal surgery. Cochrane Database Syst Rev. 2010(12): p. CD007705.

64. Parker MJ, Handoll HH, Griffiths R. Anaesthesia for hip fracture surgery in adults. Cochrane Database Syst Rev. 2004(4): p. CD000521.

65. Jorgensen H, et al. Epidural local anaesthetics versus opioid-based analgesic regimens on postoperative gastrointestinal paralysis, PONV and pain after abdominal surgery. Cochrane Database Syst Rev. 2000(4): p. CD001893.

66. Jorgensen H, et al. Effect of epidural bupivacaine vs combined epidural bupivacaine and morphine on gastrointestinal function and pain after major gynaecological surgery. Br J Anaesth. 2001;87(5):727–32.

67. Jorgensen H, et al. Effect of peri- and postoperative epidural anaesthesia on pain and gastrointestinal function after abdominal hysterectomy. Br J Anaesth. 2001;87(4):577–83.

68. Nishimori M, et al. Epidural pain relief versus systemic opioid-based pain relief for abdominal aortic surgery. Cochrane Database Syst Rev. 2012. 7: p. CD005059.

69. Llewellyn N, Moriarty A. The national pediatric epidural audit. Paediatr Anaesth. 2007;17(6):520–33.

70. Hyder N, et al. Compartment syndrome in tibial shaft fracture missed because of a local nerve block. J Bone Joint Surg Br. 1996;78(3):499–500.

71. Noorpuri BS, Shahane SA, Getty CJ. Acute compartment syndrome following revisional arthroplasty of the forefoot: the dangers of ankle-block. Foot Ankle Int. 2000;21(8):680–2.

72. Uzel AP, Steinmann G. Thigh compartment syndrome after intramedullary femoral nailing: possible femoral nerve block influence on diagnosis timing. Orthop Traumatol Surg Res. 2009;95(4):309–13.

73. Cometa MA, Esch AT, Boezaart AP. Did continuous femoral and sciatic nerve block obscure the diagnosis or delay the treatment of acute lower leg compartment syndrome? A case report. Pain Med. 2011;12(5):823–8.

74. Flagel BT, et al. Half-a-dozen ribs: the breakpoint for mortality. Surgery. 2005;138(4):717–23. discussion 723-5.

75. Pressley CM, et al. Predicting outcome of patients with chest wall injury. Am J Surg. 2012;204(6):910–3. discussion 913-4.

76. Carrier FM, et al. Effect of epidural analgesia in patients with traumatic rib fractures: a systematic review and meta-analysis of randomized controlled trials. Can J Anaesth. 2009;56(3):230–42.

77. Ho AM, Karmakar MK, Critchley LA. Acute pain management of patients with multiple fractured ribs:

a focus on regional techniques. Curr Opin Crit Care. 2011;17(4):323–7.

78. Katayama T, et al. Safety of the paravertebral block in patients ineligible for epidural block undergoing pulmonary resection. Gen Thorac Cardiovasc Surg. 2012;60(12):811–4.

79. Visoiu M, Yang C. Ultrasound-guided bilateral paravertebral continuous nerve blocks for a mildly coagulopathic patient undergoing exploratory laparotomy for bowel resection. Paediatr Anaesth. 2011;21(4):459–62.

80. Liu SS, et al. Effects of perioperative analgesic technique on rate of recovery after colon surgery. Anesthesiology. 1995;83(4):757–65.

81. Kaye AD, Urman RD, Vadivelu N. Essentials of regional anesthesia. New York: Springer; 2012.

82. Swensen JD, et al. Outpatient management of continuous peripheral nerve catheters placed using ultrasound guidance: an experience in 620 patients. Anesth Analg. 2006;103(6):1436–43.

83. Lai TT, et al. Continuous peripheral nerve block catheter infections in combat related injuries: a case report of five soldiers from Operation Enduring Freedom/Operation Iraqi Freedom. Pain Med. 2011;12(11):1676–81.

84. Marhofer P, et al. Magnetic resonance imaging of the distribution of local anesthetic during the three-in-one block. Anesth Analg. 2000;90:119–24.

Lindsay R. Higgins, Whitney K. Braddy, Michael S. Higgins, and Alan David Kaye

Introduction

Chronic pain can be defined in several different ways. Arbitrary time scales can be used to define chronic pain as pain that lasts 3–12 months. Alternatively, chronic pain may simply be defined as pain that persists beyond the expected healing time. Regardless of the definition chosen, the number of patients suffering with posttraumatic chronic pain is increasing in the United States. The reason behind this phenomenon is simply the improved survival for trauma victims. With more patients surviving major trauma, more patients later present with chronic pain. The personal and financial costs to the victims and society are staggering. In 2008, it was estimated that 100 million Americans suffer with chronic pain, and the annual cost including treatment and lost productivity may be over $600 billion dollars annually [1]. This cost is greater than the costs of heart disease and cancer combined [1]. At least one fifth of chronic pain patients identify trauma as the precipitating cause [2]. The effective diagnosis and treatment of posttraumatic chronic pain is, thus, of monumental importance in the United States.

Evaluation of Chronic Pain After Trauma

It is essential for any patient with chronic pain after trauma to receive a complete evaluation with history and physical exam. Qualification of the pain, as well as medical and surgical history, is critical components of the history. A thorough evaluation may provide important information regarding the etiology of pain and, therefore, guide its treatment. The McGill Pain Questionnaire Short form is commonly used to assess the sensory, affective, and other qualitative components of chronic pain and can be used to differentiate between neuropathic and somatic pain (Fig. 7.1).

A qualitative description of pain can provide important clues regarding the pain etiology. There are many different types of pain (Table 7.1). For example, neuropathic pain is pain that results from injury to nerve fibers and is commonly described as possessing a burning, electric, or even numb sensation. Alternatively, nociceptive pain is caused by stimulation of

L.R. Higgins, M.D., M.P.H., B.S. (✉) • W.K. Braddy, M.D.
Tulane University, Department of Anesthesiology, 1430 Tulane Avenue, New Orleans, LA 70112, USA
e-mail: lhiggins@tulane.edu; wbraddy@tulane.edu

M.S. Higgins, D.D.S.
University of Illinois Medical Center, Department of Anesthesiology, 1740 W. Taylor Street,
Chicago, IL 60612, USA

A.D. Kaye, M.D., Ph.D., D.A.B.A., D.A.B.P.M., D.A.B.I.P.P.
Department of Anesthesiology, LSU School of Medicine T6M5, 1542 Tulane Avenue, Room 656, New Orleans, LA 70112, USA

Department of Pharmacology, LSU School of Medicine T6M5, 1542 Tulane Avenue, Room 656, New Orleans, LA 70112, USA
e-mail: Alankaye44@hotmail.com

C.S. Scher (ed.), *Anesthesia for Trauma*, DOI 10.1007/978-1-4939-0909-4_7,
© Springer Science+Business Media New York 2014

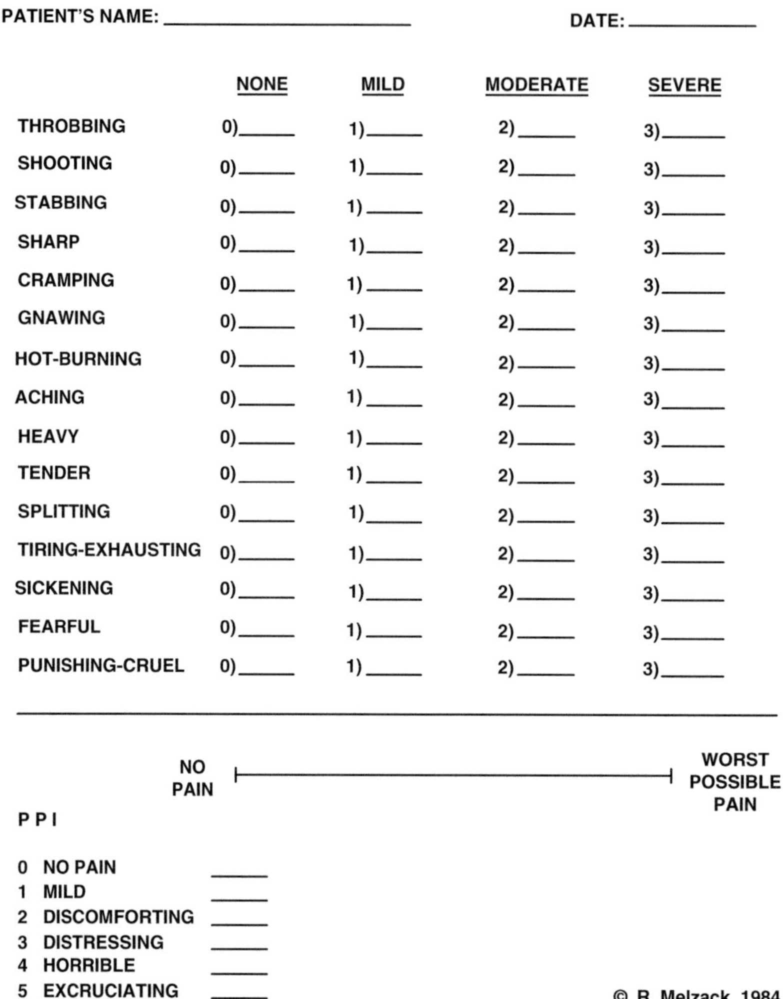

Fig. 7.1 Short-form McGill Pain Questionnaire. Items 1–11 describe sensory qualities and 12–15 describe affective qualities. Each item is ranked on a severity scale. From Melzack R, Katz J. In: Schmidt RF, Willis WD, editors. Encyclopedia of Pain. Springer; 2006. With kind permission from Springer Science and Business Media

peripheral nociceptors and is typically described as dull or aching. Distinguishing neuropathic from nociceptive pain is essential as the treatment modalities are very different.

A patient's medical and surgical history can also provide important information about the etiology of pain. For example, diseases such as diabetes or immunodeficiency states will affect wound healing and infection rates, which will influence the chronicity of pain. Further, medications may affect when and which treatment procedures may be performed safely. For example, patients who are anticoagulated may not be able to safely undergo neuraxial interventions, such as epidurals.

Lastly, a thorough physical exam will likely elucidate patterns of altered sensation, pain, and strength which can indicate the origin of pain. Evaluating extremities for temperature differences and muscular and reflex symmetry

Table 7.1 Commonly used pain terms

Neuropathic/neurogenic pain	Pain resulting from injury to or dysfunction of the central or peripheral nervous system
Nociceptive pain	Pain resulting from stimulation of nociceptive afferent nerves
Central pain	Pain resulting from injury to or dysfunction of the central nervous system
Somatic pain	Pain carried by sensory nerves
Visceral pain	Pain carried by sympathetic nerves
Neuralgia	Pain occurring in the distribution of a nerve
Radiculopathy	Loss of sensory or motor function resulting from a block to nerve conduction
Hyperalgesia	A greater than anticipated painful response to stimulation
Allodynia	Pain elicited by a stimulation that would not normally cause pain
Paresthesia	An abnormal sensation that may be provoked or spontaneous
Dysesthesia	An unpleasant and abnormal sensation that may be provoked or spontaneous
Anesthesia Dolorosa	Pain that occurs in a region of numbness

can also narrow a differential diagnosis. Using findings from the history and physical exam, radiological imaging can then be obtained to confirm diagnosis and to further guide treatment and management.

Complex Regional Pain Syndrome

CRPS is a chronic pain syndrome initiated by trauma. The injury is most commonly surgery, fracture, crush, or sprain [3]. CRPS is further categorized as CRPS-I (reflex sympathetic dystrophy) and CRPS-II (causalgia). The presentation is identical but the diagnosis of CRPS-II requires documented nerve injury.

The classic presentation is continuous pain, hyperalgesia, and allodynia in the setting of autonomic dysregulation. Acutely, this presents as edema, redness, and increased temperature. Symptoms progress over time and the affected limb develops trophic changes: contracture, loss of function, bone loss, and decreased nail and hair growth. The majority of cases resolve, but outcomes can be severe. Progressive disability is common and some patients require amputation [4].

CRPS has historically been attributed to sympathetically maintained pain and sympathetic blocks were the mainstay of therapy. However, research shows *decreased* sympathetic nervous system activity in those with CRPS [5].

Current evidence suggests that *all* CRPS involves nerve injury, as well as both peripheral and central factors [6]. The initial trauma leads to elevated inflammatory markers and acute symptoms. Persistent inflammation and pain induces peripheral and central sensitization, the mechanism for hyperalgesia and allodynia.

Much like phantom limb, the nerve injury in CRPS causes deafferentiation and decreased somatosensory cortex dedicated to the afflicted limb. Here again, the degree of cortex reutilization is associated with the degree of pain [7].

Based on this information several approaches become intuitive. With incidence estimated at 10–20 % of some orthopedic procedures, prevention is paramount. Good perioperative pain control and nerve blocks improve patient satisfaction and are shown to decrease the incidence of CRPS.

The trophic changes in chronic CRPS are due to deafferentiation (Fig. 7.2). Therefore, the goal of treatment is to enable patients to participate in physical therapy. This can be achieved with early corticosteroids, nerve blocks, or spinal cord stimulation. The resulting physical therapy increases afferent feedback and has been shown to restore somatosensory organization, decrease pain, and resolve symptoms.

Traumatic Brain Injury

According to the Centers for Disease Control and Prevention (CDC), it is estimated that 1.4 million Americans sustain traumatic brain injuries (TBIs) each year. Of those hospitalized, 43 % can expect to develop a chronic TBI-related disability [8].

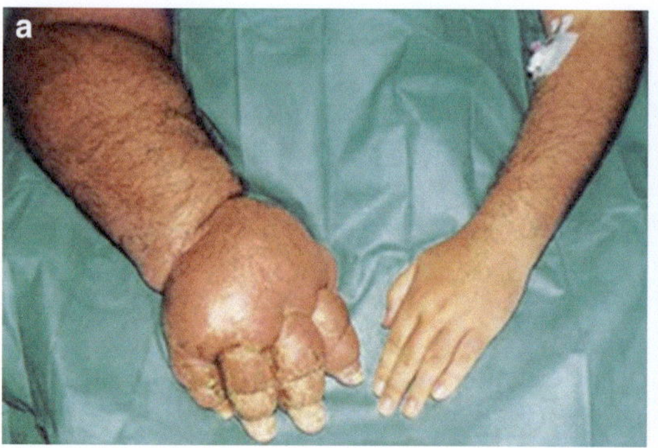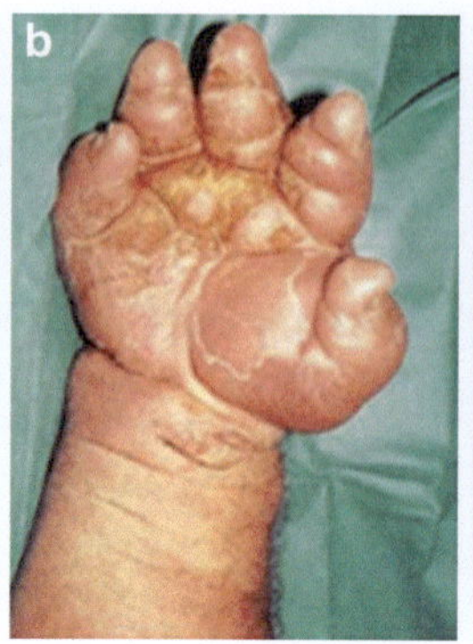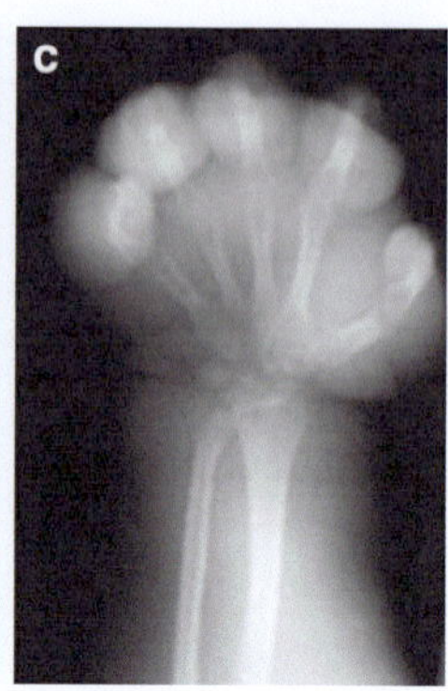

Fig. 7.2 CRPS after metacarpal fracture. This patient ultimately required amputation. From N Engl J Med, Guttmann O, Wykes V, Complex regional pain syndrome type 1, 359, p. 508. Copyright © 2008 Massachusetts Medical Society. Reprinted with permission from Massachusetts Medical Society. (**a**) Severe CRPS of the right hand and forearm in comparison to the patient's normal left side. (**b**) Closeup of the effected limb exhibiting edema, erythema, and hair loss. (**c**) Radiograph revealing the inciting injury—a nondisplaced fracture of the fifth metacarpal

The most common of these long-term sequelae is posttraumatic headache. Between 30 and 90 % of patients with mild head injury will subsequently experience posttraumatic headache [9]. Although TBI can result in pain that extends to all regions of the body, for the purposes of this discussion, we will focus on posttraumatic headache, as well as other pain syndromes that are localized to the head and neck.

The epidemiology of post-TBI pain syndromes can be difficult to describe due to variability in the definition of TBI. The CDC developed a definition of TBI and published the *Guidelines for Surveillance of Central Nervous System Injury*. These guidelines define TBI as trauma to the head that is associated with any of the following: decreased level of consciousness, amnesia, neurologic abnormalities, skull fracture, intracranial lesions, or death [10]. The leading causes of TBI in the United States are falls, motor-vehicle accidents, and assaults [10]. Certain populations are at increased risk for TBI including American Indian/Alaska Native, African Americans, extremes of age, low socioeconomic status, and male sex [10].

Traumatic brain injury can lead to pain states through mechanisms that do not directly cause injury to the brain. Sources of pain are often categorized as extracranial and intracranial. Intracranial structures that can be damaged with TBI include the intracranial arteries, cranial nerves, and the dura mater. Extracranial sources include muscle, tendons, bones, joints, skin, and peripheral nerves. Given the diversity of structures that can be injured by TBI, there is great variability in the resulting constellation of pain symptoms. However, post-TBI headache is by far the most common.

The exact mechanism for posttraumatic headache remains unclear, but it may involve physiologic aberrations, such as decreased and asymmetrical cerebral blood flow, in addition to direct trauma to tissue. Alternatively, there are some similarities in biochemical abnormalities between posttraumatic headache and migraines, so it is possible that they share a similar etiology. Other research implicates damage to the trigeminal nerve as a potential cause of posttraumatic headache. While the exact etiology of posttraumatic headache remains unclear, it is most likely multifactorial. Interestingly, the severity of TBI is indirectly related to the incidence of headache. In one study, 89 % of patients with mild TBI reported headache compared to only 18 % of those with severe TBI [11].

Posttraumatic headaches can present as tension headache, migraine, and cluster headache. Most commonly, pain is experienced similar to that of a tension headache with a tight band of pain encircling the head. This type of headache is often relieved by NSAIDS and acetaminophen. Patients who are at risk for developing migraines may subsequently unmask migraine headaches, and these are best treated by typical anti-migraine medications. It is relatively rare but cluster headaches may occur after TBI, as well.

Trauma to structures in the head other than the brain may also result in head and neck pain. For example, whiplash can result in trauma to the TMJ, occipital nerves, and cervical nerves. Whiplash injuries frequently occur after rear-end automobile collisions, and the mechanism of injury is an abrupt backward then forward motion of the head. This motion traumatizes neck muscles and ligaments. TMJ pain is the result of both hyperextension of the mandibular joint and mastoid muscle injury. Whiplash rarely causes direct trauma to the TMJ. Instead, it more commonly results in myofascial pain that can be treated with trigger point injections in the masseter, temporalis, and medial and lateral pterygoid muscles (muscles of mastication). Whiplash can occasionally cause occipital neuralgia, which is experienced as pain or diminished sensation in the upper neck, back of the head, and behind the eyes. These areas correspond to regions supplied by the greater and lesser occipital nerves. Palpation of the greater and lesser occipital nerves may reproduce the pain (Tinel's sign), and such patients may be treated effectively with occipital nerve blocks. Cervicogenic headaches are defined as headaches with any cervical origin, including both soft and bony structures. Typically, this pain originates in the back of the neck and extends to the oculofrontal--temporal area but remains unilateral. The trigeminocervical nucleus is a structure in the upper cervical spinal cord where sensory fibers of the trigeminal nerve converge with sensory fibers from the upper cervical roots, most commonly C2, C3, and C4. The result of this interaction is the possibility of referred pain between the neck, face, and head. Such pain can be treated with neurolysis of the median branch from the dorsal rami using a local anesthetic injection. Alternatively, radiofrequency ablation can be used, but this modality is more controversial.

Medical treatment for posttraumatic headache is dependent upon the characteristics of the headache. Constant headaches of a musculoskeletal origin can be treated with NSAIDS with the addition of opioids and anti-migraine medications for breakthrough pain. Commonly used anti-migraine medications include NSAIDS, caffeine, and abortive medications, such as triptans and ergot derivatives. Additional preventative medicines include beta blockers (propranolol), calcium channel blockers (verapamil), ACE-Inhibitors (lisinopril), tricyclic antidepressants, serotonin reuptake inhibitors (venlafaxine), anti-epileptics (valproate, topiramate, gabapentin), and injections of Botulinum toxin type A (Botox) in the muscles of the forehead and neck.

Unfortunately, a large percentage of posttraumatic headaches become chronic. One study reports that posttraumatic headache was reported by 44 % of patients after 6 months [12]. These chronic headaches are more difficult to treat and require treatment plans that are tailored to their individual constellation of symptoms.

Spinal Cord Injury

Trauma is the leading cause of spinal cord pain. On average, 65 % of patients who have a spinal cord injury (SCI) report having chronic pain, with about one third of those reporting severe pain [13]. Chronic pain after SCI is particularly difficult to treat, especially when it is neuropathic in nature. No treatment exists that can reliably relieve pain in the majority of patients who have chronic pain after SCI. Further treatment research is needed because currently, very few randomized controlled trials have been performed. Of those studies, few of the existing trials have had positive results [14]. As a result, very few medical treatments are available. Further, the applicability of research findings is complicated by the fact that there is a lack of a universal classification system for SCI pain. Without a universal classification system, it is difficult to conduct, interpret, and apply research findings to clinical practice. For this reason, treatment of pain following SCI is typically simply approached using a trial and error method.

In 2006, The Spinal Cord Injury Task Force of the International Association for the Study of

Table 7.2 Proposed classification of pain related to SCI

Broad type (Tier 1)	Broad system (Tier 2)	Specific structures/pathology (Tier 3)
Nociceptive	Muscoloskeletal	Bone, joint, muscle trauma or inflammation, mechanical instability, muscle spasm, repetitive overuse syndromes
	Visceral	Renal calculus, bowel, sphincter dysfunction, dysreflexic headache
Neuropathic	Above level	Compressive mononeuropathies, CPRS
	At level	Nerve root compression (including cauda equine), syringomyelia, spinal cord trauma/ischemia (transitional zone, etc.), dual level cord and root trauma (double lesion syndrome)
	Below level	Spinal cord trauma/ischemia (central dysthesia syndrome, etc.)

Reprinted by permission from Macmillan Publishers Ltd: Spinal Cord, Siddall PJ, Middleton JW, A proposed algorithm for the management of pain following spinal cord injury, 44(2):67-77, copyright 2006

Pain created a taxonomy system that organizes pain following SCI into three tiers (Table 7.2). The first tier divides SCI pain into nociceptive and neuropathic sources. The second tier subdivides nociceptive into musculoskeletal and visceral sources and subdivides neuropathic into above level, at level, and below level pain types [14]. This taxonomy system facilitates the assessment and diagnosis of spinal cord pain, which in turn directs pain management.

Nociceptive pain occurs as a result of direct stimulation of nociceptors, which are located in musculoskeletal and visceral tissues. This pain can occur as a result of processes such as trauma and inflammation. Nociceptive pain is usually characterized as dull or sharp and aching.

Neuropathic pain is due to malfunction of the nervous system resulting from either trauma or illness. Typically, the term neuropathic pain is reserved for pain that occurs due to a primary injury to the nervous system. Neuropathic pain is typically located at or near an area of abnormal sensation, and it is usually described as having a burning, shooting, or electric quality. It is far more difficult to treat neuropathic pain compared to nociceptive pain.

While nociceptive and neuropathic pains have distinctly different etiologies, it appears that both are associated with mechanisms of central plasticity [14]. Neuronal remodeling of the spinal cord and thalamus occurs as a result of amplification of excitatory neurotransmitters and suppression of inhibitory neurotransmitters [14]. The result of this stimulation is the destruction of neurons and spontaneous pain.

The first subtype of nociceptive pain is musculoskeletal pain. After SCI, acute trauma to musculoskeletal structures such as bone, muscles, and joints results in acute pain that is localized to the region of injury. In addition to acute trauma, this sort of pain may occur with overuse injuries of muscles and joints. Of note, paraplegics are much more likely than tetraplegics to experience this type of pain. Muscle spasms, which frequently occur after SCI, also fall into this category. Musculoskeletal sources of pain can be confirmed using radiographs, computerized tomography (CT), or magnetic resonance imaging (MRI).

Visceral pain is the second subtype of nociceptive pain. The quality of visceral pain is affected by the level of SCI. For example, patients with paraplegia may experience visceral pain with characteristics similar to those experienced by a person without a SCI. However, patients with tetraplegia may only have a vague sensation of discomfort. If treatments aimed at visceral pain are ineffective or if evidence of visceral pathology cannot be found, it must be considered that the pain is of a neuropathic and not visceral nature.

Above level neuropathic pain encompasses pain that is not specific to SCI. An example of above level neuropathic pain is complex regional pain syndrome (CPRS). CPRS can occur in patients without SCI, but those with SCI are more prone to its development especially in the upper extremities due to certain movements associated with wheelchair use and transfers. Another example of above level neuropathic pain is peripheral nerve compression. Modalities used to evaluate nerve compression pain include electrophysiological studies and MRI.

At level neuropathic pain results from trauma either to the nerve roots or spinal cord within two levels of the SCI. The associated pain has a dermatomal distribution that correlates to the involved spinal levels and is associated with abnormal sensations such as alloydnia and hyperaesthesia in the affected dermatomes. Nerve root pain is typically unilateral and is worsened by movement of the spine. Damage to the nerve root may occur with the primary trauma or secondary to spine instability. Evaluation with electromyographic (EMG) or somatosensory-evoked potential (SSEP) studies may show abnormalities and diagnosis is guided by radiographic, CT, and MRI imaging, which reveal compression of the foramenal nerve root compression. Although it may be difficult to distinguish between nerve root compression and spinal cord pathology, it is an important distinction because the treatments are quite different. It is important to note that syringomyelia must be ruled out when a patient presents with a delayed onset of segmental pain that is accompanied by increasing loss of sensation. MRI imaging will reveal syringomyelia if it is present.

Below level neuropathic pain often has a diffuse distribution below the level of the SCI, and it is typically constant in nature and characterized as burning, aching, or electric. Hyperalgesia is often associated with below level neuropathic pain. In some cases, it fluctuates with mood and is worsened by abrupt movements or even sudden noises. The quality of pain is also influenced by the completeness of the spinal cord lesion. Incomplete injuries are more likely to be associated with allodynia if the spinothalamic tract remains intact.

When evaluating a patient with chronic pain due to SCI, it is critical to obtain a thorough history and physical examination and to precisely document the patient's neurological examination. Imaging studies such as MRI and CT are then performed to localize the level of injury, but when the precise location remains unclear, electrodiagnostic and diagnostic nerve blocks can further localize the source of pain.

Once the etiology is precisely established, management can be tailored accordingly. Respective algorithms for the treatment of nociceptive and neuropathic pain are outlined in Figs. 7.3 and 7.4. Other third-line treatment options are outlined in Table 7.3. In addition to these treatment modalities, some research shows exercise can improve pain symptoms [15]. However, none of these treatments reliably provide relief. There is a strong need for new and more effective medical treatments. For example, Gabapentin is perhaps the most commonly prescribed medication for chronic pain, yet most patients do not experience significant relief and will eventually discontinue the medication due to lack of efficacy and side effect profile [15]. With more research and by creating a universal taxonomy to guide research, we can continue to improve diagnosis and management of chronic pain after SCI.

Phantom Limb Pain

Phantom limb pain (PLP) is traditionally associated with upper or lower extremity amputation. However, it has been described after the loss of various body parts such as the eye, tooth, tongue, breast, penis, testicle, and even internal organs. Interestingly, phantom sensation is *always* experienced after amputation. Pain is among the sensations in 50–80 % of cases.

Eighty percent of amputations are caused by vascular disease, primarily diabetes. The remaining 20 % is secondary to trauma, cancer, and congenital anomaly. The mechanism of injury is irrelevant [16]. However, there are indications that perioperative pain may affect the risk of developing PLP [17].

Of those who will develop pain, half report symptoms within 24 h of amputation and the majority declare themselves within one week. The pain is intermittent and described as

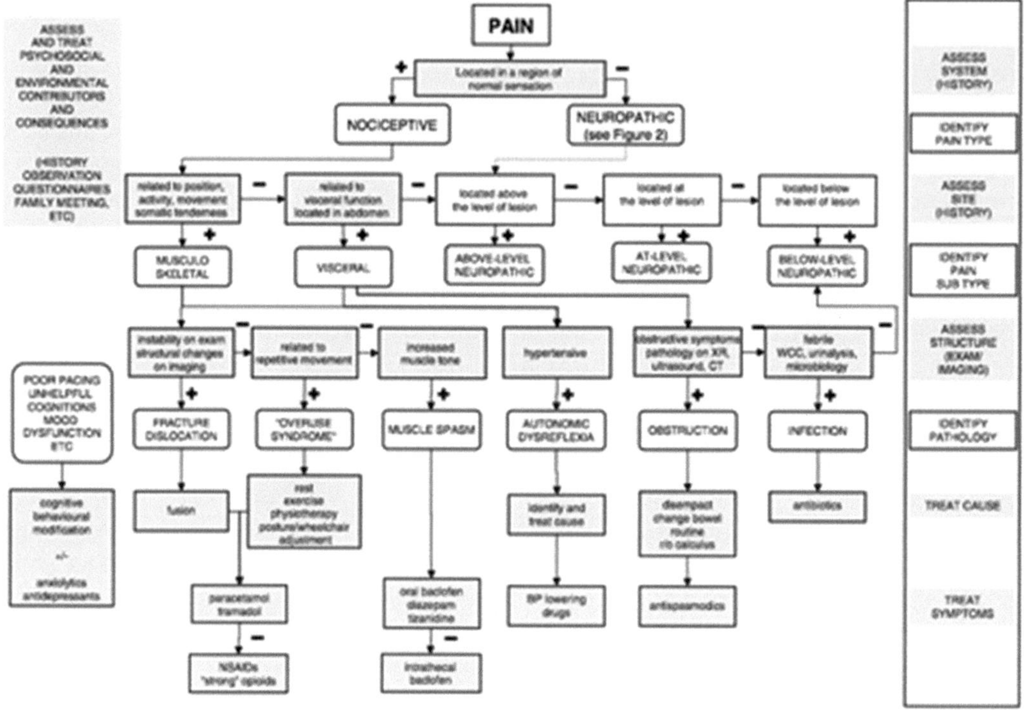

Fig. 7.3 Assessment of treatment algorithm for the management of nociceptive pain following SCI. Reprinted by permission from Macmillan Publishers Ltd: Spinal Cord, Siddall PJ, Middleton JW, A proposed algorithm for the management of pain following spinal cord injury, 44 (2):67-77, copyright 2006

cramping, burning, or shooting in the distal aspect of the amputated limb.

Peripheral and central mechanisms both appear to contribute. Severed nerve fibers at the site of amputation exhibit increased spontaneous activity. Increased signaling from these nerves leads to central sensitization of spinal cord neurons. However, stump revision and neuromectomy are ineffective treatments.

Centrally, loss of feedback from the amputated limb (deafferentiation) leads to reorganization of the prefrontal cortex. The area that previously processed input from the amputated limb becomes utilized by surrounding processing centers. A greater degree of re-utilization is associated with greater pain [18].

Presently, phantom limb is treated as neuropathic pain with moderate success. However, emphasis should be placed on prevention and re-afferentiation. We may be able to reduce the development of PLP with aggressive perioperative pain control [17].

For those already suffering, mirror box therapy [19] and advanced prostheses [20] that increase feedback may offer some benefit. Spinal cord stimulators are effective for those with intractable pain (Fig. 7.5) [21].

Posttraumatic Abdominal Pain

Trauma to the abdomen, whether from injury or surgery, can result in chronic abdominal pain. Abdominal pain following trauma can be subclassified as either a neuropathic entrapment syndrome or visceral abdominal pain.

Neuropathic entrapment syndrome occurs when direct pressure is applied to a nerve. Often the source of pressure is adhesions, inflammation, or scarring of surrounding tissues, such as the rectus sheath muscle. Neuropathic pain in the abdomen is localized to the distribution of the affected nerve and is described as sharp or tingling. Nerves that are commonly

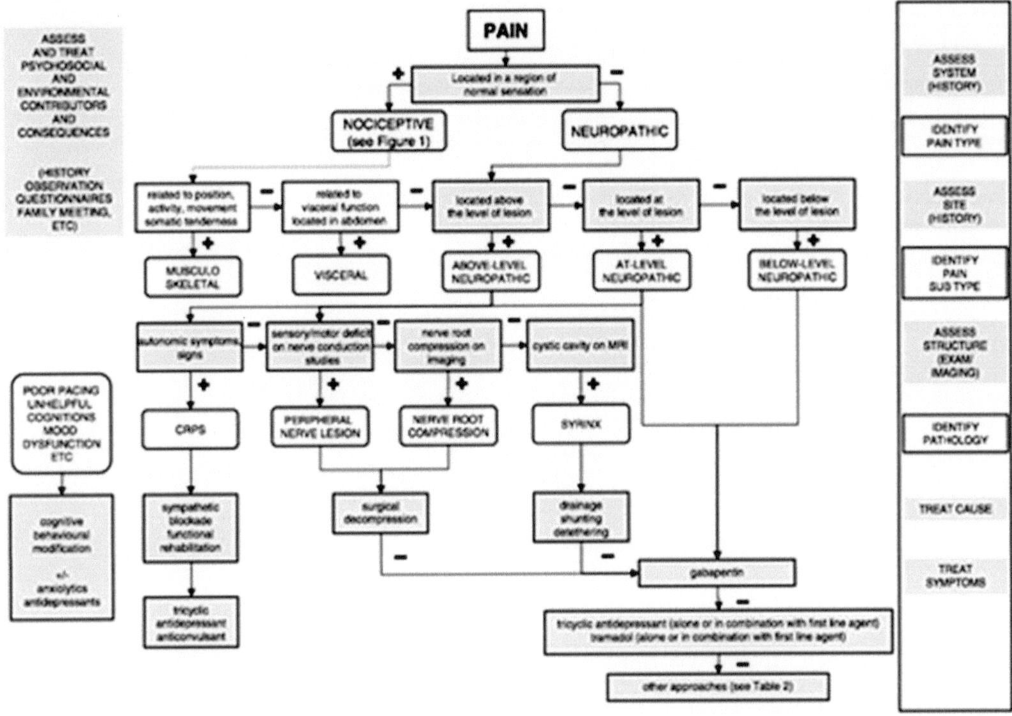

Fig. 7.4 Assessment and treatment algorithm for the management of neuropathic pain following SCI. Reprinted by permission from Macmillan Publishers Ltd: Spinal Cord, Siddall PJ, Middleton JW, A proposed algorithm for the management of pain following spinal cord injury, 44(2):67-77, copyright 2006

affected include the anterior cutaneous nerves of the lower thoracic vertebrae (T7–T12), ilioinguinal, and intercostal nerves. Conservative treatment of neuropathic abdominal pain includes medical management with gabapentin, antidepressants, opioids, and transcutaneous electrical stimulation units (TENS). Additionally, massage of the abdominal wall or steroid injections can release adhesions and free compressed nerves. More invasive options include radiofrequency ablation and cryotherapy.

Visceral abdominal pain occurs when there is direct stimulation of abdominal nociceptors as might occur with direct trauma to organs, distention of hollow structures, or with ischemia to organs. In contrast to neuropathic pain, visceral abdominal pain is poorly localized and is usually described as vague, dull, or cramping. Medical treatments are similar to those for neuropathic pain. Interventional treatments include regional anesthesia (splenic nerve blocks, celiac plexus blocks, or superior hypogastric plexus blocks), spinal cord stimulators, or intrathecal pumps, which deliver local anesthetic to the spinal canal. Alternatively, diagnostic sympathetic nerve blocks can be performed which will confirm the pain as visceral and localize it to specific nerves which can subsequently be blocked using radiofrequency ablation or alcohol injections.

Vertebral Fracture

Posttraumatic vertebral fracture is increasing in incidence in the United States. The reason for this is that the population most at risk for vertebral fracture, the elderly, is increasing in number. As a result of increased life expectancy in the United States, the elderly population is increasing. The elderly are particularly prone to vertebral fracture for two reasons. First, vertebral fractures are more likely to occur when preexisting bone disease is present. The elderly

Table 7.3 Therapeutic medications and side-effects

Treatment	Disadvantages or side effects	Special considerations
Pregabalin/gabapentin/gabapentanoid agents	Somnolence, dizziness, asthenia, dry mouth, edema, constipation	
Opioids	Constipation, drowsiness, tolerance, dependence, respiratory depression	
Mixed serotonin/noradrenaline reuptake inhibitors	Hypertensive effects, gastrointestinal disturbance, dry mouth, reduced appetite, sweating, drug–drug interactions, including serotonin syndrome	
Mexiletine	Gastrointestinal upset, cardiovascular, hematological disturbance, skin reactions	
Topiramate	Drowsiness, dizziness, ataxia, anorexia, fatigue, gastrointestinal upset, occular issues, kidney stones	
Lamotrigine	Potentially life-threatening skin rash, hepatic effects, diplopia, blurred vision, dizziness	
Dronabinol	Dizziness, drowsiness, irritability	
Older anticonvulsants	Drowsiness, dizziness, liver dysfunction, hematological effects	
Acupuncture	Invasive, vagal reactions	Effectiveness for below-level neuropathic pain uncertain
Ketamine	Dysphoria, increased secretions, increased intracranial pressure	
Propofol	Hypotension, arrhythmias, bradycardia, respiratory failure	
Alfentanil	Short-term duration, invasive, respiratory depression, bradycardia, sedation, hypotension, nausea, vomiting	
Morphine	Respiratory depression, sedation, hypotension, nausea, vomiting, constipation	Effectiveness demonstrated for mechanical allodynia
Baclofen	Reports of increased or "unmasked" neuropathic pain, sedation, rash	Stronger evidence for spasm-related pain
Intrathecal morphine and clonidine	Invasive, tolerance, hypotension, respiratory depression, drowsiness	
Subarachnoid lignocaine	Invasive, central nervous system disturbance	
Spinal cord stimulation	Invasive, infection	At-level neuropathic pain, incomplete injuries
Deep brain stimulation	Invasive, intracranial hemorrhage, infection	
Motor cortex stimulation (transcranial)	Short-term effect, infection, hemorrhage	
Motor cortex stimulation (epidural)	Invasive, infection, hemorrhage	
DREZ	Invasive, risk of further deficits, infection, hemorrhage	At-level neuropathic pain
Cordotomy	Invasive, risk of further deficits, infection, hemorrhage	

Adapted by permission from Macmillan Publishers Ltd: Spinal Cord, Siddall PJ, Middleton JW, A proposed algorithm for the management of pain following spinal cord injury, 44(2):67-77, copyright 2006

have a higher incidence of preexisting bone disease as a result of decreased bone density due to osteoporosis and chronic steroid therapy [22]. Secondly, the most common etiology of vertebral fracture are falls, which occur more frequently in the elderly. For these reasons, elderly trauma patients with vertebral pain must be closely evaluated for vertebral fracture.

In the period immediately following a vertebral injury, it is essential to obtain radiographic imaging of the spine. Identifying vertebral fractures is essential because immediate surgical intervention may be required if coexisting neurologic deficits are present. Most patients with vertebral fractures unassociated with neurologic sequelae recover fully, and the

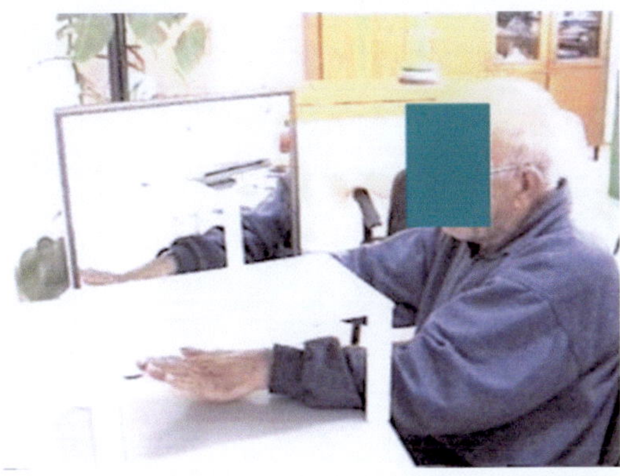

Fig. 7.5 Patient undergoing mirror therapy. Reprinted from Arch Phys Med Rehabil, 89, Gunes Yavuzer, Ruud Selles, Nebahat Sezer, Serap Sütbeyaz, Johannes B. Bussmann, Füsun Köseoğlu, Mesut B. Atay, Henk J. Stam, Mirror Therapy Improves Hand Function in Subacute Stroke: A Randomized Controlled Trial, pp. 393-8, Copyright 2008, with permission from Elsevier

mainstay of treatment is bed rest, pain control, and spine brace. However, minimally invasive treatment options are available and are becoming increasingly utilized. Vertebroplasty and kyphoplasty are percutaneous procedures that involve intraosseus injection of cement into vertebral bodies under fluoroscopic guidance. The difference between the two procedures is that kyphoplasty aims to return the vertebrae to its original height and shape. This is accomplished by inflating and then removing a balloon in the vertebral body prior to the injection of cement. Both vertebroplasty and kyphoplasty relieve pain by stabilizing the vertebrae and increasing strength. The pain relief these procedures provide is rapid, and as a result, vertebroplasty and kyphoplasty are becoming increasingly utilized (Fig. 7.6) [23].

Chronic Whiplash Syndrome

Whiplash is the descriptive term for cervical hyperextension from rapid acceleration or deceleration of the head in relation to the body [24]. This is most commonly due to rear-end motor vehicles collisions, contact sports, and

falls. The ubiquity of these mechanisms has led to enormous reporting in developed nations around the globe. The medical diagnosis is neck sprain.

The most common presenting symptoms are neck pain, stiffness, occipital headache, and thoracolumbar back pain. Serious physical injury is rare. Fifty to seventy percent of patients report complete recovery. However, 2–5 % develop chronic disability.

Chronic whiplash syndrome is symptoms that persist greater than six months. Those with rapid onset of severe pain, radiating pain, headache, preexisting spine problems, neurological signs, and hospital admission are most likely to develop chronic symptoms.

The social cost of this problem has attracted a great deal of investigation. Lack of physical findings, cultural reporting variances, and the opportunity for secondary gain complicate the discussion. Culture and expectation has a significant effect on outcome [25]. In one study, patients who were told to continue activities as usual were much better off at six-month follow-up than those who received neck immobilization and sick leave [26]. Despite widespread suggestion that secondary gain increases the rate of chronic whiplash, most data does not support this belief.

Current data indicates that treatment should be minimal. After ruling out serious injury, whiplash should be de-medicalized. Reassurance and early return to normal activities appears to be the best medicine. NSAIDS and corticosteroids are useful to assist with these goals, but soft collars and sick leave are counterproductive [27].

However, a percentage of patients do develop chronic symptoms. We have the knowledge to identify those more likely to have a poor outcome. Some suggest early aggressive treatment for these individuals. Hard collar therapy for 6–8 weeks virtually eliminates chronicity in cervical injuries. Additional research is necessary, but this approach may benefit high-risk patients with whiplash injuries (Fig. 7.7). On a societal level, better seatbelts and better headrests could drastically reduce the incidence of this injury and must be made available.

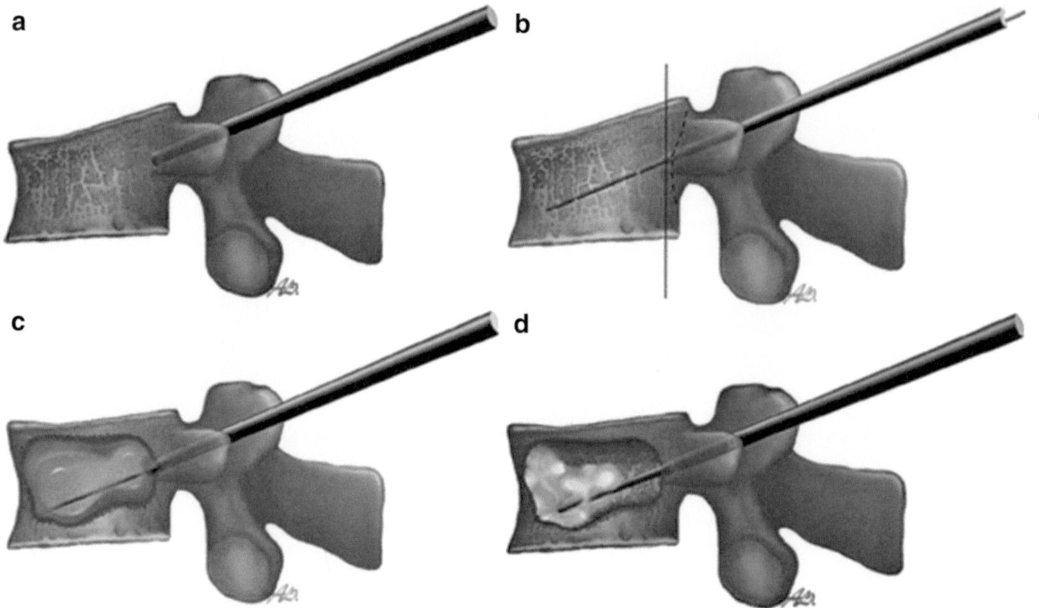

Fig. 7.6 Lateral view of balloon kyphoplasty. (**a**). The tip of the working cannula lying just within the posterior vertebral cortex (**b**), the K-wire and then the drill passed to the anterior third of the vertebral body where balloon is going to be sited (**c**). Balloon seen inflated and see the height restoration (**d**) cement being injected into the cavity created by the balloon. From Khalid Saeed, *Vertebroplasty and Kyphoplasty*, Springer, 1 January 2012. With kind permission from Springer Science and Business Media

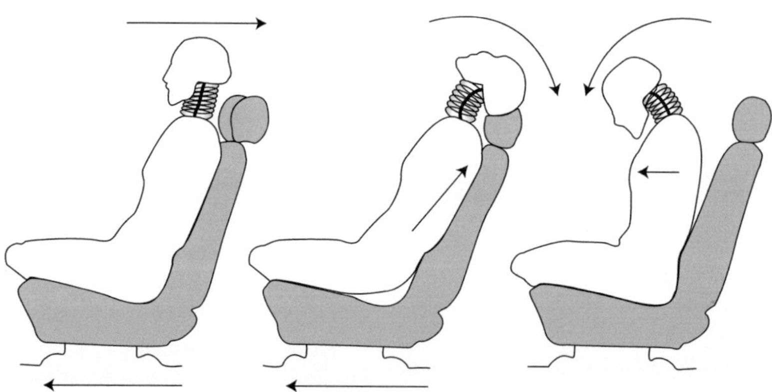

Fig. 7.7 Rear-end collision—a common mechanism of injury. Note the ineffectiveness of an improperly adjusted head restraint. From: IIHS (1997): "Special Issue: Head Restraints" [PDF, 575 KB], *Status Report* Vol.32, No.4. Website: http://www.iihs.org/externaldata/srdata/docs/sr3204.pdf. With permission from Insurance Institute for Highway Safety, Arlington, Virginia USA. www.iihs.org

In summary, traumatic injury is associated with a number of complicated pathophysiological processes that result in different chronic pain states. The clinician should appreciate mechanisms of each condition, evaluate appropriately, and provide the best therapeutic options. A good interventional pain physician and continued review of the literature made hold the greatest number of options, including interventional techniques, to optimize the disability and/or pain state of any given patient.

References

1. Gaskin D, Richard P. The economic costs of pain in the United States. J Pain. 2012;13(8):715–24.
2. Holes A, Williamson O, Hogg M, Arnold C, Prosser A, Clements J, Konstantatos A, O'Donnell M. Predictors of pain severity 3 months after serious injury. Pain Med. 2010;11:990–1000.
3. Harden RN, Bruehl S, Galer BS, Saltz S, Bertram M, Backonja M, Gayles R, Rudin N, Bughra M, Stanton-Hicks M. Complex regional pain syndrome: are the IASP diagnostic criteria valid and sufficiently comprehensive? Pain. 1999;83:211–9.
4. de Mos M, Huygen FJ, van der Hoeven-Borgman M, et al. Outcome of the complex regional pain syndrome. Clin J Pain. 2009;25:590–7.
5. Gradl G, Schürmann M. Sympathetic dysfunction as a temporary phenomenon in acute posttraumatic CRPS I. Clin Auton Res. 2005;15:29–34.
6. Oaklander AL, Rissmiller JG, Gelman LB, Zheng L, Chang Y, Gott R. Evidence of focal small-fiber axonal degeneration in complex regional pain syndrome-I (reflex sympathetic dystrophy). Pain. 2006;120:235–43.
7. Maihöfner C, Handwerker HO, Neundörfer B, Birklein F. Patterns of cortical reorganization in complex regional pain syndrome. Neurology. 2003;61:1707–15.
8. Nampiaparampil DE. Prevalence of chronic pain after traumatic brain injury. JAMA. 2008;300(6):711–9.
9. Brummett CM, Raja SN. Central Pain States. In: Benzon HT, Raja SN, Liu SS, Fishman SM, Cohen S, editors. Essentials of pain medicine. 3rd ed. New York: Elsevier-Churchill-Livingstone; 2011.
10. Corrigan JD, Selassie AW, Orman JA. The epidemiology of traumatic brain injury. J Head Trauma Rehabil. 2010;25(2):72–80.
11. Uomoto JM, Esselman PC. TBI and chronic pain: differential types and rates by head injury severity. Arch Phys Med Rehabil. 1993;74(1):61–4.
12. De Benedittis G, De Santis A. Chronic posttraumatic headache: clinical psychopathological features and outcome determinants. J Neurosurg Sci. 1983;27(3):177–86.
13. Sidall PJ, Yezierski RP, Loeser JD. Pain following spinal cord injury: clinical features, prevalence, and taxonomy. IASP Newslett. 2000;3:3–7.
14. Siddall PJ, Middleton JW. A proposed algorithm for the management of pain following a spinal cord injury. Spinal Cord. 2006;44:67–77.
15. Cardenas DD, Jensen MP. Treatments for chronic pain in persons with spinal cord injury: a survey study. J Spinal Cord Med. 2006;29:109–17.
16. Jensen TS, Krebs B, Nielsen J, Rasmussen P. Phantom limb, phantom pain and stump pain in amputees during the first 6 months following limb amputation. Pain. 1983;17:243–56.
17. Karanikolas M, Aretha D, Tsolakis I, et al. Optimized perioperative analgesia reduces chronic phantom limb pain intensity, prevalence, and frequency: a prospective, randomized, clinical trial. Anesthesiology. 2011;114:1144–54.
18. Flor H, Elbert T, Knecht S, et al. Phantom limb pain as a perceptual correlate of cortical reorganization following arm amputation. Nature. 1995;357:482–4.
19. Ramachandran VS, Altschuler EL. The use of visual feedback, in particular mirror visual feedback, in restoring brain function. Brain. 2009;132:1693–710.
20. Dietrich C, Walter-Walsh K, Preissler S, Hofmann GO, Witte OW, et al. Sensory feedback prosthesis reduces phantom limb pain: proof of a principle. Neurosci Lett. 2012;507:97–100.
21. Viswanathan A, Phan PC, Burton AW. Use of spinal cord stimulation in the treatment of phantom limb pain: case series and review of the literature. Pain Pract. 2010;10:479–84. doi:10.1111/j.1533-2500.2010.00374.x.
22. Nardi A, Ventura L, Rossini M, Ramazzina E. The importance of mechanics in the pathogenesis of fragility fractures of the femur and vertebrae. Clin Cases Miner Bone Metab. 2010;7(2):130–4.
23. McGirt M, Parker S, Wolinsky J, Witham T, Bydon A, Gokaslan Z. Vertebroplasty and kyphoplasty for the treatment of vertebral compression fractures: an evidenced-based review of the literature. Spine J. 2009;9(6):501–8.
24. Sturzenegger M, DiStefano G, Radanov BP, et al. Presenting symptoms and signs after whiplash injury: the influence of accident mechanisms. Neurology. 1994;44:688–93.
25. Ferrari R, Obelieniene D, Russell A, Darlington P, Gervais R, Green P. Laypersons' expectation of the sequelae of whiplash injury. a cross-cultural comparative study between Canada and Lithuania. Med Sci Monit. 2002;8:CR728–34.
26. Borchgrevink GE, Kaasa A, McDonagh D, Stiles TC, Haraldseth O, Lereim I. Acute treatment of whiplash neck sprain injuries. A randomized trial of treatment during the first 14 days after a car accident. Spine (Phila Pa 1976). 1998;23(1):25–31.
27. Rosenfeld M, Gunnarson R, Borenstein P. Intervention in whiplash-associated disorders: a comparison of two treatment methods. Spine. 2000;25:1782–7.

Brain Injuries: Perianesthetic Management

8

Elizabeth A.M. Frost

Historical Note

For millennia man has suffered and treated head injuries. The oldest known medical papyrus, the Edwin Smith Papyrus, dates from the seventeenth century BCE and was written in black and red hieratic, the Egyptian cursive form of hieroglyphs [1]. It was named for an American Egyptologist, Edwin Smith (1822–1906) who was born in the year that Egyptian hieroglyphic was deciphered. The authorship of the manuscript is unknown but has been attributed to writings from an even earlier time, perhaps by a priest and physician of the Old Kingdom, Imhotep (3000–2500BCE). The treatise describes 48 cases, 15 of which are head injuries, 12 facial wounds, and 7 vertebral fractures. Other cases refer to injuries of the upper thorax and shoulders. Diagnosis, management mainly by finger exploration, resulted in several treatment options that were classified as: (a) "An ailment which I will treat" (a gaping wound in the head penetrating to the bone); (b) "An ailment with which I will contend" (A gaping wound penetrating to the bone and splitting the skull);

or (c) "An ailment not to be treated" (same as the previous cases but with the addition of fever and stiffness of the neck) [2]. Therapy for the most part included immobilization for head and spinal cord injuries. Surgical stitching of wounds of the lip, throat, and shoulder was described. Dressings included the application of fresh meat (to stop bleeding) and honey (honey is still used, especially in war zones, as a type of occlusive and antiseptic dressing).

Although trephination is not mentioned in the Edwin Smith papyrus, surgical incisions of the cranium were the most common treatment for patients with head wounds, especially if they were seizing. It may have been used to clean wounds after trauma in battle [3]. Trephination was a form of primitive emergency surgery after head wounds [4] to remove shattered fragments of bone from a fractured skull, and clean out hematoma. Such injuries were typical for primitive weaponry such as slingshot projectiles and war clubs. Hippocrates, who also described the systemic effects of head injury including cardiorespiratory changes, recommended trephination and diuresis for simple skull fractures and for contusions of the brain without fractures, especially to prevent complications [4, 5].

By the nineteenth century, treatment of head injuries may have taken a step backwards. Sir Astley Cooper, consulting surgeon to Guy's Hospital in London, presented a series of lectures he had given in the operating theater at St Thomas' Hospital on the principle and practice of surgery. He wrote "trephining in concussion is now so

---

The time has been that, when the brains were out the man would die, and there be an end; but now they rise again. (Macbeth. Act 3, Scene 4;78–80 (Macbeth on seeing the ghost of Banquo))

E.A.M. Frost, M.B., Ch.B., D.R.C.O.G. (✉)
Department of Anesthesiology, Icahn Medical Center at Mount Sinai, 1 Gustave L. Levy Place, New York, NY 10029, USA
e-mail: elizabeth.frost@mountsinai.org

C.S. Scher (ed.), *Anesthesia for Trauma*, DOI 10.1007/978-1-4939-0909-4_8,
© Springer Science+Business Media New York 2014

145

completely abandoned that in the last four years I do not know that I have [performed it once whilst 35 years ago I would have performed it five or six times a year]" [6]. He recommended frequent bleeding, calomel purges, and leeches to be applied to the temporal arteries. But then head injuries in the United Kingdom may have decreased with the passing of the slingshot, the axe, and good gun control (especially among the militia).

Hope was on the way. Neurosurgery became a specialty with such luminaries as Sir William Macewen in Scotland, Sir Victor Horsley in London, Professor Fedor Krause in Germany, and Dr. Harvey Cushing in the United States [7]. Greater understanding of intracranial dynamics developed. The Monro-Kellie doctrine, a synthesis of the works of eighteenth century Scottish anatomist (Alexander Monro) and nineteenth century American physiologist (George Kellie), stated that the cranial cavity is a closed rigid box, and that the quantity of intracranial blood must change through the displacement or replacement of cerebrospinal fluid [8, 9]. Walter Cannon, an American physiologist (who coined the phrase "fight or flight") described intracranial pressure (ICP) monitoring in 1901, as an expansion of the work of Claude Bernard on homeostasis [10].

Now into the twenty-first century, we have taken from the past and refined our treatment with a better understanding of pathophysiology. While accurate diagnosis remains critical, addition of radiologic techniques has replaced manual palpation. Craniotomy, now under sterile conditions and with the benefit of anesthesia, is an improvement on trephination. The importance of controlling intracranial hypertension and cardiorespiratory perturbations, often for a prolonged period after the traumatic event, is underscored. Pharmacologic diuresis, rather than hit or miss herbal therapy, has replaced bloodletting to control intravascular volume and cerebral edema. Antibiotics appear to exert better results than honey in decreasing infection.

We do not have all the answers yet, in part because we still do not have many of the questions. But, slow as it is, given that the concern of head trauma is still with us, we have made many advances.

Scope of the Problem

Traumatic head injuries remain a major cause of death, and disability, despite the introduction of many guidelines for care. Traumatic brain injury (TBI) and head injury are often used interchangeably in the literature [11]. The classification is broad and includes neuronal, vascular, and cranial nerve injuries as well as intracranial hemorrhages, subdural hygromas among others. Further classification is made to open and close head injuries. At least 1.7 million people sustain a TBI in the United States annually and about 3 % are fatal [12, 13]. Of those individuals, about 52,000 die, 275,000 are hospitalized, and 1.365 million are treated and released from an emergency department. The number of people with TBI who are not seen in a hospital or emergency department or who receive no care is currently unknown. The current report from the CDC presents data on emergency department visits, hospitalizations, and deaths for the years 2002–2006 [12]. TBI is a contributing factor to a third of all injury-related deaths in this country. About 75 % of TBI's are concussions or other forms of mild TBI [12, 13].

The CDC has further documented TBI by age [12]:
1. Children 0–4 years, older adolescents, and adults >65 years are the most likely victims
2. 473,947 Emergency department visits for TBI are made annually by children aged 0–14 years
3. Adults aged >75 years have the highest rates of TBI-related hospitalizations and death
4. In all age groups, TBI rates are higher for males than for females
5. Males aged 0–4 have the highest rates of TBI-related emergency department visits

Direct medical costs and indirect costs such as lost productivity totaled an estimated $76.5 billion in the United States in 2000, a number that may be higher in 2013 dollars [14].

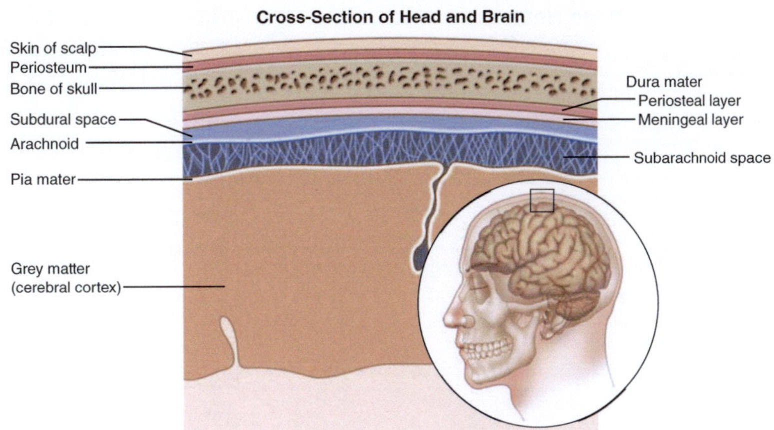

Fig. 8.1 Cross-section of the head and brain. The relative layers of the skull are illustrated

Types of Injury

Many causes are related to the wide variety of injuries. Injuries in adults tend to be due to falls, motor vehicle accidents, and assault. Falls and being struck are the most common causes of head injury in children. Assault, child, and adult abuse are most common at the extremes of age. Major cerebral dysfunction can occur with little or no apparent external injury. Force applied to the head may cause the brain to be directly injured or shaken, impacting the inner wall of the skull. The trauma can potentially cause bleeding in the spaces surrounding the brain, contuse brain tissue, or damage the nerve connections within the brain.

Skull Fractures

The cranium is made up of many fused bones that form a solid box comprised of brain tissue (84 %), cerebrospinal fluid (11 %), and blood (5 %). Any increase in one component must be offset by a decrease in another to avoid an increase in ICP. Bony fractures may or may not damage the underlying brain, depending on their location. For the most part, skull fractures are described based on their location, the appearance of the fracture, and whether the fragment is depressed. Not all bones of the cranium have the same ability to withstand trauma, with some being thinner and more fragile than others. The temporal bone, which covers the meningeal artery, is relatively thin and more easily fractured than the occipital bone and can give rise to an epidural hematoma. A fracture may be linear or have a stellate-like pattern. Gunshot and stab wounds or impaled objects cause penetrating injury and usually imply damage to the brain substance. Depressed fractures, often in children, may require surgery to elevate the fragment. Brain injury may or may not be apparent. Open fractures, when the skin above the fracture is broken, carry a much higher rate of infection (Fig. 8.1).

Basilar fractures refer to fractures of the bones at the base of the skull. Signs include bruising around the eyes (raccoon eyes) and behind the ears (Battle sign). If the fracture line extends into the bones around the facial sinuses, there is increased risk of intracranial infection. Bacteria and other miscellaneous material may also be pushed into the brain by an inappropriately placed endotracheal, nasogastric tube, or temperature probe through the nose.

Diastases fractures occur in infants and young children in whom the suture lines have not yet fused and the fontanelles remain open, allowing for widening of these suture lines.

Intracranial Bleeding

Intracranial bleeding refers to any bleeding within the skull. Intracerebral bleeding describes bleeding within the brain (Fig. 8.2). Descriptions are based upon location. Intracranial bleeding may

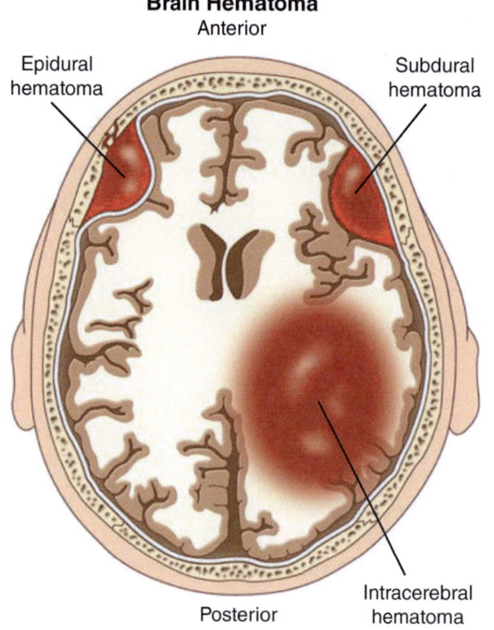

Fig. 8.2 Locations of commonly described intracerebral hemorrhage

occur with an intact skull. Thus, a plain X-ray of the skull may fail to realize the extent of injury.

Subdural hematoma is caused by rupture of bridging veins within the subdural space as brain parenchyma moves during violent head motion. It may also occur due to arterial rupture. The clot may form at the site of injury or on the opposite side of the skull (contra coup injury) usually in a deceleration injury. This injury is the most common type of TBI, occurring in about 20–40 % [15]. A lucid interval is less likely. Chronic subdural hematoma may be the result of atrophy of brain tissue as may occur in the elderly or in some disease states. As the subdural space enlarges, bridging veins are stretched and may break. Often there are no symptoms or minimal behavioral changes that may be misdiagnosed as the extension of a dementia. Asymptomatic chronic subdural hematomas often resolve spontaneously.

Epidural hematoma collect in a small area outside the dura. As a clot forms, pressure can increase rapidly, impinging on the brain and causing significant injury. Incidence is about 1 % of all head trauma admissions, but it may

also develop as a progressive lesion in up to 9 % of patients who have sustained a head injury [16]. As noted above, acute arterial epidural hematoma are most commonly caused by a blow to the temporal bones with rupture of the underlying middle meningeal artery (85 %). After a lucid interval, consciousness is often lost quickly and surgery to release the clot is urgent.

Subarachnoid hemorrhage refers to accumulation of blood within the space beneath the inner arachnoid layer of the meninges and is often associated with an intracerebral bleed. Cerebral spinal fluid (CSF) is also found in this space. Blood in this area causes significant meningeal irritation causing an almost immediate onset of severe headache, nausea, vomiting, and a stiff neck. Similar symptoms are displayed with leaking or ruptured cerebral aneurysms or arteriovenous malformation or meningitis. Treatment usually requires neuroradiologic intervention of surgery. However, days to weeks after TBI, traumatic aneurysms can form. Treatment then is more likely to be observational, especially if the aneurysm remains intact.

Intracerebral hemorrhage/cerebral contusion relate to bleeding within the brain caused by direct damage and also by resultant edema. Surgery is usually not a consideration unless the ICP is dangerously high when decompressive craniectomy may be the only choice [17].

Shear injury causes a diffuse axonal injury which is often fatal. The injury disrupts neuronal transmission. The patient is comatose with no evidence of intracerebral bleeding. MRI studies show a correlation between white matter lesions and impairment of consciousness after injury. The deeper the white matter lesions, the more profound and persistent is unconsciousness [18]. Postmortem evidence shows that about 30–40 % of individuals who die after TBI have diffuse axonal injury and ischemia [19]. The pathology is usually caused by deceleration-acceleration or lateral rotational injuries rather than direct contact. Treatment is mainly supportive.

Concussions are considered a milder form of this type of injury, although serious consequences may result in sports injuries (see below).

Fig. 8.3 An illustration of the hypoxic-ischemic cascade (Modified from Huang BY, Castillo M, Hypoxic-Ischemic Brain Injury: Imaging Findings from Birth to Adulthood, Radiographics, 28, 417–439, 2008)

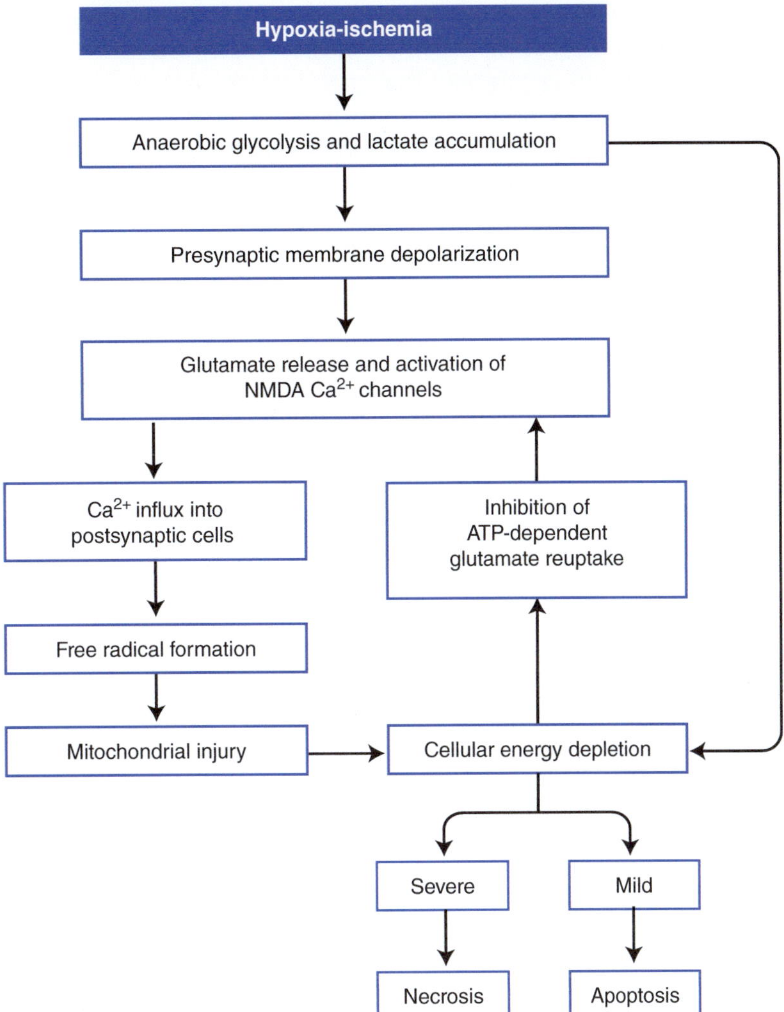

Occasionally, concussion-type symptoms may be missed. Patients may experience difficulty concentrating, mood swings, lethargy or aggression, and altered sleep habits among other symptoms.

Pathophysiology

Head injuries are classified as primary or secondary. Primary damage results from the initial blow to the head. Histologic studies done immediately after injury may show no changes, indicating that the initial injury appears to be electrical transmission failure rather than mechanical injury. The common underlying physiologic processes that result in neuronal cell death are diminished cerebral blood flow (ischemia) and reduced blood oxygenation (hypoxemia) (Fig. 8.3). Global hypoxic-ischemic insults do not affect all brain structures uniformly. Rather, certain tissues in the brain are more likely to be injured and are injured earlier than others, a concept known as selective vulnerability. The observed patterns of injury reflect dysfunction of selected excitatory neuronal circuits, which causes a complex cascade of deleterious biochemical events and, ultimately, selective neuronal death [20]. Brain ischemia causes a change from oxidative phosphorylation to anaerobic metabolism, a highly inefficient means to produce energy. Adenosine triphosphate (ATP) is rapidly depleted and lactate accumulates within cells. Normal cellular membrane function is lost. As presynaptic neuronal cell membranes depolarize, excitatory neurotransmitters—in particular, glutamate—are released. Glutamate binds predominantly to *N*-methyl-D-aspartate (NMDA) receptor-mediated calcium (Ca^{2+}) channels. Activation of NMDA receptors results in an influx of Ca^{2+} into postsynaptic neurons, and a corresponding extracellular increase in potassium. Several cytotoxic processes are triggered, including activation of membrane phospholipases and production of the oxygen-free radicals (such as nitric oxide) that damage cell membranes and constituents, especially the mitochondria. As the ATP-dependent glutamate reuptake pump fails, energy depletion is intensified resulting in cell death and/or apoptosis.

Cell death after TBI is the major cause of neurologic deficits and mortality [21]. Understanding the mechanisms of delayed posttraumatic cell loss should lead to new therapies and improved outcome. TBI induces changes in many cell types and recent work has emphasized the diversity of neuronal death phenotypes that have been defined as morphological or molecular changes [22]. The most effective neuroprotective strategies must, therefore, target multiple pathways to reflect regional and temporal changes underlying the different neuronal cell death phenotypes. Moreover, traditionally it was thought that adult neurons are in a permanent post-mitotic phase. Newer studies indicate that cell cycle constituents critically affect normal functions of the central nervous system ad also contribute to the pathophysiology of acute disorders. Cell cycle pathways are involved in mediating not only neuronal cell death, but also glial changes that play key roles in the pathophysiologic mechanisms underlying acute neurodegeneration. Thus, therapies that inhibit cell cycle may prove neuroprotective after acute insults by targeting multiple pathogenic mechanisms [23].

Rapid triage and decision-making in the treatment of TBI is challenging in "resource poor" environments such as the battlefield and developing areas of the world. Tests to guide treatment

of TBI are needed and are means to differentiate between diffuse and focal brain injury and assess the potential for determining outcome, ICP management, and responses to therapy. Several biomarkers have been identified and shown promise as prognostic indicators.

CD40L or CD154 is a membrane glycoprotein and differentiation antigen expressed on the surface of T-cells. It is part of the tissue necrotizing factor superfamily of molecules and binds T cells and antigen-presenting cells. The CD40 ligand stimulates B-cell proliferation and secretion of all immunoglobulin isotopes in the presence of cytokines CD40 ligand has been shown to induce cytokine production and in peripheral blood monocytes. It also co-stimulates proliferation of activated T-cells and this is accompanied by the production of interferon (IFN-gamma), tumor necrosis factor (TNF-alpha), and interleukin 2 (IL). In fact, sCD40L represents a central event of immune adaptive response as it acts on so many cells. Johansson et al. studied 80 trauma patients admitted to a Level I Trauma Center. High circulating sCD40L was associated with enhanced tissue and endothelial damage (injury severity score, hcDNA, Annexin V, syndecan-1 and sTM), shock (pH, standard base excess), sympathoadrenal activation (adrenaline) and coagulopathy evidenced by reduced thrombin generation (PF1.2), hyperfibrinolysis (D-dimer), increased activated partial thromboplastin time (APTT), and inflammation (IL-6) (all $P < 0.05$) [23]. A higher ISS ($P = 0.017$), adrenaline ($P = 0.049$), and platelet count ($P = 0.012$) and lower pH ($P = 0.002$) were associated with higher sCD40L by multivariate linear regression analysis. High circulating sCD40L (odds ratio [OR] 1.84 [95 % CI 1.05–3.23], $P = 0.034$), high age ($P = 0.002$), and low Glasgow Coma Score (GCS) prehospital ($P = 0.002$) were independent predictors of increased mortality.

Glial fibrillary acidic protein (GFAP) is an intermediate filament protein found in the cytoskeleton of astroglia. Recent work has indicated that GFAP may serve as a serum marker of TBI that is released after central nervous system cell damage [24]. In a study of 39 patients with TBI, persistent elevation of GFAP on day 2 was predictive of increased mortality. Excellent specificity for CT-documented brain injury was found using a cutoff point of 1 pg/mL.

A systematic review and meta analysis of randomized controlled trials and observational studies investigating the ability and accuracy of the S-100b protein in predicting prognosis after moderate or severe TBI yielded 9,228 citations, 2 randomized control trials, and 39 cohort studies [25]. Serum S-100B protein concentrations were significantly associated with poor prognosis in short-, mid-, and long-term outcomes. However, optimal thresholds for discrimination remained unclear.

Other studies have suggested that postischemic release patterns of GFAB and also S-100B protein after acute stroke may allow insight into the underlying pathophysiology and could be used in clinical stroke treatment [26].

As noted above, cerebral contusion releases leukocytes and chemokines such as the interleukins (IL2, 6, 8), monocyte chemo attractant protein, and neuron-specific enolases. While increasing levels may not be predictors of expanding contusion, these inflammatory mediators may be predictive of a poor outcome in patients with TBI in which contusions are the predominant abnormality. However, they do not distinguish those patients who will deteriorate because of contusion enlargement [27]. Another animal study confirmed an early increase in IL-6 in brain, plasma, and cerebrospinal fluid protein levels [28]. In addition, secondary posttraumatic hypoxia led to prolonged elevations in plasma IL-6. A clinical study quantified IL-6 plasma levels in patients with closed head trauma and hemorrhagic contusions during the first 6–12 h after injury. A strong correlation between IL-6 levels, volume of traumatic hemorrhage, and in-hospital course was identified [29].

Other researchers have examined the role of mitochondrial damage. The mitochondrion is a major target of TBI, as seen by increased mitochondrial activity in activated and proliferating microglia (high energy requirements and/or calcium overload) as well as increased reactive oxygen species, changes in mitochondrial permeability transition, release of cytochrome c,

caspase activation, reduced ATP levels, and neuronal death. Translocator protein (TSPO) is an 18-kDa outer mitochondrial membrane protein that interacts with the mitochondria permeability transition pore and binds to some drug ligands. TSPO levels in the brain are generally low but increase after brain injury. The use of TSPO expression as a marker of brain injury and repair has been suggested. TSPO drug ligands have been shown to participate in the control of mitochondrial respiration and function, mitochondrial steroid, and neurosteroid formation, as well as apoptosis [30].

It would seem that identification of the various biomarkers produced in the injured brain is a developing and promising tool in the management of the head-injured patients, not only for prognosis but also in treatment. Yokobori et al. have recently summarized the present status of plasma biomarkers in TBI. At present, there is insufficient evidence to support a role for diagnostic biomarkers in exactly distinguishing focal and diffuse injury or for accurate determination of raised ICP. Presently, neurofilament (NF), S100β, GFAP, and ubiquitin carboxyl terminal hydrolase-L1 (UCH-L1) seem to have the best potential as diagnostic biomarkers for distinguishing focal and diffuse injury, whereas C-tau, neuron-specific enolase (NSE), S100β, GFAP, and spectrin breakdown products (SBDPs) appear to be candidates for ICP reflective biomarkers. With the combinations of different pathophysiology related to each biomarker, a multibiomarker analysis seems to be indicated and would likely increase diagnostic accuracy. To date little research has focused on the differential diagnostic properties of biomarkers in TBI [31].

Secondary insult develops minutes to hours later due to hypotension, hypoxia, acidosis, edema, or other factors, probably accelerated by the production of free radicals. About 38 % of victims who die after head injury talked at some time following the initial insult [32]. In a review of 116 patients known to have talked at some point before dying, one or more avoidable factors were identified in 74 % and in 54 % an avoidable factor was judged certainly

Table 8.1 Several insults contributing to poor outcome after head injury

Secondary intracranial insults	Secondary systemic insults
Hemorrhage	Hypoxia
Ischemia	Hypercapnia
Intracranial hypertension	Hyperglycemia
Vasospasm	Hypotension
Infection	Hypocapnia
Seizures	Hyperpyrexia
Hydrocephalus	Anemia
Delay in diagnosis	Hyponatremia

to have contributed to death. These secondary insults have been confirmed in many more recent studies [33] (Table 8.1). Most of the patients without identifiable factors died after rapid deterioration of an expanding intracranial bleed.

Diagnosis

As noted above, symptoms range from none to coma. Common findings are headache, vomiting, seizures, and visual disturbances. The American Academy of Neurology has devised a grading scale to categorize the degree of consciousness (Table 8.2).

The Glasgow Coma Scale was designed as a prognostic indicator of outcome after head injury, but is widely used as assessment of progress or deterioration (Table 8.3) [34]. Scores range from 3 to 15. Scores <8 are considered severe injury. Confounding factors include patients who are intubated or who have eye injuries. The scale is not as readily applicable to children who have greater cerebral plasticity.

Use of the GCS makes it possible for first responders and other less trained health care workers to quickly and reliably assess injured patients. It is part of the initial evaluation, but does not indicate the diagnosis as to the cause of coma. Since it "scores" the level of coma, the GCS can be used as a standard method for any healthcare practitioner to assess change in patient

Table 8.2 American Academy of Neurology Concussion Grading Scale

Grade 1	Grade 2	Grade 3
Transient confusion	Transient confusion	…
No loss of consciousness	No loss of consciousness	Brief or prolonged loss of consciousness
Concussion symptoms or mental status change resolves in 15 min or less	Concussion symptoms or mental status change resolves in more than 15 min	…

Table 8.3 Glasgow Coma Scale

Eye opening	
Spontaneous	4
To loud voice	3
To pain	2
None	1
Verbal response	
Oriented	5
Confused, disoriented	4
Inappropriate words	3
Incomprehensible words	2
None	1
Motor response	
Obeys commands	6
Localizes pain	5
Withdraws from pain	4
Abnormal flexion posturing	3
Extensor posturing	2
None	1

status. It is a component of the Acute Physiology and Chronic Health Evaluation (APACHE) II score, the (Revised) Trauma Score, the Trauma and Injury Severity Score (TRISS) and the Circulation, Respiration, Abdomen, Motor, Speech (CRAMS) Scale, demonstrating the widespread adoption of the scale. The Glasgow outcome score considers the end result and is scored 1–5 (Table 8.4)

Other descriptive terms include "decorticate" which refers to the cortex of the brain, which deals with movement, sensation, and thinking. A flexion response may be seen on stimulation." Decerebrate" indicates that the cortex and the

Table 8.4 Glasgow Outcome Score

Score	Rating	Definition
5	Good recovery	Resumption of normal life despite minor deficits
4	Moderate disability	Disabled but independent. Can work in sheltered setting
3	Severe disability	Conscious but disabled. Dependent for daily support
2	Persistent vegetative	Minimal responsiveness
1	Death	Non survival

Table 8.5 Several risk factors identified in head injury victims

Advancing age/very young	Delay in transfer
Cardiothoracic injury	Child abuse
Alcohol abuse/male gender	Shock
Coagulation disorders	Iatrogenic
Related to injury	Delay in operation, technical errors
Incidental medication	Management errors, hypoxia, hypercarbia

brain stem that unconsciously control basic functions like breathing and heart beat may not be functioning.

Risk Factors

Several risk factors have been associated with TBI (Table 8.5).

Extremes of age—Advancing age: Several factors point to an increasing concern regarding head trauma in the elderly. As of now, 13 % of the population is >65years, a percentage that is projected to exceed 21 % by 2050 [35]. Accidental trauma at present is the fifth most common cause of death and geriatric trauma will make up 395 of trauma by 2015. In older patients, GCS < 9 is associated with a mortality rate of 80 %. Poor outcome increases 40 %/decade of life. Elderly people are more likely to sustain low energy falls and high cervical fractures are common. Traffic accidents are related to poor vision, impaired hearing, and slower response times. Thermal injuries are related to decreased smell, vision, mobility, and reaction times. Abuse and neglect are also more common in older people. Also, younger patients are more likely to receive more and better care [35]. Deceased cardiac function; by as much as 50 % means that the aging myocardium is less responsive to the catecholamine surge that is one of the first responses after TBI. Elderly patients are often maintained on beta blockers, anticoagulants, or have diabetes. Renal function may be impaired so they are less able to deal with a fluid load during resuscitation. Respiratory function, including vital capacity, the ability to cough, and oxygen saturation are decreased. Rib fractures may compound the picture. The tissue response to thyroxin is decreased. Hypotension, defined as systolic blood pressure (SBP) less than 90 mmHg, is recognized as a sign of hemorrhagic shock and is a validated prognostic indicator. The definition of hypotension, particularly in the elderly population, deserves attention. Elderly patients are more likely to present to the emergency room hypotensive and hypothermic. A recent reevaluation of what constitutes hypotension in older people has been offered. The authors considered 24,438 trauma patients to identify the model that most accurately defined hypotension for three age groups. For patients 20–49, the optimal definition of hypotension was systolic pressure of 100 mmHg. Between the ages of 50 and 69, hypotension was defined if the SBP was <120 mmHg. By 70 years, the number rose to 140 mmHg. Studies indicate that 42 % of elderly victims have increased lactate and base deficit levels with vital signs that have been considered "normal" [35, 36]. Lactate levels >4 mmol/L and/or base deficit >6 are associated with a mortality rate of 40 %. In younger individuals, mortality rates at the same values approximate 12 % [36].

Recent studies have only confirmed what was published 20 years ago: the mortality rate for blunt hade trauma in elderly patients exceeds 30 % and is six times the average in the general population. Early intensive monitoring may help uncover resuscitative or anesthetic effects that may improve outcome [37]. A review of 18,856 patients who sustained motor vehicle accidents showed a mortality rate of 2.4 % with the first

Table 8.6 General principles to follow in the management of the geriatric trauma patient

Geriatric head trauma: General guidelines
Monitor and maintain Hb near pre-injury levels
Goal-directed fluid resuscitation: pulse pressure variation as a guide, avoid excessive fluids, minimal central line catheterization
Reduce dosages of all anesthetic agents
Design a geriatric trauma care team. Manage aggressively
Be aware of under triaging

24 h [38]. Head injury, multiple trauma, and advancing age ($P = 0.0001$) were significant risk factors. General guidelines for care of the geriatric head trauma victim are summarized in Table 8.6.

Pediatric trauma: At the other extreme of age, babies are also victims of head trauma but often due to different causes. TBI is the leading cause of death in children. Hypotension, hypoxia, hyperglycemia, and fever are particularly associated with poor outcomes. Carbon dioxide reactivity and autoregulation are altered and can result in devastating cerebral ischemia or hyperemia [39]. The mechanisms for these changes are not well elucidated. Understanding the effects of TBI on a child's cerebral circulation is essential to develop protocols to improve outcome. Children who are reported to have fallen less than 4 ft are more likely to be victims of child abuse [40]. "Shaken baby" syndrome occurs mostly in children <1 year. The damage is caused by repetitive oscillations with rotational acceleration of the head. Injuries sustained include encephalopathy, retinal hemorrhages, and subdural hematomas. Fourteen to 38 % die and at least 30 % sustain neurologic sequelae [41].

Shock/Multiple trauma: The addition of major visceral or extremity injuries that cause shock significantly increases the risk of death (12–62 %), the need for rehabilitation (39–60 %), and the cost of disability [42]. These early findings have been shown again, especially concerning the number of rib fractures. Patients who had six or more rib fractures were three times more likely to die within 4 h of admission compared with patients with only one rib fracture [38]. However, especially when there is concomitant

head injury, the value of SBP, heart rate (HR), and respiratory rate (RR) have been shown to be poor predictors of outcome. The shock index (SI) is a simple calculation of the relationship between HR and SBP (HR/SBP). Normal values are around 0.6 and as the number approaches 1 or higher, there is an increased risk of shock. Some newer markers including SI × age (SIA), SBP/age (BPA1), maximum HR (220-age)-HR (minpulse, MP), and HR/maximum HR (pulse max index, PMI) have been shown to be better predictors of 48 h mortality when compared with traditional vital signs [43]. The likelihood of death was 8.4 times higher if SIA was greater than 55.

Alcohol: Several studies have looked at the severity of injuries and outcome in intoxicated patients [44, 45]. In one study of motorcycle crashes, half of the victims died before reaching hospital and alcohol was a significant factor [45]. Another study of 106 males indicated that alcohol abuse was associated with a significantly higher incidence of injuries and increased postoperative morbidity and mortality [44]. Another review of 246 patients found that alcohol intoxication combined with age >60 was associated with a higher incidence of cerebral contusions that required surgery and had a poorer prognosis [46]. However, ethanol is a systemic immunomodulator and TBI initiates a neuroinflammatory response. Goodman et al. gavaged rats with ethanol or water prior to TBI [47]. Alcohol treatment prior to TBI decreased the local neuroinflammatory response to injury. Rats given alcohol all exhibited a faster posttraumantic righting response and neurologic recovery time. Pre-injury alcohol treatment was associated with reduced levels of proinflammatory cytokines, IL-6, MCP-1 among others. Transfer of this evidence to the human setting is still debated.

Gender/Male: Complicating the issue of alcohol abuse and multiple trauma from motor cycle accidents is the question of gender as there is a higher incidence alcohol abuse and bikers among males. A recent report from the US CDC showed that death from TBI was 3.4-times more common for males versus females [48]. Males were 2.3-times more likely to have sustained injury by motor vehicle crash, 2.5-times more likely to have a TBI secondary to falls and 6.0-times more likely to be injured via firearms. However, for the most part TBI research is not only from male subjects, but data has been lacking that separates gender in analyses. Thus, there remain gaps in understanding prevention, neuroprotection, secondary injury, rehabilitation timing and therapeutics, and specific outcome remain large [49].

Delay in transfer: Debate between "stay and play" or "swoop and scoop" has been ongoing in trauma transfer. Several studies over the past 30 years indicate that prompt transfer to an appropriate facility after the initial assessment and triage yields the best results. A short scene time is possible and strong medical control and excellent support systems are essential [50]. A review of 2,067 trauma victims admissions in Finland showed that 38 % were treated at a University hospital, 26 % in large non-teaching ICUs, 20 % in mid-size ICUs, and 15 % in small ICUs. Hospital mortality was 5.6 %, broken down as 4.7 % in university ICU and 6.6 % in mid-size ICU [51]. In two subgroup analyses of severely ill trauma patients with APACHE II points >25 or SOFA score >8 points, respectively, hospital mortality was significantly lower in university ICUs. A similar study of 2,875 trauma patients in Denmark found that around 50 % of all trauma deaths occurred at the scene [52]. Increased survival of severely injured patients may be achieved by early transfer to highly specialized care. Despite these analyses and the triage and transfer guidelines that are in place in most states in the United States, compliance is far from complete.

Guidelines published by the American College of Surgeons Committee on Trauma outline criteria for the immediate transfer of moderately to severely injured patients to Level I/II Trauma Centers. Acquisition of pretransfer computed tomography (CT) scans is not required. A retrospective review of 7,713 severely injured patients who met the criteria for transfer to a level one center found that 57 % had a pretransfer CT scan. Penetrating wounds, physiologic compromise, and Injury Severity scores ≥34 were associated with fewer pretransfer CT scans, while older age and female gender were associated with more. Pretransfer CT scans were not associated with in-hospital death or worsened secondary outcomes, but increased charges by $3,761,389 ($488/person transferred with severe injuries) [53]. The authors concluded that national guidelines for the transfer of severely injured patients are followed less than half the time and pretransfer CT scans do not improve outcomes yet increase costs. The potential for further delay in appropriate care arises.

Other prehospital guidelines established by the International Brain Trauma foundation are also not followed. These guidelines state that prehospital intubation is required for all patients with TBI and GCS < 8. A Dutch study of 127 patients who met these criteria found that only 56 % were intubated and in 27 cases, no emergency medical services were involved [54].

Management of Traumatic Brain Injury

Because only about 20 % of patients with TBI require operative intervention, most of the management revolved around resuscitation and intensive care.

Initial resuscitation: Immediate care of the head-injured patient is shown in Table 8.7.

The airway: Poor airway management is consistently identified as a cause of avoidable morbidity and mortality [55]. The idea of the "golden hour" when emergent care could improve survival was developed some 40 years ago. That intubation within 1 h could decrease mortality in head-injured patients from 38 to 22 % as was described by Goldenberg and Makela in 1981 (personal communication). Following head trauma the airway may be compromised by the central lesion of shock (loss of consciousness), by direct injury causing edema, hematoma, or maxilla-facial damage or can be drug-induced (self or otherwise). If two or more of the factors listed in Table 8.8 are present, urgent intubation is indicated. Immediately following TBI there is a period of apnea. Thus, patients frequently present hypoxic and/or hypercarbic.

Table 8.7 Guidelines for immediate care of the head-injured patient

Establish and maintain an airway; auscultation to rule out pneumothorax
Normalize the cardiovascular system
Control intracranial hypertension
Appropriate fluid management; review coagulation parameters
Pain management
Temperature control
Neurologic testing; CT scans; chest X-ray, total body assessment for other injuries and bleeding

Table 8.8 Criteria for urgent intubation and ventilatory support[a]

Unconscious: GCS < 9
Respiratory rate >40/min; <10/min
Respiratory pattern irregular
Vital capacity <15 mL/kg
Maximal inspiratory force less than −20 cmH_2
VD/VT >0.5
$PaCO_2$ >45 mmHg; <25 mmHg
PaO_2 <70 mmHg on room air
% Pulmonary shunt >15 %
Mean systemic arterial pressure <80 mmHg
Maxillo-facial injuries; head and neck burns

[a]If two or more of these criteria are met, the patient is probably best managed by prompt intubation and support of respiration

The airway may be secured without any increase in ICP if intubation is performed after small doses of sedative agents. Appropriate agents include propofol (50–75 mg usually suffices), or etomidate or ketamine if the patient is hypotensive. The addition of succinylcholine (30–40 mg) is also often helpful. Initial respiratory care calls for supplemental oxygen, neutral head and neck position, clearing the mouth, inserting an airway, and reversing any narcotic depression. If pulse oximetry indicates saturation close to 95 %, controlled ventilation is not indicated and may promote aspiration. Also, it is important to auscultate the chest prior to application of positive pressure ventilation in an attempt to identify a pneumothorax which could develop a tension situation. The use of cricoid pressure is also controversial as it may obscure the view, requiring more neck extension and often does not occlude the esophagus, which often does not line up exactly behind the trachea. While application of cricoid pressure continues to be advocated, several studies conclude that although it may have a theoretical advantage during induction, there is little evidence of any benefit at this time [56, 57].

Association of neck fractures with head injury occurs in only about 7 % of patients [58]. Cervical injury is often not identified until hours or even weeks after injury. Nevertheless, trauma protocols often require that patients be transported with neck collars in place, which may do little more than engender pain in the anesthesiologist called to secure the airway. Several studies have emphasized that the need to secure the airway must take precedence. And indeed, subsequent neurologic damage related to the intubation is extremely rare [59]. Nasotracheal intubation and passage of nasogastric tubes are not recommended if there is a skull fracture, especially involving the base of the skull. Tin line stabilization from the feet to the top of the head will maintain neutral position of the head and neck. Also, use of a video laryngoscope allows for intubation with little or no neck motion. Cinefluroscopic studies of fresh cadaveric spine movement showed that cervical displacement during mask ventilation was at least twice as much as during oral or nasal intubation [60].

Cardiovascular sequelae: The importance of examining the cardiovascular system in TBI has long been recognized. Pulse examination was used as a prognostic indicator after head injury over 4,000 years ago in China [61]. As described in the Edwin Smith papyrus, the finding of a weak pulse "when the heart is too weary to speak" and a pale countenance had a poor prognosis but could still be treated, whereas a clammy appearance was "an ailment, not to be treated" [62].

The initial cardiovascular response to cerebral trauma is hypertension, tachycardia, and increased cardiac output, related to a catecholamine surge. As noted above, older patients maintained on cardiac medications who may also have decreased myocardial function may have a blunted response. Cervical spinal cord injury may also present with hypotension and bradycardia. Only in small children is the cranium relatively large enough to contain a hematoma that could result in hypotension based on the injury alone. Otherwise hypotension as the presenting feature in adults is related to systemic injuries with significant blood loss or catastrophic brain damage. SBP < 90 mmHg at the time of admission is associated with significantly increased morbidity and mortality [63]. Cushing described a combination of hypertension and bradycardia with raised ICP [64]. By the time this clinical picture presents, ICP equals diastolic pressure and the patient is usually brain dead.

Several dysrhythmic patterns have been observed. A correlation between outcome and QTc prolongation was noted. An interval of 0.44–0.49 corresponds to a mortality rate double that of patients with normal intervals and at intervals >0.5 the rate triples [65]. Myocardial damage may occur as shown by elevated creatinine phosphokinase (CPK) and myocardium brain (MB) levels. However, there does not appear to be any correlation between CPK and MB activity and electrocardiographic (EKG) changes and outcome.

Therapy is aimed at adrenergic blockade. As autoregulation is often impaired either globally or regionally, hypertension increases cerebral blood flow and thus ICP resulting in cerebral edema. Blood pressure elevations >30 % should be treated during monitoring of ICP. Maintenance of adequate cerebral perfusion pressure is essential. Beta adrenergic blockade with propranolol, esmolol, or labetalol, in increments or infusion, is indicated to reduce systemic blood pressure to <160 mmHg and diastolic pressure to <90 mmHg. Vasodilating agents such as sodium nitroprusside or nitroglycerine are not indicated. Hydralazine, 5–15 mg intravenously has also been used successfully.

Control of ICP: Uncontrolled rise in ICP is probably the most common cause of death in TBI. ICP may be increased after TBI due to brain edema, hyperemia (increased cerebral blood flow), a hematoma, or intracerebral bleed. Optimization of ICP within 24 h of injury has been shown to be the single best intervention to decrease mortality [66]. Even apparently trivial increases in ICP may result in cerebral ischemia, herniation, and pulmonary edema [67].

ICP may be measured by several means (Table 8.9). A CT scan will give a one-time estimation of brain edema.

Diffusion-weighted imaging has been used to study cerebral edema formation, but is difficult to use acutely. Radiological attenuation correlates linearly with estimated specific gravity in human tissue and thus the volume, weight, and specific gravity of any tissue can be measured by computed tomography. Lescot et al. have developed a software package (BrainView®) for Windows workstations, providing semi-automatic tools for brain analysis from DICOM images obtained from cerebral CT, The researchers found that the weight of the brain increased by an average of 82 g and the specific gravity of the contused brain also increased. They concluded that cytotoxic edema must contribute to brain edema rather than simply a breakdown in the blood brain barrier [68].

Therapy for intracranial hypertension includes diuretics (mannitol 0.25–1 g/kg), furosemide (0.25–0.5 mg/kg), head up position, improvement in oxygenation, drainage of CSF, release of intracranial hematomas, reduction of systemic hypertension, and sedation and paralysis if that is required to allow adequate ventilation. Hypertonic saline has also been shown to be as efficacious as mannitol in reducing ICP [69]. Cerebral perfusion is increased better than with normal saline and intravascular volume is stabilized more efficiently. 1-Arginine, a precursor of nitric oxide, may be added as a vasodilator. For many years hyperventilation was added. However, reduction of pCO_2 causes vasoconstriction which puts cerebral tissue at risk of ischemia. Soukup et al. studied the effects of hyperventilation on regional cerebral blood flow (rCBF) [70]. A decrease in $paCO_2$ of 20 % (that is 40–32 mmHG) resulted in a decrease in rCBF from 30 to 25 mL/100 g/min ($P = 0.001$). The partial pressure of oxygen within the brain tissue decreased from 20 to 15 mmHg ($P = 0.001$). These changes occurred

Table 8.9 Several means of measuring ICP

Type of monitor	Advantages	Disadvantages
Subdural and epidural catheters	Least invasive patients	No CSF drainage
	Easy to place	Least accurate
	Low risk of infection	Risk of bleeding
	No recalibration	
Intraventricular catheter	Most accurate	Invasive
	Drains CSF, collects for analyses	High risk of infection
	Give meds intracranially	Difficult if brain swollen or edematous
	Cost-effective	Catheter easily blocked
		Not useful for immediate monitoring
		Bleeding risk
Intraparenchymal (fiber optic transducer-tipped catheter)	Accurate	Invasive
	Not blocked by debris or clots	Cannot drain CSF
	Easy transportation of patient	Cannot be recalibrated over time, accuracy diminishes
	Use if ventricles narrowed	Expensive
		Bleeding risk
		Fragile fiber-optic cables
Subarachnoid (bolt in subarachnoid space)	Low risk of infection	Not very accurate
	Does not invade brain tissue	Blocked by swelling brain
		Needs frequent recalibration
		Risk of bleeding

CSF cerebrospinal fluid

without any changes in other vital signs. Thus, hyperventilation should be reserved only for those cases in which herniation is imminent. Modest positive end expiratory pressure may be added to improve oxygenation [71].

Opioids may release histamine and cause an increase in ICP without evidence of edema due to a direct vasodilatatory effect [72]. In cases where apparently adequate doses of diuretics have been given and ICP remains elevated, opiate infusions of boluses should be withheld.

In children especially altered autoregulation may result in hyperemia and in those circumstances a slight degree of hyperventilation might be indicated. Jugular venous bulb oxygen saturation may be used to assess whether ICP is raised due to hyperemia or edema according to the formula:

$$A - V\,DO_2 = CMRO_2/CBF$$

where >10 indicates cerebral edema and therapy is with diuretics.

($A-V\,DO_2$ is the difference in oxygen content between the radial artery and jugular bulb. $CMRO_2$ = cerebral metabolic rate of oxygen consumption.)

Fluid management: The aims of fluid resuscitation for the head-injured patient are to maintain cardiovascular stability, ensure adequate cerebral perfusion pressure, allow good tissue oxygenation, promote satisfactory operating conditions and, hopefully, provide brain protection. A major problem in initial resuscitation in the emergency room may be an overzealous team that cannulates several veins with large bore catheters and then infuses several liters of crystalloids. Certainly, administration of fluids before operative control of an injury may be ineffective, causing more bleeding by volume expansion.

The question of which fluids to give in TBI has been much debated. Crystalloids have generally been used as the first line because of ready availability and less expense. Dose-related side effects include the risk of over volume expansion and cerebral edema. Colloidal expanders include albumin and hydroxyethylstarches (HES including Hespan®, Hextend®, Voluven®, and Volvulyte®). Albumin, 5 or 25 % supplied in 100 mL aliquots, is derived from pooled human venous plasma, heated to 60° for 10 h to inactivate hepatitis viruses. It contains no isoagglutinins and thus the risk of adverse reactions is very low. Preparation charges make it significantly more expensive. HES in 0.9 % sodium chloride is a synthetic polymer derived from a waxy starch composed of amylopetin. It is supplied in 500 mL bags. Dose-related side effects include coagulopathy, renal failure, and tissue storage. The newer HES 130/0.4 (Voluven®) is said to have a lower risk of side effects [73], although these claims may not have been sufficiently validated [74]. Several reports including the SAFE (saline versus albumin fluid evaluation) study compared the use of albumin alone and saline resuscitation in head-injured patients and found a tendency to increased 24 month mortality in severely injured patients who received only albumin (up to 2 L on the first day) [75]. Less severely compromised patients tended to do better with albumin. The same authors found that albumin resuscitation produced better survival rates in sepsis patients over saline [76]. The efficacy of colloids is being currently evaluated by Myburgh et al. in a 7,000 patient multicenter randomized controlled trial that compares the effects of 6 % hydroxyethyl starch (130/0.4) to normal saline for fluid resuscitation in intensive care patients (CHEST) [77]. Two Cochrane database reviews were unable to determine that albumin reduced mortality when compared to saline in the resuscitation of patients with trauma or postoperatively [78, 79]. In a review of 3,456 patients with sepsis, administration of hydroxyethyl starch increased the need for renal replacement therapy and blood transfusion [80]. Given that colloid is significantly more expensive than crystalloid, its use has been questioned. But in all these investigations, colloid alone in significantly higher doses was compared to crystalloids. Also, the study

substance in many instances was albumin. The American Society of Anesthesiologists has advocated the combination of colloids and reduced crystalloids in the prevention of postoperative visual loss [81]. An animal study showed that isotonic crystalloids increased brain edema more than colloids at 3 and 24 h post-TBI, while blood volume was maintained by colloids but not by crystalloids [82, 83]. Oncotic pressure was reduced by crystalloids. The place of colloids may be as an adjuvant to crystalloid administration whereby the amounts infused of both may be reduced. But it is still not clear as to whether administration of colloids or a reduced volume of crystalloids results in improved patient outcome in all situations or only in certain subsets, or if the newer colloids are indeed harmful. The PRECISE RCT, now underway, may provide light on these issues [84].

The injured brain needs oxygen for survival and thus transfusion if frequently used, with residents often erring on the side of over transfusion. There is mounting evidence that blood transfusion carries many risks, not only of transmission of infection but also of antigen/antibody reactions among other consequences. Overall, adverse events from transfusions in the US account for about $17 billion adding more to the cost of each transfusion than acquisition and procedure costs combined [85]. While some complication risks depend on patient status or specific transfusion quantity involved, a baseline risk of complications simply increases in direct proportion to the frequency and volume of transfusion.

Perioperative hemoglobin determinations are far from reliable as an indicator of need to transfuse. Guidelines from the American Society of Anesthesiologists that note that transfusion is rarely needed if the Hb level is 7 g do not take the patient's age, cardiovascular state, or other comorbidities into account or even the rate of blood loss. (*Practice Guidelines for Perioperative Blood Transfusion and Adjuvant Therapies*. Last amended October 25, 2005).

Hypertonic-hyperoncotic solutions restore plasma volumes rapidly, attenuate capillary endothelial swelling, increase cardiac output,

Table 8.10 Suggested fluid replacement in TBI

Transfuse to keep Hct around 30 %
Hypertonic saline: 1–2 L to keep vital signs stable
Colloid (Volvulen®, Volvulyte® 1–2 L)
Plasmalyte (avoid 1/3 replacement for blood loss)
Normal saline
Plasma to correct coagulopathies
Avoid sugar containing solutions

restore peripheral blood flow, and release eiconosides (vasodilators) and certainly have a place in care of the patient with TBI.

Although the ideally fluid replacement has not been identified, administration of sugar containing solutions must be avoided. An injured brain cannot metabolize sugar through the usual aerobic pathways, but rather by anaerobic means which causes increase in the size of ischemic areas, especially in children [86].

A scheme for fluid management is shown in Table 8.10.

Coagulopathies: Coagulopathies are common soon after head injury and demonstration of worsening clotting studies indicates the need for repeat CT scanning [87]. Severe tissue damage coupled with systemic hypoperfusion results in a hemostatic disruption of coagulation, anticoagulation, fibrinolysis, platelets, and endo-thelium [88]. Routine tests for coagulation may be inadequate and viscoelastic modalities such as TEG and ROTEM may be required. Genet et al. compared patients with TBI and those with other severe injuries and measured biomarkers for sympathoadrenal activation, coagulation, fibri-nolysis, endothelial/cell/glycocalyx damage, and vasculogenesis [89]. They found that acute coagulopathy of shock (ACS) related more to the severity rather than the localization of injury. However, the brain is a rich source of thrombo-plastin which is released immediately during ischemia causing an early disseminated coagula-tion and fibrinolysis syndrome. Coagulation pro-file should be obtained early and repeated and, if necessary, fresh frozen plasma should be given.

Anesthetic management: As noted previously only about 20 % of TBI patients require surgery. However, when it is indicated it is usually

Table 8.11 Summary of anesthetic intraoperative management shows wide variability, according to the status of the patient

Need to maintain cardiovascular stability: Balance vasopressor with anesthetic agents
Invasive monitoring rarely indicated: unstable and place arterial cannula
Balance fluids with crystalloids, blood, and colloids; avoid overload
Balance low-dose inhalation agents in air and oxygen with narcotics
Lidocaine to reduce airway reactivity; adequate Dilantin levels; Appropriate antibiotics
Avoid nitrous oxide

emergent and due to expanding hematoma. An acute arterial epidural hematoma is the most serious and raped release often results in an almost miraculous and swift recovery. Anes-thetic care mat start with sedation and intubation in the emergency room. Most patients require CT or other radiologic procedures that also call for sedation. While it may be difficult for an anes-thetic department to also provide coverage in these off site areas, it is essential that trained healthcare providers are in attendance to allow for adequate monitoring, appropriate sedation, and resuscitation if required. A summary of anes-thetic management is shown in Table 8.11. Wide variation may be indicated according to the level of consciousness and stability of the patient. Nevertheless, some degree of sedation is neces-sary to avoid increases in ICP prior to the open-ing of the skull.

Not infrequently, patients can be safely extubated at the end of the case. Nevertheless, even in the best situation, careful postanesthetic observation is indicated.

Intensive care: Many patients require continued intubation and ventilation in an intensive care setting. Monitoring often includes cerebral oxime-try as well as ICP and cardiorespiratory monitor-ing. Fluids and electrolytes must be balances, especially sodium. Cerebral salt-wasting syn-drome (CSWS) is a rare condition manifested by hyponatremia and dehydration in response to trauma. It is due to excessive renal sodium excre-tion resulting from a centrally mediated process. It should be differentiated from the syndrome of inappropriate antidiuretic hormone (SIADH), which develops under similar circumstances and also presents with hyponatremia. The main clinical difference is that of total fluid status of the patient: CSWS leads to a relative or overt hypovolemia, whereas SIADH is consistent with a normal to hypervolemic range. Random urine sodium concentrations tend to be lower than 100 mEq/L in CSWS and greater in SIADH. If blood-sodium levels increase when fluids are restricted, SIADH is more likely. Posttraumatic hypopituitarism (PTHP) causing diabetes insipidus has been recognized for many years and is a rare occurrence. Changes in pituitary hormone secretion may be observed during the acute phase post-TBI, representing part of the acute adaptive response to the injury [90]. Moreover, diminished pituitary hormone secretion, caused by damage to the pituitary and/or hypothalamus, may occur at any time after TBI. Symptoms include extreme diuresis, which must be distinguished from the effects of overhydration or diuretic administration. It usually responds to desmopressin administration. However, diabetes insipidus related to TBI is frequently transient and can spontaneously disappear within a few days.

It is important to decrease invasive monitoring (central lines, urinary catheters, etc.) to decrease the risk of sepsis and multiple organ failure as quickly as possible. Excessive fluid administration may contribute to ventilator-associated pneumonia. All attempts should be made to discontinue supported respiration as soon as possible.

Directions for brain survival: Over the years many attempts have been made to improve survival after TBI. Barbiturate coma, while should theoretically be advantageous (it decreased ICP, decreases metabolism, and may be beneficial in regional ischemia), has not been shown to improve survival. Nevertheless, it is still used as a desperate measure. It suppresses neuronal activity but anaerobic metabolism continues as CSF levels of hypoxanthine and lactate remain elevated [91]. Barbiturate coma is associated with severe hypokalemia and abrupt discontinuation may cause hyperkalemia. It may also mask brain death. Target concentrations have not been established [92].

Hypothermia has also been used and also proved disappointing, both in adults and in children [93, 94]. However, its value may lie in the prevention of hyperthermia [93].

Decompressive craniectomy has recently been revived as a means to treat intractable intracranial hypertension [17]. Several studies in children have found fair survivals at 6 months and it appears to be a reasonable option for children with uncontrollable ICP [95]. Cranial bones are replaced at a later date with computer-designed flaps. While survival may be enhanced, older patients are still seven times more likely to have a poor functional outcome, resulting in an increased number of survivors with an unfavorable outcome [17].

Measurement of the serum biomarkers outlined earlier may help in guiding therapy such as control of cardiorespiratory parameter, fluid and electrolyte balance, and ICP.

Other recent studies have looked at on-going anticoagulant therapy in trauma victims. Unintentional discontinuation of statins may increase mortality after TBI [96]. An increasing body of evidence suggests that continuing aspirin and other antiplatelet therapy may significantly decrease the risk developing transfusion related lung dysfunction and multiple organ failure in severely injured patients [97]. Prospective clinical studies in giving trauma patients aspirin and antiplatelet therapy are now under consideration.

Guidelines

Several guidelines have been developed for the management of severe TBI by several organizations including the Brain Trauma Foundation (BTF), American Association of Neurological Surgeons, and the Congress of Neurological Surgeons [98–101]. Copies of the 3rd edn of these guidelines are available from Brain Trauma Foundation, 798 3rd Avenue, Suite 1810, New York, NY (btfinfo@braintrauma.org).

The most recent guidelines are from the Scandinavian Society and provide an evidence- and consensus-based algorithm to assist physicians in determining which patients are at higher risk for intracranial pathology, neuroimaging, and hospital admission [102]. Attention has also recently been drawn to sports-related head injuries [103, 104]. It is estimated that up to 3.8 million concussions are related to sports injuries annually in the US and some 50 % go unreported. Given that there can be serious long-term sequelae, prevention, recognition, and treatment must be reviewed, emphasizing a more individual approach with the realization that there may be no set timeline for return to play.

Conclusion

Much of the recent literature on TBI confirms what was determined years ago. There is no magic bullet yet to save the brain and basic principles must be applied. Although many guidelines have been formulated, adherence is low. Prompt and successful airway management and appropriate ventilation remain essential to good outcome after head injury. Rapid sequence induction/intubation is frequently indicated and some sedation is indicated. Normalization of cardiovascular dynamics and ICP is of equal importance. Application of cricoid pressure is probably not useful. Auscultation and chest X-ray help in the diagnosis of tension pneumothoraces, especially before positive pressure ventilation is provided. Small pneumothoraces can be managed conservatively. Identification of significant hemorrhage can be difficult in the head-injured patient when a catecholamine surge may give a falsely high blood pressure. While hypotension limits bleeding, it could worsen brain injury. The ideal initial resuscitation fluid remains controversial. Hypothermia can exacerbate bleeding and the benefit in TBI is uncertain.

References

1. Joost J, Sanchez GM, Burridge AL. The Edwin Smith Papyrus: a clinical reappraisal of the oldest known document on spinal injuries. Eur Spine J. 2010;19:1815–23.
2. Breasted JH. The Edwin Smith Surgical Papyrus: published in facsimile and hieroglyphic transliteration with translation and commentary in two volumes (University of Chicago Oriental Institute publications, v. 3-4. Chicago: University of Chicago Press, 1991) (See 1: pp. xvi, 6, 480-485, 487-489, 446-448, 451-454, 466; 2: pi. XVII, XVIIA).
3. Weber J, Czarnetzki A. Trepanationen im frühen Mittelalter im Südwesten von Deutschland—Indikationen, Komplikationen und Outcome (in German). Zentralbl Neurochir. 2001;62:10.
4. Rutkow IM. The origins of modern surgery, surgery-basic science and clinical evidence. New York: Springer; 2001. p. 2–19.
5. Adams F. The genuine works of Hippocrates translated from the Greek. London: The Sydenham Society; 1849. pp. 430, 431, 433, 455.
6. Cooper A. Lectures in the principles and practice of surgery. London: Westley; 1829. p. 119.
7. Frost EM. History of neuroanesthesia. In: Albin MS, editor. Textbook of neuroanesthesia. New York: McGraw-Hill; 1997. p. 1–20.
8. Monro A. Observations on the structure and function of the nervous system. Creech & Johnson: Edinburgh; 1783. p. 5.
9. Kelly G. Appearances observed in the dissection of two individuals; death from cold and congestion of the brain. Trans Med Chir Sci Edinb. 1824;1:84–169.
10. Cannon WB, Fraser J, Covell E. The preventive treatment of wound shock. JAMA. 1918;70:618–21.
11. McCaffrey, R. J. (Ed.) (1997). Special issues in the evaluation of mild traumatic brain injury. In *The practice of forensic neuropsychology: Meeting challenges in the courtroom*. New York: Plenum Press. pp. 71–75. ISBN 0-306-45256-1
12. Faul M, Xu L, Wald MM, Coronado VG. Traumatic brain injury in the United States: emergency department visits, hospitalizations, and deaths. Atlanta: Centers for Disease Control and Prevention, National Center for Injury Prevention and Control; 2010.
13. Centers for Disease Control and Prevention (CDC), National Center for Injury Prevention and Control. Report to Congress on mild traumatic brain injury in the United States: steps to prevent a serious public health problem. Atlanta: Centers for Disease Control and Prevention; 2003.
14. Finkelstein E, Corso P, Miller T, et al. The incidence and economic burden of injuries in the United States. New York: Oxford University Press; 2006.
15. Foulkes MA, Eisenberg HM, Jane JA, et al. The traumatic coma data bank; design, methods and baseline characteristics. J Neurosurg. 1991;75: S8–13.
16. Chen H, Guo Y, Chen SW, et al. Progressive epidural hematoma in patients with head trauma; incidence, outcome and risk factors. Emerg Med Int. 2012;2012:134905. doi:10.1155/2012/134905.
17. Honeybul S, Ho KM. The current role of decompressive craniectomy in the management of neurological emergencies. Brain Inj. 2013;27 (9):979–91 [Epub ahead of print].
18. Jenkins A, Teasdale G, Hadley MD, et al. Brain lesions detected by magnetic resonance imaging in severe head injuries. Lancet. 1986;2(8504): 445–6.

19. Miller JD, Sweet RC, Narayan R, et al. Early insults to the injured brain. JAMA. 1978;240(5):439–42.
20. Huang BY, Castillo M. Hypoxic-ischemic brain injury: imaging findings from birth to adulthood. Radiographics. 2008;28:417–39. doi:10.1148/rg.282075066.
21. Stoica BA, Faden AI. Cell death mechanisms and modulation in traumatic brain injury. Neurotherapeutics. 2010;7:3–12.
22. Stoica BA, Byrnes KR. Cell cycle activation and CNS injury. Neurotox Res. 2009;16:221–37.
23. Johansson PI, Sørensen AM, Perner A, et al. High sCD40L levels early after trauma are associated with enhanced shock, sympathoadrenal activation, tissue and endothelial damage, coagulopathy and mortality. J Thromb Haemost. 2012;10(2):207–16.
24. Lumpkins KM, Bochicchio GV, Keledjian K, et al. Glial fibrillary acidic protein is highly correlated with brain injury. J Trauma. 2008;65(4):778–84. doi:10.1097/TA.0b013e318185db2d.
25. Mercier E, Boutin A, Lauzier F, et al. Predictive value of S-100B protein for prognosis in patients with moderate and severe traumatic brain injury; a systematic review and meta-analysis. BMJ. 2013;346:f1757.
26. Herrmann M, Vos P, Wunderlich M, et al. Release of glial tissue-specific proteins after acute stroke. Stroke. 2000;31:2670–7.
27. Rhodes J, Sharkey J, Andrews P. Serum IL-8 and MCP-1 concentration do not identify patients with enlarging contusions after traumatic brain injury. J Trauma. 2009;66(6):1591–7.
28. Chatzipanteli K, Vitarbo E, Alonso OF, et al. Temporal profile of cerebrospinal fluid, plasma and brain interleukin -6 after normothermic fluid percussion brain injury; effect of secondary hypoxia. Ther Hypothermia Temp Manag. 2012;2(4):167–75.
29. Antunes AA, Sotomajor VS, Sakamoto KS, et al. Interleukin-6 plasma levels in patients with head trauma and intracerebral hemorrhage Asian. J Neurosurg. 2010;5(1):68–77.
30. Papadopoulos V, Lecanu L. Translocator protein (18 kDa) TSPO: an emerging therapeutic target in neurotrauma. Exp Neurol. 2009;219(1):53–7.
31. Yokobori S, Hosein K, Burks S, Sharma I, Gajavelli S. Biomarkers for the clinical differential diagnosis in traumatic brain injury—a systematic review. CNS Neurosci Ther. 2013;19(8):556–65. doi:10.1111/cns.12127 [Epub ahead of print].
32. Rose J, Valtonen S, Jennett B. Avoidable factors contributing to death after head injury. BMJ. 1977;2:615–8.
33. Rangel-Castilla L, Wyler AR Closed head trauma. Medscape Reference. http://emedicine.medscape.com/article/2518340overview. Accessed May 31, 2013.
34. Teasdale G, Jennett B. Assessment of coma and impaired consciousness. A practical scale. Lancet. 1974;2(7872):81–4.
35. Banks SE, Lewis MC. Trauma in the elderly: considerations for anesthetic management. Anesthesiol Clin. 2013;31(1):127–39.
36. Edwards M, Lev E, Mirocha J, et al. Defining hypotension in moderate to severely injured trauma patients: raising the bar for the elderly. Am Surg. 2010;76(10):1035–8.
37. Stevens WC, Dhanaraj VJ. Characteristics of elderly patients affecting outcome from trauma. Anesthesiology. 1992;77(3A):1089.
38. Lien YC, Chen CH, Lin HC. Risk factors for 24 hour mortality after traumatic rib fractures owing to motor vehicle accidents: a nationwide population-based study. Ann Thorac Surg. 2009;88(4):1124–30.
39. Philip S, Udomphorn Y, Kirkham FJ, et al. Cerebrovascular pathophysiology in pediatric traumatic brain injury. J Trauma. 2009;67(2 Suppl):S128–34.
40. Chadwick DL, Chin S, Salerno C, et al. Deaths from falls in children: how far is fatal. J Trauma. 1991;31(10):1352–5.
41. Vitale A, Vicedomi ID, Vega GR, et al. Shaken baby syndrome: pathogenetic mechanism, clinical features and preventive aspects. Minerva Pediatr. 2012;64(6):641–7.
42. Siegel JH, Gens DR, Mamantov T, et al. Effect of associated injuries and blood volume replacement on death, rehabilitation and disability in blunt traumatic brain injury. Crit Care Med. 1991;19(10):1252–68.
43. Bruijns SR, Guly HR, Bouamra O, et al. The value of traditional vital signs, shock index, and age-based markers in predicting trauma mortality. J Trauma Acute Care Surg. 2013;74(6):1432–7.
44. Sonne NM, Tonneson H. The influence of alcoholism on outcome after evacuation of subdural hematoma. Br J Neurosurg. 1992;6(2):125030.
45. Carrasco CE, Godinho M, Berti de Azevedo Barros M, et al. Fatal motorcycle crashes: a serious public health problem in Brazil. World J Emerg Surg. 2012;7 Suppl 1:S1–5.
46. Chrastina J, Hrabovsky D, Riha I, et al. The effect of age, alcohol intoxication and type of brain injury on the prognosis of patients operated for craniocerebral trauma. Rozhi Chir. 2013;92(3):135–42.
47. Goodman MD, Makley AT, Campion EM, et al. Preinjury alcohol exposure attenuates the neuro-inflammatory response to traumatic brain injury. J Surg Res. 2013;184(2):1053–8.
48. Adekoya D, Thurman DJ, White DD, Webb KW. Surveillance for traumatic brain injury deaths—United States, 1989-1998. MMWR Surveill Summ. 2000;51(10):1–14.
49. Hirschberg R, Weiss D, Zafonte R. Traumatic brain injury and gender: what is known and what is not. Future Neurology. 2008;3(4):483–9.
50. Spaite DW, Tse DJ, Valenzuela TD, et al. The impact of injury severity and prehospital procedures on scene time in victims of major trauma. Ann Emerg Med. 1991;20(12):1299–305.

51. Ala-Kokko TI, Ohtonen P, Koskenkari J, et al. Improved outcome after trauma care in university-level intensive care units. Acta Anaesthesiol Scand. 2009;53(10):1251–6.

52. Meisler R, Thomson AB, Abildstrom H, et al. Triage and mortality in 2875 consecutive trauma patients. Acta Anaesthesiol Scand. 2010;5492:218–23.

53. Mohan D, Barnato AE, Angus DC, et al. Determinants of compliance with transfer guidelines for trauma patients: a retrospective analysis of CT scans acquired prior to transfer to a level 1 trauma center. Ann Surg. 2010;251(5):946–51.

54. Franschman G, Peerdeman SM, Greuters S, et al. Prehospital endotracheal intubation in patients with severe traumatic brain injury: guidelines versus reality. Resuscitation. 2009;80(10):1147–51.

55. Harris T, Davenport R, Hurst T, et al. Improving outcome in severe trauma: trauma systems and initial management: intubation, ventilation and resuscitation. Postgrad Med J. 2012;88(1044):588–94.

56. Butler J, Sen A. Towards evidence-based emergency medicine; best BETs from the Manchester Royal Infirmary. BET 1: cricoids pressure in emergency rapid sequence induction. Emerg Med J. 2013;30(2):163–5.

57. Loganathan N, Liu EH. Cricoid pressure: ritual or effective measure? Singapore Med J. 2012;53(9):620–2.

58. Redan JA, Livingston DH, Bartholomew J, et al. The value of intubating and paralyzing patients in the emergency patient. J Trauma. 1991;31(3):371–5.

59. Grande CM, Barton CR, Stene JK. Appropriate techniques for airway management of emergency patients with suspected spinal cord injury. Anesth Analg. 1988;76:710–8.

60. Hauswald M, Sklar DP, Tandberg D, et al. Cervical spine movement during airway management0cine-fluroscopic appraisal in human cadavers. Am J Emerg Med. 1991;9:535–8.

61. Veith I. The Yellow Emperor's classic of internal medicine (trans). Berkeley: University of California; 1973. p. 159–60.

62. Breasted JH. The Edwin Smith Papyrus Chicago. Chicago: University of Chicago Press; 1930. p. 113–78.

63. Tolani K, Bendo AA, Sakabe T. Anesthetic management of head trauma. In: Newfield P, Cottrell JE, editors. Handbook of neuroanesthesia. Philadelphia: Wolters Kluwer; 2012. p. 100.

64. Cushing H. The blood-pressure reaction of acute cerebral compression, illustrated by cases of intracranial hemorrhage: a sequel to the Mutter lecture 1901. Am J Med Sci. 1903;125(6):1017–43.

65. Miner ME, Allen SJ. Cardiovascular effects of severe head injury. In: Frost E, editor. Clinical anesthesia in neurosurgery. Boston: Butterworth; 1984. p. 372–4.

66. Rubicsek S. Mortality after TBI ASA Annual Meeting 2008: A366. Eur J Anaesthesiol Suppl. 2008;42:110–4. doi:10.1017/S0265021507003304.

67. Nishikawa T. Risk management for neurosurgical anesthesia. Masui. 2009;58(5):545–51.

68. Lescot T, Degos V, Puybasset L. Does the brain become heavier or lighter after trauma? Eur J Anaesthesiol Suppl. 2008;42:110–4. doi:10.1017/S0265021507003304.

69. Sell SL, Avila MA, Yu G, Vergara L, et al. Hypertonic resuscitation improves neuronal and behavioral outcomes after traumatic brain injury plus hemorrhage. Anesthesiology. 2008;108(5):873–81. doi:10.1097/ALN.0b013e31816c8a15.

70. Soukup J, Bramsiepe I, Brucke M, et al. Evaluation of a bedside monitor of regional CBF as a measure of CO_2 reactivity in neurosurgical intensive care patients. J Neurosurg Anesthesiol. 2008;20(4):249–55. doi:10.1097/ANA.0b013e31817ef487.

71. Young N, Rhodes JK, Mascia L, et al. Ventilatory strategies for patients with acute brain injury. Curr Opin Crit Care. 2010;16(1):45–52. doi:10.1097/MCC.0b013e32833546fa.

72. Hocker SE, Fogelson J, Rabinstein AA. Refractory intracranial hypertension due to fentanyl administration following closed head injury. Front Neurol. 2013;4:3. doi:10.3389/fneur.2013.00003.

73. James MF. The role of tetrastarches for volume replacement in the perioperative setting. Curr Opin Anaesthesiol. 2008;21(5):674–8.

74. Hartog CS, Bauer M, Reinhart K. The efficacy and safety of colloid resuscitation in the critically ill. Anes Analg. 2011;112(1):156–64.

75. Myburgh J, Cooper DJ, Finfer S, et al. (SAFE Study Investigators). Saline or albumin for fluid resuscitation in patients with traumatic brain injury. N Engl J Med. 2007;357(9):874–84.

76. Finfer S, McEvoy S, Bellomo R, et al. (SAFE Study Investigators). Impact of albumin compared to saline on organ function and mortality of patients with severe sepsis. Int Care Med. 2011;37(1): 86–96.

77. Myburgh J, Li Q, Heritier S, et al. Statistical analysis plan for the crystalloid versus hydroxyethyl starch trial (CHEST). Crit Care Resusc. 2012;14(1):44–52.

78. Alderson P, Bunn F, Lefebvre C, et al. Human albumin solution for resuscitation and volume expansion in critically ill patients. Cochrane Database Syst Rev. 2004;18(4):CD001208.

79. Perel P, Roberts I, Ker K. Colloids versus crystalloids for fluid resuscitation in critically ill patients. Cochrane Database Syst Rev. 2013;2: CD000567. doi:10.1002/14651858.

80. Haase N, Perner A, Hennings LI, et al. Hydroxyethyl starch 130/0.38–0.45 versus crystalloid or albumin in patients with sepsis: a systematic review with meta-analysis and trial sequential analysis. BMJ. 2013;346:f839. doi: 10.1136/bmj.f839

81. American Society of Anesthesiologists Task Force on Perioperative Blindness. Practice advisory for perioperative visual loss associated with spine surgery. Anesthesiology. 2006;104:1319–28.

82. Jungner M, Gründe PO, Mattiasson G, Bentzer P. Effects on brain edema of crystalloid and albumin fluid resuscitation after brain trauma and hemorrhage in the rat. Anesthesiology. 2010;112(5):1194–203. doi:10.1097/ALN.0b013e3181d94d6e.

83. Drummond JC. Colloid osmotic pressure and the formation of posttraumatic cerebral edema. Anesthesiology. 2010;112(5):1079–81. doi:10.1097/ALN.0b013e3181d94e53.

84. McIntyre L, Fergusson DA, Rowe B, et al. The PRECISE RCT: evolution of an early septic shock fluid resuscitation trial. Transfus Med Rev. 2012;26 (4):333–41. doi:10.1016/j.tmrv.2011.11.003.

85. Shander A, Hofmann A, Gombotz H, Theusinger OM, Spahn DR. Estimating the cost of blood: past, present, and future directions. Best Pract Res Clin Anaesthesiol. 2007;21:271–89.

86. Michaud LJ, Rivera FP, Longstreth WT, et al. Elevated initial blood glucose levels and; poor outcome following severe brain injuries in children. J Trauma. 1991;31(10):1356–62.

87. Stein SC, Young GS, Taucci RC, et al. Delayed brain injury after head trauma: significance of coagulopathy. Neurosurgery. 1992;30(2):160–5.

88. Frith D, Brohi K. The pathophysiology of trauma-induced coagulopathy. Curr Opin Crit Care. 2012;18 (6):631–6.

89. Genét GF, Johansson PI, Meyer MA, et al. Trauma-induced coagulopathy: standard coagulation tests, biomarkers of coagulopathy, and endothelial damage in patients with traumatic brain injury. J Neurotrauma. 2013;30(4):301–6. doi:10.1089/neu.2012.2612.

90. Bondanelli M, Ambrosio MR, Zatelli MC, et al. Hypopituitarism after traumatic brain injury. Eur J Endocrinol. 2005;152:679–91.

91. Stover JF, Pleines UE, Morganti-Kossmann MC, et al. Thiopental attenuates energetic impairment but fails to normalize cerebrospinal fluid glutamate in brain-injured patients. Crit Care Med. 1999;27(7):1351–7.

92. Neil MJ, Dale MC. Hypokalaemia with severe rebound hyperkalaemia after therapeutic barbiturate coma. Anesth Analg. 2009;108(6):1867–8. doi:10.1213/ane.0b013e3181a16418.

93. Cairns CJ, Andrews PJ. Management of hyperthermia in traumatic brain injury. Curr Opin Crit Care. 2002;8(2):106–10.

94. Adelson PD, Wisniewski SR, Beca J, et al. Comparison of hypothermia and normothermia after severe traumatic brain injury in children (Cool Kids): a phase3, randomized controlled trial. Lancet Neurol. 2013;12(6):546–53.

95. Shoja MM, Chern JJ. Decompressive craniectomy. J Neurosurg Pediatr. 2013;11(3):358. doi:10.3171/2012.7.PEDS12178. Epub 2013 Jan 11.

96. Orlando A, Bar-Or D, Salottolo K, Levy AS, et al. Unintentional discontinuation of statins may increase mortality after traumatic brain injury in elderly patients: a preliminary observation. J Clin Med Res. 2013;5(3):168–73. doi:10.4021/jocmr1333w.

97. Harr JN, Moore EE, Johnson J. Antiplatelet therapy is associated with decreased transfusion-associated risk of lung dysfunction, multiple organ failure, and mortality in trauma patients. Crit Care Med. 2013;41 (2):399–404. doi:10.1097/CCM.0b013e31826ab38b.

98. Brain Trauma Foundation; American Association of Neurological Surgeons; Congress of Neurological Surgeons. Guidelines for the management of severe traumatic brain injury. Neurotrauma. 2007;24 Suppl 1:S1–106.

99. Bullock MR, Chesnut R, Ghajar J, Surgical Management of Traumatic Brain Injury, et al. Surgical management of acute subdural hematomas. Neurosurgery. 2006;58(3 Suppl):S16–24.

100. Badjatia N, Carney N, Crocco TJ, et al. Guidelines for prehospital management of traumatic brain injury 2nd edition. Brain Trauma Foundation; BTF Center for Guidelines Management. Prehosp Emerg Care. 2008;12 Suppl 1:S1–52. doi:10.1080/10903120701732052.

101. Adelson PD, Bratton SL, Carney NA, et al. Guidelines for the acute medical management of severe traumatic brain injury in infants, children, and adolescents. Chapter 19. The role of anti-seizure prophylaxis following severe pediatric traumatic brain injury. Pediatr Crit Care Med. 2003;4(3 Suppl):S72–5.

102. Unden J, Ingebrigtsen T, Romner B, et al. Scandinavian guidelines for initial management of minimal, mild, and moderate head injuries in adults: an evidence and consensus-based update. BMC Med. 2013;11:50. doi:10.1186/1741-7015-11-50. Pub on line Feb 2103.

103. Harmon KG, Drezner JA, Gammons M, et al. American Medical Society for Sports Medicine position statement: concussion in sport. Br J Sports Med. 2013;47(1):15–26.

104. Mitka M. Guideline: tailor appraisal of concussion during sports. JAMA. 2013;309(15):1577.

Anesthesia for Cervical Spinal Cord Injury

9

Apolonia E. Abramowicz and Maria Bustillo

Incidence and Causes of Spinal Cord Injury

The February 2013 National Spinal Cord Injury Statistical Center at the University of Birmingham, Alabama publication reports that approximately 12,000 new cases of spinal cord injury (SCI) occur annually in the United States, not including those who die at the scene of the accident [67]. The figure is an approximation as no studies on the incidence of SCI have been carried out since the 1990s. The National Spinal Cord Injury Database compiles data on an estimated 13 % of new SCI cases in the USA reported to federally funded Model System Centers. Since 2010, 52.2 % of patients reported to the database were categorized as having either incomplete (40.6 %) or complete (11.6 %) tetraplegia at discharge. The term quadriplegia has been largely abandoned; tetraplegia should be used instead. Of note, only less than 1 % of injuries resulted in complete neurologic recovery, but the percentage of incomplete tetraplegia has increased, while complete tetraplegia has decreased. Based on these figures, it may be inferred that approximately 6,000 persons annually suffer cervical spinal cord injury with some degree of neurological impairment. Vehicular accidents and falls account for the majority of the SCIs (65 %), with falls causing more injuries than in the past. Sports injuries and violence are currently responsible for a declining share of SCI and account for 23.5 % of the injuries. Males constitute 80.7 % of all SCI cases, and although the average age at injury is presently 42.6 years, almost half of injuries occur between the ages of 16 and 30. Alcohol is a major factor in 25 % of SCI [17]. The decrease in life expectancy after SCI is due primarily to pneumonia and septicemia. Advances in urologic management have decreased the incidence of renal failure as the leading cause of mortality. The annual cost of healthcare and living expenses in tetraplegia decreases from a high of $1 million in the first year after injury to $110,000 per year thereafter [67].

Of all patients with complete cervical spinal cord injury, approximately 10 % will regain some sensory function and another 10 % will regain some motor function, but 80 % will not improve.

In victims of severe blunt trauma, injury to the cervical spine occurs in 1.8 % of cases. Patients with head trauma are more likely to have a cervical spinal cord injury. The most common level of injury is the C2 vertebra, followed by C6 and C7 [31]. Spinal Cord Injury Without Radiologic Abnormalities (SCIWORA) occurs most commonly in pediatric patients whose elastic spines have more cartilaginous elements, in adults with acute disc prolapse and in patients with cervical spondylosis.

A.E. Abramowicz, M.D. (✉) • M. Bustillo, M.D.
Department of Anesthesiology, Montefiore Medical Center, Albert Einstein College of Medicine,
111 East 210th Street, New York, NY 10467, USA
e-mail: apabramo@montefiore.org

C.S. Scher (ed.), *Anesthesia for Trauma*, DOI 10.1007/978-1-4939-0909-4_9,
© Springer Science+Business Media New York 2014

Penetrating or blunt trauma to the neck with injury to the vertebral artery may result in cervical spinal cord infarction. The vertebral artery supplies the cervical spinal cord through its single anterior and two posterior branches which descend from the skull base. Additionally, segmental branches of the vertebral arteries provide collateral flow. Penetrating ballistic trauma to the neck (from explosions and gunshot wounds) carries a very high mortality rate. In a study of 90 British Iraq and Afghanistan war casualties, it was associated with cervical spine and/or cord injury in 20 soldiers (22 %). Of those, only 6 (6.6 %) survived to reach hospital care, but 3 of them died of their wounds and only 1 (1.8 %) of the 49 survivors who reached surgical care had an unstable cervical spine injury and lived until emergency surgical spinal intervention; 2 others (3.7 %), despite spinal cord contusion, had spinal fractures not deemed unstable [77].

Of interest to anesthesiologists are perioperative cervical spinal cord injuries. Hindman et al. studied cervical spine injuries reported to the ASA Closed Claims Database and associated with surgery under general anesthesia [38]. Cervical spinal cord injuries ($n = 37$) occurred mostly in men (73 %), in the absence of preexisting spinal trauma (81 %) and instability (76 %) and were permanent and disabling. In the study, 81 % of patients had preoperative nontraumatic anatomic abnormalities such as cervical spinal stenosis and 65 % underwent surgery on the cervical spine. The authors hypothesize that cervical spondylosis, much more prevalent than spinal instability, appears to confer a susceptibility to cord injury related to positioning (Fig. 9.1) and perhaps systemic hypotension, as 24 % of patients had surgery in the sitting position [38, 49]. Cord injury was attributed to airway instrumentation in only 11 % of patients. Ahn and Fehlings of the influential Toronto Spine Program have reviewed 84 papers on perioperative spinal cord injury published between 1966 and 2008, in an attempt to identify patients at risk and in order to propose evidence-based approaches for prevention and improvement of outcomes [3]. The overall incidence of perioperative SCI for surgery on the spine at all levels is estimated by the authors to vary between 0 to a frightening 3 %. The more common medical causes of spinal instability include Rheumatoid Arthritis, Down syndrome, and hypermobile transition zones between fused regions of the cervical spine, as in Klippel–Feil syndrome. The authors advocate "a careful fiberoptic intubation without hyperextension as an important consideration to prevent SCI" and "careful control of the spine" during positioning. Little quality evidence to support this recommendation is given. Nevertheless, the authors list hyperextension of the neck during intubation and positioning in patients with severely tight cervical canals, as well as in those with nontraumatic spinal instability as the "potential" cause of perioperative SCI. A large population of patients could be at risk, as the authors list those with congenital stenosis, diffuse idiopathic skeletal hyperostosis, ossified posterior longitudinal ligament (OPLL), but also those with severe spondylosis of the lumbar spine which correlates with spondylosis of the cervical spine. Kudo described two older women with transient tetraplegia after general anesthesia with endotracheal intubation for retinal detachment and lumbar fusion surgery, respectively, and who recovered after a few hours; postoperative MRI revealed cervical spondylosis with severe spinal canal narrowing [47]. Systolic blood pressure varied between 85 and 150 mmHg. The widely quoted and highly recommended editorial by McLeod in the *British Journal of Anaesthesia* published in 2000 addresses the issue of spinal cord injury and direct laryngoscopy [61]. It emphasizes the importance of positioning and its impact on spinal cord perfusion during prolonged periods of immobility in the perioperative period, in addition to the common sense approach to the selection of the technique of airway instrumentation for the purpose of establishing mechanical ventilation in all patients with cervical spine disease; mechanical instability of the cervical spine is but one risk factor for spinal cord injury during anesthetic care.

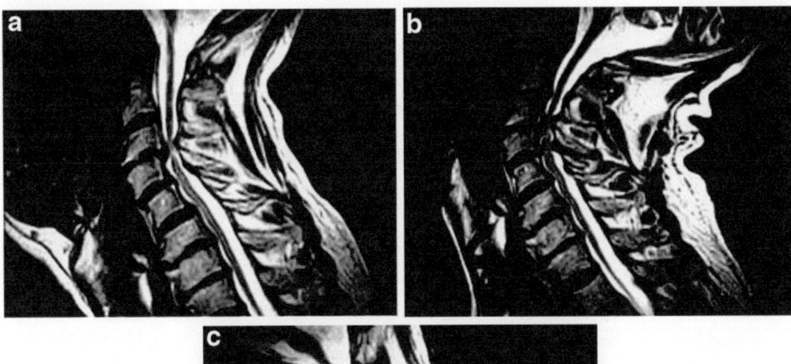

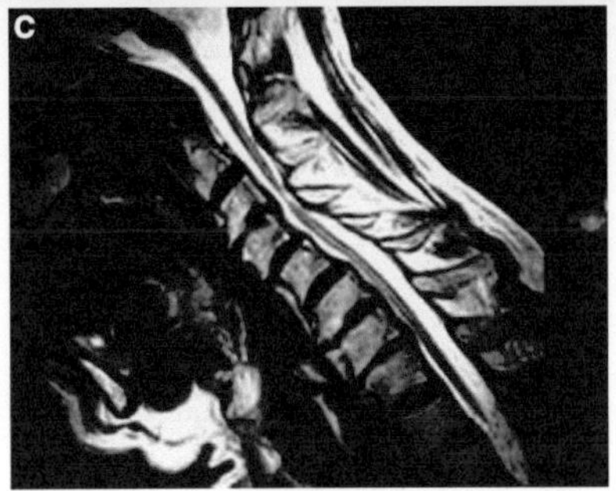

Fig. 9.1 Sagittal MRI scans of the cervical spine; (**a**) showing ventral spinal cord compression from disc herniation at C3–C4 and vertebral body osteophytes. Note the compression of the spinal cord in extension (**b**) that is diminished flexion (**c**). (From Shedid D, Benzel EC: Cervical Spondylosis Anatomy: Pathophysiology and Biomechanics, Neurosurgery 60;S1-7-S1-13, 2007)

Classification of Spinal Cord Injury

The acute management of a patient with cervical spinal cord injury begins with neurological assessment and culminates in a functional outcome that often depends on the deficits at presentation. In 2000, the American Spinal Injury Association (ASIA) has promulgated its International Standards for Neurological Classification of Spinal Cord Injury which has been universally adopted as the best scoring system for the neurological assessment of adult patients with acute SCI. The acute neurological assessment may be hindered by concomitant head injury, drug effects, and the presence of an artificial airway. Nevertheless, the ASIA Impairment Scale (AIS) is considered the most accurate and reproducible neurological assessment tool in acute SCI [4] (Fig. 9.2). The AIS replaces the similar, but older and less stringently defined Frankel scale, while retaining the same injury categories. The AIS is a five level scale, where level E (Normal) implies recovered normal neurological function in someone with an initial spinal cord injury clinical presentation, and level A (Complete) implies lack of motor and sensory function in the sacral segments S4–S5. Level B is a Sensory Incomplete injury, where sensory but no motor function is preserved below the neurological level, and levels C and D reflect Incomplete Motor injury, with D level patients having better strength than C. The "neurological level" of injury is defined as the first spinal segmental level which shows loss of function. In addition, ASIA classifies incomplete spinal cord injuries into five types: central cord syndrome, where function of the upper limbs is more impaired than the lower limbs, the Brown-Sequard syndrome, where only one side of the cord is lesioned and the anterior cord syndrome, where the motor function is absent but the sensory function is spared. Finally, distal spinal injuries may result in conus medullaris and cauda equina syndromes.

The term "spinal shock" means transient absence of all reflex neurologic activity below the level of injury; sensorimotor activity is absent as well. Patients have flaccidity of bowel and bladder, priapism is common; the reflex arcs below the level of injury, for example the bulbocavernosus reflex, recover within days to weeks.

The term "neurogenic shock" describes the symptoms of vasodilatation with hypotension, bradycardia, and hypothermia which result from the interruption of the sympathetic nervous system

a

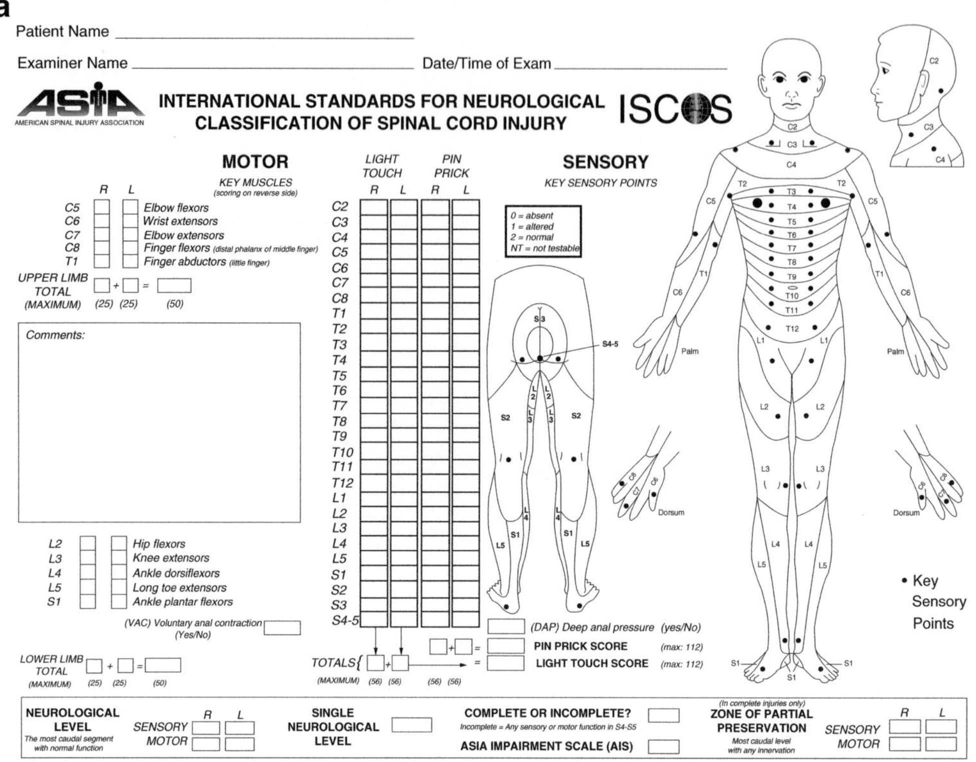

b

Muscle Function Grading

0 = total paralysis

1 = palpable or visible contraction

2 = active movement, full range of motion (ROM) with gravity eliminated

3 = active movement, full ROM against gravity

4 = active movement, full ROM against gravity and moderate resistance in a muscle specific position.

5 = (normal) active movement, full ROM against gravity and full resistance in a muscle specific position expected from an otherwise unimpaired peson.

5* = (normal) active movement, full ROM against gravity and sufficient resistance to be considered normal if identified inhibiting factors (i.e. pain, disuse) were not present.

NT = not testable (i.e. due to immobilization, severe pain such that the patient cannot be graded, amputation of limb, or contracture of >50% of the range of motion).

ASIA Impairment (AIS) Scale

☐ **A = Complete.** No sensory or motor function is preserved in the sacral segments S4-S5.

☐ **B = Sensory Incomplete.** Sensory but not motor function is preserved below the neurological level and includes the sacral segments S4-S5 (light touch, pin prick at S4-S5: or deep anal pressure (DAP)), AND no motor function is preserved more than three levels below the motor level on either side of the body.

☐ **C = Motor Incomplete.** Motor function is preserved below the neurological level**, and more than half of key muscle functions below the single neurological level of injury (NLI) have a muscle grade less than 3 (Grades 0-2).

☐ **D = Motor Incomplete.** Motor function is preserved below the neurological level**, and <u>at least half</u> (half or more) of key muscle functions below the NLI have a muscle grade ≥ 3.

☐ **E = Normal.** If sensation and motor function as tested with the ISNCSCI are graded as normal in all segments, and the patient had prior deficits, then the AIS grade is E. Someone without an initial SCI does not receive an AIS grade.

**For an individual to receive a grade of C or D, i.e. motor incomplete status, they must have either (1) voluntary anal sphincter contraction or (2) sacral sensory sparing <u>with</u> sparing of motor function more than three levels below the motor level for that side of the body. The Standards at this time allows even non-key muscle function more than 3 levels below the motor level to be used in determining motor incomplete status (AIS B versus C).

NOTE: When assessing the extent of motor sparing below the level for distinguishing between AIS B and C, the **motor level** on each side is used; whereas to differentiate between AIS C and D (based on proportion of key muscle functions with strength grade 3 or greater) the **single neurological level** is used.

Steps in Classification

The following order is recommended in determining the classification of individuals with SCI.

1. Determine sensory levels for right and left sides.

2. Determine motor levels for right and left sides.
   Note: in regions where there is no myotome to test, the motor level is presumed to be the same as the sensory level, if testable motor function above that level is also normal.

3. Determine the single neurological level.
   This is the lowest segment where motor and sensory function is normal on both sides, and is the most cephalad of the sensory and motor levels determined in steps 1 and 2.

4. Determine whether the injury is Complete or Incomplete. (i.e. absence or presence of sacral sparing)
   If voluntary anal contraction = **No** *AND all S4-5 sensory scores =* **0** *AND deep anal pressure =* **No,** *then injury is COMPLETE. Otherwise, injury is incomplete.*

5. Determine ASIA Impairment Scale (AIS) Grade:
   Is injury <u>Complete</u>? If **YES,** AIS=A and can record ZPP (lowest dermatome or myotome on each side with some preservation)

   NO ↓

   Is injury motor <u>Incomplete</u>? If **NO,** AIS=B (Yes=voluntary anal contraction OR motor function more than three levels below the motor level on a given side, if the patient has sensory incomplete classification)

   YES ↓

   Are <u>at least</u> half of the key muscles below the single <u>neurological</u> level graded 3 or better?

   NO ↓ AIS=C   **YES** ↓ AIS=D

If sensation and motor function is normal in all segments, AIS=E
Note: AIS E is used in follow-up testing when an individual with a documented SCI has recovered normal function. If at initial testing no deficits are found, the individual is neurologically intact; the ASIA Impairment Scale does not apply.

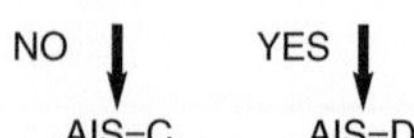

Fig. 9.2 (**a**) ASIA spinal cord injury classification and assessment; (**b**) ASIA impairment scale

control of hemodynamics in acute cervical and high thoracic spinal cord injury. At the time of injury, there is an initial sympathetic surge of brief duration, with hypertension and potential for subendocardial ischemia, arrhythmias, and "neurogenic" pulmonary edema.

Autonomic hyperreflexia manifests as severe hypertension with reflex bradycardia. It occurs after spinal reflexes have returned, usually after 4–6 weeks of injury. It is common in patients with spinal cord injury lesions above T6. It occurs classically when bladder or bowel distension but also other somatic or visceral triggers stimulate the sympathetics within the spinal cord below the level of injury. As the descending central inhibitory pathways are disrupted, the splanchnic and peripheral bed vasoconstriction below the level of injury remains unopposed and causes severe hypertension, which may be life-threatening. Loss of consciousness, seizures, and hemorrhagic stroke may occur. Compensatory baroreceptor-mediated vasodilatation is present above the level of injury; the vasomotor center activates the vagal parasympathetics and severe bradycardia ensues. Patients are well aware of the episodes; in addition to the pounding headache, they experience anxiety, malaise, nausea, flushing, and sweating above the level of injury and nasal congestion.

The Spinal Cord Independence Measure (SCIM), since 2007 in its third iteration, hence III, is the preferred functional assessment tool used by clinicians involved in the care and follow-up of patients with spinal cord injuries [16]. It evaluates three subscales of self-care, respiration and sphincter management, and mobility for a total score of 0–100. It quantifies the patient's ability to perform everyday tasks and the impact of the disability on the patient's medical condition; in that it is vastly superior to neurological improvement measures which rely on assessing the dermatomal or myotomal level of the lesion.

The injury to the cervical spine may be categorized as atlanto-occipital, atlanto-axial, high (C3, C4), and low cervical.

Management of the Cervical Spinal Cord-Injured Patient

The primary traumatic injury of the spinal cord results from spinal cord compression and contusion. The main elements of treatment comprise immediate resuscitation and stabilization of vital organ function, prevention of cord injury propagation from spinal displacement and ischemia, surgical management and neuroprotective strategies which target the putative inflammatory, neurotoxic and oxidative local processes commonly called "secondary spinal cord injury," the pathophysiology of which has not been elucidated. It is believed that neuroprotection must be applied within a short period of time after injury; the length of this therapeutic window is yet to be defined. It is important to remember that additional injuries are frequently associated with SCI. Although in many ways unique, SCI patients' initial management should follow the ATLS primary and secondary surveys so that no other important injuries are overlooked. In March of 2013, the Congress of Neurological Surgeons has published an update to the 2002 Guidelines for the Management of Acute Cervical Spine and Spinal Cord Injuries [34]. Reflecting the lack of good quality studies of cardiopulmonary management of SCI patients in the intervening decade, there is no change in the pertinent recommendations relative to the 2002 Guidelines. Explicitly excluding anesthesia citations in its updated review, the guideline on Acute Cardiopulmonary Management offers three level III (based on case series) recommendations: in SCI, patients should be managed in an intensive care unit and "systolic blood pressure below 90 mmHg should be corrected when possible and as soon as possible," the mean arterial blood pressure should be kept between 85 and 90 mmHg for the first 7 days after acute SCI and finally all monitoring devices necessary to detect cardiac, hemodynamic, and respiratory dysfunction should be used.

Cervical Spinal Immobilization After Injury

Victims of blunt trauma with either multiple injuries or isolated head injury, those with altered mental status for any reason, and those who have pain over the spine or severe pain from an associated injury (severe enough to be "distracting" and hence obscuring neck pain) are presumed to have spinal instability and are therefore considered at risk for motion-induced secondary spinal cord injury. Patients with motor or sensory deficits have spinal cord injury which may be aggravated by spine motion. The standard element of management, which starts at the scene of the injury, is spinal immobilization. It is continued until spinal instability resulting from disk and ligament disruption, facet joint subluxation, or bone fracture has been ruled out, ideally in less than 24 h. In general, spinal immobilization consists of a rigid cervical collar, supports (sand bag) on both sides of the head and a backboard with multiple straps which attach the patient to the board and restrain the movement of the entire body. Specific clearance protocols vary, with good quality, fine-cut computed tomography reviewed by an experienced radiologist being recommended by the State of NY [67]. It has been known for over 20 years that patients with spinal cord injury should be transferred to a specialty SCI center as soon as possible, as it results in a decrease of acute care length and in the incidence of preventable respiratory complications and pressure ulcers [63]. In addition, the incidence of paralysis in patients with acute spinal cord injury admitted to a specialized trauma center is significantly lower. In a study of discharge files of 4121 patients with traumatic spinal cord injury, Macias found that when the American College of Surgeons' guidelines are followed and patients are admitted to a level I or II trauma center, the adjusted odds ratio for paralysis at discharge was significantly lower (0.67 at $p < 0.001$), while mortality remained unchanged. Higher surgical volume was associated with reduced paralysis; the authors

conjecture that was possibly due to greater use of spinal surgery [54].

The efficacy of cervical spinal immobilization with various devices has been measured primarily in normal human volunteers using different methods [81] such as clinical assessment, plumblines, radiography, cinematography, computed tomography, and MRI, generating a normative body of knowledge. SCI patients have not been well studied yet. The difficulty is in establishing what constitutes a neutral neck position and in quantifying movement between individual vertebral segments. The "neutral" position has been defined as the "normal anatomic position of the head and torso that one assumes when standing and looking ahead" [85]. Alternatively, De Lorenzo, in a MRI study of 19 adults found that a slight degree of flexion, equivalent to a 2 cm occiput elevation, produces a favorable increase in the size of the spinal canal at C5 and C6, regions of frequent unstable cervical spine injury [23]. These findings indicate that some degree of occipital padding is required in adults strapped to a board to achieve neutral positioning of the head and neck relative to the torso. Body habitus and muscular development must be taken into account when determining the thickness of padding.

The safety record of the cervical collar and rigid board immobilization is far from perfect. Tightly applied cervical collars have been associated with intracranial pressure elevation by 4.5 mmHg [21, 45]. The length of time a patient with SCI spends on a rigid board increases the risk of early decubitus ulcers, probably after only a 2 h period. Transient marginal mandibular nerve palsy from pressure from a hard cervical collar has been reported, as has skin breakdown over the occiput. Spinal immobilization increases the risk of aspiration and may restrict respiratory function. It has been reported that the presence of a rigid Philadelphia® Collar and backboard restricts ventilation by 15 % [90]. Contraindications to the use of spinal immobilization include penetrating trauma to the spine as it increases the death rate twofold relative to non-immobilized patients, because it delays transport and definitive management of the associated injuries, more life-threatening than SCI. Likewise, it is contraindicated in ankylosing spondylitis, as spinal immobilization may cause neurological deterioration.

Manual in-line stabilization (MILS) is an acceptable cervical spine stabilization technique when the rigid collar interferes with endotracheal intubation by preventing mouth opening. In fact, it is recommended by current ATLS guidelines. After the anterior portion of the collar has been removed, the maneuver is performed by an assistant standing at the patient's side, facing either the feet or the head. The assistant's hands rest on the sides of the patient's head and act as lateral and anti-extension supports, by applying just enough pressure to oppose the atlanto-occipital extension and, to a lesser extent at the C1–C2 joint, occurring during direct laryngoscopy. In addition, when traumatic disruption of the alignment of the subaxial (below C2) vertebrae is present, airway instrumentation may cause vertebral motion, i.e. distraction and or subluxation, distal to the atlanto-occipital junction. MILS would not be expected to prevent this cause of spinal motion. This has been confirmed in a variety of cadaver studies [55, 56]. MILS significantly degrades laryngoscopic view and as a result direct laryngoscopy transmits higher pressure on the tissues adjacent to the unstable vertebral segments, perhaps even doubling it [56, 84, 88]. Illustrating the caveats of theoretical recommendations is a case report of CT-documented odontoid fracture reduction as a result of cranio-cervical motion during emergency direct laryngoscopy with MILS [71]. Despite mounting evidence that MILS, which has been adopted in the 1980s as an off-shoot of "manual in-line traction" and only on the basis of the efficacy of cervical immobilization during general care, may extend the time to intubation with resultant hypoxia, intubation failure, and airway complications, it is still considered a recommended immobilization maneuver during urgent airway instrumentation in un-cleared or unstable cervical spine, when the cervical collar must be opened [55].

Airway Management in Cervical Spinal Cord Injury

Emergency airway management may be required in patients with high cervical cord injury due to acute respiratory failure, or to protect the airway in the setting of coexisting head trauma or polytrauma. Because of the lack of diaphragmatic function, injury above C3 is lethal unless rescue ventilation is rapidly established; these patients will be intubated in the field by emergency personnel. The issues related to spinal cord protection through cervical spine immobilization during airway instrumentation have been discussed above. Further controversies include the choice of intubation technique, airway adjuncts, the utility and role of cricoid pressure, and the place of bag-mask ventilation during rapid sequence induction in SCI. In addition, the emergency setting presents challenges related to the necessity of promptly securing the airway without previous airway examination, the risk of aspiration, lack of patient cooperation, hemodynamic instability, preexisting hypoxemia, craniofacial injuries and airway compromise from prevertebral tissue swelling or hematoma [18, 32]. The recently updated ASA Practice Guidelines for Management of the Difficult Airway (Fig. 9.3) include a difficult airway algorithm which now incorporates the use of supra-glottic devices as rescue ventilation tools or intubation conduits, and video-laryngoscopes; this algorithm does not specifically address the problems of the cervical spine-injured patient, but should be followed whenever unexpected difficulties are encountered despite airway management planning [6].

Although bag-mask ventilation is contraindicated in the classic rapid sequence induction scenario because of the risk of gastric distension and the resulting increased risk of aspiration, it is even more problematic when protecting the cervical spine is an additional concern. Older studies on human cadavers concluded that chin lift and jaw thrust and mask ventilation caused more cervical spine displacement than other airway procedures, notably than

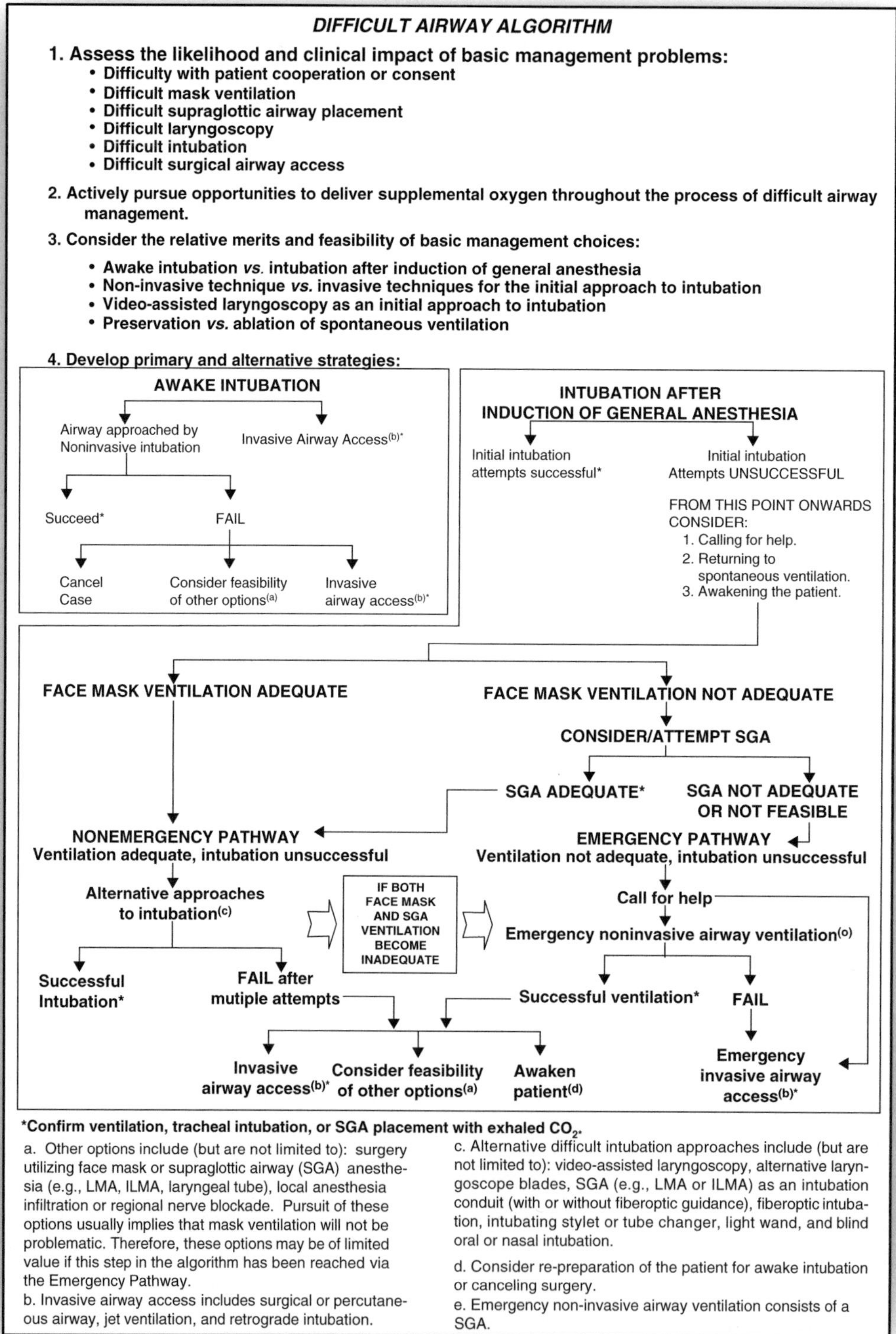

Fig. 9.3 ASA Practice Guidelines for Management of the Difficult Airway. (From Anesthesiology. 2013 Feb;118(2):251-70. Practice guidelines for management of the difficult airway: an updated report by the American Society of Anesthesiologists Task Force on Management of the Difficult Airway. Apfelbaum JL, Hagberg CA, Caplan RA, Blitt CD, Connis RT, et al.)

direct laryngoscopy (DL) [8, 37]. Two newer studies showed that the displacement is either comparable to DL in human cadavers with posteriorly destabilized C3, or of smaller magnitude in healthy patients with anatomically normal airways and with MILS simulation [14, 91]. Lacking more convincing data, it is probably safe to assume that in the absence of factors suggesting difficulty with mask ventilation, it is an acceptable maneuver in cervical spinal injury. Since proper preoxygenation in the setting of emergency intubations in not always possible, and since the benefit of the correction of hypoxemia may in some circumstances outweigh the risk of aspiration, it appears that gentle mask ventilation could be acceptable, when necessary, from the standpoint of cervical cord protection.

Cricoid pressure (Sellick's Maneuver) aims to occlude the lumen of the esophagus between the cricoid cartilage and the C5–C6 level of the cervical spine by applying external pressure to the cricoid cartilage in an attempt to reduce aspiration of passively regurgitated stomach contents. The effect of the maneuver on spine motion was examined in human cadavers with intact cervical spine and was found to be modest. When utilized in a cervical spinal injury patient, a bimanual technique may be safer, with one hand under the neck, counteracting the downward pressure on the cricoid cartilage. Recent trauma emergency tracheal intubation guidelines removed cricoid pressure during rapid sequence induction as a level 1 recommendation as there is doubt it decreases the incidence of aspiration in the emergency room setting, while having been shown to worsen the laryngoscopic view and impair mask ventilation efficacy in that setting [60]. Similarly, the 2010 American Heart Association Guidelines for Cardiopulmonary Resuscitation and Emergency Cardiovascular Care state that "routine use of cricoid pressure during airway management of patients in cardiac arrest is no longer recommended." The comprehensive review of the efficacy of cricoid pressure and its potential to interfere with airway management techniques has been included in the 2010 Scandinavian Practice Guidelines on General Anesthesia for Emergency Situations by the working group of the Scandinavian Society of Anesthesiology and Intensive Care Medicine. In light of the lack of scientific evidence of its effectiveness, numerous reports questioning its efficacy and its potential for airway distortion and obstruction, even when applied properly, resulting in more difficult laryngoscope insertion, glottis visualization and reduced tidal volumes with increased airway pressures during mask ventilation, cricoid pressure can be used based on individual judgment of the anesthesiologist but is not recommended [41]. In US hospitals with anesthesia residency programs, cricoid pressure remains commonly used by anesthesiologists during rapid sequence induction [28].

There is no evidence-based recommendation for the choice of tracheal intubation technique in cervical SCI. The available data do not include outcome trials [79]. Despite a large volume of publications addressing surrogate end-points of vertebral angulation, anterior and posterior displacement of the spine, atlanto-occipital and atlanto-axial extension in normal patients and injured spine cadaver models with and without MILS simulation, using a myriad of airway devices, we are left with the unsatisfying conclusion that individual judgment must guide us in the selection of intubation technique and airway adjuncts. Awake fiberoptic intubation has theoretical advantages in that little spinal movement occurs during visualization and intubation, although topical anesthesia of the trachea commonly results in coughing. In addition, a neurological evaluation can be performed after intubation, and after the patient is positioned awake, with muscle tone aiding in avoiding potentially harmful motion. Awake fiberoptic intubation may not be practical in the uncooperative or unstable patient or a patient with a soiled airway. Failed awake intubation carries its own morbidity. Since the publication of Crosby's exhaustive Airway Management in Adults after Cervical Spine Trauma paper, many new airway devices have been studied in anesthetized healthy patients and established human cadaver models with one standardized type of injury [19]. The research continues to focus on the

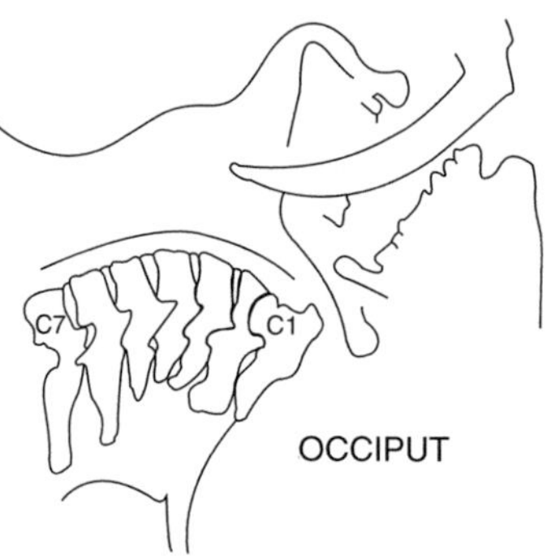

Fig. 9.4 Impact of Macintosh blade laryngoscopy on cervical spine movement. From Crosby ET. Anesthesia for cervical Spinal Cord Injury, Anesthesiology 2006;104(6):1293-318

mechanical effects of various devices and compares the measurable displacement they cause (Fig. 9.4). Brimacombe reported that in his cadaver model with C3 instability, the Combitube did worst and only nasal intubation over a fiberoptic bronchoscope produced no spinal movement [14]. The standard LMA and fiberoptic intubation through the intubating laryngeal mask had intermediate motion scores. We also know that the Torchlight® blind Intubating Lighted Stylet causes 57 % less motion than a Macintosh blade direct laryngoscopy (DL) at the Occiput-C1, C1–C2, C2–C5, and C5-thoracic segments studied in anesthetized patients, that the GlideScope® decreases only the C2–C5 segment motion by 50 % but at the expense of a 62 % prolongation of the duration of intubation, which, 8 years of experience with it later, might no longer be a valid finding [10, 91]. Robitaille reported that the GlideScope® improved glottic visualization during intubation with MILS in normal patients, but did not decrease the degree of extension at the occiput or motion at the rostral C spine relative to Macintosh DL [80]. Lately, Kill compared the GlideScope® to Macintosh DL in anesthetized normal patients without MILS [44]. He found that the GlideScope reduced movement of the cervical spine, particularly in the hands of more experienced operators, while improving the intubation success rate. Curiously, the rigid fiberscope Bonfils® Stylet caused less extension at the atlanto-occipital, C1–C2, and C3–C4 levels, but not C2–C3, than the Macintosh DL [82]. The rigid but malleable Shikani Optical Stylet®,

however, did not reduce motion at C1–C2 segment, but did better by 52 % than Macintosh DL at the other levels studied [93]. We also know that compared to Macintosh DL, the Airtraq® decreases cervical spinal motion by an average of 66 %, but not at the C1–C2 junction [92].

Aziz reviewed the use of video-assisted intubation in the management of patients with artificially applied MILS. The papers compare the intubation success rate, Intubation Difficulty Scale, intubation time or laryngeal view obtained using the different video laryngoscopes and Aitraq® versus DL, or in one case, versus GlideScope® [9]. The findings favor video laryngoscope use and are summarized in Table 9.1. Video laryngoscopes decrease intubation difficulty in patients with cervical spine immobilization and may be easy to learn. The author concludes that in the absence of neurologic outcome data, intubation techniques which maximize success rates during MILS are likely to gain acceptance.

Elective airway management in spinal cord injury patients undergoing surgery creates favorable conditions for unhurried airway topicalization and awake fiberoptic intubation. The nasal route is favored by some, but the oral route allows placement of a larger tube and avoids the risk of septic complications from bacteremia during nasal instrumentation and from sinusitis, if the patient must remain intubated after surgery. Sedation is optional and must take into account the patient's injury level, respiratory reserve, and baseline blood pressure. If a halo is in place, difficulty in securing the

Table 9.1 Compilation of studies of videolaryngoscopy and intubation performance

Author	Device	Control	Sample	Outcome assessed	Major findings
Malik MA Br J Anaesth 2008	GlideScope (Veraton, Bothell, WA) Airway Scope AWS (Pentax, Hoya, Japan)	DL	120	Laryngeal view IDS intubation time success rate	Improved laryngeal view and IDS Slower intubation time. No difference in success
Maharaj CH Anesthesiology 2007	Airtraq (Prodol, Vizcaya, Spain)	DL	40	IDS intubation attempts laryngeal view	Reduced number of intubation attempts. Improved IDS. Improved laryngeal view
Smith CE Anesthesiology 1999	WuScope (Pentax, Orangeburg, NY)	DL	87	IDS laryngeal view, intubation attempts	Improved IDS and laryngeal view. No difference in success or number of attempts
Malik MA Br J Anaesth 2009	Airway Scope (AWS)	DL	90	IDS, laryngeal view	Improved IDS and laryngeal view.
Enomoto Y Br J Anaesth 2008	Airway Scope (AWS)	DL	203	Laryngeal view, intubation time, success rate	Improved laryngeal view, increased success rate, faster intubation time
Liu EH Br J Anaesth 2009	Airway Scope (AWS)	GlideScope	70	IDS, intubation time, success rate within a defined time interval	Faster Intubation time, lower IDS, improved laryngeal view, and higher intubation success with AWS
McElwain J Br J Anaesth 2011	Airtaq, C-MAC (Karl Storz, Tuttlingen, Germany)	DL	90	IDS success rate. laryngeal view. hemodynamic stability	Reduced IDS, improved laryngeal view with Airtraq

Modified with permission from Aziz M. Use of video-assisted intubation devices in the management of patients with trauma. Anesthesiol Clin. 2013 Mar;31(1):157-66
DL direct laryngoscopy, *IDS* Intubation Difficulty Scale Score

airway should be anticipated, as access to the airway is limited and glottic visualization may be hindered by the relatively flexed position of the head. Alternatively, some centers perform fiberoptic intubation after induction of anesthesia. The advantage of this approach is that coughing-induced spine motion is prevented, but a jaw thrust might be necessary. As in emergency situations, general anesthesia followed by an intubation technique other than flexible fiberoptic is acceptable as long as MILS is maintained. The choice depends on specific airway characteristics, practitioner's expertise, and patient's preference and ability to cooperate [53].

Respiratory Management

Patients with cervical spinal cord injury have intercostal muscle weakness or paralysis and rely on diaphragmatic function for ventilation. The level of respiratory dysfunction correlates with the level of injury; forced vital capacity (FVC) may be severely decreased. The main inspiratory muscles are the diaphragm, innervated by the C3–C5 nerves and the intercostal muscles, innervated by the T2–T11 nerves. Without simultaneous intercostal muscle contraction, the contraction of the diaphragm sucks in the anterior chest wall, causing paradoxical chest wall movement. The accessory inspiratory muscles are the sternocleidomastoid and the trapezius muscles, innervated by the accessory nerve (cranial nerve XI), and the scalene muscles, innervated by the C3–C8 nerves. Forced expiration requires abdominal muscle contraction; their innervation is provided by the T6–T12 nerves. Injuries above C3 cause instant apnea; survivors are ventilator-dependent unless a diaphragm stimulator is used. Injuries at C4 (the fifth cervical nerve originates between the C4 and C5 vertebrae) or above often result in immediate respiratory failure. Because of abdominal muscle paralysis and low VC, cough is ineffective. Restricted ventilation and impaired clearance of airway secretions predispose to atelectasis, pneumonia, and respiratory failure which occur on average within 4 days of injury and are the leading causes of death in SCI patients. Reduced lung volume and atelectasis reduce lung compliance, increasing the work of breathing. Rapid, small tidal volume breathing, barely exceeding the volume of dead space, is inefficient and may further contribute to diaphragmatic fatigue. Monitoring FVC is an objective way of assessing ventilation; values below 12–15 mL/kg indicate the need for assisted ventilation. Noninvasive ventilation may help reduce the work of breathing by improving lung compliance; BiPAP is usually required and can be considered before endotracheal intubation. Patients with a FVC below 25 % of predicted value have a high incidence of respiratory failure requiring mechanical ventilation. In a case series, all patients with complete SCI at C5 or above required a tracheostomy; of those with a C6 injury or below, 79 % required intubation and 50 % eventually required tracheostomy [83]. FVC increases approximately by 9 % per decreasing level of injury. Interestingly, patients with adequate alveolar ventilation and normal p_aCO_2 often have relative hypoxemia, likely because of ventilation perfusion mismatch occurring immediately after SCI. Maintaining the supine position has advantages for respiratory function in acute cervical SCI at all levels: the abdominal contents push the diaphragm higher into the chest, decrease its radius of curvature (make it less flat), which causes more efficient contractions. Supine FVC and FEV_1 are larger compared to seated values [24]. Abdominal binding is useful in improving diaphragmatic mechanics as well. Regardless of the level of injury, FVC improves after 5 weeks and doubles 3 months after injury. Over time, developing spasticity of the intercostal and abdominal muscles minimizes paradoxical, "seesaw" pattern of abdominal and chest wall excursions on inspiration and contributes to improvement of respiratory function [87]. The expiratory function and therefore the ability to cough also improves over time, as the pectoralis major

muscle's clavicular portion contraction helps raise the intrathoracic pressure. Interruption of sympathetic innervation to the lungs appears to have physiological significance due to heightened cholinergic tone and may explain obstructive airway changes, common in tetraplegic patients. There is good responsiveness to the anticholinergic Ipratropium bromide inhalation. When instituting mechanical ventilation for purely restrictive respiratory failure without associated lung pathology, larger than the usual "lung protective" tidal volumes have been advocated to decrease atelectasis and accelerate weaning [24]. In consideration of these facts an arterial blood gas must be obtained as quickly as possible, supplemental oxygen should be given to all patients with an acute cervical SCI and mechanical ventilation, noninvasive or invasive, should be considered in all patients with C4 or C5 lesions, even if they appear compensated. Meticulous attention to optimization of respiratory function and clinical pathways for respiratory management decrease mortality from SCI and may prevent some aspects of secondary spinal cord injury. Anesthesiologists should be aware that in patients with acute cervical SCI, immediate extubation after anesthesia close to the time of injury should not be contemplated.

Hemodynamic Management

Patients with acute cervical spinal cord injury often present with neurogenic shock manifesting as hypotension due to the loss of sympathetic vasomotor tone with decreased preload related to blood pooling; associated bradycardia is due to the loss of function of cardiac accelerator fibers and contributes to decreased cardiac output. Despite lack of evidence beyond case series reports, it is believed that aggressive blood pressure management in the face of potentially disrupted spinal cord blood flow autoregulation is important in preventing secondary spinal cord injury and leads to improved functional outcomes. The 2013 updated Acute Cardiopulmonary Management of Patients with Cervical Spinal Cord Injuries guideline remains unchanged from its first version from 11 years ago. As an option, or level III recommendation, it calls for restoration of systolic blood pressure to above 90 mmHg as quickly as possible and maintenance of mean arterial pressure between 85 and 90 mmHg for 7 days after injury. Between 60 and 85 % of patients with complete high SCI have a systolic blood pressure below 90 mmHg; the average BP on admission was 66 mmHg in a series of patients with ASIA A injury. This incidence may be lower in patients with lower levels of injury and incomplete injuries. Similarly, in 71 % of severely injured patients, heart rate was below 45 beats per minute for at least one day but this was present in only 35 % of patients with milder, incomplete injuries [83]. Patients with cervical spinal cord injury are at risk for life-threatening episodic and recurrent hemodynamic instability for up to 10–14 days after injury; asystole has been described with tracheal suctioning. The highest risk involves the most injured patients; stable hemodynamic function at presentation is not a predictor of lack of complications. Persistent orthostatic hypotension is present in 29 % of chronically injured tetraplegic patients. Because up to 30 % of SCI patients may have multiple trauma and hemorrhage, it is important to identify hypovolemia as the coexisting cause of hypotension [11]. Since reflex tachycardia does not occur in the neurogenic shock period, bradycardia does not rule out hypovolemia. The initial management of neurogenic shock is volume expansion; if fluid resuscitation alone does not raise the systolic blood pressure above 90 mmHg, vasopressors should be added. Treatment of bradycardia should be undertaken simultaneously; sinus node slowing may be profound enough to produce hypotension and even cardiac arrest. Hypotensive patients who do not respond to Atropine require temporary pacing; up to 17 % of patients with complete injury required pacing in another case series [83]. Among 37 acute SCI patients with neurogenic shock admitted to one institution, adrenal insufficiency was identified in 22 % of cases; there was no correlation with the duration of vasopressor use to maintain the MAP at 85–90 mmHg [74]. The choice of vasopressor

for neurogenic shock has not been well studied. In a review of vasopressor use in patients with acute spinal cord injury, arterial and central line placement is recommended; dopamine is favored over phenylephrine because of concern for bradycardia, and vasopressin is suggested as a reasonable choice [65]. Others use norepinephrine or epinephrine [24, 40]. Vasopressors may have deleterious effects in case of concurrent brain injury. Dopamine may impair hepato-splanchnic oxygenation; β-receptor agonists and exogenous catecholamines have recently come under scrutiny as a cause of stress-induced cardiomyopathy (SIC) (takotsubo cardiomyopathy) [1]. The cardiomyopathy is characterized by transient left ventricular apex akinesia with hypercontractile basal segments of the heart in the absence of coronary artery disease, associated with significant left ventricular dysfunction. SIC has been described after traumatic brain injury, status epilepticus, subarachnoid hemorrhage and in cases of neurogenic pulmonary edema [22]. SIC has been attributed to a catecholamine surge or sympathetic nervous system activation in the setting of acute neurological injury. SIC has been described in a male patient with chronic C5 tetraplegia 10 days after removal of a spinal opioid pump, demonstrating that systemically elevated catecholamines, presumably from opioid withdrawal, can cause SIC in the absence of an intact nervous system [78]. The patient recovered after a week of extracorporeal membrane oxygenation. Lethal neurogenic pulmonary edema with severe acute cardiomyopathy has been described in a chronic incomplete C5 injury patient after two episodes of autonomic hyperreflexia presumed to be only the second such report [15]. Catecholamines could be harmful in spinal cord injury patients with cardiac dysfunction and/or pulmonary edema. It appears that the association of neurogenic pulmonary edema with SIC is being diagnosed more often as cardiac echocardiography is used in cases of acute decompensation following a neurological injury. In the absence of evidence that blood pressure augmentation in the week following acute spinal cord injury is unsafe, this Cervical SCI recommendation should probably be followed.

Temperature Management

Vasodilatation impacts temperature regulation and predisposes to hypothermia in low ambient temperatures. Conversely, hyperthermia may easily occur in high temperatures because sweating below the level of injury is impaired. Patient temperature must be closely monitored and warming devices, including fluid warmers, should be used.

Thromboembolism

Patients are at high risk within hours, because of immobility. Prophylaxis should be instituted within 72 h of injury (level II recommendation, 2013 Guidelines). In patients who are not candidates for anticoagulation and/or sequential compression devices, vena cava filters are recommended (level III recommendation).

Gastrointestinal System

Acute SCI causes ileus and delayed gastric emptying, which may persist for 2–3 weeks. Pulmonary aspiration is a risk, especially since patients are positioned supine to optimize pulmonary function.

Steroids in the Treatment of Cervical Spinal Cord Injury and Therapeutic Hypothermia

As of March 2013, large dose methylprednisolone should not be used in acute spinal cord injury patients. Until now, as the only widely used neuroprotective therapy, steroid administration has been the mainstay of treatment of blunt spinal cord injury since the NASCIS (National Acute Spinal Cord Injury Study) II and III trials of the 1990s [12, 13]. Both studies have been repeatedly criticized for serious methodological and statistical analysis flaws, but steroid use has continued in the face of lack of other treatment

options for a devastating injury in predominantly young, healthy patients [64]. For this reason, and despite evidence of harmful effects of steroids, and just a hint of benefit measured only in minor improvements across many muscle groups, but not in functional neurological improvement, the 2002 Guidelines for the Management of Acute Cervical Spine and Spinal Cord Injuries recommended methylprednisolone for either 24 or 48 h as an option. Methylprednisolone is the only steroid studied by NASCIS; it was never approved by the FDA for this indication. In March 2013, the Congress of Neurological Surgeons (CNS) and the American Association of Neurological Surgeons (AANS) published their updated Guidelines [35, 39]. There is now level I evidence that high-dose steroids are harmful, but only level III evidence of inconsistent benefits of steroids in acute blunt SCI; the updated guideline unequivocally recommends against the use of methylprednisolone in these patients [5]. The adverse effects attributable to steroids include increased incidence of pneumonia, sepsis, GI complications, thromboembolism, hyperglycemia and finally, acute corticosteroid myopathy. This iatrogenic entity tends to improve spontaneously over 6–8 months and its resolution is thought to perhaps underlie some of the motor function improvement observed in the NASCIS studies.

There has been an increasing interest in the use of therapeutic mild or modest (33 °C) hypothermia after acute spinal cord injury, along with some anecdotal reports of its efficacy. In the 2010 clinical case series of systemic hypothermia in cervical SCI from the Miami Project to Cure Paralysis at the University of Miami, 14 patients with complete (ASIA grade A) cervical spinal cord injuries were cooled using venous femoral endovascular heat exchange cooling catheters to maintain the core temperature at 33 °C for 48 h, with rewarming at the rate of 0.1 °C per hour, over a 24 h period. Improvement in one AIS grade or better occurred in 42.8 % of the patients within three months; a very significant improvement compared to data reported for spontaneous recovery from other trials [51]. As none of the patients showed improvement over the first

2 weeks after injury, misclassification of the severity of injury either due to spinal shock or sedative administration seems not to be at issue in this report. A more recent publication from the same group describes a prospective cohort of 21 additional ASIA grade A patients managed with the same hypothermia protocol [26]. They report late improvement of at least one ASIA grade in 35.5 % of cases; most observed complications were respiratory and included pneumonia in 60 % of patients and pulmonary edema in 43 %. Thromboembolic complications with two pulmonary embolisms occurred in 14 % of patients, which does not represent an excess of these events despite the use of a femoral venous cooling catheter system. The same group has reviewed the current state of knowledge on hypothermia in SCI and reports that a randomized trial of systemic hypothermia with 17 centers participating and the intent to recruit 200 patients is being planned [2]. At this time, although advances in endovascular cooling technology allow the institution of hypothermia with minimal delay which is important for the effectiveness of neuroprotective strategies, moderate hypothermia is not a proven therapeutic modality in acute spinal cord injury.

Timing of Surgery

Issue is now actively debated, but it is far from resolved. The current surgical management trend of acute cervical SCI patients favors early decompression and stabilization of the cervical spine. Logistical difficulties with early intervention in this patient population, because of delayed transfers to specialized centers and patient eligibility due to coexisting injuries or morbid conditions, are common. The term "early surgery" is therefore usually arbitrarily defined as surgery occurring within 24 h of injury. The best evidence in favor of early surgery comes from a multicenter, prospective, but nonrandomized cohort study of 313 patients with acute cervical SCI who underwent definitive open surgical decompression and fixation with instrumentation of the cervical spine [29]. The

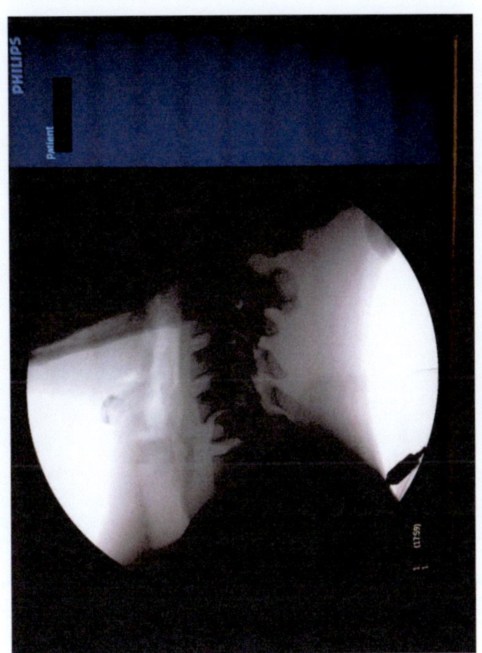

Fig. 9.5 Jumped bilateral facets X-ray. Courtesy of Dr. John Houten

study concluded that surgery prior to 24 h after SCI is safe and is associated with improved neurologic outcome, defined as at least two grade ASIA impairment scale (AIS) improvement at 6 months of injury. Despite a debate as to the significance of the results for surgical practice standards, there is a definite momentum towards early decompression/fusion in SCI patients; this may be performed via an anterior, posterior, and combined approach [72]. This change is of importance to anesthesiologists, because of the complexities of intraoperative management of patients with neurogenic shock and the ensuing necessity for urgent evaluation and optimization of these patients.

A subset of patients with acute SCI present with cervical facet dislocation (Fig. 9.5). Although relatively rare among patients with cervical spine trauma, facet dislocation, especially if bilateral, results in spinal cord injury in up to 90 % of patients. The injury occurs during high-velocity neck hyper-flexion with slippage of the upper vertebra lower facets relative to the upper facets of the lower vertebra; as a result, the diameter of the spinal canal is decreased,

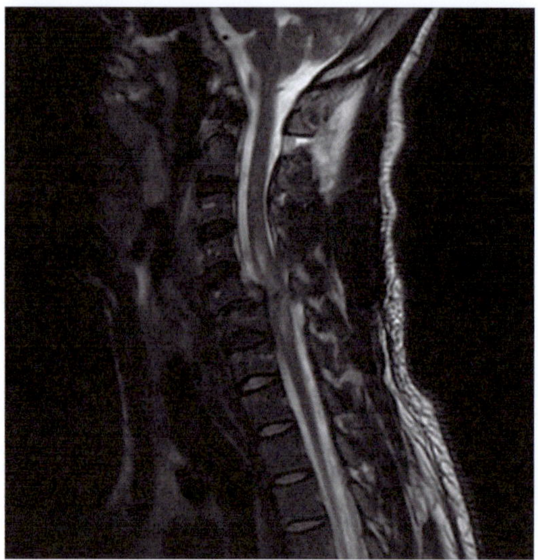

Fig. 9.6 MRI of cervical spinal cord after bilateral facet dislocation at C5, C6 level. Courtesy of Dr. John Houten

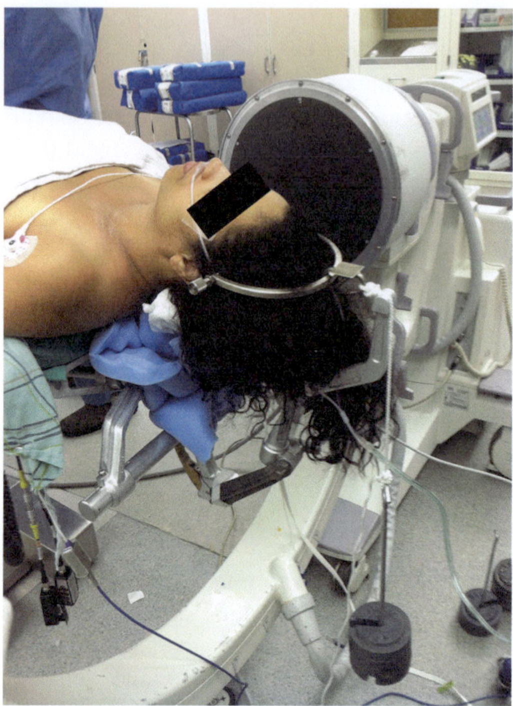

Fig. 9.7 Skeletal traction to reduce facet dislocation. Courtesy of Dr. John Houten

compressing the spinal cord and causing cord contusion (Fig. 9.6). These patients often undergo urgent skeletal traction and closed reduction of the dislocation, as rapid restoration of the alignment of the spine may, in certain cases, lead to immediate neurological recovery and is therefore advocated as a means of prompt decompression of the spinal cord [94]. Skull tongs are placed under local anesthesia, and weights are sequentially added via a pulley system to distract and realign the cervical spine; this is sometimes done at the bedside (Fig. 9.7). In patients breathing spontaneously, the pain the procedure causes is usually treated with intravenous opioids. In some instances, closed reduction is performed in the operating room under general anesthesia; if unsuccessful, it may be immediately converted to an open, surgical reduction (Figs. 9.8 and 9.9).

Surgical Interventions

Anesthetic implications vary depending on the surgical access. Anterior approaches are either open cervical for anterior discectomy and plate fusion, or percutaneous for odontoid fractures. Cervico-medullary junction decompression is carried out through a trans-oral approach. Minimally invasive spine surgery is making inroads—an endonasal endoscopic approach for odontoid and C1 arch resection has been described. Posterior approaches involve laminectomy decompression with fixation, usually with lateral mass screws and rods, for subaxial injuries and atlanto-axial-occipital fusion. A minority of patients will be placed in a halo vest after surgery.

Complications of Surgery of Relevance to Anesthesiologists

The most common complication of the *anterior cervical approach* to spinal fusion is transient dysphagia. The most dangerous complication is postoperative hematoma; the reported incidence of clinically apparent hematoma is 0.2–5.6 %. Wound drainage does not completely safeguard against this complication. Approximately half of postoperative hematomas require emergency

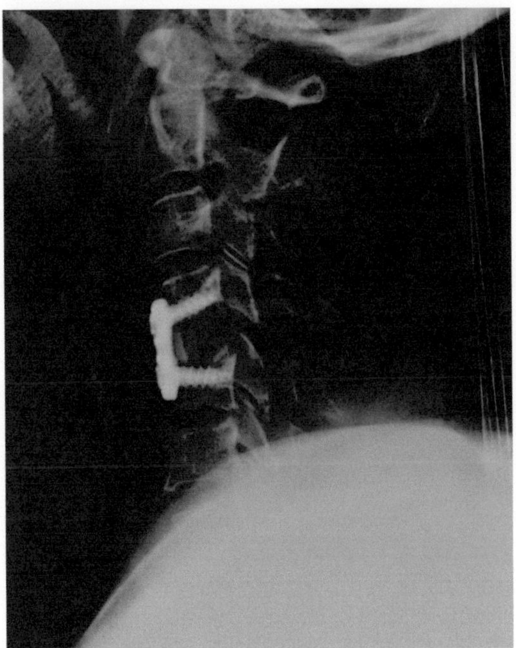

Fig. 9.8 Anterior reduction and fusion of facet dislocation. Courtesy of Dr. John Houten

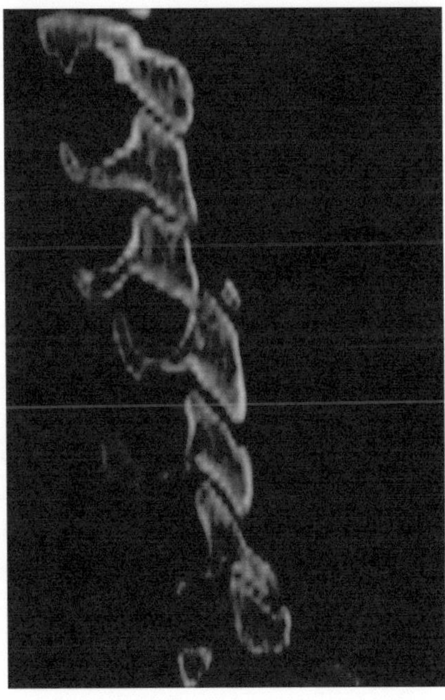

Fig. 9.9 *Arrow* points to cervical facet dislocation—CT
scan. Courtesy of Dr. John Houten

surgical evacuation, due to complaints of
dyspnea despite normal oxygenation, overt
respiratory compromise, worsening dysphagia,

and hematoma expansion associated with neck
pain [30]. When a postoperative neck hematoma
is present, difficulties securing the airway may
occur despite a reassuring initial intubation
course. This may be due to either direct airway
compression with luminal impingement and
deviation, or more ominously, because of airway
edema. The edema is thought to occur as blood
collects in the anterior neck and hinders venous
and lymphatic outflow. The swelling of the
arytenoids and the epiglottis may be present,
even when the total volume of hematoma is low
[73]. Thought should be given to either
attempting to visualize the glottis or performing
the endotracheal intubation awake. Opening the
wound under local anesthesia to decompress the
hematoma may facilitate intubation.

Symptomatic recurrent laryngeal nerve palsy
is another common complication of the anterior
approach with an incidence of 1.1–3.1 % in
large patient series from the last 20 years [30].
Asymptomatic, and presumably transient,
recurrent laryngeal nerve dysfunction is much
more common. The vagus and the recurrent
laryngeal nerves are not visualized during
surgery. The cause of recurrent laryngeal
neuropraxia and paralysis has been attributed to
nerve stretch and compression between the
surgical retractor and the endotracheal tube
balloon, observed anatomically in cadaveric
investigations [46]. In a clinical study by the
same authors, deflating the endotracheal cuff
and re-inflating it after retractor blade placement,
which presumably allows the endotracheal tube
to "recenter" itself in the larynx, decreased the
rate of temporary vocal cord paralysis from 6.4 to
1.69 % [7]. The highest rate of vocal cord
dysfunction has been observed after surgery at
T1 level, while C7 had a rate of 3.9 %. Higher
surgical levels were associated with an incidence
of 1.3 % at C5 and 2.2 % at C6 in the same case
series. Trauma as the indication for surgery was
not associated with an increased incidence of
recurrent laryngeal nerve palsy. The importance
of this observation is that recurrent laryngeal
nerve injury may occur in cervical spine
fractures, especially if the injury involves lower
vertebrae. Indeed, in a report of two patients with

C6–C7 and C7–T1 fracture dislocation, respectively, and who presented with dysphonia, recurrent laryngeal nerve injury presumed to be caused by the injury was confirmed preoperatively [33]. The left-sided approach is theoretically more protective of the recurrent laryngeal nerve, because the left nerve has a longer loop and is better protected within the tracheo-esophageal groove. Most right-handed surgeons prefer the right-sided approach however. Several studies refute the superiority of the left-sided approach [43]. A high level of suspicion for recurrent laryngeal nerve injury in cervical spine injuries should arise when hoarseness or dysphonia is evident in awake, talking patients. Anterior surgery in patients with preexisting recurrent laryngeal nerve injury should be performed from the approach ipsilateral to the injury to prevent bilateral nerve paralysis. Recurrent laryngeal nerve EMG monitoring to prevent intraoperative nerve damage, although commonly used, has not been systematically studied in anterior cervical spinal fusion. The 2013 Guidelines for Improving Voice Outcomes after Thyroid Surgery recommend intra-operative recurrent laryngeal nerve EMG monitoring to identify the nerve as an option only, emphasizing the importance of proper placement of the laryngeal electromyography endotracheal tube.

Rare complications of the anterior approach to spine surgery are esophageal and pharyngeal perforation (with possibly subcutaneous emphysema), dural perforation and CSF leakage, vertebral artery injury, Horner's syndrome, and neurological deterioration.

The posterior approach necessitates prone positioning with the attendant risk of neurological injury in unstable cervical spine injuries during rotation from the supine position. This may be minimized by the use of a cervical collar with manual in-line stabilization during manual patient transfer, awake self-positioning in neurologically intact patients after intubation, or via the "Jackson table" technique, where the patient is transferred to the table supine with the usual immobilization precautions, then secured to the table which is then rotated 180°. Continuous electrophysiological monitoring may be utilized before and immediately after positioning prone. A pin head-fixation device is commonly used in posterior cervical spine surgery. It has a potential to cause excessive neck motion during both patient transfer and while it is being secured to any operating table, including the Jackson table.

Paraspinal muscle dissection and laminectomy may cause blood loss, although this is seldom very significant at the cervical level. Vertebral artery injury is a very rare but potentially important cause of blood loss and intra-operative neurological injury.

Prolonged spine surgery may cause rhabdomyolysis, and when performed in the prone position, it is a risk factor for peri-operative visual loss, especially in the male, obese patients positioned on a Wilson frame [20, 75].

Improper positioning may cause outright compression of the inferior vena cava and severely decreased preload. Prone positioning decreases blood pressure and cardiac output in anesthetized patients, likely because of a decrease in venous return and decreased cardiac compliance [27]. The hemodynamic effects of prone positioning depend on the type of positioner used. The Jackson table and the longitudinal bolsters have the least effect on cardiac function by echocardiography performed immediately after positioning when adequate fluid replacement is provided after turning the patient prone [25]. Because it is important to minimize venous engorgement of the orbital content and the airway in the prone position, some degree of head-up tilt is necessary. This may contribute to a decrease in venous return and cardiac output, even when using the Jackson table. The hemodynamic changes occurring in the prone position are expected to have more clinical significance in the elderly, those with chronic cardiovascular comorbidities, and patients with neurogenic shock. The hemodynamic effects of the prone position have anesthetic implications: the plasma concentration of Propofol is increased when cardiac output is lower, presumably because of decreased drug clearance [50]. Therefore, if needed, the choice of vasopressor must take into account its effect not just on the blood pressure, but also the cardiac output and by extension, on the hypnotic effect of Propofol [66]. In general, hemodynamic management in the prone position has not been well studied; CVP does not predict fluid responsiveness and correlates poorly with left ventricular end-diastolic volume, especially in the prone position [58].

The rare occurrence of venous air, fat, and bone fragment embolism must be considered in cases of sudden hemodynamic instability [27]. The increasingly common direct spinal wound application of powdered Vancomycin to prevent postoperative infection, intended to maximize local antibiotic concentration without high plasma levels, may nevertheless result in circulatory collapse as in the intravenous route of administration [57].

The respiratory effects of the prone position are positive in terms of lung volumes, preferential blood flow to dependent lung areas and ultimately, improved ventilation/perfusion matching leading to the utilization of the prone or near-prone position in the mechanically ventilated ARDS patients. Surgery on the cervical spine in the prone position involves the use of large radiographic equipment like a C-arm, or more commonly now an O-ring CT scanner which is manipulated in close proximity to the endotracheal tube. The risk of accidental extubation has to be anticipated as this complication has been reported. A recent case report reviews the airway management options should this occur [89]. Additional causes of airway loss in the prone position include endotracheal tube obstruction by bloody secretions or inspissated secretions; reinforced endotracheal tube malfunction with obstruction has been reported as well [76]. Although turning the patient supine in an emergency may be delayed by the need to remove instrument constructs from the wound, having a stretcher available at all times is a basic prone patient-operative safety feature. Airway rescue maneuvers in the prone position may include tube reinsertion over a flexible fiberoptic bronchoscope, ventilation and intubation through an LMA, aspiration of secretions and clearing the tube lumen with an arterial embolectomy catheter [27].

Neurophysiological Monitoring During Cervical Spinal Decompression with Fusion and Instrumentation

Intra-operative neurophysiological monitoring (IOM) is widely used in spine surgery in the hope of the early detection of iatrogenic neurological insults related to the mechanical stress of positioning, surgical manipulation, and cord perfusion from hypotension. The risk of neurological injury during cervical spine surgery, although ever-present and potentially devastating, has not been well quantified.

Because the dorsal and ventral portions of the cord have separate blood supply, simultaneous monitoring of the somatosensory (SSEPs) and transcranial myogenic electrical motor-evoked potentials (MEPs), as well as spontaneous electromyography (EMG) from relevant muscle groups, is usually performed, and is called multimodal IOM. SSEPs monitor the sensory dorsal column-medial lemniscus pathway, recording subcortical or cortical responses to stimulation of a peripheral nerve. Because SSEP acquisition requires signal averaging, the temporal summation provides a reading with some delay, sometimes of a few minutes duration, depending on the number of averages needed. The time interval between the stimulus applied to the peripheral nerve and the evoked response is called latency, while the size of the response is its amplitude. The alert or warning criteria differ, and many clinical papers do not report them, but a decrease in amplitude of more than 50 % and increase in latency by 15 % or more are considered significant changes that must be communicated to the surgical and anesthesia teams. SSEPs can localize the site of injury or ischemia more exactly than the MEPs provided the sensory pathway is affected, as recordings can be monitored from both the cerebral cortex and subcortical sites. MEPs assess the entire motor axis. Electrical stimulation with high-frequency trains of high voltage is applied percutaneously over the motor cortex and compound muscle action potentials (CAMPs) are recorded from muscle groups of interest. MEPs cause patient movement during stimulation, although this can be minimized by stimulus voltage adjustment, and as a result can only be assessed periodically. The warning criterion for MEPs varies. Some centers use an all-or-none criterion; others consider an 80 % reduction in amplitude at any one recording site to be an alert value. Another way of quantifying the alert value for MEPs is establishing a minimum stimulus threshold value that results in CAMPs; an increase in the threshold of 100 V is considered a warning [48]. MEPs may trigger seizures, albeit very rarely. Volatile anesthetics and nitrous oxide decrease the amplitude of MEPs and interfere with the ability to monitor MEPs, and are therefore proscribed. Spontaneous EMG allows continuous monitoring of selective nerve root function throughout the surgery. MEP and EMG monitoring precludes the use of muscle relaxants during surgery on practical grounds.

The American Academy of Neurology and the American Clinical Neurophysiology Society analyzed twelve studies meeting pre-defined quality and enrolment size criteria in an effort to determine whether spinal cord IOM predicts adverse surgical outcomes [70]. On this basis, the published evidence-based guideline concludes that "IOM is established as effective to predict an increased risk of the adverse outcomes of paraparesis, paraplegia and quadriplegia in spinal surgery." This conclusion assumes, in the authors' opinion, that a "knowledgeable professional clinical neurophysiologist supervisor" is responsible for the IOM, as opposed to IOM "conducted by a technician alone or by an automated device." Armed with the knowledge that well-conducted IOM has an excellent, if not perfect, predictive value for the most severe neurological complications, we still do not know whether the use of IOM prevents neurological injury in spine surgery. There are no guidelines addressing this issue. A firm consensus exists only for scoliosis surgery. There is data addressing the sensitivity and specificity of modern multimodal IOM, but it does not specifically address surgery in spinal

cord-injured patients. In general, the reported sensitivity and specificity of IOM in cervical spine surgery in the last decade, that is since myogenic MEP monitoring has become an integral part of IOM, is between 95 and 100 % [48]. However, as discussed previously, warning criteria vary and measures of neurological outcome are also variable. A retrospective analysis of 200 consecutive cervical spine surgery cases managed with IOM included 40 traumatic spine injury patients; it reports a specificity of 100 % of SSEPs and MEPs, and a sensitivity of 100 % of the combination of SSEPs and MEPs for detecting impending neurological injury [52]. Of note, the SSEPs were primarily useful in alerting of a malposition of the arm and, in one instance, of the need to raise the blood pressure while the MEP alerts were caused by hypotension and in one case, graft malposition.

Filling the void of information on the preventive value of IOM on intraoperative neurological injury is a simulation model which evaluates the cost-benefit of IOM, assuming a 5 % baseline neurologic complication rate, a cost of IOM of $1,535 per case, a prevention rate of an IOM alert of 52 % in 10,000 surgeries, and a lifetime cost of lost wages and health care of an intraoperative incomplete neurologic deficit involving either the spinal cord or nerve roots of $900,000 [69]. The simulation predicts considerable cost-savings if IOM is used; 2.3 million dollars would be saved for each 100 spine surgeries. The savings would occur even if the risk of neurological injury were 1 %, although only $3,500 per procedure would be saved, and even if the prevention rate were far lower than the one assumed. There being no economic or outcome down-side to poor specificity, the focus should be on the sensitivity of the IOM techniques used. In summary, the cost-benefit is most favorable if IOM is used in patients with severe underlying pathology and those undergoing high-risk procedures, and if there is corrective action in response to an IOM alert. This certainly applies to patients with incomplete spinal cord injury.

Pain Associated with Spinal Cord Injury

The SCI Guidelines have a new level I recommendation: the clinical assessment of Pain in SCI patients should be performed, preferably using the International Spinal Cord Injury Basic Pain Dataset to evaluate the severity of pain as well as physical and emotional functioning [42].

Pain associated with spinal cord injury is common; its prevalence is estimated at 80 %. Chronic pain of SCI interferes with the ability to achieve maximal functional recovery and degrades the quality of life. It may also lead to severe depression. Pain may be neuropathic or nociceptive, or both. Nociceptive pain may be related to spasticity and painful muscle spasms, as well as overuse of the arms and shoulders; it responds to standard pain management protocols. Neuropathic pain below the level of injury is more common in tetraplegics, but overall there is no relationship between the presence of pain and the completeness or level of the lesion [86]. In addition to its high prevalence, neuropathic pain associated with spinal cord injury is resistant to conventional pharmacological treatment and is therefore debilitating; there is also a tendency for the pain to worsen over time. In most patients the pain is spontaneous, but can also manifest as allodynia and hyperalgesia. The central neuropathic pain of SCI has several subsets determined by pain location: above, at, and below the level injury. It is believed that different mechanisms of abnormal neural activity and inflammation at spinal and supraspinal levels are involved in these pain subsets. Central neuropathic pain differs from peripheral neuropathic pain. Efficacy would therefore be expected from distinct treatment combinations; however the lack of understanding of the pathophysiology of central neuropathic pain hinders the development of pharmacological regimens targeted to central neuropathic pain processes. Certain drugs, such as tricyclic antidepressants, commonly used in peripheral neuropathic pain are not as effective in SCI patients and they may be poorly tolerated in patients with incomplete injuries because of urinary retention; bladder distension is a known trigger of autonomic hyperreflexia. Opioids are commonly utilized, but with only a 30 % longer-term response rate. Intrathecal opioids have been used in combination with intrathecal clonidine and baclofen and with ziconotide, a selective N-type calcium channel blocker [36]. Newer research however indicates that in the acute phase of injury, opioids may exacerbate injury-induced excitotoxic damage to neurons and cause glial activation in the spinal cord and may actually promote the development of pain after spinal cord injury by activating central sensitization pathways. In addition, in the setting of spinal cord injury opioids may negatively impact recovery of locomotor function through the same mechanisms [95]. Oral gabapentin shows some promise. Daily intravenous ketamine infusions have been added to oral gabapentin with some success; the improvement is transient and disappears some two weeks after the infusions are stopped. Neither deep brain stimulation nor dorsal column spinal cord stimulation is effective in SCI pain; combinations have not been studied [62].

In summary, the recommended SCI pain assessment tools should bring about more standardized information about pain syndromes, their time course and help design treatment modalities in more homogenous groups of patients and analyze their effectiveness, perhaps enhancing the understanding of the pathophysiological processes underlying SCI pain.

Anesthetic Technique Specific to Spinal Cord Injury

Little is known about the short- and long-term effects of specific anesthetic agents in the setting of acute spinal cord injury. Knowledge of the respiratory and cardiovascular implications of SCI is essential in managing an anesthetic in a spinal cord-injured patient. The presence of coexisting injuries and the risk of aspiration must be taken into account. Chiefly however, the anesthesiologist should do no harm and focus on preventing secondary spinal cord injury by maintaining spinal alignment during airway instrumentation to the extent dictated by its urgency and by ensuring adequate spinal cord perfusion. The newest guidelines of the Congress of Neurological Surgeons provide some guidance in the form of target blood pressure values, albeit at a low level of evidence.

The prolific group from Korea led by K.Y. Yoo has published a dozen papers in European and American anesthesiology journals over the last decade, examining the effects of laryngoscopy and intubation on cardiovascular responses, as well as anesthetic requirements for endotracheal intubation and prevention of autonomic hyperreflexia, in acutely and chronically spinal cord-injured patients [96, 97]. Summarizing their findings, cardiovascular responses to intubation are blunted in tetraplegic patients, irrespective of the time since injury: blood pressure does not increase and may fall, heart rate does increase, but to a lesser extent than in paraplegics. Norepinephrine levels do not increase at intubation in acute tetraplegia, but do so mildly after 4 weeks of injury. Predictably, the arousal response to intubation, measured by BIS values, is no different in SCI patients than in non-injured controls.

Succinylcholine is a drug with a very fast onset of action. It is ideally suited for emergency endotracheal intubations. Its administration poses the risk of hyperkalemic cardiac arrest in susceptible patients. Spinal cord injury with tetraplegia involves the majority of the body's muscle mass. Denervation causes upregulation of acetylcholine receptors at the muscle membrane within hours of immobilization. The appearance of extrajunctional receptors takes about 12 h. The extrajunctional receptors will in turn upregulate, since denervation persists. Within 48–72 h of injury, this upregulation may be critical enough to cause lethal hyperkalemia after succinylcholine administration to tetraplegic patients. As long as the paralysis persists, these patients are potentially at risk for hyperkalemia after succinylcholine administration [59]. It is worth noting that Yoo's group has used succinylcholine

in the cohort of 214 acute and chronic SCI patients described in the reference, seemingly without ill effect [97].

Research in acute spinal cord injury must lead to a better understanding of the "secondary injury" processes, allowing for focused neuroprotection strategies. Some candidate interventions might be metalloproteinase inhibition by Minocycline or sodium channel blockade by Riluzole. The North American Clinical Trials Network (NACTN) for Treatment of Spinal Cord Injury is currently enrolling patients for a prospective evaluation of the natural history of spinal cord injury managed in selected, specialized centers. This work is likely to provide us with new best practices and of importance to anesthesiologists, test the emerging evidence that ultra-rapid spine decompression and fusion improves neurological outcome. The NIH funding for spinal cord injury research remains flat at about $79 million US$ annually, of which approximately $5 million is allocated to the longitudinal patient follow-up by NACTN [68].

Other research focuses on axonal growth and re-myelination, synapse formation, and the use of central nervous system stem cells in spinal cord injury repair. Although the body of knowledge about the injury and its healing is growing, the promise of a cure for SCI is as yet unfulfilled.

Acknowledgments The authors wish to thank Dr. John K. Houten, Professor of Clinical Neurological Surgery, Albert Einstein College of Medicine, Chief, Division of Spinal Neurosurgery, Montefiore Medical Center, Bronx, NY for graciously making available to us and giving us permission to reprint the images of cervical facet dislocation, cord compression, skeletal traction and anterior cervical fusion. We thank Ms. Samantha Rawana for her expert and cheerful assistance with copyright compliance and manuscript submission and Mr. James Sweeney for making everything appear in the required dpi resolution.

References

1. Abraham J, Mudd JO, Kapur NK, Klein K, Champion HC, Wittstein IS. Stress cardiomyopathy after intravenous administration of catecholamines and beta-receptor agonists. J Am Coll Cardiol. 2009;53(15):1320–5. doi:10.1016/j.jacc.2009.02.020.

2. Ahmad F, Wang MY, Levi AD. Hypothermia for acute spinal cord injury-a review. World Neurosurg. 2013;pii:S1878–8750(13):00015–6. doi: 10.1016/j.wneu.2013.01.008. [Epub ahead of print]

3. Ahn H, Fehlings MG. Prevention, identification, and treatment of perioperative spinal cord injury. Neurosurg Focus. 2008;25(5):E15. doi:10.3171/FOC.2008.25.11.E15.

4. American Spinal Injury Association [Internet]. Atlanta: International Standards for Neurological Classification of Spinal Cord Injury Exam Sheet. 2013. http://www.asia-spinalinjury.org/elearning/ISNCSCI.php. [Revised 2013 Feb].

5. Anderson, Pauline. New CNS/AANS Guidelines Discourage Steroids in Spinal Injury. Medscape [Internet]. 2013. http://www.medscape.com/viewarticle/781669.

6. Apfelbaum JL, Hagberg CA, Caplan RA, Blitt CD, Connis RT, Nickinovich DG, et al. Practice guidelines for management of the difficult airway: an updated report by the American Society of Anesthesiologists Task Force on Management of the Difficult Airway. Anesthesiology. 2013;118(2):251–70. doi:10.1097/ALN.0b013e31827773b2.

7. Apfelbaum RI, Kriskovich MD, Haller JR. On the incidence, cause, and prevention of recurrent laryngeal nerve palsies during anterior cervical spine surgery. Spine (Phila Pa 1976). 2000;25(22):2906–12.

8. Aprahamian C, Thompson BM, Finger WA, Darin JC. Experimental cervical spine injury model: evaluation of airway management and splinting techniques. Ann Emerg Med. 1984;13(8):584–7.

9. Aziz M. Use of video-assisted intubation devices in the management of patients with trauma. Anesthesiol Clin. 2013;31(1):157–66. doi:10.1016/j.anclin.2012.10.001. Epub 2012 Nov 3.

10. Aziz MF, Healy D, Kheterpal S, Fu RF, Dillman D, Brambrink AM. Routine clinical practice effectiveness of the Glidescope in difficult airway management: an analysis of 2,004 Glidescope intubations, complications, and failures from two institutions. Anesthesiology. 2011;114(1):34–41. doi:10.1097/ALN.0b013e3182023eb7.

11. Bernhard M, Gries A, Kremer P, Böttiger BW. Spinal cord injury (SCI)—prehospital management. Resuscitation. 2005;66(2):127–39.

12. Bracken MB, Shepard MJ, Collins WF, Holford TR, Young W, Baskin DS, et al. A randomized, controlled trial of methylprednisolone or naloxone in the treatment of acute spinal-cord injury. Results of the Second National Acute Spinal Cord Injury Study. N Engl J Med. 1990;322(20):1405–11.

13. Bracken MB, Shepard MJ, Holford TR, Leo-Summers L, Aldrich EF, Fazl M, et al. Administration of methylprednisolone for 24 or 48 hours or tirilazad mesylate for 48 hours in the treatment of acute spinal cord injury. Results of the Third National Acute Spinal Cord Injury Randomized Controlled Trial National Acute Spinal Cord Injury Study. JAMA. 1997;277(20):1597–604.

14. Brimacombe J, Keller C, Künzel KH, Gaber O, Boehler M, Pühringer F. Cervical spine motion during airway management: a cinefluoroscopic study of the posteriorly destabilized third cervical vertebrae in human cadavers. Anesth Analg. 2000;91(5):1274–8.

15. Calder KB, Estores IM, Krassioukov A. Autonomic dysreflexia and associated acute neurogenic pulmonary edema in a patient with spinal cord injury: a case report and review of the literature. Spinal Cord. 2009;47(5):423–5. doi:10.1038/sc.2008.152. Epub 2009 Jan 13.

16. Catz A, Itzkovich M, Tesio L, Biering-Sorensen F, Weeks C, Laramee MT, et al. A multicenter international study on the Spinal Cord Independence Measure, version III: Rasch psychometric validation. Spinal Cord. 2007;45(4):275–91. doi:10.1038/sj.sc.3101960. Epub 2006 Aug 15.

17. CDC.gov [Internet]. Atlanta: Centers for Disease Control and Prevention; 2010. http://www.cdc.gov/traumaticbraininjury/scifacts.html. [Updated 2010 Nov 4].

18. Cleiman P, Nemeth J, Vetere P. A significant cervical spine fracture: think of the airway. J Emerg Med. 2012;42(2):e23–5. doi:10.1016/j.jemermed.2008.07.027. Epub 2009 Jan 6.

19. Crosby ET. Airway management in adults after cervical spine trauma. Anesthesiology. 2006;104(6):1293–318.

20. Dakwar E, Rifkin SI, Volcan IJ, Goodrich JA, Uribe JS. Rhabdomyolysis and acute renal failure following minimally invasive spine surgery: report of 5 cases. J Neurosurg Spine. 2011;14(6):785–8. doi:10.3171/2011.2.SPINE10369. Epub 2011 Mar 18.

21. Davies G, Deakin C, Wilson A. The effect of a rigid collar on intracranial pressure. Injury. 1996;27(9):647–9.

22. Davison DL, Terek M, Chawla LS. Neurogenic pulmonary edema. Crit Care. 2012;16(2):212. doi:10.1186/cc11226.

23. De Lorenzo RA, Olson JE, Boska M, Johnston R, Hamilton GC, Augustine J, et al. Optimal positioning for cervical immobilization. Ann Emerg Med. 1996;28(3):301–8.

24. Denton M, McKinlay J. Cervical cord injury and critical care. Contin Educ Anaesth Crit Care Pain. 2009;9(3):82–6.

25. Dharmavaram S, Jellish WS, Nockels RP, Shea J, Mehmood R, Ghanayem A, et al. Effect of prone positioning systems on hemodynamic and cardiac function during lumbar spine surgery: an echocardiographic study. Spine (Phila Pa 1976). 2006;31(12):1388–93. discussion 1394.

26. Dididze M, Green BA, Dalton Dietrich W, Vanni S, Wang MY, Levi AD. Systemic hypothermia in acute cervical spinal cord injury: a case-controlled study. Spinal Cord. 2013;51(5):395–400. doi:10.1038/sc.2012.161. Epub 2012 Dec 18.

27. Edgcombe H, Carter K, Yarrow S. Anaesthesia in the prone position. Br J Anaesth. 2008;100(2):165–83. doi:10.1093/bja/aem380.

28. Ehrenfeld JM, Cassedy EA, Forbes VE, Mercaldo ND, Sandberg WS. Modified rapid sequence induction and intubation: a survey of United States current practice. Anesth Analg. 2012;115(1):95–101. doi:10.1213/ANE.0b013e31822dac35. Epub 2011 Oct 24.

29. Fehlings MG, Vaccaro A, Wilson JR, Singh A, Cadotte WD, Harrop JS, et al. Early versus delayed decompression for traumatic cervical spinal cord injury: results of the Surgical Timing in Acute Spinal Cord Injury Study (STASCIS). PLoS One. 2012;7(2):e32037.

30. Fountas KN, Kapsalaki EZ, Nikolakakos LG, Smisson HF, Johnston KW, Grigorian AA, et al. Anterior cervical discectomy and fusion associated complications. Spine (Phila Pa 1976). 2007;32(21):2310–7.

31. Goldberg W, Mueller C, Panacek E, Tigges S, Hoffman JR, Mower WR, et al. Distribution and patterns of blunt traumatic cervical spinal injury. Ann Emerg Med. 2001;38(1):17–21.

32. Grissom TE, Varon AJ. Airway management controversies in trauma care. ASA Newslett. 2013;77(4):12–4.

33. Gulsen S, Yilmaz C, Calisaneller T, Caner H, Altinors N. Preoperative functional assessment of the recurrent laryngeal nerve in patients with cervical vertebra fracture: case report. Neurosurgery. 2009;64(1):E191–2; discussion E192. doi: 10.1227/01.NEU.0000336328.59216.08.

34. Hadley MN, Walters BC. Introduction to the guidelines for the management of acute cervical spine and spinal cord injuries. Neurosurgery. 2013;72 Suppl 2:5–16. doi:10.1227/NEU.0b013e3182773549.

35. Hadley MN, Walters BC, Aarabi B, Dhall SS, Gelb DE, et al. Clinical assessment following acute cervical spinal cord injury. Neurosurgery. 2013;72 Suppl 2:40–53. doi:10.1227/NEU.0b013e318276edda.

36. Hama A, Sagen J. Combination drug therapy for pain following chronic spinal cord injury. Pain Res Treat. 2012;2012:840486. doi:10.1155/2012/840486. Epub 2012 Mar 18.

37. Hauswald M, Sklar DP, Tandberg D, Garcia JF. Cervical spine movement during airway management: cinefluoroscopic appraisal in human cadavers. Am J Emerg Med. 1991;9(6):535–8.

38. Hindman BJ, Palecek JP, Posner KL, Traynelis VC, Lee LA, Sawin PD, et al. Cervical spinal cord, root, and bony spine injuries: a closed claims analysis. Anesthesiology. 2011;114(4):782–95. doi:10.1097/ALN.0b013e3182104859.

39. Hurlbert RJ, Hadley MN, Walters BC, Aarabi B, Dhall SS, Gelb DE, et al. Pharmacological therapy for acute spinal cord injury. Neurosurgery. 2013;72 Suppl 2:93–105. doi:10.1227/NEU.0b013e31827765c6.

40. Jia X, Kowalski RG, Sciubba DM, Geocadin RG. Critical care of traumatic spinal cord injury. J Intensive Care Med. 2013;28(1):12–23. doi:10.1177/0885066611403270. Epub 2011 Apr 11.

41. Jensen AG, Callesen T, Hagemo JS, Hreinsson K, Lund V, Nordmark J, et al. Scandinavian clinical practice guidelines on general anaesthesia for emergency situations. Acta Anaesthesiol Scand. 2010;54(8):922–50. doi:10.1111/j.1399-6576.2010.02277.x.

42. Jensen MP, Widerström-Noga E, Richards JS, Finnerup NB, Biering-Sørensen F, Cardenas DD. Reliability and validity of the International Spinal Cord Injury basic pain data set items as self-report measures. Spinal Cord. 2010;48(3):230–8. doi:10.1038/sc.2009.112. Epub 2009 Sep 29.

43. Kilburg C, Sullivan HG, Mathiason MA. Effect of approach side during anterior cervical discectomy and fusion on the incidence of recurrent laryngeal nerve injury. J Neurosurg Spine. 2006;4(4):273–7.

44. Kill C, Risse J, Wallot P, Seidl P, Steinfeldt T, Wulf H. Videolaryngoscopy with glidescope reduces cervical spine movement in patients with unsecured cervical spine. J Emerg Med. 2013;44(4):750–6. doi:10.1016/j.jemermed.2012.07.080. Epub 2013 Jan 22.

45. Kolb JC, Summers RL, Galli RL. Cervical collar-induced changes in intracranial pressure. Am J Emerg Med. 1999;17(2):135–7.

46. Kriskovich MD, Apfelbaum RI, Haller JR. Vocal fold paralysis after anterior cervical spine surgery: incidence, mechanism, and prevention of injury. Laryngoscope. 2000;110(9):1467–73.

47. Kudo T, Sato Y, Kowatari K, Nitobe T, Hirota K. Case Report Post Operative transient tetraplegia in two patients caused by cervical spondylotic myelopathy. Anaesthesia. 2011;66(3):213–6. doi:10.1111/j.1365-2044.2010.06562. Epub 2011 Jan 25.

48. Lall RR, Lall RR, Hauptman JS, Munoz C, Cybulski GR, Koski T, et al. Intraoperative neurophysiological monitoring in spine surgery: indications, efficacy, and role of the preoperative checklist. Neurosurg Focus. 2012;33(5):E10. doi:10.3171/2012.9.FOCUS12235.

49. Lanier WL, Warner MA. New perioperative cervical injury: medical and legal implications for patients and anesthesia providers. Anesthesiology. 2011;114(4):729–31. doi:10.1097/ALN.0b013e3182104884.

50. Leslie K, Wu CY, Bjorksten AR, Williams DL, Ludbrook G, Williamson E. Cardiac output and propofol concentrations in prone surgical patients. Anaesth Intensive Care. 2011;39(5):868–74.

51. Levi AD, Casella G, Green BA, Dietrich WD, Vanni S, Jagid J, et al. Clinical outcomes using modest intravascular hypothermia after acute cervical spinal cord injury. Neurosurgery. 2010;66(4):670–7. doi:10.1227/01.NEU.0000367557.77973.5F.

52. Li F, Gorji R, Allott G, Modes K, Lunn R, Yang ZJ. The usefulness of intraoperative neurophysiological monitoring in cervical spine surgery: a retrospective analysis of 200 consecutive patients. J Neurosurg

Anesthesiol. 2012;24(3):185–90. doi:10.1097/ANA. 0b013e318255ec8f.

53. Liu EH, Goy RW, Tan BH, Asai T. Tracheal intubation with videolaryngoscopes in patients with cervical spine immobilization: a randomized trial of the Airway Scope and the GlideScope. Br J Anaesth. 2009;103(3):446–51. doi:10.1093/bja/aep164. Epub 2009 Jun 19.

54. Macias CA, Rosengart MR, Puyana JC, Linde-Zwirble WT, Smith W, Peitzman AB, Angus DC. The effects of trauma center care, admission volume, and surgical volume on paralysis after traumatic spinal cord injury. Ann Surg. 2009;249(1):10–7. doi:10. 1097/SLA.0b013e31818a1505.

55. Manoach S, Paladino L. Manual in-line stabilization for acute airway management of suspected cervical spine injury: historical review and current questions. Ann Emerg Med. 2007;50(3):236–45. Epub 2007 Mar 6.

56. Manoach S, Paladino L. Laryngoscopy force, visualization, and intubation failure in acute trauma: should we modify the practice of manual in-line stabilization? Anesthesiology. 2009;110(1):6–7. doi:10.1097/ ALN.0b013e318190b27b.

57. Mariappan R, Manninen P, Massicotte EM, Bhatia A. Circulatory collapse after topical application of vancomycin powder during spine surgery. J Neurosurg Spine. 2013;19(3):381–3.

58. Marik PE, Baram M, Vahid B. Does central venous pressure predict fluid responsiveness? A systematic review of the literature and the tale of seven mares. Chest. 2008;134(1):172–8. doi:10.1378/chest.07-2331.

59. Martyn JA, Richtsfeld M. Succinylcholine-induced hyperkalemia in acquired pathologic states: etiologic factors and molecular mechanisms. Anesthesiology. 2006;104(1):158–69.

60. Mayglothling J, Duane TM, Gibbs M, McCunn M, Legome E, Eastman AL, et al. Emergency tracheal intubation immediately following traumatic injury: an Eastern Association for the Surgery of Trauma practice management guideline. J Trauma Acute Care Surg. 2012;73(5 Suppl 4):S333–40. doi:10. 1097/TA.0b013e31827018a5.

61. McLeod ADM, Calder I. Spinal cord injury and direct laryngoscopy—the legend lives on. Br J Anaesth. 2000;84(6):705–9.

62. Mehta S, Orenczuk K, McIntyre A, Willems G, Wolfe DL, Hsieh JT, et al. Neuropathic pain post spinal cord injury part 1: systematic review of physical and behavioral treatment. Top Spinal Cord Inj Rehabil. 2013;19(1):61–77. doi:10.1310/sci1901-61.

63. Middleton PM, Davies SR, Anand S, Reinten-Reynolds T, Marial O, Middleton JW. The pre-hospital epidemiology and management of spinal cord injuries in New South Wales: 2004–2008. Injury. 2012;43(4):480–5. doi:10.1016/j.injury.2011.12.010. Epub 2012 Jan 11.

64. Miller SM. Methylprednisolone in acute spinal cord injury: a tarnished standard. J Neurosurg Anesthesiol.

2008;20(2):140–2. doi:10.1097/01.ana.0000314442. 40952.0d.

65. Muzevich KM, Voils SA. Role of vasopressor administration in patients with acute neurologic injury. Neurocrit Care. 2009;11(1):112–9. doi:10. 1007/s12028-009-9214-z. Epub 2009 Apr 22.

66. Myburgh JA, Upton RN, Grant C, Martinez A. Epinephrine, norepinephrine and dopamine infusions decrease propofol concentrations during continuous propofol infusion in an ovine model. Intensive Care Med. 2001;27(1):276–82.

67. National Spinal Cord Injury Statistical Center. Facts and figures at a glance. Birmingham, AL: University of Alabama at Birmingham; 2013.

68. New York state in-hospital cervical spine clearance guidelines in blunt trauma [Internet]. New York: New York State Department of Health. 2013. http://www. health.ny.gov/professionals/ems/state_trauma/ resources.htm.

69. Ney JP, van der Goes DN, Watanabe JH. Cost-benefit analysis: intraoperative neurophysiological monitoring in spinal surgeries. J Clin Neurophysiol. 2013;30 (3):280–6. doi:10.1097/WNP.0b013e3182933d8f.

70. Nuwer MR, Emerson RG, Galloway G, Legatt AD, Lopez J, Minahan R, et al. Evidence-based guideline update: intraoperative spinal monitoring with somatosensory and transcranial electrical motor evoked potentials: report of the Therapeutics and Technology Assessment Subcommittee of the American Academy of Neurology and the American Clinical Neurophysiology Society. Neurology. 2012;78(8):585–9. doi:10. 1212/WNL.0b013e318247fa0e.

71. Ostermeier A, Danz S, Unertl K, Grasshoff C. Risking or saving the patient's neck-relocation of an odontoid fracture by direct laryngoscopy and manual in-line stabilization during resuscitation. Resuscitation. 2011;82(1):137–8. doi:10.1016/j.resuscitation.2010. 09.479. Epub 2010 Nov 2.

72. O'Toole JE. Timing of surgery after cervical spinal cord injury. World Neurosurg. 2013;pii:S1878–8750 (13)00289–1.doi 10.1016/j.wneu.2013.02.024. [Epub ahead of print]

73. Palumbo MA, Aidlen JP, Daniels AH, Thakur NA, Caiati J. Airway compromise due to wound hematoma following anterior cervical spine surgery. Open Orthop J. 2012;6:108–13. doi:10.2174/ 1874325001206010108. Epub 2012 Mar 5.

74. Pastrana EA, Saavedra FM, Murray G, Estronza S, Rolston JD, Rodriguez-Vega G. Acute adrenal insufficiency in cervical spinal cord injury. World Neurosurg. 2012;77(3–4):561–3. doi: 10.1016/j. wneu.2011.06.041. Epub 2011 Nov 7.

75. Lee LA, Roth S, Todd MM, Posner KL, Polissar NL, Postoperative Visual Loss Study Group. Risk factors associated with ischemic optic neuropathy after spinal fusion surgery. Anesthesiology. 2012;116(1):15–24. doi:10.1097/ALN.0b013e31823d012a.

76. Rajkumar A, Bajekal R. Intraoperative airway obstruction due to dissection of a reinforced endotracheal tube

in a prone patient. J Neurosurg Anesthesiol. 2011;23 (4):377. doi:10.1097/ANA.0b013e31822cf882.

77. Ramasamy A, Midwinter M, Mahoney P, Clasper J. Learning the lessons from conflict: pre-hospital cervical spine stabilisation following ballistic neck trauma. Injury. 2009;40(12):1342–5. doi:10.1016/j.injury. 2009.06.168. Epub 2009 Jul 17.

78. Redfors B, Shao Y, Omerovic E. Stress-induced cardiomyopathy in a patient with chronic spinal cord transection at the level of C5: endocrinologically mediated catecholamine toxicity. Int J Cardiol. 2012;159(3):e61–2. doi:10.1016/j.ijcard.2011.12. 025. Epub 2012 Jan 10.

79. Robitaille A. Airway management in the patient with potential cervical spine instability: continuing professional development. Can J Anaesth. 2011;58 (12):1125–39. doi:10.1007/s12630-011-9597-0. Article in English, French. Epub 2011 Oct 27.

80. Robitaille A, Williams SR, Tremblay MH, Guilbert F, Thériault M, Drolet P. Cervical spine motion during tracheal intubation with manual in-line stabilization: direct laryngoscopy versus GlideScope videolaryngoscopy. Anesth Analg. 2008;106(3):935–41. doi:10.1213/ane.0b013e318161769e.

81. Roozmon P, Gracovetsky SA, Gouw GJ, Newman N. Examining motion in the cervical spine I: imaging systems and measurement techniques. J Biomed Eng. 1993;15(1):5–12.

82. Rudolph C, Schneider JP, Wallenborn J, Schaffranietz L. Movement of the upper cervical spine during laryngoscopy: a comparison of the Bonfils intubation fibrescope and the Macintosh laryngoscope. Anaesthesia. 2005;60(7):668–72.

83. Ryken TC, Hurlbert RJ, Hadley MN, Aarabi B, Dhall SS, Gelb DE, et al. The acute cardiopulmonary management of patients with cervical spinal cord injuries. Neurosurgery. 2013;72 Suppl 2:84–92. doi:10.1227/NEU.0b013e318276ee16.

84. Santoni BG, Hindman BJ, Puttlitz CM, Weeks JB, Johnson N, Maktabi MA, et al. Manual in-line stabilization increases pressures applied by the laryngoscope blade during direct laryngoscopy and orotracheal intubation. Anesthesiology. 2009;110 (1):24–31. doi:10.1097/ALN.0b013e318190b55.

85. Schriger DL, Larmon B, LeGassick T, Blinman T. Spinal immobilization on a flat backboard: does it result in neutral position of the cervical spine? Ann Emerg Med. 1991;20(8):878–81.

86. Siddall PJ, McClelland JM, Rutkowski SB, Cousins MJ. A longitudinal study of the prevalence and characteristics of pain in the first 5 years following spinal cord injury. Pain. 2003;103(3):249–57.

87. Theron A, Ford P. Management of acute cervical spine injury. Anaesthesia. 2008;24(1):30–4.

88. Thiboutot F, Nicole PC, Trépanier CA, Turgeon AF, Lessard MR. Effect of manual in-line stabilization of the cervical spine in adults on the rate of difficult orotracheal intubation by direct laryngoscopy: a randomized controlled trial. Can J Anaesth. 2009;56 (6):412–8. doi:10.1007/s12630-009-9089-7. Epub 2009 Apr 24.

89. Thiel D, Houten J, Wecksell M. Accidental tracheal extubation of a patient in the prone position. Anesthesia & Analgesia Case Reports. 2014;2(2):20–22.

90. Totten VY, Sugarman DB. Respiratory effects of spinal immobilization. Prehosp Emerg Care. 1999; 3(4):347–52.

91. Turkstra TP, Craen RA, Pelz DM, Gelb AW. Cervical spine motion: a fluoroscopic comparison during intubation with lighted stylet, GlideScope, and Macintosh laryngoscope. Anesth Analg. 2005; 101(4):1011.

92. Turkstra TP, Pelz DM, Jones PM. Cervical spine motion: a fluoroscopic comparison of the AirTraq Laryngoscope versus the Macintosh laryngoscope. Anesthesiology. 2009;111(1):97–101. doi:10.1097/ ALN.0b013e3181a8649f.

93. Turkstra TP, Pelz DM, Shaikh AA, Craen RA. Cervical spine motion: a fluoroscopic comparison of Shikani Optical Stylet vs Macintosh laryngoscope. Can J Anaesth. 2007;54(6):441–7.

94. Wilson JR, Vaccaro A, Harrop JS, Aarabi B, Shaffrey C, Dvorak M, et al. The impact of facet dislocation on clinical outcomes after cervical spinal cord injury: results of a multicenter North American prospective cohort study. Spine (Phila Pa 1976). 2013;38 (2):97–103. doi:10.1097/BRS.0b013e31826e2b91.

95. Woller SA, Hook MA. Opioid administration following spinal cord injury: Implications for pain and locomotor recovery. Exp Neurol. 2013. pii: S0014–4886(13)00091–5. doi: 10.1016/j.expneurol. 2013.03.008. [Epub ahead of print]

96. Yoo KY, Jeong CW, Kim SJ, Jeong ST, Shin MH, Lee J. Cardiovascular and arousal responses to laryngoscopy and tracheal intubation in patients with complete spinal cord injury. Br J Anaesth. 2009; 102(1):69–75. doi:10.1093/bja/aen317. Epub 2008 Nov 5.

97. Yoo KY, Jeong CW, Kim SJ, Jeong ST, Kwak SH, Shin MH, et al. Altered cardiovascular responses to tracheal intubation in patients with complete spinal cord injury: relation to time course and affected level. Br J Anaesth. 2010;105(6):753–9. doi:10.1093/bja/ aeq267. Epub 2010 Oct 5.

Anna Clebone

Introduction

As airway experts, anesthesiologists are frequently involved in the management of patients with facial trauma. The successful management of facial trauma is crucial for both the immediate goals of airway control and cessation of hemorrhage, and the long-term goals of restoring function and cosmetic appearance. The skilled use of both routine and advanced airway maneuvers can decrease morbidity and improve outcomes in these patients, while an understanding of facial anatomy and common patterns of injury can guide interventions.

As a perioperative physician, the anesthesiologist's comprehensive knowledge of associated injuries can help to prevent further injury. Facial fractures, in particular, are associated with a 23 % incidence of head injury [1] and a 6 % incidence of critical comorbidities [2]. Frequently encountered, life-threatening complications include shock from hemorrhage, lung injury requiring drainage of the chest via thoracostomy, and head trauma necessitating craniotomy [2]. After the patient's airway is protected, therefore, the underlying facial injuries sometimes become a lesser priority to more emergent secondary injuries.

A. Clebone, M.D. (✉)
Department of Anesthesiology and Perioperative Medicine, Case Western Reserve University, University Hospitals, 11100 Euclid Avenue, LKS 5007, Cleveland, OH 44106, USA
e-mail: Anna.Clebone@UHhospitals.org

Epidemiology

The most common cause of traumatic facial fracture is motor vehicle accident, accounting for more than half of these injuries as reported in one large study of over a 1,000 patients [3]. In another study of over 20,000 injuries, victims of traffic accidents were more likely to suffer facial bone fractures or soft tissue injury [4]. In those patients with facial fractures, those who had been riding a motorcycle at the time of injury had the highest incidence of associated injuries [3]. In children, play was the cause of more than 50 % of craniomaxillofacial injuries [5].

Initial and Emergency Room Management

The initial management of any trauma patient begins with the Advanced Trauma Life Support (ATLS) protocol. The principle of "airway, breathing, circulation" is particularly relevant in facial trauma patients, due to the proximity of the injury to the airway. Further complicating management is the potential for these patients to be unconscious or inebriated. In a patient with an altered mental status, even a minor facial injury can cause mechanical obstruction of the airway from blood, secretions, or a foreign body, for example, as a tooth or bone fragment obstructing the airway. Oftentimes, urgent management will be required before the arrival of airway or

C.S. Scher (ed.), *Anesthesia for Trauma*, DOI 10.1007/978-1-4939-0909-4_10,
© Springer Science+Business Media New York 2014

resuscitation equipment. In the field, airway obstruction can be managed by putting the patient into a position where he is lying on his side, and (in the absence of suspected spinal cord injury), with his neck extended into sniffing position, while waiting for help and equipment to arrive. Occasionally, inward displacement of the jaw itself will be contributing to the obstruction, in which case grasping and pulling forward either the broken mandible or maxilla can result in relief of airway obstruction and subsequent ability to oxygenate and ventilate. The use of manual realignment of facial fracture segments in the field can also assist in controlling bleeding, especially in cases of severe LeFort fractures [6]. Failure to quickly optimize the airway and improve oxygenation can further complicate management, due to the fact that hypoxemia is a cause of acute delirium and an uncooperative, combative patient.

Examination

Associated injuries are not always immediately apparent. It is crucial to look for physical signs that may indicate imminent loss of the patient's airway, which include drooling, loss of gag reflex, stridor, or cyanosis. Subtle changes may be indicative of larger injuries. Even with minor facial injuries, airway obstruction can occur from unexpected sources. Obvious signs of injury cannot be relied upon exclusively, for example, soft tissue injury may be minor even in a major facial fracture and may be particularly misleading in blunt trauma.

The initial exam should also include a careful inspection of the mouth to determine if any teeth, tooth fragments, fillings, or dentures are missing. If so, the possibility of these foreign bodies being lodged in the bronchi or lungs must be considered and evaluated.

Airway Management

Among all trauma patients, maxillofacial injury patients may present with the most challenging airway problems. Difficulties can exist with (1) spontaneous ventilation, due to depressed consciousness and concomitant brain injury; (2) mask ventilation, due to the potential for altered facial soft tissue and bony structures; and (3) intubation, due to the extent of trauma present. It may be difficult to visualize the patient's vocal cords during laryngoscopy due to bleeding, airway swelling, hematoma, or the presence of a foreign body. The early use of intravenous steroids may aid in lessening the airway and facial swelling that can occur. Infrequently, disruption of the larynx or trachea itself can occur with facial trauma. Those patients with burn injuries that may involve the airway present an increased level of concern, due to the potential for friability of tissues and airway edema that may evolve after the initial injury.

Once a decision is made that a patient's airway must be secured, a plan should be established for the induction of general anesthesia. A rapid sequence intubation utilizing succinylcholine with etomidate is most commonly chosen, because of the decreased risk of aspiration of gastric contents, due to minimization of time between the loss of airway reflexes and securing of the airway. A risk exists, however, of complete airway compromise when muscle relaxant is used, because the patient's respiratory drive is taken away. Etomidate is problematic as well, due to the associated inhibition of steroid synthesis from its binding to beta hydroxylase, leading to immunosuppression, which may be hazardous in the septic or polytrauma patient. A newer agent, carboetomidate, may replace etomidate in the future due to its decreased binding to beta hydroxylase and decreased inhibition of steroid synthesis [7].

An alternate plan allows the patient to breathe spontaneously under general anesthesia by means of either an inhalation induction, or the use of induction agents that will avoid the cessation of respirations, such as a combination of dexmedetomidine and a judicious dose of propofol. Although risky, the use of an inhalation induction has been reported for the uncooperative trauma patient with facial fractures. Inhalation inductions have been reported for the uncooperative trauma patient [8]. There remains, however the possibility of aspiration of gastric contents, especially in trauma patients who may have eaten recently, or who may have decreased gastric mobility. Additionally, collapse of laryngeal soft tissue may occur with the onset of general anesthesia, leading to airway compromise during an inhalation induction.

The vast majority of facial trauma patients requiring intubation will be wearing a rigid collar for immobilization of the cervical spine. Several techniques for maintaining this immobility during intubation of the trachea have been described. In one study, the view of the patient's larynx was poor (a grade 3 or 4) in 22 % of patients undergoing direct laryngoscopy with in-line manual stabilization, and in 64 % of patients with the use of sandbags, tape, and rigid collar, suggesting that in-line manual stabilization is the better option if cervical spine protection can be maintained [9]. This may be due to the fact that incidental restriction of mandible mobility occurs from this rigid collar. In those cases in which clinicians are unsure if manual in-line stabilization can be preserved (e.g., out of hospital environment), video laryngoscopy may be of benefit during intubation while a rigid collar is kept in place [10].

Associated Injuries

In one study of 339 children under the age of 15 with facial fractures, 11 % had associated injuries of the limbs, head and neck, or chest, 3.5 % had head and neck injuries that were classified as severe, and 3.2 % had a brain injury [11]. This low incidence of intracranial injuries may be due to the inherent stability of the bony structures of the face, which helps to protect the brain and the skull [12]. Cranial protection during mandibular injury, for example, occurs because force is dispersed along a normal vector, typically leading to fracture of only the mandible without extension to the skull base [12]. If, however, the midface receives an impact, shearing forces predominate, which can rip apart the facial and cranial bones. Therefore, in midfacial trauma, fracture of the skull base is a common occurrence [12].

Even in the absence of frank intracranial injury associated with facial trauma, concussion is a concern, due to transmitted forces. Afrooz et al., in a review of 691 pediatric patients who presented with facial fracture but without obvious head injury, found that almost one-third met the diagnostic criteria for concussion [13]. The type of fracture involved was relevant; those patients with nasal and mandibular fractures had a lower rate of concussion than those children with orbital or maxillary fractures [13]. In adults, as well, in a separate retrospective study of 772 patients, the presence of a midface injury was associated with trauma to the central nervous system [14]. The clinician should, therefore, have a higher rate of suspicion for head injury in those patients with orbital or maxillary bony injuries, and appropriate follow-up should be performed. The early treatment of traumatic brain injury can improve outcome in both pediatric and adult populations. Young children under 2 years old may, in particular, benefit from intensive interventions following an associated brain injury [15]. In one small study of 122 patients up to age 12, infants with traumatic brain injury classified as "moderate" had outcomes that were worse compared with children over the age of 2 who also had a moderate injury [15]. Further complicating the treatment of traumatic brain injury is the fact that, in many cases of craniofacial fractures, an appropriate diagnosis is not made despite the presence of symptoms [16].

Dental Injuries

The presence of dental injuries should always be considered in a patient with facial trauma. An avulsed or fractured tooth can easily become dislodged causing bleeding that can increase the difficulty of airway management. A completely displaced tooth or fragment can be aspirated and become lodged in the patient's airway. The incidence of dental injury coexisting with maxillofacial fracture is high, occurring in 42 % in one recent retrospective series of 473 patients, with avulsion being the most frequent type of injury, and the incisor the most common tooth injured [17]. Increased vigilance is required in children [18] and adults [19] with mandibular fractures, due to the high incidence of concomitant dental injury.

Vascular Injuries and Hemorrhage

It is commonly, although incorrectly, thought that facial injuries pose an insignificant risk of bleeding. Approximately one tenth of patients with facial trauma may require resuscitation secondary to hemorrhage, and a fifth of those patients with massive hemorrhage will die [20]. The extensive vascular network of the face increases the danger of massive hemorrhage [21]. Bleeding is exacerbated because no valves exist in the veins of the head and neck [6]. The type of trauma that occurred influences outcome, with blunt leading a greater incidence of unsuppressed hemorrhage than penetrating (2.3 % vs. 1.43 %) [21]. The location of injury predicts the vessels involved. Midface fractures are associated with disruptions to the internal maxillary artery, which branches from the external carotid artery [20]. Nasal fractures can lead to disturbance of the anterior and posterior ethmoidal arteries, which branch from the internal carotid artery [20]. Bleeding after midface fractures can be particularly assiduous to control due to difficulty accessing the internal maxillary artery in its intraosseous path [20].

The anesthesiologist plays a critical role in managing blood loss and coagulopathy in patients with facial fracture and massive hemorrhage. Ongoing bleeding can be due to inadequate surgical hemostasis, requiring further surgical exploration or angiographic embolization of vessels. It is important to also consider the possibility of trauma-associated coagulopathy, which requires the use of blood products and antifibrinolytics. The trauma patient has several factors which predispose to coagulopathy. A large amount of bleeding and need for large volume fluid resuscitation may cause a dilutional coagulopathy and environmental exposure may lead to hypothermia. Use of a

thromboeleastogram (TEG) can be invaluable in deciphering if coagulopathy is a significant contributor to ongoing bleeding [22]. The amount and rate of bleeding can guide decision making when considering if angiographic intervention and embolization are needed.

Due to the extensive vascularity of the head and neck, the possibility exists for an extension of initial bleeding to a site remote from the original trauma. Subarachnoid hemorrhage and death have occurred following blunt facial and neck trauma as a result of internal carotid artery disruption [23]. In a case reported by Salvatori et al., the initial findings, facial bruising and midline fracture of the mandible, were not suggestive of such extensive injury [23]. This case is illustrative of the fact that, in all traumas, the possibility of associated injuries is real and must be thoroughly considered.

Intraoperative Management

Submental Intubation

Innovative techniques can be used in patients with facial trauma to achieve intubation of the trachea and decrease morbidity. For many facial injuries, visualization of the surgical field is improved by using an alternate to the oral route of endotracheal intubation. Placement of an airway device or tube in the nose is contraindicated in many patients after facial trauma because of preexisting nasal injury or the potential for accidental intracranial placement if a basal skull fracture exists concomitantly. In light of these difficulties, the submental and retromolar routes to intubation have recently gained popularity as alternatives to tracheostomy.

Submental intubation involves creating a surgical airway in the submental area, through the floor of the mouth (Fig. 10.1). The procedure begins after a routine orotracheal intubation is performed. After the incision is made, the circuit connector is removed from the tip of the endotracheal tube, and the top of the endotracheal tube is pulled through the incision, reconnected to the circuit, and re-sutured. Although it is an

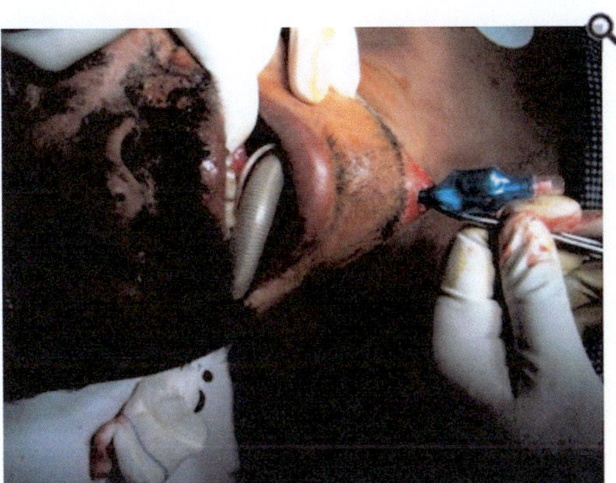

Fig. 10.1 Submental intubation. The endotracheal tube is being taken out through the submental incision. With kind permission from Springer Science + Business Media: J Maxillofac Oral Surg, Submental Intubation: An Alternative and Cost-Effective Technique for Complex Maxillofacial Surgeries, 9, 2010, 266–269, Chiradip Kar and Srijon Mukherjee

infrequently used technique, few complications have occurred with submental intubation, as described in several recent case series [24–27] which included a total of 68 patients. Postoperatively, the single complication observed in these series was minor (a superficial infection) [26]. Intraoperatively, attention must be paid to the surgical field to avoid endotracheal tube compression and deviation, which can result in increased airway pressures [27]. In these case series, submental intubation was used successfully for a wide range of types of facial injury, including mandibular and maxillary fracture, and was especially useful in patients requiring maxillo-mandibular fixation [28].

Retromolar Intubation

Retromolar intubation is a less invasive method of intubation that can achieve both the goal of a secured airway and the objective of avoiding the surgical site, providing room for a surgical repair of both nasal and jaw deformities [29]. This technique works particularly well in patients with a maxillary, LeFort II, or zygomatic fracture [29]. Typically, a slightly smaller endotracheal tube (6.5–7.0 French in adults) is used for oral endotracheal intubation. Subsequent to intubation, the endotracheal tube is manipulated so that it passes into the space which is behind the last molar and in front of the ascending ramus of the mandible [29]. In a patient with severe trismus as well as altered jaw occlusion, this can be used as an alternative means of intubation by utilizing the fiberoptic scope to pass through the retromolar space and provide a route to the trachea [30]. Securing of the endotracheal tube typically occurs via the surgical team placing wire around both the endotracheal tube and the last molar present [31]. Retromolar intubation can be particularly advantageous in pediatric and preteen patients, due to the fact that the back molars have not yet erupted, and therefore a larger space exists in which to place the endotracheal tube [31]. Although this technique can provide excellent operating conditions and the avoidance of a surgical airway, care must be taken intraoperatively that the lumen of the tube does not become mechanically compressed. Constriction of the lumen of the endotracheal tube will rarely result in increased airway pressures [29], this complication did not occur in one case series of 48 pediatric patients with maxillofacial trauma and retromolar intubation [31].

Airway Fire

The combination of oxidizer, ignition, and fuel during surgery and anesthesia presents a risk for airway fire. According to the American Society of Anesthesiologist's Practice Advisory, surgery for facial trauma is "high-risk" when an electrosurgical or electrocautery device is used, due to the proximity of the ignition and fuel sources to oxygen [32]. Head and neck surgery was the procedure involved in 95 % of malpractice claims associated with monitored anesthesia care, and 20 % of these claims were for burn injuries [33].

When an airway fire is detected, it is imperative to disconnect the circuit to cease flow of gas into the circuit, remove the endotracheal tube and any fuel sources from the airway, and extinguish the fire with water. After stopping the fire, ventilation must be restarted, preferably by mask while the patient's airway is assessed [32].

Although the step of removing the endotracheal tube is appropriate in most cases, a special concern exists with an airway fire that takes place in the setting of facial trauma due to concomitant airway edema or bleeding. Those factors lead to a greater risk of impossible ventilation upon extubation. In several case reports in which an endotracheal tube was used, the additional presence of a tracheostomy opening or an unimpeded oropharynx (i.e., in a nasal or submental intubation) allowed for venting of flame with the resulting injury reported as minor [34, 35]. In specific cases in which subsequent intubation may be impossible and the flame is immediately extinguished, the risk of removing the endotracheal tube may outweigh the benefit.

Previous Facial Trauma

Patients with previous facial trauma presenting for subsequent anesthetics require special consideration due to the potential for significantly altered airway structures. A full evaluation of the airway and knowledge of a patient's current anatomical abnormalities is necessary. A flexible nasal scope, utilized in the preoperative area after local topicalization, can provide valuable information as to if obstructions to endotracheal tube or supraglottic airway (LMA) placement exist, or if friable tissue is present, as described by Rosenblatt et al. [36].

Ankylosis of the tempromandibular joint (TMJ) can occur posttraumatically and is of particular concern to the anesthesiologist due to the subsequent limitations in mouth opening that may occur [37]. The purpose of the TMJ is to serve as a hinge which allows for the opening and closing of the mouth. The position of the TMJ is between the condylar process of the mandible and the articulating fossa of the temporal bone of the cranium. When trauma occurs, the potential exists for these two bones to fuse as the injury heals, or for the ligaments surrounding the TMJ to calcify, restricting mouth opening [38]. Several techniques have

been described to secure the airway in this challenging situation. Classically, a fiberoptic scope is passed either orally or nasally in a patient who is either (1) awake with excellent airway topicalization or (2) under general anesthesia and breathing spontaneously. In the pediatric patient, however, an awake intubation is typically not possible due to limited patient cooperation. Additionally, due to the small size of the pediatric fiberoptic scope, the visual field is limited, and locating the vocal cords can be challenging. Several alternate methods of intubation in the anesthetized pediatric patient with TMJ ankylosis have been described (see Table 10.1). Due to the fact that the patient is anesthetized, all of these approaches carry a risk of apnea, bronchospasm, and laryngospasm, with the subsequent inability to oxygenate and ventilate. Additionally, the placement of a supraglottic airway such as an LMA via the oral route may be impossible. Regardless of which technique is utilized to secure the airway, in these patients with severely limited mouth opening, equipment for performing an emergent tracheostomy, as well as a surgeon experienced in this technique, should be immediately available. It should also be kept in mind that when instrumenting the nose, the potential for epistaxis is non-negligible, and may cause further airway compromise [39, 40].

For high-risk situations, a combination of anesthetic techniques can be helpful. Tsui et al. report a 9-year-old with developmental delay, scarring from burns to the face, decreased mouth opening, poor neck mobility, and previous difficult intubation requiring the use of a supraglottic airway for ventilation who presented for further reconstruction [43]. Nebulized lidocaine, 4 % was used after an inhalation induction to blunt airway reflexes as a fiberoptic intubation was performed [43]. The delivery of lidocaine was achieved through a nebulizer with a connection through a T-piece adapter to the inspiratory limb of a circle system (oxygen flow rate 4 L/min) [43]. Although this patient was anesthetized uneventfully, it is important to keep in mind that this technique carried the risk of multiple complications, including complete obstruction

Table 10.1 Case reports of intubation for pediatric patients with severely limited mouth opening secondary to TMJ ankylosis

Author	Age	Respirations	Anesthesia	Intubation technique
Mohan [38]	12 years	Spontaneous	TIVA	Standard, after a normal oral aperture was achieved surgically via condylectomy with an unsecured airway
Kundra [41]	14 months	Spontaneous	Inhaled anesthetic through the nasal endotracheal tube	An adult fiberoptic laryngoscope was placed in one side of the nose as a camera to view the patient's vocal cords, while a much smaller endotracheal tube was pushed through the other side of the nose and visualized with the scope as it passed through the glottis
Vas [42]	24 days to 9 years	Spontaneous	Ventilation and inhaled anesthetic through an airway placed in one nostril	"Semi-blind" nasal intubation technique. Air bubbles generated from the patient's glottis were visualized through the small interincisor gap and the endotracheal tube was pushed through the second nostril towards those bubbles. The tongue was pulled gently out of the way using a McGill forceps, and visualization was achieved via a small fiberoptic light placed in the buccal mucosa. Many of these patients could only be ventilated in the lateral position due to complete airway obstruction when supine

of the airway, coughing or airway obstruction with subsequent laryngospasm, as well as the possibility of cardiac compromise or apnea due to the depth of anesthesia required during an inhalation induction.

Vision

Rapid and skillful perioperative anesthesia management is essential in cases of sight-threatening, but treatable ocular trauma. Eye injuries can be missed when considering apparently life-threatening concomitant facial and systemic trauma [44]. Quick recognition and appropriate treatment of eye injuries, however, can be vision saving. It is important to recognize when the eye is likely to be involved in a given instance of facial trauma. A portion of the orbital bone is fractured in every case of maxillary LeFort II or III fracture, as well as in those cases of zygomatic fracture or nasal fracture which involve the ethmoidal bone. The structures in the region of the eye are complex. Seven different facial bones make up the portions of the bony structure surrounding the eye, which is known as the

orbit. These include the frontal, maxillary, palatine, zygomatic, lacrimal, ethmoid, and sphenoid bones.

The outermost layer of the eye is the sclera, which completely surrounds the eye, except in the area immediately in front of the lens, which is called the cornea. The gap between the lens and the cornea is known as the anterior chamber and is filled with the aqueous humor. The space behind the lens contains the vitreous body. A laceration involving a tear in either the sclera or the cornea is known as an open globe injury. Surgery will involve the extraction of any foreign materials, as well as an attempt to return parts of the aqueous and vitreous humor that may have been extruded back into the globe, and a closure of the original laceration. In patients with open globe injuries, the preservation of vision is threatened by both the extent of injury and the potential for infection. In ocular trauma, a breach of the protective cover of the eye can occur. When bacteria and fungi track into the vitreous and aqueous humor, an inflammatory condition known as posttraumatic endophthalmitis can occur, which can lead to retinal detachment and vision loss. The probability of infection can be decreased by early operative repair, typically within 24 h of injury, as well as by the use of antibiotics.

The two types of ocular trauma require opposite approaches. A penetrating trauma to the eye should be immediately treated surgically with closure of the tear in an attempt to avoid extrusion of ocular contents and infection [44]. Blunt trauma, if severe, is more complex, causing both soft tissue damage and bony fracture, however, treatment is often not emergent unless the injury is vision-threatening, or the globe is open [44]. In one series of 588 patients with orbital fractures after blunt trauma, almost 90 % had a periorbital hematoma, ~14 % were associated with retrobulbar hemorrhage, and one-fifth had visual abnormalities, with all but two patients suffering from an optic nerve injury [45]. When associated with a visual disturbance, a retrobulbar hematoma can lead to blindness if not promptly surgically evacuated [46].

Unanticipated ocular comorbidities can occur secondary to craniofacial fracture. In one case which involved compound facial fractures, the combination of a fracture of the skull base and a subarachnoid hemorrhage resulted in increasing intraocular pressure and proptosis 2 weeks after the initial injury [47]. This was found to be due to the progressive tracking of cerebrospinal fluid underneath the periosteum of the orbit [47]. A careful follow-up and consideration of the original injury is necessary when evaluating ocular issues.

In addition to carefully evaluating for coexisting injuries, the preoperative exam in ocular trauma patients must include documentation of visual acuity, as well as a record of extraocular muscle function. The anesthetic plan must be based on the cooperation of the patient, the extent of the injury and procedure planned, and the need to control intraocular pressure. Minor ocular trauma such as an eyelid laceration or corneal abrasion may not require general anesthesia if the patient is otherwise amenable to treatment with local anesthesia or a nerve block. The presence of a ruptured globe is a relative contraindication to a peribulbar or retrobulbar block, due to the pressure on the eye during injection. General anesthesia is required if the surgeon requires the globe to remain completely still.

When inducing general anesthesia for an ocular trauma patient with an open globe, the anesthesiologist should attempt to mitigate increases in intraocular pressure. A normal intraocular pressure is 10–22 mmHg, which is increased when hypercarbia or hypertention occur, or when a Valsalva maneuver is performed. A hematoma behind the eye, as well as manual pressure on the eye by the anesthesiologist during mask ventilation, can also increase extraocular pressure and cause injury. Although a theoretical risk exists of extrusion of the vitrous or aqueous bodies and loss of vision when intraocular or extraocular pressures are increased, there is no evidence and only anecdotal reports that state that an eye fell out due to an anesthetic [48].

Vomiting, coughing, or sudden movement can be harmful. In most trauma centers, a rapid sequence induction is performed with etomidate and succinylcholine. The theoretical risk of extrusion of intraocular contents due to the increase in intraocular pressure that occurs with succinylcholine must be weighed against the risk of aspiration when succinylcholine is not utilized. A sufficient depth of anesthesia should be ensured prior to laryngoscopy in order to minimize increases in blood pressure [49]. Propofol and thiopental (if available) can be used as induction agents due to the fact that both decrease intraocular pressure; however, propofol may be a better choice due to the fact that it also decreases the incidence of postoperative nausea and vomiting. The use of a rapidly acting narcotic, such as fentanyl 1–2 µg/kg, and an agent that blunts airway reflexes, such as lidocaine, can also assist in the avoidance of systemic hypertension, which may lead to further increases in intraocular pressure.

Recent research has explored the addition of remifentanil to blunt the rise in intraocular pressure associated with laryngoscopy and intubation [50]. In adults who received a dose of propofol 2 mg/kg for the induction of anesthesia, the addition of remifentanil 4 µg/kg led to a decrease in intraocular pressure of 39 % immediately after induction, which persisted throughout direct laryngoscopy and the placement of an endotracheal tube, regardless of whether or not the patient moved or coughed [51]. Dexmedetomidine 0.6 µg/kg, in one study, when used in conjunction with thiopental, attenuated the rise in intraocular pressure that is typically associated with intubation [52]. These studies, however, were performed in patients undergoing non-opthalmic surgery. Further research will be needed to determine if these results apply to patients with ocular trauma. Ketamine should be avoided if possible in ocular trauma patients, due to its tendency to cause eyelid spasm, nystagmus, postoperative vomiting, as well as increased intraocular pressure, although the latter may not be a significant factor at low doses under 2 mg/kg [53].

The goal during the maintenance of general anesthesia is to avoid increases in intraocular pressure. This should include an adequate depth of anesthesia to prevent spikes in blood pressure, as well as the maintenance of normocapnia. Muscle relaxation should also be used to ensure adequate operating conditions and decrease the likelihood of bucking or coughing intraoperatively. Placing the patient in a head-up position can facilitate venous drainage from the eye, which will contribute to maintaining a normal intraocular pressure. The anesthesiologist must also be attentive to hemodynamic changes during surgery. Hypotension can ensue from blood loss due to associated injuries, if not treated appropriately. Pressure on the eye or pulling on the ocular muscles during surgery can cause bradycardia, due to the oculo-cardiac reflex (stimulation of the afferent trigeminal nerve leading to a vagal response at the sinoatrial node of the heart).

Prior to the emergence of general anesthesia, gastric contents should be evacuated using an orogastric tube. Agents that decrease the likelihood of airway irritation on emergence, such as lidocaine or fentanyl, should also be given before extubation. According to a consensus guideline by the Society for Ambulatory Anesthesia, opthlamic surgery is a risk factor for postoperative nausea and vomiting [54]. An antinausea agent, such as ondansetron 0.1 mg/kg (up to 4 mg), should be administered before emergence.

Nasal Injuries

The most frequent site of facial injury is the nose. Frequently, nasal fractures will be reduced in the emergency room under sedation. A risk exists of airway obstruction in the patient with altered consciousness. Bleeding may into the hypopharynx from the nose during this procedure. A safer alternative, especially if more than minimal sedation is required, is to reduce the fracture in the operating room under general anesthesia, with the trachea protected by a cuffed endotracheal tube.

Maxillary Injuries

The upper jaw is also known as the maxilla. The classification scheme for maxillary fractures delineated in 1901 by Rene Le Fort is still in widespread use today. Although the large number of midfacial bones, as well as their potential for commutation during impact allows for numerous permutations, this basic classification of three types of fractures remains relevant. The labeling of LeFort fractures begins from the lowest part of the maxilla, with Type I, with Types II and III involving progressively higher portions of the midface (Figs. 10.2, 10.3, and 10.4). On imaging, fractures of specific portions of the facial skeleton provide information as to the type of LeFort fracture present (see Table 10.2). A fracture of the pterygoid process is pathognomic for the presence of at least one of the three types of LeFort fracture [55].

The need for emergent airway management is common in patients with LeFort fractures. Over a quarter of patients with LeFort fractures require emergent endotracheal intubation or tracheostomy, as reported in one study of 117 patients by Thompson et al. [56]. Information on the kind of LeFort fracture present can be useful in predicting the need for control of the airway. In the series published by Thompson et al., those patients with

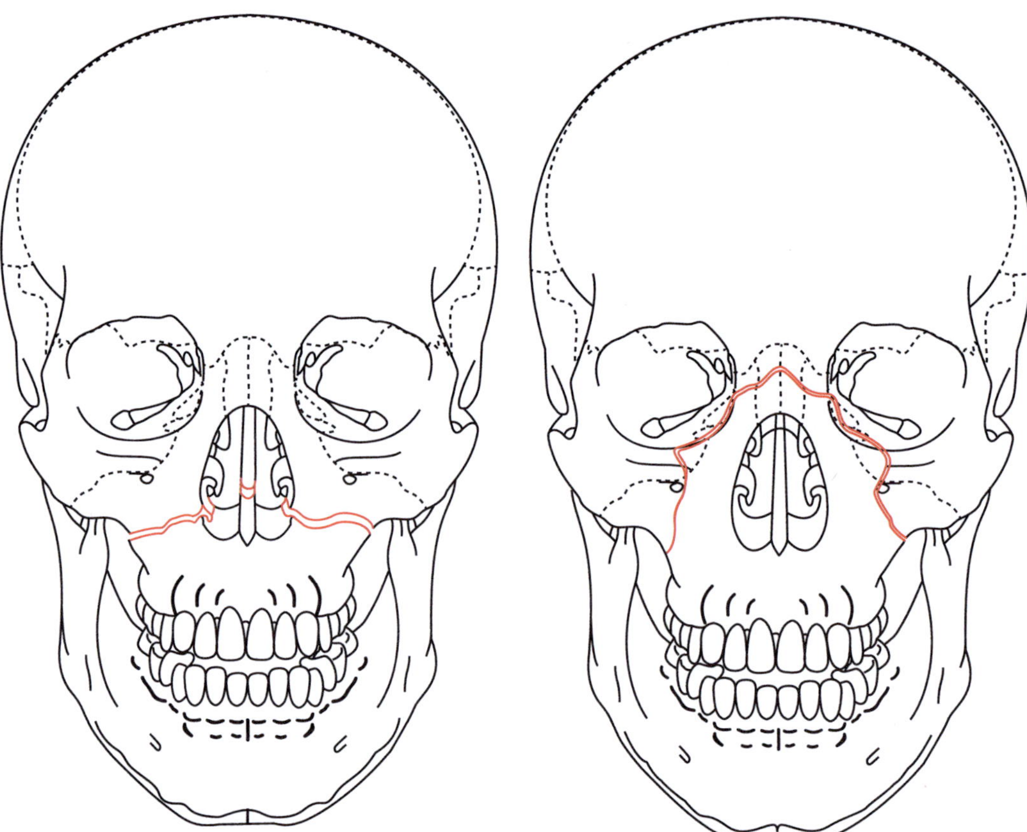

Fig. 10.2 LeFort I. From manual of internal fixation in the Cranio-Facial Skeleton, Joachim Prein, ed., Berlin: Springer Verlag, 1998

Fig. 10.3 LeFort II. From manual of internal fixation in the Cranio-Facial Skeleton, Joachim Prein, ed., Berlin: Springer Verlag, 1998

high grade (LeFort III) fractures were more likely to require immediate airway management [56]. Other predictors of the need for intubation or tracheostomy included further facial fractures, such as a mandible fracture or concomitant injuries of the larynx, pharynx, or cranium [56].

Although airway compromise is common in patients with LeFort fractures, its origin can occur from a variety of sources, both obvious and obscure. The result of a LeFort facture is a dislodgement of the maxillary bones posteriorly and inferiorly towards the oropharynx. Consequentially, bleeding can obscure the upper airway, leading to an urgent requirement for endotracheal intubation or tracheostomy [57]. As every anesthesiologist knows, even the presence of a correctly placed endotracheal tube does not guarantee a secure airway. The patency of an endotracheal tube is easily compromised by kinking or obstruction of the lumen, or by mechanical compression. Joo et al. described compression of a nasotracheal tube externally by the posterior displacement of pieces of a LeFort II and III fracture [58]. Carefully pulling the midface forward relieved the airway obstruction in this case [58]. Fortunately, the endotracheal tube utilized was unreinforced; when a reinforced tube becomes kinked, it is impossible to unbend, and replacement of the tube is mandated. The initial performance of a tracheostomy instead of a nasotracheal intubation, while not without risk, would have prevented this compression of the endotracheal tube. Additionally, the nasal route of intubation can be problematic in

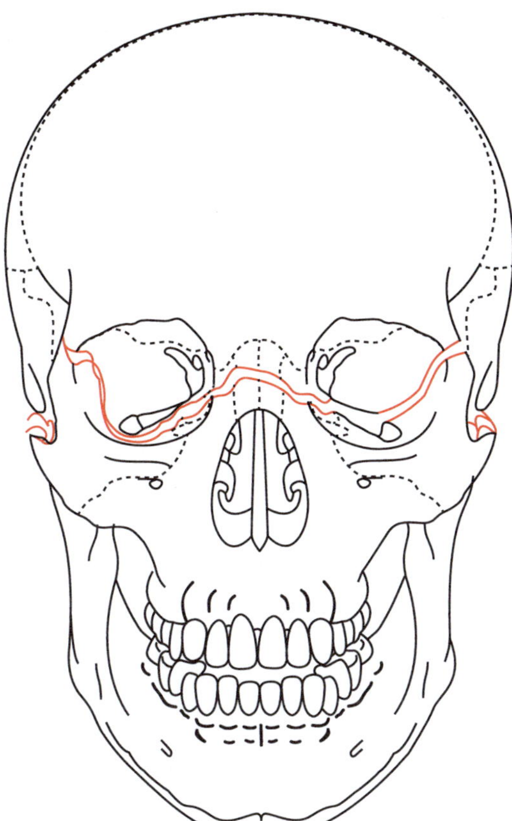

Fig. 10.4 LeFort III. From manual of internal fixation in the Cranio-Facial Skeleton, Joachim Prein, ed., Berlin: Springer Verlag, 1998

patients with LeFort II or LeFort III fractures, due to the risk of intracranial placement of the endotracheal tube if the cribriform plate is fractured.

Airway compromise can also occur from unexpected sources. Maxillary fracture, specifically of the antral wall, has been reported to lead to retropharyngeal emphysema and severe airway compromise [59]. The mechanism of airway compromise in this case is introduction of air into connective tissue, dissecting the fascial planes.

Another mechanism of limited mouth opening and difficult airway management is trismus, which is of particular concern in patients with maxillary fractures. Extending up from the maxilla is the zygomatic process, which is one of the bones of the cheek. When trauma occurs to the side of the cheek, a zygomatic arch fracture can

occur. Bleeding and swelling into the masseter muscle can occur as a result, leading to trismus and difficulty securing the airway.

Mandibular

The stability built into the facial skeleton reaches ideal form in the lower jaw bone, the mandible [12], which is the most durable and largest bone in the face. Due to the prominent position of the mandible on the face, it is also the most common site of fracture [60]. The mandible is made up of three parts. The most anterior, horizontal section is called the "body" of the mandible, which is flanked on each side by a column called a "rami." The angle of the mandible is the area joining the body and rami on each side. At the top of each ramus are two rounded processes which jut upwards with a U-shaped concavity in-between. The coronoid process sits anteriorly and the condyloid process lies posteriorly. The condyloid process serves as a hinge which joins the cranium to the mandible at the tempromandibular joint (TMJ). The body of the mandible itself consists of the symphysis as its centermost portion. Fractures will often distribute exclusively along the mandibular bone, in many cases without disrupting the base of the skull [12]. Care must be taken, however, to elucidate the extent of the mandibular injury; the maximal impact to the bone may occur far from the site of injury [12]. For example, blunt force on the chin, which can occur in a car crash, often transmits force through the angle and up the rami of the mandible, fracturing the condylar or coronoid process. In one study by King et al., of 225 mandible fractures at a single center, the most common types of fractures were parasymphyseal (35 %), body (21 %), and angle (15 %) [61]. Similar demographics were found by Natu et al., in a review of 66 patients with mandibular fractures, with parasymphyseal fractures as the most common type [62]. Due to the high frequency, it is particularly important to consider the possibility of a concomitant subcondylar fracture in those patients with a parasymphyseal fracture [61, 62]. In contrast, in children, the condylar process was

Table 10.2 LeFort fractures

Class	Shape	Location	Exam signs	Radiologic signs	Complications
LeFort I	Horizontal	Separating the part of the maxilla that contains the upper teeth from the rest of the face	The dento-alveolar segment of the maxilla can be manually displaced separately from the rest of the maxilla [55]	Fracture of the lateral margin of the nasal fossa [55]	Airway obstruction
LeFort II	Triangular	Across the cheekbones and the lower portion of the orbits	The piece of the face containing both the nose and the upper teeth can be physically shifted out of plane, separate from the skull [55]	Fracture of the inferior orbital rim [55]	Airway obstruction
LeFort III	"W"-shaped	Through the lateral and lower walls of the orbit	The piece of the face containing both the nose and the upper teeth can be physically shifted out of plane, separate from the skull [55]	Fracture of the zygomatic arch [55]	Can involve the ethmoidal bone and cribriform plate, sometimes with leak of cerebrospinal fluid "CSF rhinorrhea"

the most frequently fractured mandibular site, followed by the symphysis [63].

In military injuries, the mandible is the bone that is most often fractured in craniomaxillofacial trauma [64]. In a recent review of 391 soldiers from Iraq and Afghanistan, with mandibular injuries, at least two separate fracture sites were found in 51 %, and multiple facial fractures were found in 46 % [64].

As with all injuries, the initial physical exam is of importance. Areas of paresthesia and tenderness should be determined, along with the presence of any loose teeth. The inferior alveolar nerve runs through the core of the mandible, therefore paresthesia in its distribution (the lip and chin) is suggestive of mandibular fracture. Trismus can be a complicating factor in mandibular trauma as well. A hematoma underneath the tongue is suggestive of mandibular fracture. Due to the fact that the mandible provides support for the tongue, the tongue itself can obstruct the airway when this support structure is disrupted (Fig. 10.5).

Bone immobilization is a key principle in successful mandibular fracture healing. For fractures of the jaw, intermaxillary fixation is often used. In this technique, wires are utilized in order to keep the fragments immobile; however, this renders the airway inaccessible if the

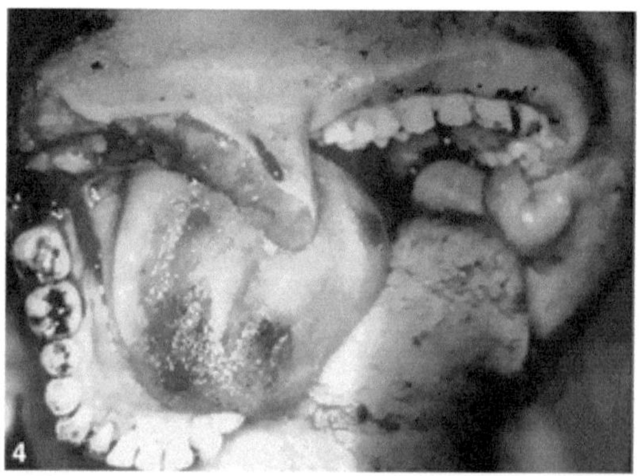

Fig. 10.5 Avulsion of the anterior mandibular segment. With kind permission from Springer Science + Business Media: Aesthetic Plast Surg, Multidisciplinary and multistage treatment of complex facial trauma: case report, 26, 2002, 40-3, Nagler RM, Peled M, Laufer D

patient has difficulties with ventilation or obstruction. Good postoperative care is essential, including appropriate doses of narcotics to avoid hypopnea, as well as the treatment of nausea to prevent vomiting and subsequent airway obstruction from stomach contents. Traditionally, the presence of wire cutters by the bedside was thought to mitigate this risk, by providing an immediate means of cutting the wires used for the intramaxillary fixation, and therefore accessing the airway. A study by Goss et al., however, showed that more than 30 seconds was required for jaw release to be accomplished by surgeons who performed intermaxillary fixation, and over 2 minutes was needed by experienced hospital staff [65].

In mandibular fractures specifically, airway management can be further complicated by trismus. A block of the inferior alveolar branch of the mandibular division of the trigeminal nerve (a "mandibular nerve block") can relieve trismus and increase mouth opening in certain patients, such as those with pain or muscle spasm. In patients with adequate mouth opening after these nerve blocks, an awake fiberoptic intubation can potentially be avoided [66]. The inferior alveolar branch can be anesthetized by feeling for the posterior ramus of the mandible and injecting medially, in the middle of the pterygoid fossa in between the medial and lateral pterygoid muscles. The risks of a mandibular nerve block must be weighed against the benefits. In the more common use of these blocks for dental practice, the complication rate is not negligible; approximately 0.15–0.54 % of patients have a transitory injury to their lingual and inferior alveolar nerves and up to 0.01 % have lasting damage to these structures [67].

A nasal endotrachial tube is commonly requested for mandibular fracture patients to improve visualization of the surgical field. A high level of caution is required before placing any object into the nose in a patient with traumatic injury. Most concerningly, in patients with a fracture to the cribriform plate, an endotrachial tube or nasogastric tube could inadvertently be placed intracranially, with catastrophic results. Also critically, a nasal injury may be coexisting or hemorrhage may lead to coagulopathy.

In controlling postoperative pain and swelling, non-pharmacologic interventions should also be considered. Treating the area of fracture with cold packs or a localized cooling device can be beneficial [68]. In one study, continuous cooling (12 h/day) after bilateral mandibular fracture repair led to decreased swelling of the face and pain when using a specialized mask which circulated chilled water [68]. In patients with mandibular fracture, especially in patients who have undergone prolonged intramaxillary fixation, eating is limited to a liquid diet, and nutritional status may be a concern. In severe or pediatric cases, total parenteral nutrition may be required.

Pediatrics

Children recover from facial fractures more easily than adults due to differences in the structure of their bones and teeth. In the pediatric population, bone is less likely to fracture, and when it does break, it heals faster [69]. The resiliency of pediatric bone is due to its mechanical tendency to deform before breaking [70]. The frontal sinuses are delayed in normal childhood development and begin to form at 8 years of age; therefore, frontal bone fractures are unusual in children [71]. When facial fractures do occur in children, the bone elasticity and suture flexibility inherent in pediatric patients are typically protective and fractures occur with little displacement [72]. Due to the rapidity of healing, fractures in children should be reduced in fewer than 5 days, so that the healing does not occur in a maligned position.

Teeth that are lost are usually primary teeth, and permanent teeth will regrow in time [73]. Misalignment of the teeth postfracture is therefore a less common complication in children [73].

Infants with facial fractures present a special concern, due to the fact that children under 6 weeks of age, and sometimes up to 6 months, are "preferential nasal breathers" [74]. Any obstruction of the nares by bleeding, soft tissue injury, or bone fracture could quickly lead to airway obstruction in the infant. Although many infants will initiate mouth breathing after a period of nasal obstruction, often by crying, this reflex is not reliable, and oxygen desaturation may occur in the interim [74]. Use of an oral airway may be necessary in the unconscious, but spontaneously breathing infant, or after the induction of general anesthesia before the airway is secured. The infant's reliance on the diaphragm to achieve tidal volumes is also problematic in cases of trauma. Mask ventilation or swallowed air can inflate the abdomen, which greatly decreases lung excursion, leading to difficulty with ventilation. Even during periods of respiratory distress, it may be necessary to manually decompress the stomach with an orogastric tube in infants in order to achieve acceptable ventilation.

Pain Management

After facial trauma surgery, causes of postoperative pain include both soft tissue injury and bone pain. Likely due to the variability in facial trauma injuries and methods of surgical repair, no randomized controlled trial has been performed on the best practices for pain management after these surgeries.

Fear of deformity or loss of essential functions may also contribute to a patient's perception of pain after facial trauma surgery. These worries make adequate analgesia even more essential. Facial trauma patients may also need social and psychiatric support to aid in coping with their injury.

Use of narcotic medications is often required, but it should be balanced with use of "opioid sparing" adjuvants such as NSAIDS, acetaminophen, and localized interventions (lidocaine patches, ice packs) unless a specific contraindication exists. The early use of neuropathic agents should be considered, although additional research still needs to be done on the use of these medications for specific types of trauma. Opioids, in particular, should be used with caution in facial trauma due to the possibilities of injury to the airway, blood in the oropharynx, and impaired level of consciousness, all of which can contribute to airway obstruction. A facial trauma patient who may present initially with the ability to ventilate and oxygenate can quickly become hypoxic with the addition of opioids due to any or all of these factors. The neurologic exam is also important in facial fracture patients due to the possibility of concomitant brain injury. Narcotics can interfere with the neurologic examination of a patient, limiting a patient's ability to cooperate, as well as artificially shrinking the size of a patient's pupils,

interfering with the accuracy of the neurologic exam.

Regional Anesthesia

Regional anesthesia often provides the advantage of improved analgesia. Oftentimes, less opioid is needed, decreasing narcotic side effects such as sedation, respiratory depression, itching, and nausea. Narcotics can be particularly dangerous in a facial trauma patient, given the difficulties of airway management due to the altered anatomy, and potentially limited mouth opening, jaw mobility, and neck movement. The use of nerve blocks to control postoperative pain for facial trauma surgery is limited, however, by the concern for needle trauma to nerves, vascular structures, or intracranial contents. Given the potential for high levels of toxicity due to the proximity of these vessels to the brain, this concern is understandable. As a higher level of comfort and skill with regional anesthesia occurs, and "real-time" imaging techniques such as ultrasound guidance improve, however, these techniques will become more popular. Head and neck blocks for children have been described in a detailed article by Dr. Suresh of Northwestern Children's Hospital [75].

References

1. Zandi M, Seyed Hoseini SR. The relationship between head injury and facial trauma: a case-control study. Oral Maxillofac Surg. 2013;17(3):201–7.
2. Tung TC, Tseng WS, Chen CT, Lai JP, Chen YR. Acute life-threatening injuries in facial fracture patients: a review of 1,025 patients. J Trauma. 2000;49(3):420–4.
3. Kostakis G, Stathopoulos P, Dais P, Gkinis G, Igoumenakis D, Mezitis M, et al. An epidemiologic analysis of 1,142 maxillofacial fractures and concomitant injuries. Oral Surg Oral Med Oral Pathol Oral Radiol. 2012;114(5 Suppl):S69–73.
4. Gassner R, Tuli T, Hachl O, Moreira R, Ulmer H. Craniomaxillofacial trauma in children: a review of 3,385 cases with 6,060 injuries in 10 years. J Oral Maxillofac Surg. 2004;62(4):399–407.
5. Gassner R, Tuli T, Hachl O, Rudisch A, Ulmer H. Cranio-maxillofacial trauma: a 10 year review of

9,543 cases with 21,067 injuries. J Craniomaxillofac Surg. 2003;31(1):51–61.

6. Asensio JA, Trunkey DD, ScienceDirect (Online service). Current therapy of trauma and surgical critical care. Philadelphia: Mosby/Elsevier; 2008. Available from: http://www.sciencedirect.com/science/book/9780323044189.

7. Shanmugasundararaj S, Zhou X, Neunzig J, Bernhardt R, Cotten JF, Ge R, et al. Carboetomidate: an analog of etomidate that interacts weakly with 11beta-hydroxylase. Anesth Analg. 2013;116(6):1249–56.

8. Smith CE, Fallon WF. Sevoflurane mask anesthesia for urgent tracheostomy in an uncooperative trauma patient with a difficult airway. Can J Anaesth. 2000;47 (3):242–5.

9. Heath KJ. The effect of laryngoscopy of different cervical spine immobilisation techniques. Anaesthesia. 1994;49(10):843–5.

10. Aoi Y, Inagawa G, Hashimoto K, Tashima H, Tsuboi S, Takahata T, et al. Airway scope laryngoscopy under manual inline stabilization and cervical collar immobilization: a crossover in vivo cinefluoroscopic study. J Trauma. 2011;71(1):32–6.

11. Thoren H, Schaller B, Suominen AL, Lindqvist C. Occurrence and severity of concomitant injuries in other areas than the face in children with mandibular and midfacial fractures. J Oral Maxillofac Surg. 2012;70(1):92–6.

12. Barash PG. Clinical anesthesia. Philadelphia: Wolters Kluwer; 2009. Available from: http://ovidsp.ovid.com/ovidweb.cgi?T=JS&NEWS=n&CSC=Y&PAGE=booktext&D=books&AN=01429405.

13. Afrooz PN, Grunwaldt LJ, Zanoun RR, Grubbs RK, Saladino RA, Losee JE, et al. Pediatric facial fractures: occurrence of concussion and relation to fracture patterns. J Craniofac Surg. 2012;23(5):1270–3.

14. Pappachan B, Alexander M. Correlating facial fractures and cranial injuries. J Oral Maxillofac Surg. 2006;64(7):1023–9.

15. Anderson V, Catroppa C, Morse S, Haritou F, Rosenfeld J. Functional plasticity or vulnerability after early brain injury? Pediatrics. 2005;116 (6):1374–82.

16. Puljula J, Cygnel H, Makinen E, Tuomivaara V, Karttunen V, Karttunen A, et al. Mild traumatic brain injury diagnosis frequently remains unrecorded in subjects with craniofacial fractures. Injury. 2012;43 (12):2100–4.

17. Zhou HH, Ongodia D, Liu Q, Yang RT, Li ZB. Dental trauma in patients with maxillofacial fractures. Dent Traumatol. 2013;29(4):285–90.

18. Iso-Kungas P, Törnwall J, Suominen AL, Lindqvist C, Thorén H. Dental injuries in pediatric patients with facial fractures are frequent and severe. J Oral Maxillofac Surg. 2012;70(2):396–400.

19. Roccia F, Boffano P, Bianchi FA, Ramieri G. An 11-year review of dental injuries associated with maxillofacial fractures in Turin. Italy Oral Maxillofac Surg. 2013;17(4):269–74.

20. Yang WG, Tsai TR, Hung CC, Tung TC. Life-threatening bleeding in a facial fracture. Ann Plast Surg. 2001;46(2):159–62.

21. Khanna S, Dagum AB. A critical review of the literature and an evidence-based approach for life-threatening hemorrhage in maxillofacial surgery. Ann Plast Surg. 2012;69(4):474–8.

22. Grassetto A, Saggioro D, Caputo P, Penzo D, Bossi A, Tedesco M, et al. Rotational thromboelastometry analysis and management of life-threatening haemorrhage in isolated craniofacial injury. Blood Coagul Fibrinolysis. 2012;23(6):551–5.

23. Salvatori M, Kodikara S, Pollanen M. Fatal subarachnoid hemorrhage following traumatic rupture of the internal carotid artery. Leg Med (Tokyo). 2012;14 (6):328–30.

24. Badjate SJ, Shenoi SR, Budhraja NJ, Ingole P. Transmylohyoid orotracheal intubation: case series and review. J Clin Anesth. 2012;24(6):460–4.

25. Shetty PM, Yadav SK, Upadya M. Submental intubation in patients with panfacial fractures: a prospective study. Indian J Anaesth. 2011;55(3):299–304.

26. Caron G, Paquin R, Lessard MR, Trépanier CA, Landry PE. Submental endotracheal intubation: an alternative to tracheotomy in patients with midfacial and panfacial fractures. J Trauma. 2000;48(2):235–40.

27. Caubi AF, Vasconcelos BC, Vasconcellos RJ, de Morais HH, Rocha NS. Submental intubation in oral maxillofacial surgery: review of the literature and analysis of 13 cases. Med Oral Patol Oral Cir Bucal. 2008;13(3):E197–200.

28. Davis C. Submental intubation in complex craniomaxillofacial trauma. ANZ J Surg. 2004;74 (5):379–81.

29. Lee SS, Huang SH, Wu SH, Sun IF, Chu KS, Lai CS, et al. A review of intraoperative airway management for midface facial bone fracture patients. Ann Plast Surg. 2009;63(2):162–6.

30. Truong A, Truong DT. Retromolar tracheal intubation in a pediatric patient with a difficult airway and bilateral nasal stenoses. Can J Anaesth. 2012;59 (8):809–10.

31. Habib A, Zanaty OM. Use of retromolar intubation in paediatric maxillofacial trauma. Br J Anaesth. 2012;109:650–1.

32. Apfelbaum JL, Caplan RA, Barker SJ, Connis RT, Cowles C, Ehrenwerth J, et al. Practice advisory for the prevention and management of operating room fires: an updated report by the American Society of Anesthesiologists Task Force on Operating Room Fires. Anesthesiology. 2013;118(2):271–90.

33. Rinder CS. Fire safety in the operating room. Curr Opin Anaesthesiol. 2008;21(6):790–5.

34. Chee WK, Benumof JL. Airway fire during tracheostomy: extubation may be contraindicated. Anesthesiology. 1998;89(6):1576–8.

35. Ng JM, Hartigan PM. Airway fire during tracheostomy: should we extubate? Anesthesiology. 2003;98 (5):1303.

36. Rosenblatt W, Ianus AI, Sukhupragarn W, Fickenscher A, Sasaki C. Preoperative endoscopic airway examination (PEAE) provides superior airway information and may reduce the use of unnecessary awake intubation. Anesth Analg. 2011;112(3):602–7.

37. Benaglia MB, Gaetti-Jardim EC, Oliveira JG, Mendonca JC. Bilateral temporomandibular joint ankylosis as sequel of bilateral fracture of the mandibular condyle and symphysis. Oral Maxillofac Surg. 2014;18(1):39–42.

38. K M, Rupa LM, Krishna Murthy SG, P G G, U B. Anaesthesia for TMJ Ankylosis with the Use of TIVA, Followed by Endotracheal Intubation. J Clin Diagn Res. 2012;6(10):1765–7.

39. Morimoto Y, Sugimura M, Hirose Y, Taki K, Niwa H. Nasotracheal intubation under curve-tipped suction catheter guidance reduces epistaxis. Can J Anaesth. 2006;53(3):295–8.

40. Watanabe S, Yaguchi Y, Suga A, Asakura N. A "bubble-tip" (Airguide) tracheal tube system: its effects on incidence of epistaxis and ease of tube advancement in the subglottic region during nasotracheal intubation. Anesth Analg. 1994;78(6):1140–3.

41. Kundra P, Vasudevan A, Ravishankar M. Video assisted fiberoptic intubation for temporomandibular ankylosis. Paediatr Anaesth. 2006;16(4):458–61.

42. Vas L, Sawant P. A review of anaesthetic technique in 15 paediatric patients with temporomandibular joint ankylosis. Paediatr Anaesth. 2001;11(2):237–44.

43. Tsui BC, Cunningham K. Fiberoptic endotracheal intubation after topicalization with in-circuit nebulized lidocaine in a child with a difficult airway. Anesth Analg. 2004;98(5):1286–8. Table of contents.

44. Fleisher LA. Anesthesia and uncommon diseases. 5th ed. Philadelphia, PA: Saunders; 2006. 658 p.

45. Karabekir HS, Gocmen-Mas N, Emel E, Karacayli U, Koymen R, Atar EK, et al. Ocular and periocular injuries associated with an isolated orbital fracture depending on a blunt cranial trauma: anatomical and surgical aspects. J Craniomaxillofac Surg. 2012;40 (7):e189–93.

46. Brucoli M, Arcuri F, Giarda M, Benech R, Benech A. Surgical management of posttraumatic intraorbital hematoma. J Craniofac Surg. 2012;23(1):e58–61.

47. Rha EY, Kim JH, Byeon JH. Posttraumatic delayed cranio-orbital cerebrospinal fluid leakage: case report. J Plast Reconstr Aesthet Surg. 2013;66(4):563–5.

48. Amadasun FE, Isesele TO. Vitreous humour extrusion after suxamethonium induction of anaesthesia in a polytraumatized patient: a case report. Case Rep Med. 2010;2010:913763.

49. Bakke EF, Hisdal J, Semb SO. Intraocular pressure increases in parallel with systemic blood pressure during isometric exercise. Invest Ophthalmol Vis Sci. 2009;50(2):760–4.

50. Robin J, Alexander R. Remifentanil obtunds intraocular pressure rises associated with suxamethonium. Br J Anaesth. 2008;101(3):432. author reply 432–3.

51. Hanna SF, Ahmad F, Pappas AL, Mikat-Stevens M, Jellish WS, Kleinman B, et al. The effect of propofol/remifentanil rapid-induction technique without muscle relaxants on intraocular pressure. J Clin Anesth. 2010;22(6):437–42.

52. Mowafi HA, Aldossary N, Ismail SA, Alqahtani J. Effect of dexmedetomidine premedication on the intraocular pressure changes after succinylcholine and intubation. Br J Anaesth. 2008;100(4):485–9.

53. Halstead SM, Deakyne SJ, Bajaj L, Enzenauer R, Roosevelt GE. The effect of ketamine on intraocular pressure in pediatric patients during procedural sedation. Acad Emerg Med. 2012;19(10):1145–50.

54. Gan TJ, Meyer TA, Apfel CC, Chung F, Davis PJ, Habib AS, et al. Society for Ambulatory Anesthesia guidelines for the management of postoperative nausea and vomiting. Anesth Analg. 2007;105 (6):1615–28. table of contents.

55. Rhea JT, Novelline RA. How to simplify the CT diagnosis of Le Fort fractures. AJR Am J Roentgenol. 2005;184(5):1700–5.

56. Thompson JN, Gibson B, Kohut RI. Airway obstruction in LeFort fractures. Laryngoscope. 1987;97(3 Pt 1):275–9.

57. Ng M, Saadat D, Sinha UK. Managing the emergency airway in Le Fort fractures. J Craniomaxillofac Trauma. 1998;4(4):38–43.

58. Joo DT, Orser BA. External compression of a nasotracheal tube due to the displaced bony fragments of multiple LeFort fractures. Anesthesiology. 2000;92 (6):1830–2.

59. Azenha MR, Yamaji MA, Avelar RL, de Freitas QE, Laureano Filho JR, de Oliveira Neto PJ. Retropharyngeal and cervicofacial subcutaneous emphysema after maxillofacial trauma. Oral Maxillofac Surg. 2011;15(4):245–9.

60. Boffano P, Roccia F, Gallesio C, Karagozoglu KH, Forouzanfar T. Bicycle-related maxillofacial injuries: a double-center study. Oral Surg Oral Med Oral Pathol Oral Radiol. 2013;116(3):275–80.

61. King RE, Scianna JM, Petruzzelli GJ. Mandible fracture patterns: a suburban trauma center experience. Am J Otolaryngol. 2004;25(5):301–7.

62. Natu SS, Pradhan H, Gupta H, Alam S, Gupta S, Pradhan R, et al. An epidemiological study on pattern and incidence of mandibular fractures. Plast Surg Int. 2012;2012:834364.

63. Yamamoto K, Matsusue Y, Horita S, Murakami K, Sugiura T, Kirita T. Maxillofacial fractures in children. J Craniofac Surg. 2013;24(1):153–7.

64. Zachar MR, Labella C, Kittle CP, Baer PB, Hale RG, Chan RK. Characterization of mandibular fractures incurred from battle injuries in Iraq and Afghanistan from 2001-2010. J Oral Maxillofac Surg. 2013;71 (4):734–42.

65. Goss AN, Chau KK, Mayne LH. Intermaxillary fixation: how practicable is emergency jaw release? Anaesth Intensive Care. 1979;7(3):253–7.

66. Heard AM, Green RJ, Lacquiere DA, Sillifant P. The use of mandibular nerve block to predict safe anaesthetic induction in patients with acute trismus. Anaesthesia. 2009;64(11):1196–8.

67. Hillerup S, Jensen R. Nerve injury caused by mandibular block analgesia. Int J Oral Maxillofac Surg. 2006;35(5):437–43.

68. Rana M, Gellrich NC, von See C, Weiskopf C, Gerressen M, Ghassemi A, et al. 3D evaluation of postoperative swelling in treatment of bilateral mandibular fractures using 2 different cooling therapy methods: a randomized observer blind prospective study. J Craniomaxillofac Surg. 2013;41(1):e17–23.

69. Lindaman LM. Bone healing in children. Clin Podiatr Med Surg. 2001;18(1):97–108.

70. Yu J, Dinsmore R, Mar P, Bhatt K. Pediatric maxillary fractures. J Craniofac Surg. 2011;22(4):1247–50.

71. Shah RK, Dhingra JK, Carter BL, Rebeiz EE. Paranasal sinus development: a radiographic study. Laryngoscope. 2003;113(2):205–9.

72. Imahara SD, Hopper RA, Wang J, Rivara FP, Klein MB. Patterns and outcomes of pediatric facial fractures in the United States: a survey of the National Trauma Data Bank. J Am Coll Surg. 2008;207 (5):710–6.

73. Maqusi S, Morris DE, Patel PK, Dolezal RF, Cohen MN. Complications of pediatric facial fractures. J Craniofac Surg. 2012;23(4):1023–7.

74. Bergeson PS, Shaw JC. Are infants really obligatory nasal breathers? Clin Pediatr (Phila). 2001;40 (10):567–9.

75. Suresh S, Voronov P. Head and neck blocks in infants, children, and adolescents. Paediatr Anaesth. 2012;22(1):81–7.

Thoracic and Abdominal Injuries

11

Levon M. Capan and Sanford M. Miller

Injuries to the thorax and the abdomen—the torso—contribute significantly to trauma-related mortality and morbidity. While the vulnerability of the closely organized vital organs to injury in this region plays an important role in morbidity and mortality, the noncompressible nature of hemorrhage in this area also contributes immensely to otherwise preventable trauma deaths. While it is estimated that one fourth of trauma deaths is secondary to chest trauma alone and claims about 16,000 lives per year [1], hemorrhage in the torso (thorax, abdomen, and pelvis) also results in a mortality of as much as 70–80 % after otherwise survivable noncerebral and noncardiac injuries in both civilian and military populations [2]. The overall mortality from exsanguination, which remains second to central nervous system (CNS) injury as a cause of death, primarily originates from injuries of the thorax, abdomen, and pelvis; there has been a reduction in death from extremity bleeding because of effective control with tourniquets or topical hemostatic agents, but not from torso bleeding. With increasing use of anticoagulant agents for prophylaxis and management of cardio- and cerebrovascular disorders, bleeding-related mortality from truncal injuries is probably more frequent. For example, the predominant injury site in patients with cardiovascular disease who died after trauma in one study was chest in 15 % and abdomen in 3 % of instances; head and neck was the injury site in 69 % of patients [3].

In 2008, of the more than 42 million injury-related emergency room visits in the United States only 4 % were due to torso injuries; the corresponding percentages for upper extremity injuries, lower extremity injuries, head and neck injuries, and vertebral injuries were 18 %, 15 %, 14 %, and 5 %, respectively [4]. Other diagnoses such as poisoning, adverse effects, ill-defined conditions, and mental disorders made up the remaining injury-related emergency room admissions [4]. Thus, although torso injuries represent a relatively small percentage of the emergency room load, they appear to cause a greater proportion of morbidity and mortality than other injuries.

Up to 80 % of thoracic injuries coexist with other injuries in major trauma patients, but they require major surgery and anesthesia relatively infrequently. Yet undetected, relatively minor thoracic injuries may result in life-threatening events during surgery for associated injuries or intensive care management of the multiple trauma patient. Pneumothorax and hemothorax are perfect examples of this clinical situation. On the other hand, because of their sometimes silent nature, even major thoracic injuries (e.g., esophageal, diaphragmatic, and airway trauma) may be missed if appropriate diagnostic

L.M. Capan, M.D. (✉) • S.M. Miller, M.D.
NYU Medical Center and Bellevue Hospital Center,
550 First Avenue, New York, NY 10016, USA
e-mail: levon.capan@nyumc.org

C.S. Scher (ed.), *Anesthesia for Trauma*, DOI 10.1007/978-1-4939-0909-4_11,
© Springer Science+Business Media New York 2014

measures are not utilized. Abdominal and pelvic injuries are present in 9–14 % of hospitalized blunt trauma victims with a mortality rate of about 10 %, but more than one-third of the most severely injured hospitalized patients are likely to have abdominal and/or pelvic injuries, and their mortality increases to 21–50 % if there is a simultaneous severe brain or thoracic injury, since the increased need for fluids and transfusion increases brain and pulmonary edema [5]. While it is difficult to predict intra-abdominal organ involvement in penetrating trauma, in blunt injuries, the spleen is the most commonly injured organ followed by the retroperitoneal organs and the liver [5].

Thoracic Trauma

Although penetrating weapons may inflict severe damage, generally blunt thoracic injuries have a higher overall mortality and morbidity because of a greater likelihood of multisystem involvement. Nevertheless, the coexistence of many vital organs with different functions in the small thoracic cavity makes trauma to the chest a potential cause of serious consequences [1] (Table 11.1). Shock produced by thoracic trauma has three components. The pulmonary component is caused by airway, lung, and/or diaphragmatic injuries and is responsible for hypoxia and hypercarbia. Hemorrhage from the chest wall, thoracic vessels, and sometimes the heart is responsible for the hypovolemic component, and cardiac injuries in the form of pericardial tamponade, myocardial contusion, or valvular disruption are responsible for the cardiogenic component of shock. Sometimes they may be present simultaneously, resulting in the so-called thoracic shock. Each of these components must be considered during management of shock caused by thoracic injuries (Fig. 11.1).

Management of the patient with chest injury involves (a) initial evaluation and resuscitation, (b) relatively minor surgical interventions such as placement of chest tubes for removal of air or blood from the pleural space, (c) definitive surgical repair of injured thoracic organs, and

Table 11.1 Potential mechanisms of life-threatening adverse consequences caused by thoracic trauma

Mechanism	Pathology
Airway obstruction	Airway injuries
	Blood and secretions
Hypoxia/Hypercarbia	Hemothorax
	Pneumothorax
	Pulmonary contusion
Hemorrhage	Chest wall vessel injury
	Pulmonary/Hilar vessel injury
	Cardiac injury
	Thoracic great vessel injury
Myocardial failure	Cardiac contusion
	Valvular injury
	Septal injury
Pericardial tamponade	Hemopericardium

(d) intensive care. The timing of surgical interventions can be categorized in three periods: (a) immediately upon arrival in the emergency department, (b) urgently within few hours of arrival, and (c) delayed after the first day in the hospital [6]. The goals of management are different in each of these time windows: immediate intervention is done for resuscitative purposes, urgent intervention provides definitive repair of injured organs, and delayed intervention is for repair of missed injuries. Of course, the patient's physiologic status and the diagnosis of the clinical condition are the main factors in deciding the type of care. The anesthesiologist's function in each of these phases is to assist in resuscitation, to administer anesthesia for urgent and delayed surgery, and to provide care in the intensive care unit. The remaining part of this section will provide information relating to management strategies for each of these phases.

Resuscitation Phase

Management in this phase is according to the Advanced Trauma Life Support (ATLS) guidelines. Prompt tracheal intubation followed by positive pressure ventilation and positive end expiratory pressure (PEEP), if necessary, should be established in patients who are unconscious, unable to protect their airway, or are in

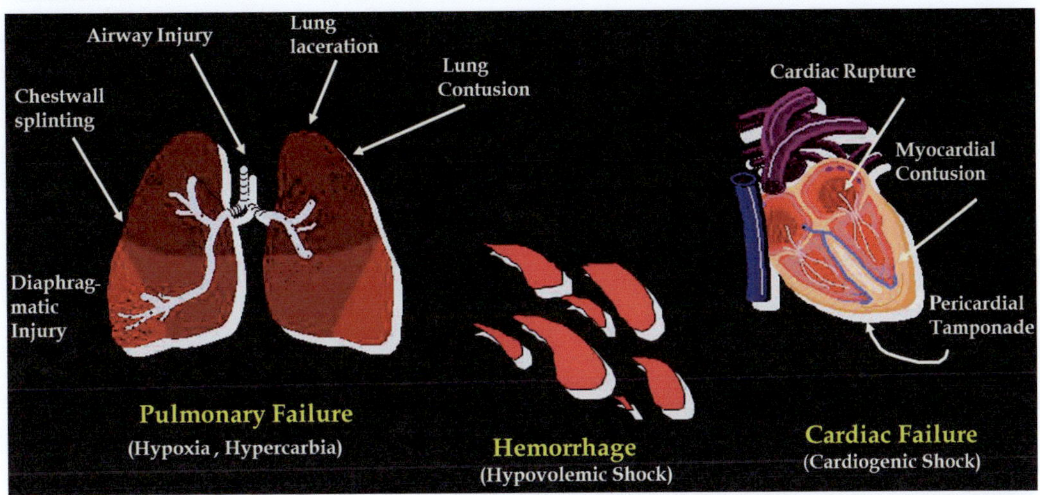

Fig. 11.1 Three main components of shock in thoracic injuries, hemorrhage, airway/pulmonary and cardiac abnormalities, and their etiology. More than one component may be present simultaneously, leading to the condition of "thoracic shock"

respiratory distress. Large bore intravenous lines should be secured both above and below the diaphragm for administration of fluids and blood products as deemed necessary. The chest wall should be inspected during spontaneous breathing for paradoxical movement suggestive of flail chest or for open sucking chest wounds. The latter must be treated immediately by an occlusive dressing and a chest tube. Respiratory distress, impaired oxygenation, and hemodynamic instability may be caused by pneumothorax and/or hemothorax necessitating immediate decompression with a 14 gauge needle, and tube thoracostomy after auscultation of the chest in unstable patients.

The clinical diagnosis of pneumothorax is difficult. Decreased breath sounds on the affected side may not be appreciated in a noisy environment such as the emergency department. Elevated airway pressure in intubated and ventilated patients may be attributed to other pulmonary abnormalities such as airway obstruction, atelectasis, diffuse inflammatory lung disease, or mainstem intubation. Likewise hypoxia, hypercarbia, or hypotension may be attributed to other causes. Neck vein distension may not be present in a hypovolemic patient, and

finally, tracheal deviation may be difficult to appreciate. Nevertheless, the presence of these signs in the trauma patient should raise a strong suspicion of pneumothorax. In hemodynamically stable patients with adequate oxygenation, additional radiographic or ultrasonographic evaluation can be obtained to confirm the diagnosis. In the hypotensive and hypoxic patient time should not be wasted in waiting for these evaluations; after rapid auscultation of the lung fields and elimination of other causes of decreased or absent breath sounds unilaterally or bilaterally a needle thoracostomy should be performed and the pleural air evacuated with a 14 gauge needle-catheter assembly introduced either at the second intercostal space at the midclavicular line or the fifth intercostal space at the midaxillary line. A large-bore (28–36 F) chest tube may be introduced following this procedure for continuous drainage, which may serve not only for evacuation of air but also of blood; hemothorax may be present in up to 20 % of patients with chest trauma [7]. Although some reports recommend observation without placing a chest tube after needle aspiration in pneumothoraces classified by CT according to their size, from miniscule to limited anterior to

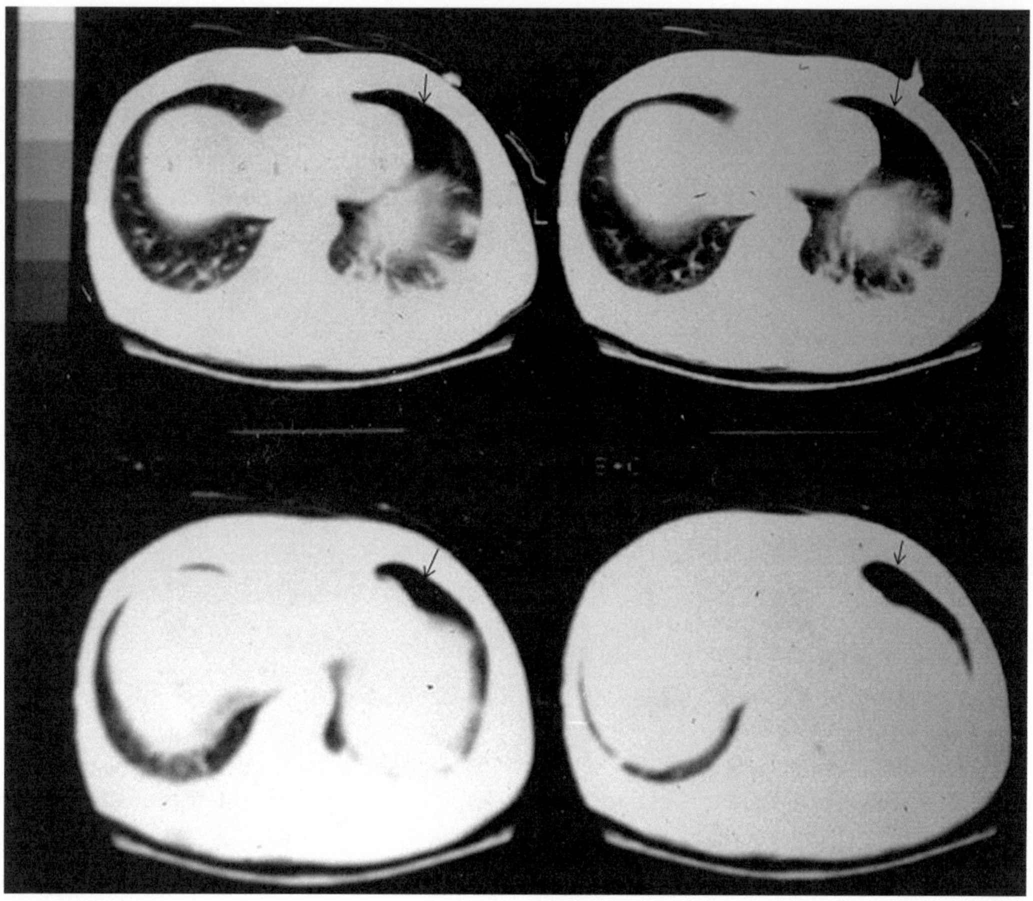

Fig. 11.2 Computed tomography image of the chest showing pleural accumulation of air in the anteromedial sulcus of the lung (*arrow*) in caudal cuts. Occult pneumothorax could not be detected in the supine plain chest film

anterolateral [8, 9], there is ample evidence that after traumatic pneumothorax the possibility of developing a life-threatening tension pneumothorax is high, especially when general anesthesia or positive pressure ventilation will be administered [7, 10, 11]. Reluctance to place a chest tube stems from concerns related to increased pain, decreased lung expansion, and infection. There is some evidence to suggest that using smaller pigtail catheters may be less painful [12]. Also an effective multimodal pain management strategy may decrease pain-related complications of the chest tube. For prevention of infection, a recent meta-analysis demonstrated that antibiotic prophylaxis using various generations of cephalosporins decreased the overall incidence of chest tube-related

pulmonary infection [13]. However, this favorable effect was prominent in patients with penetrating trauma but not in a relatively small number of blunt trauma patients [13].

It is now well established that computed tomography (CT) scans are far superior to plain radiographs in demonstrating traumatic lesions of the chest (Fig. 11.2) [14]. Occult pneumothorax is the term used for pneumothorax not appearing on a plain chest film but detectable on CT scan image [9]. Part of the reason for the low diagnostic ability of a plain chest film for pneumothorax is the fact that concern for hypovolemia and hypotension, and the presence of vertebral injuries, precludes upright positioning of these patients, which is ideal for visualizing the air in the pleural space [14]. In the supine position the "deep sulcus sign," which results from the tendency of pleural air to track in the lateral and caudal regions, is usually the diagnostic radiographic sign of life-threatening tension pneumothorax [14]. In severely injured patients CT evaluation must be initiated as soon as a physiologic stability is established. Considering that the radiation level delivered by CT is about six times greater than that of plain chest radiograms and may contribute to an increase in malignancies later in life, unnecessary use of CT should be avoided and evaluation with plain chest films considered in patients who are injured by low-risk mechanisms. Plain films may also be useful in unstable patients who cannot tolerate transport to the CT unit.

Because of its simplicity and portability, sonographic diagnosis of posttraumatic pneumothorax has gained popularity during the past 10–15 years. A linear ultrasound probe with a frequency range of 5–10 MHz is placed over the second intercostal space at the midclavicular line or at the fourth or fifth intercostal space at the anterior axillary line to detect two important signs: lung sliding and comet tail artifacts. Lung sliding is the movement of the visceral over the parietal pleura that normally occurs when there is no air between the two pleural surfaces. Comet tail artifacts are generated by the visceral pleura and are longitudinal echogenic lines moving back and forth over the lung fields (Fig. 11.3). Neither lung sliding nor comet tail artifacts appear when there is air between the layers of the pleura. Another ultrasound sign that further improves the capability of this technique to diagnose occult pneumothorax is the "lung point" which is obtained in a special mode called "time-motion mode" and clearly differentiates normal lung from collapsed lung if the probe is placed in the transitional zone between the normal lung and pleural air. The normal lung underlying the probe has a normal granular pattern whereas the pneumothorax appears in a horizontal line pattern (Fig. 11.3). The absence of lung sliding has 100 % sensitivity and 78 % specificity [15]. The "lung point" sign is very specific and, if present, is pathognomonic for pneumothorax [15].

Ultrasound diagnosis of pneumothorax is most helpful for the anesthesiologist perioperatively, especially intraoperatively in patients who are having surgery for associated injuries and are suspected to have pneumothorax. Rather than waiting for radiographic evaluation, applying an ultrasound probe over the chest provides a timely diagnosis. Ultrasound examination of the chest may also be helpful in diagnosing pleural effusion, pneumonia, pulmonary embolism, and rib fractures [16]. There are some pitfalls with this technique that may lead to inaccurate diagnosis of pneumothorax. By stopping the movement of the left lung, a right bronchial intubation may be interpreted as pneumothorax. Also bilateral pneumothoraces may be missed, possibly because no difference may be observed between the two lungs. Likewise occult pneumothoraces may show intermittent or partial lung sliding and thus may not be recognized.

Emergency department (ED) thoracotomy should be considered in patients who arrive or become pulseless during resuscitation. Overall, the neurologically intact survival rate is about 10–15 % after this procedure; the best results are obtained in patients who have sustained isolated penetrating chest injury [17, 18]. Among penetrating mechanisms, stab wounds are more likely to respond than gunshots [18]. Although patients sustaining blunt injuries in thoracic or non-thoracic regions are considered to be unresponsive to emergency room thoracotomy [19], recent data from the Western Trauma Association have demonstrated that injury mechanism alone is not a predictor of futility for this procedure and 9 % of the survivors in their series were blunt trauma victims [20]. They found that the duration of the prehospital cardiopulmonary resuscitation (CPR) is an important determinant of survival; if this period exceeds 10 min after blunt trauma or 15 min after penetrating trauma without response should herald a fatal outcome [20]. Likewise they demonstrated that asystole during presentation to ED in the absence of pericardial tamponade is a predictor of a lack of response to resuscitative thoracotomy [20]. Considering the microbial contamination risks to the

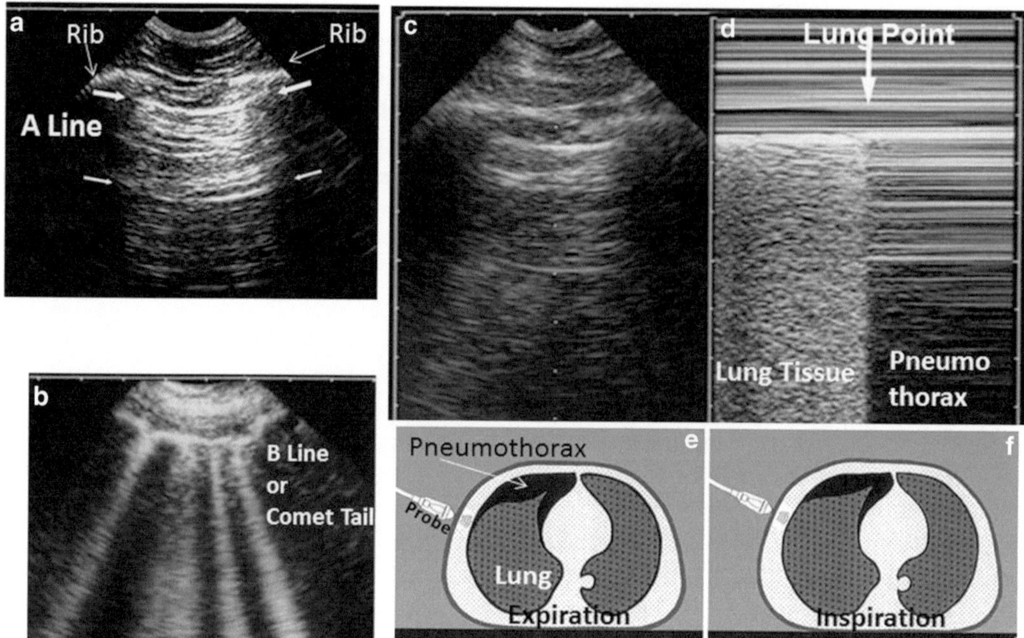

Fig. 11.3 Ultrasound images of normal lung (**a**, **b**) and pneumothorax (**c**, **d**). (**a**) Image obtained by a longitudinally placed ultrasound probe over the intercostal space showing proximal and distal ribs and the A lines (*thick* and *thin arrows*) which are echogenic *horizontal lines* appearing at same distances as the distance between the probe and the first A line. (**b**) Comet tail artifacts or B lines originate from the pleura and are vertically oriented, well-defined, laser beam like lines that continue up to the edge of the screen and erase the A lines. (**c**) real-time mode frozen image without comet tail artifacts. (**d**) Time-motion mode image showing the homogeneous granular pattern of normal lung on the left and the motionless horizontal lines of pneumothorax on the right. The line between these two patterns is called "lung point" which, if seen, is a definite evidence of pneumothorax. (**e**) Lung point may be seen when there is a relatively small volume of pneumothorax and during expiration pleural air comes under one side of the ultrasound probe producing a time-motion image that shows a granular pattern (normal lung) on one side and a horizontal line pattern (pneumothorax) on the other side of the screen. (**f**) During inspiration with expansion of the lung, entire lung tissue is under the probe and a normal granular appearance may be obtained with time-motion image. It should be emphasized that diagnosis of pneumothorax with ultrasound relies primarily on the movement of the lung rather than frozen images. Thus lung sliding and comet tail artifacts which are produced by the movement of the lung are the most commonly utilized features. Reprinted from Lichtenstein D, Meziere G, Lascols N et al. Ultrasound diagnosis of occult pneumothorax. Critical Care Medicine 2005; 33:1231–38

provider and the expense of such a futile procedure, it is generally accepted that ED thoracotomy should not be attempted for these patients. The therapeutic benefits of emergency department thoracotomy are control of hemorrhage, open cardiac massage, which is more effective in hypovolemic trauma victims than closed compression, evacuation of cardiac tamponade, cross-clamping of the descending aorta to limit distal bleeding, cross-clamping of the pulmonary hilum in the case of air embolism or massive bronchopleural fistula, and the possibility of infusion of fluids into the right atrial appendage with large bore tubing.

Historically, pericardiocentesis was recommended to relieve pericardial tamponade. However the therapeutic effectiveness of this procedure is low in the presence of clotted blood in the pericardial sac. Its diagnostic benefit in comparison to focused assessment with sonography for trauma (FAST) is also minimal. Thus in relatively stable patients, diagnosis and removal of pericardial blood is performed with a subxiphoid incision and creation of pericardial

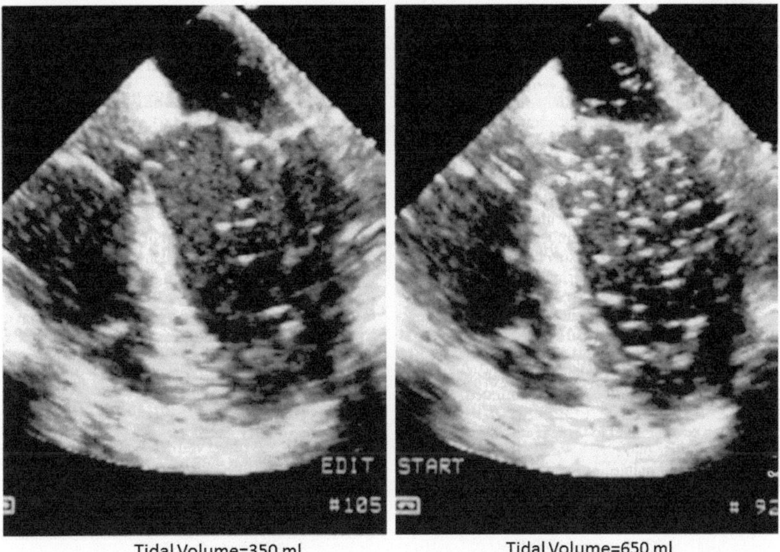

Fig. 11.4 Transesophageal echocardiography images showing the effect of ventilation with low (350 mL) and high (650 mL) tidal volumes on the quantity of gas bubbles in the left cardiac chambers of a trauma patient. Higher tidal volume with higher inspiratory pressure produced a greater quantity of gas bubbles in the left ventricle. Reprinted with permission of the American Thoracic Society. Copyright © 2014 American Thoracic Society. Saada M, Goarin J-P, Riou B, Rouby J-J, Jacquens Y, Guesde R, Viars P. Systemic gas embolism complicating pulmonary contusion. Diagnosis and management using transesophageal echocardiography. American Journal of Respiratory and Critical Care Medicine. 1995;152:812–5. Official Journal of the American Thoracic Society

window, preferably under general anesthesia, or by ED thoracotomy if the patient is in extremis. Currently, a transdiaphragmatic pericardial window is created laparoscopically under direct vision. Apart from being easier and safer, this approach permits evaluation of the abdomen with minimal morbidity and no mortality [21].

Air embolism is a well-known but rare complication of penetrating chest trauma and results from a fistulous connection between a bronchiole and pulmonary venules [22]. It is unlikely to occur in spontaneously breathing victims because the pressure gradient between the two structures is in favor of the pulmonary vessels and is the cause of hemoptysis in some patients. With positive pressure ventilation, reversal of the gradient results in massive venous air embolism which may become arterial in the presence of patent foramen ovale or by passage of air through pulmonary capillaries into the left heart and the systemic circulation [22]. Arterial air embolism is usually manifested by sudden lateralizing neurologic symptoms and profound hypotension or cardiac arrest [22]. Depending on the amount of air entry in the arterial system, multiple air bubbles or froth may be noticed in blood withdrawn from the arterial line. The condition should be suspected in penetrating chest trauma victims with hemoptysis, and ventilation should be achieved with the lowest possible airway pressures (Fig. 11.4) [23]. Interestingly, animal studies have shown that increasing bronchial pressure increases the pressure on the venules, but that the gradient increases in favor of the bronchus and promotes further embolization [22].

In the operating room, TEE, if available and applicable, can permit adjusting the tidal volume based on observation of the density of air bubbles in the cardiac chambers (Fig. 11.4) [23]. However, this may not be easy because the pulmonary edema that frequently occurs in these patients tempts one to use high airway pressures and PEEP [24]. In the emergency department, resuscitative thoracotomy may be performed and immediate twisting of the lung after division of the inferior pulmonary ligament may occlude the hilar vessels and prevent further embolization. A similar surgical maneuver can be applied in the operating room if needed. The appropriateness of resuscitative thoracotomy for this purpose, however, is questioned [22]. Otherwise the only other useful measure is to occlude the main stem bronchus of the suspected side of embolization with a double lumen tube or a bronchial blocker [22].

Air embolism is unlikely to occur after blunt thoracic trauma, although it has been described after pulmonary contusion [23]. It can also happen after a penetrating injury without lung involvement; a case report described a venous air embolism after a tangential gunshot wound to the chest [24]. Unlike air embolism after lung injury, which is often associated with severe hemodynamic and oxygenation abnormalities, these injuries are relatively stable and permit less aggressive measures, such as the use of hyperbaric oxygen. Ground transportation to hyperbaric oxygen treatment facilities is preferred over air transport given the fact that air bubbles enlarge at high altitudes [24].

Urgent Thoracotomy

As mentioned above, only an estimated 15–30 % of chest injuries require operative intervention. Most trauma to the chest involves air or blood leak into the pleural space, which is treated with chest tubes; these must be placed under strictly sterile conditions at an accurate depth into the pleural space to prevent complications such as inadequate drainage of air or blood, empyema, and fibrous tissue formation over the lung surface necessitating prolonged antibiotic treatment and decortication during later phases of management. The indications for operating room surgical intervention are shown in Table 11.2. Of these only a few, such as major bleeding and massive air leak from the chest tube, hemodynamic deterioration, cardiac tamponade, and air embolism require rapid transport to the operating room. The rest of the problems require urgent

Table 11.2 Indications for surgical intervention for chest trauma

Drainage of blood in excess of 1,000–1,500 mL upon insertion of the chest tube
Drainage of blood from the chest tube in excess of 200–300 mL/h for several hours
Hemodynamic deterioration attributed to intrathoracic organ injury
Cardiac tamponade
Intrathoracic or thoracic outlet great vessel injury
Massive air leak from the chest tube
Tracheal or bronchial injury
Esophageal injury
Retained hemothorax
Traumatic cardiac valvular and aneurysmal lesions
Traumatic diaphragmatic hernia
Traumatic aortic disruption (currently the majority of these lesions are treated with endovascular approach)
Tracheoesophageal fistula
Posttraumatic empyema

surgery but only when the patient is in stable condition.

Bleeding

An estimated 300,000 cases of traumatic hemothorax occur in the United States per year; the majority are caused by chest trauma [25]. As an indication for thoracotomy, initial chest tube drainage of 1,000–1,500 mL of blood and continuing drainage of 200–300 mL/h [25] must be assessed with caution in some clinical conditions. Parenchymal bleeding from the low pressure pulmonary circulation is usually tamponaded by complete expansion of the lung, rendering thoracotomy unnecessary. Likewise, substantial drainage in patients receiving anticoagulant drugs and with coagulopathy secondary to associated brain injury precludes thoracotomy because a controllable bleeding site will not be found and surgery will be counterproductive. Finally, when the transport time to a trauma center is prolonged, accumulated blood in the pleural space may result in significant initial chest tube drainage, but should not indicate surgery.

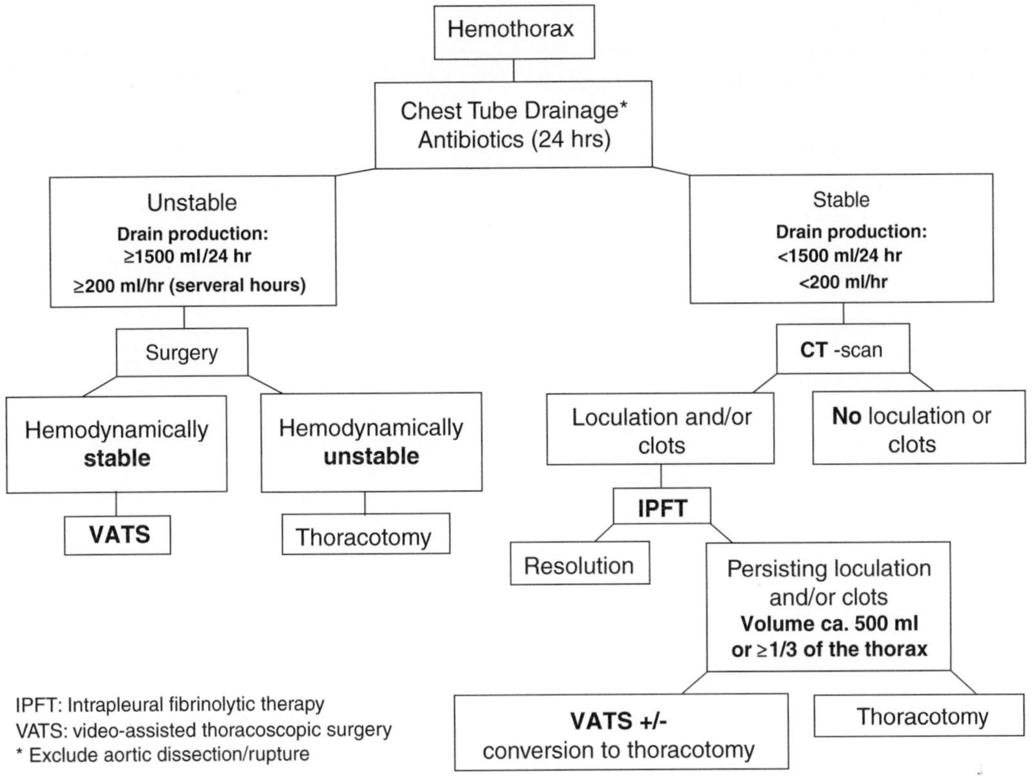

Fig. 11.5 Algorithm for management of hemothorax. Reprinted from Respiratory Medicine, 104, Boersma WG, Stigt JA, Smit HJM, Treatment of hemothorax, pp. 1583–7, Copyright 2010, with permission from Elsevier

Decision making for management of hemothorax is based on the volume of drainage from the chest tube and the hemodynamic stability of the patient. A management algorithm is shown in Fig. 11.5. Surgery involves video-assisted thoracoscopic surgery (VATS) or thoracotomy necessitating lung isolation. Replacement of blood volume with blood products and fluids is an important task of the anesthesiologist during surgery for acute hemorrhage. The surgical approach in the later phase involves evacuation of residual clots and lysis of adhesions and loculated effusions to prevent empyema or fibrothorax. Surgery in this phase is indicated if the estimated volume of pleural blood is greater than 500 mL or it is filling more than 30 % of the hemithorax. A reliable assessment of blood volume in the pleural cavity can be made by CT rather than plain chest film.

Nonsurgical management of loculated blood clots in the pleural cavity may be performed by instilling intrapleural fibrinolytic agents such as urokinase, streptokinase, or TPA [25].

Pulmonary and Airway Injuries

Massive air leak is defined as one that is present during both inspiration and expiration. It may be caused by major pulmonary parenchymal lacerations and by thoracic airway injuries that prevent complete expansion of the lung, and thus decrease effective tidal volume and ventilation. Indications for operative intervention following a lung injury, bleeding, or air leak are more common following penetrating than blunt injuries [6]. On the other hand, penetrating injuries usually require simpler operations, such as suturing, wedge resection, or tractotomy, which involves dissecting along the trajectory of a weapon to identify and ligate injured vessels individually [6].

Lobectomy or pneumonectomy is more likely to be performed for blunt lung injuries that are more severe and diffuse [6]. These procedures have very high (50–100 %) mortality and should be considered only when there is no other alternative [6, 26, 27]. The development of acute pulmonary hypertension, which is probably secondary to shock induced thromboxane and neutrophil activity on the pulmonary vascular bed, contributes to this early postoperative mortality. One fourth of these patients also develop arrhythmias, usually in the form of atrial fibrillation, complicating the clinical outcome. Perihilar lung injuries usually cause hemorrhagic shock and are treated by placing a hilar clamp and twisting the lung after dividing the inferior pulmonary ligament [6]. Isolation of the injured lung using a double lumen endobronchial tube or bronchial blocker is essential not only to facilitate exposure but also to prevent complications such as contamination of the uninjured lung and loss of tidal volume.

Tracheobronchial injuries typically occur on the posterior wall within 3–5 cm proximal and/or distal to the carina. These are relatively infrequent injuries, occurring more commonly after blunt trauma, irrespective of the mechanism of injury. They may present in varying clinical forms including pneumothorax, subcutaneous and/or mediastinal emphysema, hemoptysis, loss of tidal volume, and sometimes airway obstruction. Often they are accompanied by pulmonary contusion, atelectasis, and/or aspiration with resulting shunting and hypoxemia. Mechanical ventilation in the presence of airway injury may be difficult and at times impossible. Perforation may spare the pleura and involve the mediastinum, producing massive emphysema. Often these injuries are missed only to be recognized after recovery from the acute injury. Complete bronchial transection may present with the falling or dropped lung sign on the chest radiograph, in which the lung falls away from the hilum (Fig. 11.6) [28]. Diagnosis is made

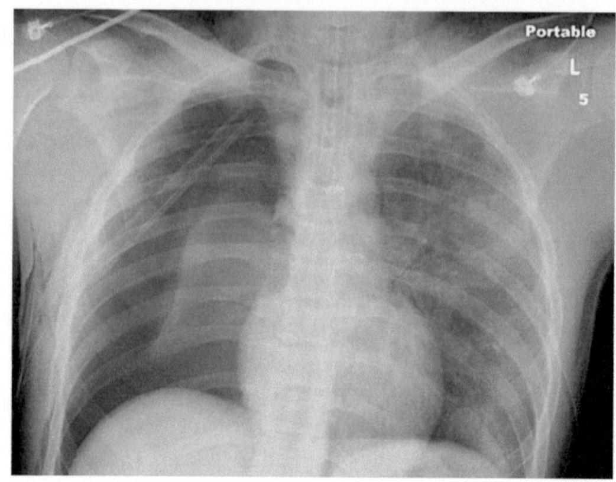

Fig. 11.6 Chest radiograph of a patient with multiple injuries and complete transection of the right main stem bronchus. There is a complete fallen or dropped lung sign with a large pneumothorax and lung collapse suggesting transection of the right main stem bronchus. Walker JL, Wiersjh J, Benson C, Young HA, Dearmond DT and Johnson SB, Perfusion (27), pp. 34–8, copyright 2011. Reprinted by permission of SAGE

based on clinical findings, chest radiography, or CT and confirmed by rigid or flexible bronchoscopy. Establishment of adequate ventilation is the first goal of management. Positive pressure ventilation should be avoided if satisfactory air exchange is achieved with spontaneous breathing. Tracheal intubation, if necessary, must be done under direct vision using fiberoptic bronchoscopic (FOB) guidance to avoid entry of the endotracheal tube into the tracheobronchial wall defect, producing total airway obstruction. In this way the tube can be placed distal to the injury. This procedure alone may be sufficient for spontaneous healing proximally if the injury is small and well contained (Fig. 11.7) [29]. Signs of healing are cessation of air leak from the chest tube, full expansion of the lung, and no need for positive pressure ventilation. After obtaining these signs, withdrawing the tube and inspecting the area with FOB can confirm the situation.

Bronchial injuries can be managed with a double lumen endobronchial tube. The bronchial lumen is placed in the intact bronchus under direct vision with FOB guidance. Severe injuries with deformed airways filled with blood and secretions and separation of the tracheobronchial

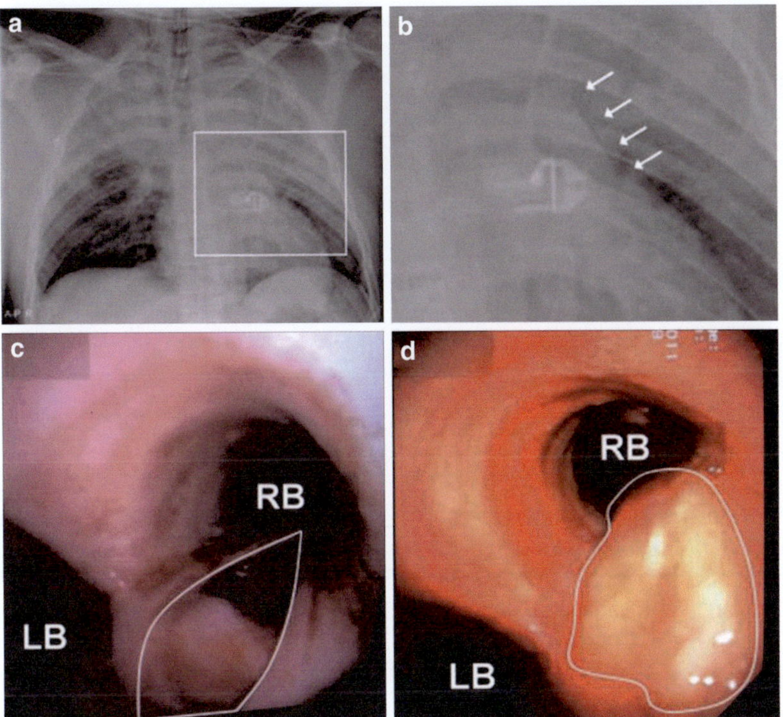

Fig. 11.7 (**a**) Chest radiograph of a patient after blunt high energy chest trauma. Radiolucent line on the left of the cardiac silhouette marked with a square shape suggests pneumomediastinum; (**b**) Enlarged image of the radiolucency marked with *arrows*; (**c**) Bronchoscopic view of the distal tracheal and right main stem bronchus tear; (**d**) 2 weeks later bronchoscopic appearance of the granulation tissue showing spontaneous healing. Reproduced by permission from Brakman M, Buddingh KT, Smit M, Struys MMRF, Ziljstra JG and van Meurs M. A 28-year old man with air in the mediastinal space after a car accident. Anesthesiology 2012;117:878

wall may not be manageable with an endobronchial tube. In these patients, ventilation for emergency surgery is continued using a single lumen tube while the leak from the chest tube is monitored. After thoracotomy a sterile single lumen tube is placed into the intact side by the surgeon to replace the tracheal tube and is brought out through the incision and connected to a ventilator [28]. Prophylactic antibiotics, humidified air, careful frequent suctioning, and bronchoscopy at regular intervals are necessary. Sepsis and airway obstruction are the most important threats to these patients and require active monitoring after surgery. Postoperative positive pressure ventilation should be stopped as soon as possible, or if not possible, ventilation should be applied distal to the surgical site by advancing the tube below the repair. Jet

ventilation and rarely, extracorporeal membrane oxygenation may be considered.

Cardiopulmonary support may be needed in patients with multiple injuries, transected bronchus, and severe lung contusion with hypoxemia [28]. Traditionally veno-venous cardiopulmonary support is provided by placing one cannula into the femoral vein and another into the internal jugular. A dual lumen veno-venous cannula has recently been made available, eliminating the inconvenience of placing two separate cannulae (Elite Dual Lumen One lumen V-V Cannula, Avalon Laboratories, Grand Rapids, MI). The cannula is placed via an internal jugular vein using the Seldinger technique under TEE guidance; one leg of the cannula is directed into the inferior vena cava and the other close to the tricuspid valve. Blood from the inferior vena cava is oxygenated by a cardiopulmonary support assembly and returned to the right atrium via the second lumen [28]. The system requires the use of systemic heparinization which is a concern that should be weighed against the severity of hypoxemia.

Cardiac Injuries

Emergent intervention is indicated for cardiac injuries presenting as herniation, bleeding, or cardiac tamponade. Cardiac herniation from the pericardial defect may occur infrequently, potentially causing cardiac strangulation with severe hemodynamic depression and possible cardiac arrest. Immediate thoracotomy for reduction of cardiac herniation is indicated; while preparations are made for surgery, the patient should be kept on the side contralateral to the presumed herniation [30].

Penetrating injuries within the cardiac window, defined as the quadrangle between two perpendicular lines dropped from the midclavicular points to the last ribs, are very likely to cause cardiac trauma. Although penetrating trauma can injure any cardiac structure, the right ventricle is injured most frequently because of its anterior position. Small puncture wounds of the ventricle heal spontaneously in most instances, but bleeding from atrial tears usually does not stop. Gunshot wounds of the ventricles always bleed. Depending on the size and shape of the pericardial defect, blood extravasating from the heart may escape into the pleural space or remain in the pericardial sac. Blunt injuries may also cause cardiac injury involving any of the cardiac structures, but they most frequently cause damage in the form of myocardial contusion and pericardial tamponade. Although chronically the pericardium can accommodate several hundred milliliters of fluid, as little as 50 mL of blood acutely may result in pericardial tamponade [1]. Accumulation of blood in the pericardium decreases the stroke volume and increases the heart rate. The poor compliance of the pericardium allows pressure to build up within the sac which may compress the epicardial vessels, and cause myocardial ischemia, especially in patients with preexisting coronary disease whose myocardial demand is already increased because of compensatory tachycardia. The systolic blood pressure shows paradoxical changes during spontaneous breathing. During inspiration, with decreasing intrathoracic pressure, diastolic filling increases, causing leftward shift of the septum and thus decreasing the capacity of the left ventricle and the stroke volume, which is reflected in the systemic blood pressure as a reduction known as "pulsus paradoxus" [1].

A dusky, plethoric face, distended neck veins, hypotension, and muffled heart sounds suggest the presence of pericardial tamponade. Muffled heart sounds are difficult to detect in a busy and noisy emergency department. Pericardiocentesis, once used to diagnose hemopericardium, is rarely used now because of its invasive nature and high rate of inaccuracy. Currently transthoracic echocardiography or FAST examination is used for diagnosis. The appearance of pericardial blood during FAST confirms the diagnosis. However, the sensitivity of FAST decreases in the presence of massive hemothorax [6]; the small amount of blood remaining in the pericardial sac during hemorrhage into pleural space is still capable of producing tamponade, but may be difficult to detect by FAST [6].

If bilateral chest tubes do not improve the clinical picture in this situation, the decision may be made to perform a thoracotomy. Severe hemodynamic depression calls for a resuscitative thoracotomy, while stable patients are moved to the operating room for a subxiphoid pericardial window with or without laparoscopy [21], or formal thoracotomy under general anesthesia. Anesthesia should be induced after preparation and draping of the field. Intravenous fluids should be increased to optimize preload before induction; the heart rate must be kept fast and the afterload increased. Ketamine is commonly recommended for this purpose. Positive pressure ventilation must be applied judiciously as excessive airway pressures may compromise

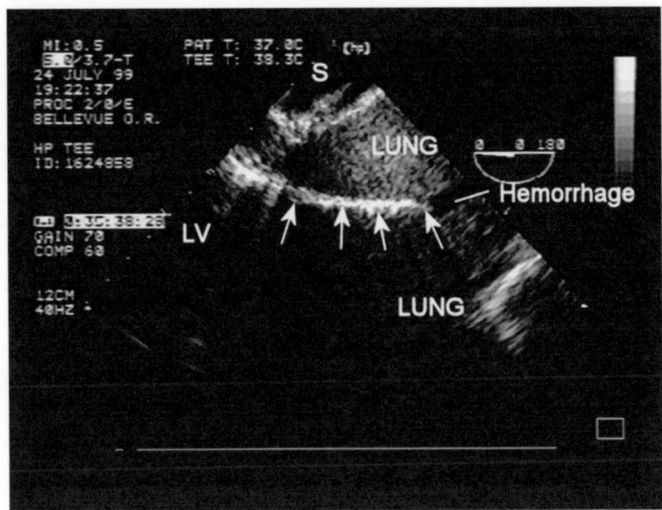

Fig. 11.8 Transesophageal echocardiography (TEE) image of a patient who, after a suicide attempt by stabbing himself at the left fourth intercostal space at the parasternal region, was brought to the emergency room and emergently transported to the operating room without any radiographic evaluation. Transgastric TEE view shows the impaling knife in close proximity to the pericardium overlying the left ventricle. The tip of the knife is in the lung parenchyma causing some bleeding. *S* Stomach, *LV* Left Ventricle; *arrows* depict the knife. The credit line should be: Navparkash S Sandhu and Levon M Capan, Role of Transesophageal Echocardiography in Management of Thoracic Stab Wound, Journal of Perioperative Echocardiography, 2014

hemodynamics by further increasing inflow occlusion between the right atrium and ventricle. In penetrating injuries, an efflux of blood after opening the pericardium suggests cardiac injury and necessitates definitive surgery via a sternotomy. Immediate repair is indicated in injuries with cardiac wall defects, coronary artery injuries, and great vessel injuries. Coronary artery injuries occur in about 2 % of penetrating cardiac trauma. The left anterior descending artery is the most commonly injured coronary vessel. The type of injury varies; laceration, thrombosis, dissection, and fistula formation to an adjacent vein or a cardiac chamber have all been reported [30, 31]. Electrocardiogram and troponin changes may suggest myocardial infarction [32]. While percutaneous coronary angioplasty may be used for treatment, in patients undergoing thoracotomy, injuries to the proximal two thirds of the artery are bypassed whereas those in the distal third are ligated. Intracardiac lesions such as septal defects, valve injuries, and ventricular aneurysms can be repaired electively with the use of cardiopulmonary bypass. It should be emphasized that acute traumatic valve insufficiency and septal defects become symptomatic more rapidly than chronic abnormalities. Acute mitral insufficiency may rapidly progress to pulmonary hypertension and edema, acute aortic insufficiency may cause excessive left ventricular wall stress, and septal defects may cause right ventricular and pulmonary artery dilation. Immediate chest radiographs may be normal in these patients, but echocardiography will provide the diagnosis [30].

Atrial wounds and right and left ventricular wounds that are not in the vicinity of the coronary arteries can be controlled by finger pressure followed by appropriate suturing. Wounds near the coronary arteries can also be closed with sutures under careful electrocardiographic and echocardiographic monitoring to avoid myocardial ischemia. Intraoperative transesophageal echocardiography (TEE) is extremely useful, not only to monitor intravascular volume and myocardial wall motion abnormalities but also to recognize intracardiac injuries and to follow the course of impaling foreign bodies in the chest (Fig. 11.8). Indeed many patients with penetrating chest injuries

Table 11.3 Common clinical, radiographic, and ultrasound features of thoracic aortic injuries

Clinical	Radiographic	Spiral computed Tomography	Ultrasound
Increased arterial pressure and pulse amplitude in upper extremities	Widened mediastinum	Mediastinal hematoma	Intimal flap
	Blurring of the aortic contours	Aortic wall	Turbulent flow
	Widened paraspinal interfaces	irregularity	Dilated aortic isthmus
Decreased arterial pressure and pulse amplitude in	Left apical cap	Intimal flap	Acute false aneurysm
	Opacified aortopulmonary window	False aneurysm	Intraluminal medial flap
lower extremities	Broadened paratracheal stripe	Pseudocoarctation	Hemothorax
Absent or weak left radial artery pulse	Displacement of the left	Intramural hematoma	Hemomediastinum
Osler's sign: discrepancy between	main-stem bronchus	Intraluminal clot or	
left and right arm blood pressure	Displaced SVC	medial flap	
Retrosternal or interscapular pain	Rightward deviation of the		
Hoarseness	esophagus and trachea		
Systolic flow murmur over	Nasogastric tube shift		
the precordium or medial to	Left hemothorax		
the left scapula	Sternal and/or upper rib		
Neurologic deficits in the lower	fractures		
extremities	Lung contusion		
	Pneumothorax		

Reproduced with permission from Capan LM, Miller SM, Gingrich KJ. Trauma and burns. In Barash PG, Cullen BF, Stoelting RK, Cahalan MK, Stock MC, Ortega R. Clinical anesthesia, seventh edition, Wolters Kluwer, Lippincott Williams & Wilkins, Philadelphia, 2013; pp. 1490–1534

from various types of weapons may be transported emergently to the operating room without any radiographic evaluation. In these circumstances TEE is the only available imaging method that permits diagnosis of the type of injury. In stable patients with penetrating and blunt cardiac injuries multidetector CT provides the most accurate and valuable initial information [33].

Blunt Thoracic Aortic Injury

Damage to the aorta is the most commonly encountered great vessel injury after blunt trauma. These injuries are responsible for at least one third of the trauma-related fatalities at the scene after motor vehicle and pedestrian auto collisions, and they are likely to be accompanied by various associated thoracic and intra-abdominal organ injuries [34]. The isthmus—the junction between the free and fixed portions of the descending aorta just distal to the left subclavian artery—is involved in the majority of cases and results in an 80 % mortality in the first hour following injury. The isthmus is anchored by the ligamentum arteriosum and the left mainstem bronchus, fixing the aorta distally and making it vulnerable to traction and tearing. Less frequent injuries of the thoracic aorta occur at its root and at the level of the diaphragm, which are also points of fixation and thus prone to shearing during rapid change of velocity. If all three layers of the vascular wall are torn, sudden death at the accident scene is usually unavoidable. Patients who arrive to the hospital have only one or two layers injured with continuity of blood flow maintained by the adventitial layer or the surrounding mediastinal fibrous tissues. Those with only intimal injuries may present with intramural hematoma, mural thrombus, or intimal flap. When the medial layer is also injured, the motion of the flap with each cardiac cycle can be observed on TEE. Patients with mild adventitial injuries consisting of partial transection, mediastinal bleeding, and intraluminal obstruction may present with pseudoaneurysm. The absence of thrombus formation or any other change in or around the vessel that prevents further bleeding is likely to result in rapid death from exsanguination.

The presenting signs, symptoms, radiographic, CT, and ultrasound findings of blunt thoracic aortic injuries are shown in Table 11.3.

Table 11.4 The Vancouver simplified classification of blunt thoracic aortic injuries

Grade	Vancouver simplified classification
1	Intimal flap, thrombus, or intramural hematoma <1 cm
2	Intimal flap, thrombus, or intramural hematoma >1 cm
3	Pseudoaneurysm (simple or complex, no extravasation)
4	Contrast extravasation (with or without aneurysm)

Reprinted from Journal of Thoracic and Cardiovascular Surgery, 144, Lamarche Y, Berger FH, Nicolaou S, Bilawich A-M, et al. Vancouver simplified grading system with computed tomographic angiography for blunt aortic injury, pp. 347–54, Copyright 2012, with permission from Elsevier

There may be no clinical findings in the emergency department. Only 20–30 % of patients with mediastinal widening actually have a thoracic aortic injury, although the negative predictive value of the finding is 98 %. Measuring the left mediastinal width (≥6 cm) and its fraction of the total mediastinal width (≥0.6) may increase the specificity and positive predictive value of the plain film [35]. Multidetector CT scans are capable of providing an excellent definition of traumatic aortic injury. These scanners, with volume-rendered image reconstruction techniques, produce CT angiography images that permit reliable noninvasive diagnosis and have practically eliminated the need for biplanar aortography or digital subtraction angiography. Better definition of the extent of the injury with this technology has allowed the establishment of a noninvasive classification of the severity of aortic injuries, and based on that classification, the formulation of treatment. TEE is also capable of providing reliable information and is capable of diagnosing subadventitial aortic injuries that require intervention [36]. However, CT is used in the majority of instances in awake patients. Introducing a TEE probe under these circumstances may be impractical and undesirable because of the danger of aortic rupture secondary to cardiovascular stimulation. The possibility of an intercurrent esophageal injury is another reason for not introducing a TEE probe in these patients. However, considering that esophageal injury is relatively rare, intraoperative TEE may be especially useful for the anesthesiologist to diagnose an aortic injury when associated injuries require immediate surgery without time for CT examination of the chest.

Many classification systems of blunt thoracic aortic injuries are proposed based on CT angiography findings [37–40]. These are relatively similar; they divide the injuries into four categories. The simplified Vancouver Classification system is shown in Table 11.4. A simpler classification based on TEE findings is also available and classifies traumatic aortic injury into three categories: a grade 1 injury consists of an intramural hematoma, limited intimal flap and/or mural thrombus; a grade 2 injury consists of subadventitial rupture, injury to the media, altered aortic geometry and/or a small hemomediastinum; a grade 3 injury consists of transsection with massive blood extravasation, intraluminal obstruction causing pseudocoarctation, and ischemia (Fig. 11.9) [41]. Of these, grade 1 injuries can be treated nonoperatively with serial follow-ups with TEE or CT [41]. Grade 2 and 3 injuries require immediate or delayed surgery based on clinical findings [41]. Severity grading may also be accomplished by criteria involving TEE measurement of maximum aortic diameter, the ratio between injured and normal aortic diameters, the depth of pseudoaneurysm, the esophagus-to-aortic isthmus distance, the aortic isthmus-to-left visceral pleural distance, and the presence of hemothorax [41].

Prioritization of surgery when multiple injuries are present depends on the hemodynamic and neurologic status of the patient. Although the aorta should be repaired as early as possible, unless it is leaking, control of active hemorrhage

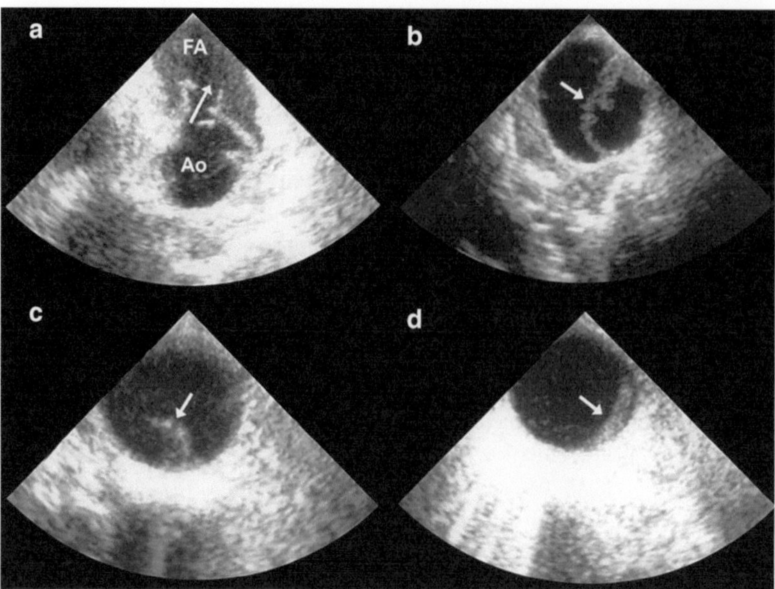

Fig. 11.9 Transesophageal echocardiographic appearances of three grades of traumatic aortic injury. (**a**) Grade 3 injury. Adventitia of the aortic wall is damaged and false aneurysm (FA) is communicating (*arrow*) with the aortic lumen (Ao). (**b**) Grade 2 injury. Large medial flap moves back and forth during each cardiac cycle. Adventitia is intact. (**c, d**) Grade 1 injury. Intimal flap (**c**) and intramural hematoma (**d**) (shown with *arrows*) without hemomediastinum or alteration of aortic geometry. Reprinted with permission from Goarin J-P, Cluzel P, Gosgnach M, et al. Evaluation of transesophageal echocardiography for diagnosis of traumatic aortic injury. Anesthesiology 2000;93:1373–7

from other sites and drainage of an intracranial hematoma not only have a higher surgical priority but also preclude heparinization needed for aortic repair. In most instances, a blood clot between the aorta and the mediastinal pleura occludes the vessel. Any disturbance of the tamponaded region may reinitiate bleeding. A rapid flow of blood in a large artery tends to pull the endothelium into the stream and thus may rupture an injured vessel that is sealed with a clot or hematoma. Such an increase in the aortic blood flow is usually caused by increased myocardial contractility; every effort should be made to prevent increased cardiac contractility and hypertension. Decreasing the aortic wall shear stress, which may dislodge a clot formed over the injured segment, should be the initial goal. This can be achieved by decreasing myocardial contractility with β-blocker agents. Other hypotensive agents may not be as effective for this purpose.

Major changes have occurred in the management of blunt aortic injuries during the past 15 years, resulting in improved early outcomes (Table 11.5). Blunt thoracic injury is now being diagnosed with contrast-enhanced CT angiography, which has replaced aortography and the less invasive TEE. Likewise endovascular thoracic repair has supplanted open surgery as the primary surgical treatment [42]. Nevertheless aortography is still being used intraoperatively in patients undergoing endovascular stenting. An alternative to aortography in this setting is the use of intravascular ultrasound. Additionally, more patients (Grade 1 and sometimes 2) are being treated conservatively, and in this nonoperatively treated group, risk-adjusted mortality has decreased over time [43].

Endovascular aortic repair has gained popularity for two reasons: it is minimally invasive and is associated with fewer early complications—such as paraplegia, stroke,

Table 11.5 Change in the management of blunt thoracic aortic injuries from 1997 to 2007

	AAST$_1$		AAST$_2$	
	$N = 253$		$N = 193$	
Diagnosis				
Aortagram	220	(87 %)	16	(8 %)
CT Scan	88	(35 %)	180	(93 %)
TEE	30	(12 %)	2	(1 %)
Repair				
Open	207	(100 %)	68	(35 %)
Endovascular	–		125	(65 %)
Outcomes				
Mortality	53/241	(22 %)	25/193	(13 %)
Paraplegia				
All patients	18	(9 %)	2	(2 %)
Open repair	18	(9 %)	2	(3 %)
Endovascular	0		1/125	(1 %)
Renal failure	18	(9 %)	17	(9 %)
Repair site complication	1/207	(1 %)	25/125	(20 %)

AAST$_1$, American Association for the Surgery of Trauma 1997 Study
AAST$_2$, American Association for the Surgery of Trauma 2007 Study
TEE, Transesophageal echocardiogram
Reproduced with permission from Demetriades D, Velmahos GC, Scalea TM et al. Diagnosis and treatment of blunt thoracic aortic injuries: changing perspectives. J Trauma 2008;64:1415

bleeding, or death—than are encountered after open thoracotomy [44]. The procedure is tolerated well and can be performed even in patients with significant associated injuries [45]. The anesthetic management is also simpler than that required for open repair. Patients should be monitored with a right radial artery cannula in case the left subclavian artery is covered by the stent. A central line is usually placed for administration of vasoactive drugs. Although monitored anesthesia care with combined sedation and local anesthesia is utilized in some centers, it is the authors' preference to administer general anesthesia to these patients. Embolization of aortic atheromas may occur; in anesthetized patients TEE may help to visualize these prior to stent deployment. Cerebral oximetry may also inform the clinician of possible embolization when a decrease in O_2 saturation occurs. Transcranial Doppler also can be useful for this purpose but it is not practical intraoperatively. During aortography and stent deployment, ventilation may have to be stopped and systemic blood pressure may have to be lowered to a mean of 60 mmHg. Endoleak, a leak between the graft and the

vascular wall, is one of the early recognized complications. Long-term complications and survival compared to open repair are not clearly known at this time. It is possible that graft failure may occur from aging of the stent material and maturing and enlargement of the thoracic aorta over time.

At present, repair of blunt thoracic injuries via the traditional left thoracotomy is a rare procedure. In the authors' institution, an open repair has not been performed for the past 3 years. If it is performed, lung isolation with a double lumen endobronchial tube should be provided to facilitate surgical exposure and prevent contamination of contralateral lung by blood. The endobronchial tube should be inserted only after visualizing the orifice of the left main stem bronchus; a pseudoaneurysm encroaching on the bronchus may be ruptured if the tube is blindly forced into the bronchus. Further, partial heparinization, and at times, partial left heart bypass by left atriofemoral or femoral–femoral conduits are required to decompress the left heart and perfuse the distal aorta and the spinal cord during the "clamp and sew" technique.

The "clamp and saw" technique involves placement of clamps just distal to the origin of the left subclavian artery and below the injured segment. Debridement of the vessel wall and reanastomosis of the aorta is then performed rapidly and the clamps are released. The systemic blood pressure, blood lactate, and K^+ should be monitored; elevation of K^+ should be treated with insulin and glucose. Paraplegia, one of the dreaded complications of this technique, occurs in about 9 % of patients and is attributed to the ischemia of the spinal cord caused by decreased anterior spinal artery blood flow which originates from the left subclavian artery, and the spinal branches of the aorta, such as the Adamkiewicz artery [46]. Thus a short clamp time is essential to prevent this complication. Anastomosis can be performed in as little as 7–9 min in uncomplicated cases. The incidence of excessive bleeding, mortality, and morbidity is very high with this technique. Some surgeons used shunting between the proximal aorta and the vessel distal to the clamp for perfusion of the spinal cord and the lower extremities with some but not substantial beneficial effects.

Great Vessel Injuries

Major branches of the thoracic aorta—the left subclavian, left common carotid, and innominate arteries—are mostly damaged by penetrating trauma. They may be injured by stab wounds at the base of the neck directed down into the chest or gunshot wounds anywhere in the neck or the chest [6]. These victims infrequently reach the operating room because most expire at the scene from exsanguination [47]. Those who reach the emergency department may present in conditions varying from near stable to complete hemodynamic deterioration. A transmediastinal gunshot wound or the presence of a wound at the base of the neck should raise the suspicion of injury to these vessels [6]. Presenting symptoms include hemothorax, pericardial tamponade, external bleeding, pulse deficit in the distribution of the affected vessel, brachial plexus injury, stroke, coma, and/or the presence of a thrill or bruit at

the base of the neck. There may be mediastinal widening or an apical cap observed on chest radiography. The presence of a distal pulse does not rule out injury to these vessels because blood flow may be maintained through perivascular tissues allowing flow in spite of complete transection of the vascular wall. Likewise, the absence of bleeding or hematoma may be due to complete vascular thrombosis or an intimal flap, again not ruling out injury to the vessel. Patients presenting in extremis may be diagnosed during emergency department thoracotomy or an urgent thoracotomy in the operating room. In patients who are hemodynamically stable or responsive to resuscitation the diagnosis is made by CT angiography and conventional angiography in the operating room [48].

Anesthetic management may involve massive transfusion and treatment of possible associated complications such as coagulopathy, hypothermia, hyperkalemia, or hypocalcemia; lung isolation preferably with a double lumen tube; hemodynamic optimization with fluids and vasoactive agents; titration of anesthetic agents; and advanced cardiac life support, if needed. Because of their proximity to injured vessels, injuries to the recurrent laryngeal nerve, phrenic nerve, and vagus may occur as a result of both trauma and surgery. Consequences of these injuries should be considered if there are postoperative airway or pulmonary complications.

Esophageal Injuries

Esophageal injuries are insidious and difficult to recognize in the presence of more overt clinical manifestations of associated injuries. Yet when missed, they may be complicated by severe mediastinitis, with potentially high morbidity and mortality. They may result from blunt or penetrating trauma. Blunt injuries are usually caused by a direct blow to the neck or the chest producing a sudden increase in intraluminal pressure and a burst lesion [6]. Penetrating injuries may be caused by stab wounds or gunshot wounds to the neck or the chest. Gunshot injuries primarily involve the cervical esophagus; only

1 % of these wounds involve the intrathoracic esophagus [6]. Clinical manifestations depend on the location, size, time of diagnosis, and degree of contamination; symptoms are nonspecific and may be present in less than 80 % of victims. Odynophagia, dysphagia, chest or back pain, or hematemesis are the initial symptoms. Blood draining from a nasogastric tube placed in the emergency department should raise the suspicion of esophageal injury. During auscultation of the chest, one may be able to hear Hamman's sign, a crunch with each heart beat, which suggests the presence of mediastinal emphysema. An initial chest radiograph may show mediastinal emphysema, much smaller in size than that caused by airway perforation, and some pleural effusion. Definitive diagnosis is made by CT, which demonstrates a collection near the esophagus, followed by esophagoscopy and barium esophogram. When both esophagoscopy and esophogram are used, the diagnostic capability may be almost 100 % [1, 6]. If the diagnosis is missed, the clinical picture may change within a few days to fever, drainage of pus from the chest tube, hemodynamic instability, and disorientation in some patients [49]. Secretions from an injury to the cervical esophagus drain into the deep cervical fascia which is connected to the mediastinum. Secretions from the proximal two thirds of the thoracic portion of the esophagus drain into the right pleural cavity, causing effusion or empyema. Drainage from the distal third of the esophagus produces left-sided effusion. Finally, perforation of the most distal segment of the esophagus produces free abdominal air, peritonitis, or subdiaphragmatic abscess if the diagnosis is delayed [1].

Anesthetic management of these injuries involves prevention of aspiration of gastric fluid and the barium used for the esophogram, management of sepsis and possible septic shock, lung isolation if possible, and postoperative intensive care.

Diaphragmatic Injuries

Lateral crashes and deceleration of greater than 40 km/h in vehicular accidents, and head-on impacts on a seat-belted driver are the likely mechanisms of this injury [50, 51]. Diaphragmatic injuries are more common on the left side than on the right which is protected by the liver [1, 51]. Often small diaphragmatic injuries may go unrecognized, to be diagnosed few days to years later [1]. Because these injuries are frequently missed, their clinical presentation may be divided into three phases [51]. The acute phase, from the initial insult to apparent recovery from injury; the latent phase, characterized by the entrance of intra-abdominal contents into the thorax, at any time from the traumatic event to a few weeks later; and the obstructive phase, presenting as strangulation of the herniated contents within 3 years after injury. Obviously the clinical presentations of each of these phases vary, but in almost all of these situations the risk of perioperative regurgitation is high. Injuries of greater than 6 cm in length are likely to permit abdominal contents into the thoracic cavity and cause compression of the lung, producing abnormal gas exchange; or of the heart, causing dysrhythmias or hypotension as well as gastric or intestinal obstructive symptoms [51]. These issues may also set the stage for severe regurgitation and aspiration of gastric contents after induction of anesthesia [51]. Diaphragmatic herniation may be suspected when the distal end of a nasogastric tube in the stomach appears above the diaphragm on the chest radiograph [52]. When difficulty of visualization occurs, insufflation of air via the nasogastric tube may optimize the image [52]. Definitive diagnosis can be made by contrast-enhanced CT scan. When herniation is absent, diagnosis and repair can be made by video-assisted thoracoscopy or laparoscopy. Lung isolation with a blocker or double lumen tube may be necessary for the former procedure.

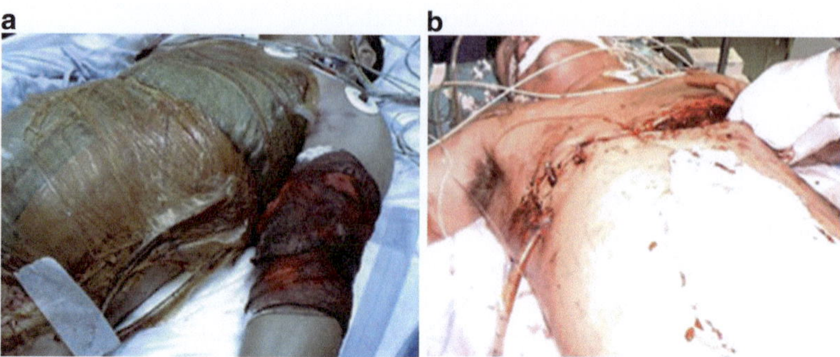

Fig. 11.10 (**a**) Patient with thoracic and abdominal injuries left with open chest and abdomen after a damage control procedure. The packed chest is covered with silastic and then sealed with towels and sterile clear plastic adhesive. (**b**) Covering materials are removed and chest cavity is explored

Delayed Thoracotomy

Delayed repair may be indicated for four reasons: (a) debridement and irrigation of a chest deliberately left open during emergency surgery; (b) to repair injuries that could not be managed initially because of a need to manage life-threatening higher priority injuries; (c) to repair injuries that require heparinization, which would complicate the management of other injuries during the initial period; and (d) to repair wounds missed during the initial stage. Delayed thoracotomy, defined as surgery after 24 h following trauma, is performed to repair intracardiac injuries, traumatic aortic rupture, and missed injuries to evacuate a retained hemothorax with or without decortication and to drain posttraumatic empyema. The incidence of posttraumatic empyema in patients with retained hemothorax was found to be 27 % in a recent study [53]. Rib fractures, severe injury [injury severity score (ISS) >25], and additional interventions to evacuate the hemothorax were found to be independent predictors. No relationship between use or choice of antibiotics and development of empyema could be demonstrated [53].

The concept of leaving the abdominal cavity open during a damage control procedure to prevent postoperative compartment syndrome has also been applied to severe chest injuries (Fig. 11.10) [54]. The chest is left open for two reasons: (a) most of these patients return to OR, often several times, at 1 or 2 day intervals in order to repair less life-threatening injuries or for a "second look" at an originally repaired injury and (b) to prevent thoracic compartment syndrome which may be caused by edema of the intrathoracic organs when the chest is closed. The combination of high airway pressures, ineffective ventilation, and hypotension secondary to cardiac and major vessel compression leads to rapid demise. Leaving the chest open prevents these problems. This was done initially by using multiple towel clips attached to the fascia on both sides of the wound after packing the chest. Fascial closure, even with towel clips, can increase intrathoracic pressure. Currently the packed chest is covered with silastic or other nonadhesive material and then sealed with sterile clear plastic adhesive. Upon return to the OR, these materials are removed and the appropriate surgery performed. Often these patients present themselves to the OR intubated eliminating the need for formal induction and tracheal intubation. General anesthesia with tracheal intubation should be administered in extubated patients after careful evaluation of hemodynamic and intravascular volume status, oxygenation, renal function, and electrolytes.

Intracardiac injuries include insufficiency of aortic, mitral, and tricuspid valves, and atrial or ventricular septal defects. As mentioned above, severe acute traumatic insufficiency of the mitral and aortic valves is poorly tolerated: increased ventricular wall stress may rapidly progress into pulmonary edema necessitating early surgery. However, these injuries are rare, and often mild to moderate valvular insufficiency is tolerated well, allowing elective surgical correction.

Ventricular septal defects can be recognized by increased pulmonary vascularity with a normal heart size on the chest radiograph. The diagnosis should be confirmed by echocardiography. A traumatic atrial septal defect may be missed during the initial evaluation but can also be recognized by echocardiography.

The consequences of an improperly placed chest tube for hemothorax are resorption of the pleural blood with time, infection (posttraumatic empyema), and fibrothorax. Blood in the pleural space is a powerful culture medium and thus antibiotic prophylaxis does not compensate for an improperly placed chest tube. If drainage ceases in the presence of radiographic and preferably CT evidence of fluid in the pleural cavity, placement of another tube is unlikely to effectively drain the clotted blood. Video-assisted thoracoscopy or thoracotomy should be considered, especially after a penetrating injury. Frequently, hemothorax forms a fibrous layer over the visceral pleura that restricts effective expansion of the lung and necessitates decortication. Complete removal of this fibrous tissue from the lung surface provides adequate lung expansion. Chest tubes placed after decortication should be removed as early as safely possible to prevent infection.

Thoracic Injuries Requiring Nonsurgical Management

Blunt trauma to the chest may produce injuries of the lung and heart that require supportive nonsurgical care. The presence of these injuries may complicate the anesthesia administered for surgery of both thoracic and nonthoracic trauma. Their presence without the requirement for surgery necessitates admission to the intensive care unit to optimize hemodynamic status and pulmonary gas exchange.

Flail Chest and Pulmonary Contusion

Flail chest develops if more than three adjacent ribs are broken in at least two sites, or when rib fractures are associated with sternal fracture(s) or costochondral separation at three adjacent levels.

For many years, it was thought that the gas exchange abnormalities in this situation were caused by the paradoxical breathing in the injured hemithorax created by the pleural pressure differential across the unsupported chest wall. It is now clear that morbidity is largely a result of pulmonary dysfunction secondary to underlying lung contusion. A reduction in lung volume secondary to splinting and the development of hemo- or pneumothorax in some cases also contributes to morbidity.

Rib fractures are primarily caused by compression forces; shear forces and blast injury may also be responsible. The degree of rib deformation caused by a broad compressive impact determines the extent of chest wall injury. Cadaver studies have demonstrated that in adults 20 % deformation of chest wall produces isolated rib fractures, whereas 40 % deformation results in a flail chest [55].

Pulmonary contusion results from direct compressive and shear forces. The mechanism of the resulting gas exchange abnormality is as follows: the impact producing the rib fractures is transferred to the underlying lung causing alveolar disruption, interstitial and intra-alveolar hemorrhage, and atelectasis. Within hours pulmonary edema ensues as the permeability of the pulmonary capillaries increases. As a result of an inflammatory reaction, after 18–24 h cellular debris, proteinaceous material, and blood start to fill the lung architecture. All of these changes cause increased elastic recoil of the lung, decreased functional residual capacity (FRC) and diminished lung compliance, resulting in increased work of breathing, which in turn causes respiratory fatigue and gradual respiratory insufficiency progressing to failure (Fig. 11.11) [55, 56]. As the muscular effort to expand the chest increases, paradoxical motion of the flail chest also increases. In addition to this inflammatory response, the quality and quantity of pulmonary surfactant is decreased in pulmonary contusion.

It is crucially important that this situation is recognized as early as possible in order to apply therapeutic measures to prevent, or at least minimize, the occurrence of pulmonary complications such as atelectasis, retained secretions, tracheobronchitis, pneumonia, and/or

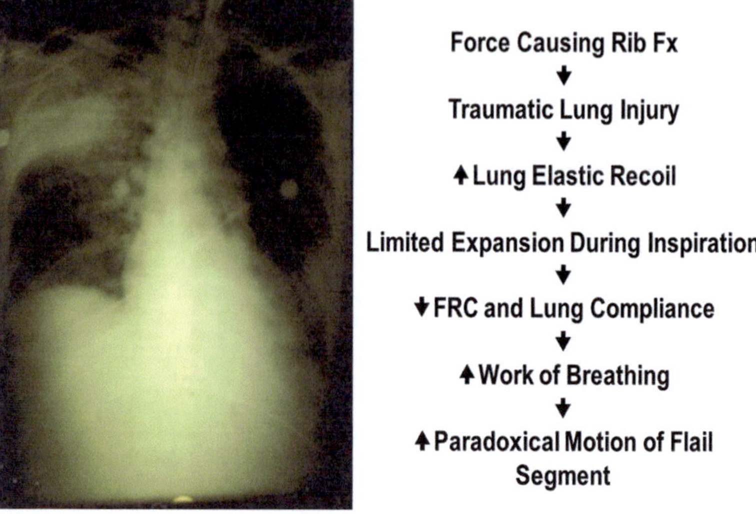

Fig. 11.11 Chest radiograph of a patient with flail chest and severe pulmonary contusion (*left panel*). Mechanism of development of pulmonary contusion after rib fractures (*right panel*)

respiratory failure. Treatment after development of these complications is difficult and the likelihood of acute respiratory distress syndrome (ARDS) increases. The estimated mortality rate of pulmonary contusion is as high as 25 %; development of ARDS increases mortality to 50 % [57, 58]. Older age (>65), three or more rib fractures, preexisting, especially cardiopulmonary, disease, and development of pneumonia are also risk factors for mortality after pulmonary contusion [59].

Although flail chest should be easy to recognize with the help of physical examination and chest radiography, in some instances it may not be detected early enough. Shallow breathing interferes with adequate physical examination, while abnormalities on plain chest x-rays develop late. Although they may precede the changes seen on chest films, alterations in arterial blood gases may still develop late and may not be detected if the patient is on supplemental oxygen. As much as possible, these patients should be managed breathing room air with close supervision and continuous monitoring with pulse oximetry. If O_2 saturation drops, the patient should be followed with periodic blood gas measurements and treated accordingly. The PaO_2/FIO_2 ratio may be a helpful indicator, and when it drops below 300 in a previously healthy patient, treatment should be initiated because the likelihood of ARDS increases in these patients. It should be emphasized that the PaO_2 alone cannot predict

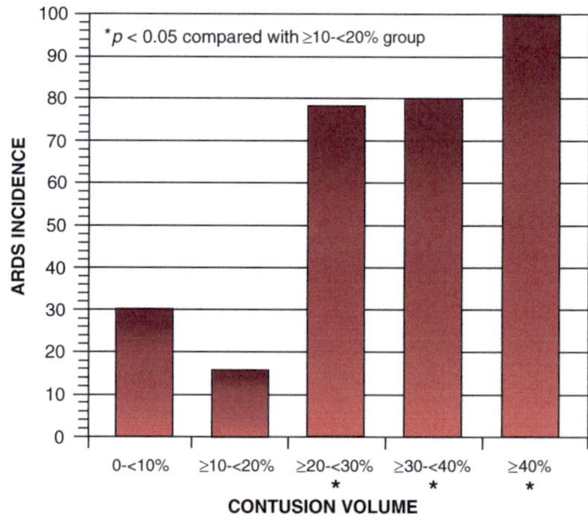

Fig. 11.12 Relationship between the contusion volume and the likelihood of development of Acute Respiratory Distress Syndrome (ARDS). Contusion volume greater than 20 % or greater of total lung volume predicts the development of ARDS. Reproduced with permission from Miller PR, Croce MA, Bee TK, Qaisi WG, Smith CP, Collins GL, Fabian TC. ARDS after pulmonary contusion: accurate measurement of contusion volume identifies high-risk patients. J Trauma 2001; 51:223–8; discussion 229–30

the contusion volume. Likewise, the extent of the flail is not predictive of the amount of contusion. A plain chest radiograph or, most accurately, 3D CT can determine contusion volume and predict the likelihood of ARDS and the need for ventilator support. A contusion volume greater than 20 % increases the likelihood of ARDS (Fig. 11.12) [60]. Recently a semiautomated computer program has been designed to analyze pulmonary CT scans and provide an objective indication of the fraction of contused lung in relation to the total lung volume [61]. Using this method, an admission lung contusion ratio $\geq 24\%$ was found to predict the development of ARDS and pneumonia later during hospitalization, confirming earlier findings [61].

Ventilator-associated pneumonia is considered a "never event" by the Centers for Medicare and Medicaid Services, and a "ventilator bundle" consisting of stress ulcer prophylaxis, deep venous thrombosis prophylaxis, elevation of the head of the bed, and daily cessation of sedation for weaning assessment is recommended to prevent this complication. A study conducted in patients with pulmonary contusion demonstrated that, although it should be applied as a universal preventive measure, the ventilator bundle did not prevent pneumonia in these patients [62]. Male sex and chest injury severity were the two independent factors determining the development of pneumonia [62].

Until the middle 1970s it was thought that routine tracheal intubation and ventilation of these patients improved outcome. Trinkle and colleagues [63] were the first to demonstrate that routine intubation and ventilation increased the likelihood of pneumonia, infection, and multiorgan failure in these patients. The current understanding is to avoid tracheal intubation unless patients are exhibiting respiratory difficulties and the PaO_2 is <60 mmHg in a patient spontaneously breathing room air or <80 mmHg if O_2 is administered by mask or nasally, $PaCO_2$ is >50 mmHg, $A\text{-}aDO_2$ is 350 mmHg at FIO_2 1.0, and PaO_2/FIO_2 ratio is <200 mmHg [56, 63]. Additionally, severe shock, head injury, need for anesthesia and surgery, airway compromise, and preexisting cardiopulmonary disease are indications for tracheal intubation and mechanical ventilation.

There are, however, other ventilator maneuvers that may be applied to improve gas exchange and prevent complications. Early use of continuous positive airway pressure (CPAP) by mask decreases the work of breathing and prevents respiratory fatigue and the complications associated with it. If there is an inadequate response to CPAP, tracheal intubation and airway pressure release ventilation (APRV) can be used. Basically this mode of ventilation is applied to spontaneously breathing intubated patients. With APRV the CPAP applied for a short period of time is brought from a high level, such as 10–12 cmH_2O, to about 5–6 cmH_2O to provide ventilation. This is done by a device with a flow generator that maintains continuous positive pressure in the system as it exits through a threshold resistor valve. The patient breathes spontaneously with this high CPAP. A time-controlled threshold resistor valve placed at the end of the system periodically lowers the CPAP for a short period of time. Thus this system is similar to volume-controlled inverse ratio ventilation except that it allows the patient to breathe spontaneously. In other words, APRV utilizes a long period of positive pressure and a very short period of lower but not zero pressure while the patient breathes spontaneously. The advantages of this mode of ventilation over volume-controlled inverse ratio ventilation or intermittent mandatory ventilation, are improved V/Q matching, improved oxygenation, lower sedation requirement, lower peak airway pressures, and a reduced incidence of ventilator-associated pneumonia that otherwise occurs in up to 30 % of ventilated patients with pulmonary contusion [64, 65]. APRV is also safe and effective in optimizing oxygenation and CO_2 removal when patients are transitioned from another mode of ventilation [66]. There is, however, some data to suggest that it may take longer to wean patients from APRV than from conventional volume-cycled ventilation with daily 30–60 min trials of spontaneous breathing [67].

If the patient is not able to breathe spontaneously, the choice is to use conventional mechanical ventilation with PEEP titrated to oxygenation and hemodynamic response. As discussed above, one of the objectives in the management of pulmonary contusion is to prevent progression into ARDS. Although there is no proof that the use of low-volume ventilation with PEEP, which has been shown to improve outcome in ARDS, can also be beneficial in patients with severe pulmonary contusion, most centers use the same ventilation strategy even though pulmonary contusion is usually unilateral. This strategy may also be beneficial in reducing ventilator-induced lung injury which is thought to be secondary to alveolar collapse and reopening, "atelectrauma" [55].

In unilateral contusion with severe hypoxemia unresponsive to conventional ventilation with PEEP, independent lung ventilation can be tried. In this mode, each lung is ventilated separately with two synchronized ventilators via a double lumen endobronchial tube. There is also some evidence that the life-threatening hypoxia caused by bilateral lung contusion can be managed successfully using High Frequency Jet Ventilation (HFJV), and, as described more recently, with High Frequency Oscillatory Ventilation (HFOV). Multiple combinations of convection and diffusion responsible for air movement in HFOV maintains consistent high airway pressures preventing cyclic alveolar collapse or "atelectrauma" and provides more rapid improvement in oxygenation than with conventional ventilation [68, 69]. This mode of ventilation may also enhance cardiac performance, which may be compromised as a result of contusion or ischemia. Finally in desperate situations, extracorporeal membrane oxygenation (ECMO) has been used for a few days with some success.

There have been several studies about the place of surgical fixation of rib fractures in the management of flail chest and pulmonary contusion. A recent meta-analysis reviewing a total of 753 patients in 11 manuscripts suggests that, compared to nonoperative treatment, surgical fixation results in substantial decreases in ventilator days, development of pneumonia, intensive care unit days, mortality, septicemia, tracheostomy rate, and chest deformity [70]. Although few, prospective randomized studies support the

beneficial effect of a surgical approach [71]. Surgical fixation has also been shown to be cost-effective compared to conservative care [72]. Although the final decision in this regard waits for the results of more prospective randomized studies, the current understanding is that patients with severe multiple rib fractures and substantially diminished muscular support for the floating segment will benefit from surgical fixation [73]. This approach may also be beneficial for patients with decreased cardiopulmonary reserve [73].

A practice management guideline published by the Eastern Association for the Surgery of Trauma also emphasizes three additional aspects of care [74]. First is to refrain from overzealous fluid administration; second is to provide adequate pain control; and third is to apply respiratory care in the form of frequent tracheobronchial suctioning with or without FOB guidance, airway humidification, bronchodilators, and chest physiotherapy. It is clear that in the setting of multiple trauma and hemorrhage, fluid restriction may have deleterious effects. While adequate fluid resuscitation to provide optimal perfusion is essential, excess intravascular volume may jeopardize healing by accumulating within the lung tissue. Monitoring fluid status not only by systemic blood pressure, but also using many other indices such as systolic pressure variation, pulse pressure variation, urine output, filling pressures, blood lactate, base excess/deficits, and even with TEE may be helpful for this purpose.

Rib fractures, even without flail chest, cause significant morbidity owing to pain and subsequent atelectasis from hypoventilation. In patients with pulmonary contusions, especially in the elderly, the deleterious effects of pain are increased. Aggressive pain control applied early after the injury using multimodal analgesia appears to reduce the incidence of respiratory failure, pulmonary sepsis, and subsequent mortality [75]. In our experience, the most effective pain management technique is continuous thoracic epidural analgesia with

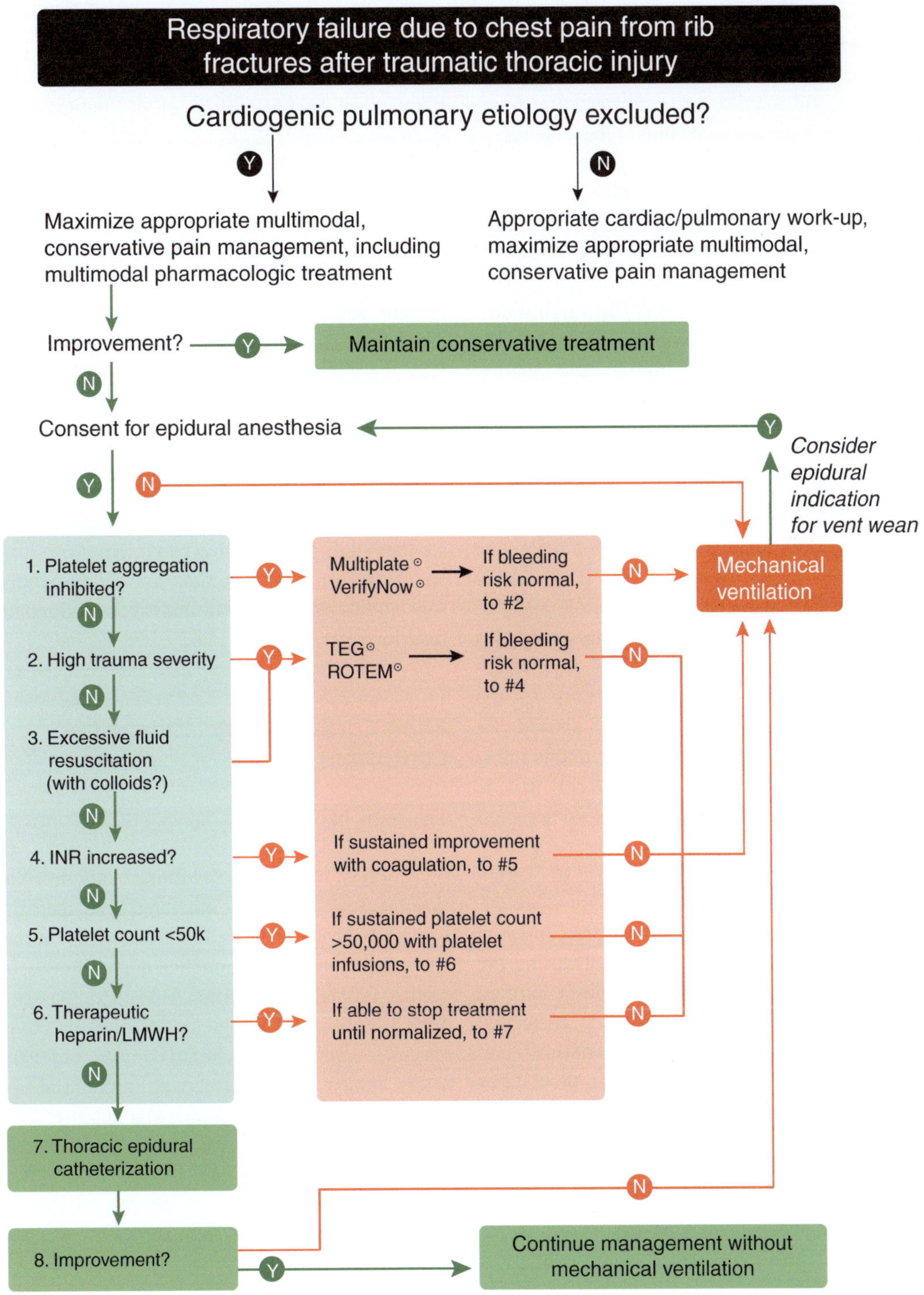

Fig. 11.13 Proposed decision-making process in management of pain-induced respiratory insufficiency or failure after traumatic fractures of the ribs. Cardiogenic and pulmonary causes of respiratory failure and various causes of coagulopathy should be ruled out before attempting epidural analgesia. However, epidural may

a low concentration of bupivacaine (0.125–0.25 %) placed at the dermatomal level of the injury and infused at a rate of 4–8 mL/h with careful monitoring of pain level and systemic blood pressure. It should be considered when more than three or four ribs are fractured [76]. Prior to attempting epidural analgesia however, pulmonary and cardiogenic causes of respiratory failure and the various causes of coagulation abnormalities must be eliminated, while analgesia is provided by multimodal techniques (Fig. 11.13) [75]. Unfortunately concomitant spine or other injuries, and inability of the patient to consent to the procedure often preclude this treatment. Continuous thoracic paravertebral block with ultrasound guidance may also be considered a part of multidimensional pain management that can effectively replace epidural analgesia [76]. This technique may also be useful alone when rib fractures are unilateral and patients exhibit intolerance to parenteral nonopioid and opioid analgesics [77]. Multiple intercostal blocks, though effective, are labor intensive, uncomfortable for the patient and short-lasting; they should be repeated at least twice a day. Continuous intercostal nerve block inserted lateral to the paraspinous muscles has been shown to avert these problems and to improve pulmonary function and pain control and to decrease the length of hospital stay [78].

Although flail chest and pulmonary contusion do not require surgical management during the immediate phase of trauma, anesthesia is often administered to these patients for associated injuries. It is not uncommon that arterial blood gases may deteriorate during these procedures because of progression of the contusion. Frequent monitoring of blood gases levels along with proper ventilator management, fluid resuscitation, and respiratory care should be utilized as outlined above. The long-term outlook for

trauma patients with blunt chest injuries has been recently investigated. Leone et al. [79] from France demonstrated that 6 months after blunt chest trauma, 70 % of the patients had decreased physical function and six-minute walk distance, and at least one abnormal pulmonary function test. Sixty percent of patients had an abnormal chest CT which did not correlate with an admission $PaO_2/FiO_2 < 200$, although abnormal pulmonary function tests did. At 12 months follow-up, an increase in forced vital capacity and physical performance was noted. However, physical performance remained less than that recorded before injury. This data suggest that it takes at least 12 months after injury for a multiple trauma patient with blunt chest injury to regain reasonable physical performance and pulmonary function. This is confirmed by another study which followed patients with lung contusion for 12–48 months and demonstrated substantial recovery and improved pulmonary function tests [80].

Blunt Cardiac Injury (Myocardial Contusion)

The term blunt cardiac injury (BCI), formerly called myocardial contusion, refers to myocardial damage involving myofibrillar disintegration, edema, bleeding, or necrosis. Clinically it presents as EKG changes, cardiac enzyme abnormalities, complex dysrhythmias, or cardiac failure. By definition, BCI encompasses a wide variety of pathologic conditions, including varying degrees of myocardial damage; coronary artery injury; cardiac free-wall, interatrial- or interventricular septal, or valvular rupture; and, when impalement by a fractured sternum or rib occurs, penetrating cardiac injury from blunt trauma [81]. Not all of these injuries are caused by myocardial damage from direct mechanical

Fig. 11.13 (Continued) be used while the patient is being ventilated to provide analgesia and to facilitate weaning from the ventilator. *INR* International Normalized Ratio, *LMWH* low molecular weight heparin, Multiplate® = MEA = multiple electrode aggregometry; ROTEM® = rotational thromboelastometry; TEG® = thromboelastography; VerifyNow® = whole blood turbidimetric platelet aggregometry. Reproduced by permission from Ahn Y, Gorlinger K, Alam H, Eikerman M. Anesthesiology 2013;118:701–8

trauma; they may occur indirectly as a result of coronary occlusion or exacerbation of preexisting coronary artery disease by the stress of trauma. Catecholamine activity following injury, pain, severe CNS injury, and hemorrhagic shock can also produce cardiac lesions, manifested by EKG abnormalities and troponin release, in the absence of direct impact to the heart.

In major trauma, multiple injuries frequently coexist with BCI. The perioperative physician must be able to anticipate cardiac-induced hemodynamic and rhythm abnormalities; determine the contribution of cardiac trauma to the overall circulatory abnormality caused by hemorrhage, hypothermia, acid–base and electrolyte abnormalities, or various other causes; and based on these findings implement the most appropriate management.

It is infrequent that major cardiac complications occur and require treatment as a result of blunt injury to the heart. However, they may be fatal when they do happen. Often they are difficult to diagnose. The presence of first rib fracture, hemothorax, and free air in the thorax on the chest radiograph suggest the presence of BCI.

As in pulmonary contusion, BCI may be produced by direct precordial impact, crush injury of the chest causing compression of the heart between the sternum and the spine, shearing forces, and blast injuries. Chest pain, angina responding to nitroglycerine, dyspnea, chest wall ecchymosis, and fractures of ribs and/or sternum are some of the suggestive clinical findings. Sternal fracture alone, however, does not predict BCI. EKG, blood troponin I level, and echocardiography are the principal diagnostic tools. In rare instances when ischemic, valvular and septal injuries are suspected, coronary angiography or ventriculography may be indicated.

A 12-lead EKG was considered the best screening test until recently. However, it has been shown that EKG alone cannot rule out BCI [82]. Nonspecific changes such as tachycardia, bradycardia, or occasional atrial or ventricular premature contractions occur in a majority of patients, and usually do not require treatment. Sometimes these arrhythmias appear 12–24 h after the injury. More serious abnormalities such as ST segment or T wave changes, conduction delays, and complex atrial and ventricular dysrhythmias occur less frequently and often require treatment. Although sensitive, the EKG is not specific. Because of its anterior position, the right ventricle is injured more frequently than the left. Thus standard leads, which primarily detect left-sided abnormalities, may miss some right heart events. Nevertheless, right-sided EKG leads (V4R) also did not help diagnose BCI [82]. Delayed (>24 h) serious EKG abnormalities may very rarely occur. However, if these compromising conditions exist, patients should be monitored in a telemetry ward or intensive care unit for at least 24 h. Troponin I measurement is recommended to improve the negative predictive value of EKG to 100 % [82]. If the EKG is abnormal, continuous cardiac monitoring, serum troponin I concentration 6 and 12 h after the injury in hemodynamically stable patients, and echocardiography in hemodynamically unstable patients, should be obtained.

Because of their low specificity, serum creatine kinase (CK) and creatine kinase MB (CK-MB) determinations, tests performed routinely in the past to diagnose myocardial contusion, are no longer performed. Skeletal muscle, colon, lung, liver, and pancreatic tissue contain both CK and CK-MB. Thus in multiple trauma, a positive value may not indicate cardiac injury. Troponin I, on the other hand, is specific for cardiac muscle. However, negative levels of CK-MB or troponin I do not rule out clinically relevant BCI, because in many cardiac trauma patients muscle disintegration is not significant enough to release detectable enzyme levels; yet even a small area of myocardial damage can cause dysrhythmias if it is in a critical location.

Echocardiography may be helpful in many ways in BCI. It provides information about myocardial function (wall motion abnormalities, increased end-diastolic wall thickness), cardiac structural abnormalities (echo-dense areas on the ventricular walls, valve malfunction, hemopericardium, intracardiac thrombi), cardiac preload (end-diastolic area), systolic cardiac function (fractional ventricular area change), and air embolism (air bubbles in the cardiac chambers, patent foramen ovale). Echocardiography can help not only in the diagnosis of BCI, but also in hemodynamic management. Dysrhythmias, unexplained hypotension, and/or heart failure are definite indications for TTE or TEE.

TEE is a much more valuable monitor than TTE, whose usefulness is limited by mechanical ventilation, pleural effusion, pneumothorax, and difficulty in placing the patient in left lateral decubitus position. Furthermore, myocardial contusion, hemopericardium, valvular lesions, hemomediastinum, and aortic rupture are more likely to be recognized with TEE than with TTE. Nevertheless, it is important to eliminate esophageal injury before attempting TEE in chest trauma patients.

BCI increases surgical and anesthetic risk. Although most patients with cardiac chamber perforation do not reach the hospital, some, especially those with atrial lesions, may arrive in the operating room. Thus preoperative information about the nature of the injury is important. An increased incidence of intraoperative dysrhythmias and hypotension in patients with preoperatively diagnosed myocardial contusion has been reported, although it is not entirely clear whether these occurrences were caused by the myocardial injury itself or resulted from the complications of associated injuries. The duration of the effects of BCI is also a relevant issue for the anesthesiologist, since many trauma patients present for surgery days to months after injury. In the vast majority of patients, dysrhythmias last no more than a few days. Ventricular wall motion abnormalities may persist for up to a year, but any increased risk of perioperative complications appears to last for no more than 1 month. An intracardiac thrombus, a well-known complication of myocardial contusion, may be present for more than 1 year after injury, further emphasizing the need for preoperative echocardiography even well after the accident.

The clinical presentation of patients with BCI varies; sometimes more than one compromising condition may be present in the same patient. Orliguet et al. proposed an algorithm describing the management principles for each of these scenarios (Fig. 11.14). Dysrhythmias appear to respond readily to antiarrhythmic agents. Hypotension may be caused by hypovolemia, pump failure, or both. Fluid loading, with monitoring of cardiac function by echocardiography or right heart catheterization, improves hypovolemia. Pump failure is usually caused by right ventricular dysfunction exacerbated by increased pulmonary vascular resistance due to pulmonary contusion, aspiration of gastric contents, or ARDS. An initial right ventricular-free wall dilatation, which results in tricuspid insufficiency, may be followed by leftward ventricular septal shift, which alters the geometry and compliance of the left ventricle, increasing left ventricular filling pressure and decreasing cardiac output. This should by no means be a signal to decrease fluid loading. On the contrary, volume replacement should continue with concomitant use of inotropes and pulmonary vasodilators such as amrinone or milrinone. Positive-pressure ventilation may also be adjusted to minimize intrathoracic pressure and thus right ventricular afterload. As mentioned in the pulmonary contusion section, HFJV or HFOV with its relatively low mean airway pressure may be beneficial in these circumstances. As shown in the algorithm, hemopericardium is treated by surgical drainage. If used, anticoagulants should be stopped. Myocardial infarction and valvular, septal, and coronary vascular injuries are treated in the same way as they would be in the absence of trauma. Of course, severe trauma may dictate surgery before angioplasty, coronary artery bypass, repair of injured cardiac valves, or closing of a septal defect.

Rarely, pump failure may be unresponsive to pharmacologic measures and require cardiac assistance. The ventricular balloon pump has been used in these rare cases of BCI. However, in most patients dysfunction originates from the right ventricle. Thus, if assistance is needed, biventricular assist devices would be preferable.

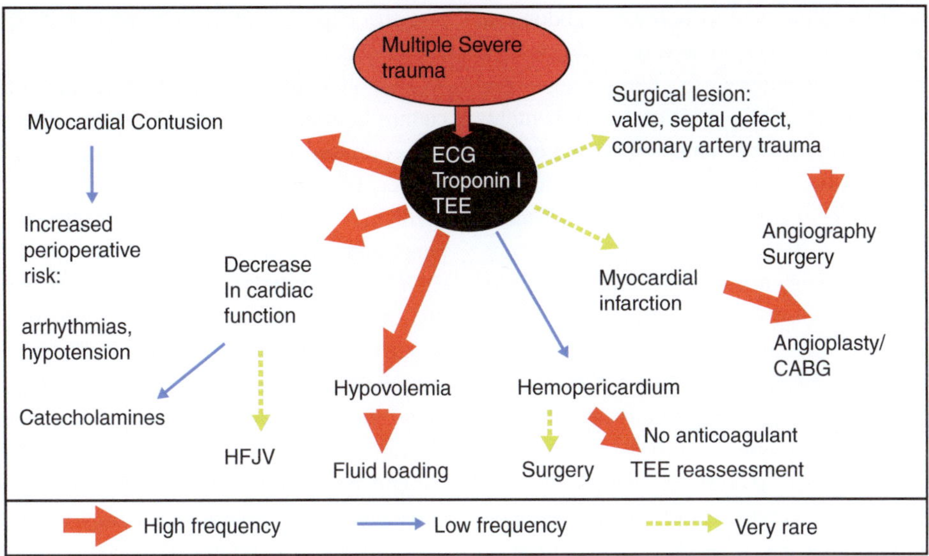

Fig. 11.14 Decision-making tree for management of various clinical scenarios caused by blunt cardiac injury (BCI). Electrocardiogram (ECG), Troponin I, and transesophageal or transthoracic echocardiography (TEE or TTE) are the tools for evaluation. *Arrows* represent the frequency of occurrences of each clinical condition and the frequency of management methods. *Thick arrows* high frequency, *thin arrows* low frequency, and *dotted arrows* rare occurrences. *CABG* coronary artery bypass graft, *HFJV* high frequency jet ventilation. Adapted with permission from Orliaguet G, Ferjani M, Riou B. The heart in blunt trauma. Anesthesiology 2001;95:544

Commotio cordis (agitated heart) is characterized by malignant ventricular arrhythmias such as tachycardia, fibrillation, and even cardiac arrest often resulting in death if not treated. Like BCI, it is caused by a sudden blow to the chest, in this case during the 10–20 ms period of the T-wave upstroke, but it is not associated with any structural cardiac abnormality. It usually occurs to players during contact sports like football or hockey, or recreational games. Commotio cordis is usually managed at the accident scene and consists of defibrillation in patients with ventricular tachyarrhythmias. In those sustaining cardiac arrest, advanced cardiac life support should be instituted [83].

Abdominal Injuries

The abdomen may be injured by both blunt and penetrating trauma, producing solid organ, hollow viscus, and vascular injuries. Motor vehicle accidents and falls are the most common causes of blunt trauma, whereas stab and gunshot wounds are the most common etiologies of penetrating trauma in the civilian population. Intra-abdominal injuries involving intra- and retroperitoneal organs and hemoperitoneum are responsible for the majority of hemorrhage-related deaths from trauma; bleeding is second to head injury as a cause of trauma deaths in the United States [84]. The pattern of injury varies with the cause; blunt trauma produces mostly solid organ damage, primarily involving the spleen and the liver, and only infrequently produces hollow viscus injury, whereas penetrating trauma can injure any of the intra-abdominal organs. Often blunt abdominal trauma is accompanied by injuries to other regions such as the head, spine, thorax, pelvis, and extremities which further complicate management and worsen the outcome [85]. Penetrating injuries, especially gunshot wounds, may involve multiple intra- and extra-abdominal organs, but they are usually located in the vicinity of the original injury. Both blunt and penetrating abdominal injuries may cause severe physiologic disturbances secondary to hemorrhage and peritoneal spilling of gastrointestinal contents [85]. As in injuries of many other anatomical regions, alcohol and illegal drugs play an important role in the occurrence of abdominal injuries [86].

Surgical management of abdominal injuries has evolved over the past three decades. The concept of "Selective Surgical Conservatism" has largely replaced the old concept of mandatory emergency surgical exploration of blunt and penetrating abdominal injuries, unless the presenting clinical picture is complicated by hemodynamic instability, peritonitis, or evisceration, in which case surgical exploration is indicated without delay. Selective surgical conservatism involves nonoperative management by careful evaluation and performing surgery on a timely manner only on those who actually demonstrate signs of injuries that are not amenable to nonoperative treatment. Advanced technology for the diagnosis and treatment of these patients permits application of this concept to clinical practice and avoidance of nontherapeutic laparotomies which may be associated with a complication rate up to 41 %, including small bowel obstruction, ileus, pneumothorax, wound infection, myocardial infarction, iatrogenic visceral injury, and death [87–89]. Nevertheless, minor errors of diagnosis and clinical judgment that delay operative treatment, which is considered a failure of this approach, also may potentially result in major complications that may be fatal in some cases [90]. Patient selection for nonoperative management is essential. Penetrating trauma victims with high ISSs, liver or spleen injury, and a requirement for transfusion are likely to fail the nonoperative approach. In blunt abdominal trauma patients, nonoperative failure is predicted by advanced age, low admission systolic pressure, higher ISS, lower Glasgow coma scores (GCS), metabolic acidosis, and a requirement for transfusion [91]. It is important to have a reliable CT capability and well-established management protocols prescribing observation, serial physical examinations,

and the expected clinical responses to specific CT findings [88].

Hemodynamically unstable trauma patients cannot be transported to a CT suite; the evaluation is limited to physical examination and FAST to decide about surgery. Physical evaluation involves evaluating for evisceration in penetrating trauma, abdominal wall ecchymosis such as the seat belt sign in blunt trauma, abdominal distention, tenderness, and/or guarding. The absence of abdominal distension does not rule out abdominal bleeding. As much as 1 L of blood may accumulate before even a minor change in girth occurs. Additionally, the diaphragm moves upward, allowing more blood to accumulate in the peritoneal cavity without any major change in abdominal circumference. It is more likely for hemorrhagic shock to develop before distension. Physical examination is often unreliable because of patient agitation, distracting injuries, neurologic abnormalities, and factors such as sedation, paralysis, and tracheal intubation. FAST is more accurate than physical examination [92]. However, FAST is operator dependent and as a diagnostic tool it is inferior to multidetector CT evaluation [93]. It has good specificity but only moderate sensitivity. It can diagnose injuries causing intraperitoneal fluid accumulation but not those without it and cannot determine the severity of organ injury [93]. In hemodynamically unstable patients its sensitivity further decreases [93]. Although serial FAST examinations may decrease the risk of false negative results, the limited time to make decisions in unstable patients diminishes the value of this option. Combining the findings of physical examination with those obtained by FAST may improve diagnosis and decision making [92]. The advantages of FAST over CT are completion of the study in one-third the time with less cost and without the danger of radiation [93].

FAST screening is performed by placing a 3.0–5.0 MHz ultrasound probe over the subxiphoid area to detect pericardial fluid, the right upper quadrant to detect blood in the hepatorenal pouch, the left upper quadrant for visualizing perisplenic blood, and above the pubic symphysis to detect blood in the rectovesical pouch [92].

In hemodynamically stable patients the diagnosis of penetrating abdominal trauma is relatively straightforward. Stab wounds may be evaluated with multidetector CT evaluation for anterior injuries to detect peritoneal fluid or organ injury [94]. Alternatively, tractotomy or local wound exploration can be performed to determine whether the peritoneum is involved. Laparoscopy or laparotomy may be indicated after a positive tractotomy. A diaphragmatic knife injury is unlikely to be recognized with CT; laparoscopy is indicated for its evaluation [94]. The unpredictable course of bullets in the body often necessitates laparoscopy and sometimes exploratory laparotomy after a gunshot wound to the abdomen. Although the use of selective nonoperative management for penetrating abdominal injuries is increasing, with a parallel decline in nontherapeutic laparotomies, a recent study using the North American National Trauma database demonstrated 21 and 15 % failure rate of this approach for gunshot wounds and stab wounds, respectively. As mentioned above, patient selection, serial physical examinations during the observation period, and accurate CT interpretations may reduce the failure rate of nonoperative management.

In hemodynamically stable blunt abdominal trauma patients helical CT is commonly used after physical examination of the abdomen. It is reported to have a high sensitivity (97–98 %) and specificity (97–99 %) [92], but in spite of its very high sensitivity for solid organ injuries, its accuracy in blunt bowel and mesenteric injuries is not as high as the commonly used four-slice multidetector CT [95]. With the use of contemporary 64-slice devices, the accuracy of detection of bowel and mesenteric injury has increased [96].

There is some concern about overusing the CT scan for diagnosis of blunt abdominal injuries, as only 20 % of tests are positive and only 3 % indicate surgical intervention [92]. This in the face of increased cost and the risk of contrast induced nephropathy and radiation injuries. The recommended guidelines for using abdominal CT, though not concrete, are positive physical examination, abdominal wall contusions, multiple rib fractures, or visualization of intraperitoneal fluid with FAST [97]. Using a combination of physical examination, FAST, and laboratory tests may reduce the need for further CT evaluation [92].

Laparoscopy is an excellent diagnostic tool in hemodynamically stable blunt and penetrating abdominal trauma patients [98]. Although general anesthesia is needed, it is minimally invasive and decreases the nontherapeutic laparotomy rate and its complications to approximately 1 % [98]. It also allows repair of diaphragmatic, bladder and solid organ injuries. The strengths and weaknesses of currently used diagnostic tools for abdominal trauma are summarized in Table 11.6 [99].

Thoracoabdominal Trauma

Thoracoabdominal trauma is defined as injury that involves both the thoracic and abdominal cavities with or without affecting the diaphragm [100]. These injuries are also characterized as "double jeopardy," given that they involve two anatomic cavities, and their serious nature, complex clinical presentation, and high morbidity and mortality [100, 101].

Patients with penetrating thoracoabdominal injuries are a major challenge for the trauma surgeons and anesthesiologists in all phases of care because of the frequent associated diagnostic and therapeutic pitfalls. Table 11.7, which summarizes some of the clinical characteristics of these injuries from three clinical series, attests to their challenging nature [100–102]. They may result from stab, gunshot, or shotgun wounds. Often they require CPR and tracheal intubation in the field, and resuscitative thoracotomy in the emergency department or the operating room. They frequently present with low revised trauma and high ISSs [101, 102]. Approximately two-thirds of these patients are relatively easy to manage, and laparotomy and closed chest thoracostomy suffices for their care [101, 102]. The remaining one third can tax the diagnostic

Table 11.6 Diagnostic tools in abdominal trauma: strengths and weaknesses

Diagnostic tool	Strength	Weakness
Physical examination	Expeditious, safe, and inexpensive; potential for serial examination	Diagnosis of specific injury (e.g., diaphragm)
Diagnostic peritoneal lavage	Expeditious, safe, and inexpensive	Diagnosis of diaphragmatic injury, hollow viscus injury, retroperitoneal injury; can be oversensitive and nonspecific
Computed tomography	Evaluation of peritoneum and retroperitoneum	Diagnosis of diaphragmatic injury, hollow viscus injury
	Staging of solid-organ injury	Expensive; controversial need for contrast
Ultrasonography	Expeditious, safe, and inexpensive; accurate for free peritoneal fluid	Diagnosis of diaphragmatic injury, hollow viscus injury, penetrating injury, good specificity, but moderate sensitivity
	Potential for serial examinations	Less accurate in the presence of large retroperitoneal hematomas
Laparoscopy	Diagnosis of peritoneal penetration, diaphragmatic injury	Diagnosis of hollow viscus injury, retroperitoneal injury
	Evaluation of bleeding or solid-organ injury	Expensive
	Potential for therapy	
Video-assisted thoracic surgery	Evaluation of lung, diaphragm, mediastinum, chest wall, and pericardium; potential for treatment	Requires operating room; expensive Diagnosis of abdominal injuries

Reprinted from J Am Coll Surg, 189, Villavicencio RT, Aucar JA, Analysis of laparoscopy in trauma, p. 11, Copyright 1999, with permission from Elsevier

and resuscitative abilities of both anesthesiologists and surgeons [101, 102]. The most important preoperative difficulty centers around deciding on which cavity to explore. Often these patients present with unstable hemodynamic and oxygenation status and cannot be safely transported to a CT scan. This, coupled with the need for rapid transport to the operating room for surgical control of injuries, often permits little time for thorough evaluation. Preoperative evaluation of these patients includes history taking; information about the trajectory of the weapon; physical examination of both the thorax and the abdomen; radiographic evaluation; and bedside sonography (EFAST). The remaining part of the evaluation continues in the operating room during the surgical intervention and requires close communication between the anesthesiologist and the surgeon [101, 102].

Inaccurate selection of the thorax or the abdomen as the first anatomical region for surgery occurs in up to 44 % of cases (Table 11.7) [102]. Termed "inaccurate surgical sequencing," this phenomenon is defined as surgically entering a cavity in which there is either no injury or an injury which is less severe than the one in the unopened region [100]. Accurate sequencing is defined as first opening the cavity which contains the most severe or lethal injury [100]. Inaccurate sequencing under these circumstances has negative and possibly devastating implications: prolongation of operating time in a severely compromised patient, promoting the vicious cycle of hypothermia, acidosis, and coagulopathy, and potential mortality [101, 102].

Several pitfalls in this setting cause inaccurate surgical sequencing. Misleading chest tube output, the unreliable nature of physical signs such as abdominal tenderness, persistent hypotension giving the impression that it is caused by the abnormality in the cavity to which surgery is targeted, injuries missed during early evaluation that manifest intraoperatively, or attributing hypotension to bleeding when it is caused by cardiac or other factors [102].

Unreliable chest tube drainage can occur in several ways. Obstruction of the tube by kinking, intraluminal clot, or contact with tissues may direct the clinician's suspicion to the abdomen,

Table 11.7 Clinical features of penetrating thoracoabdominal injuries in three surgical series

	Hirshberg et al. (1995)	Asensio et al. (2002)	Clarke et al. (2011)
	N = 228	N = 254	N = 16
Injury type	GSW, Stab, SGW	GSW, Stab, SGW	Stab
Field CPR	–	14 %	–
Field intubation	–	10 %	–
Resuscitative thoracotomy	10 %	20 %	–
RTS	8.6 ± 2.4	6.04	–
ISS	42 ± 6.8	27	–
Combined laparotomy and thoracotomy	36 %	29 %	100 %
EBL (overall)	–	3,000 mL	–
EBL (combined laparotomy and thoracotomy)	–	6,827 mL	–
Inaccurate surgical sequencing	23 %	44 %	25 %
Negative thoracotomy	22 %	22 % (13 % without resuscitative thoracotomy)	–
Negative laparotomy	11 %	11 %	25 %
Missed injuries	9 %	4 %	25 %
Mortality from missed injuries	–	67 %	–
Reoperation rate for missed injuries	15 %	16 %	–
Reoperation rate for damage control surgery	14 %	–	–
Overall mortality rate	20 %	31 %	19 %
Mortality rate in patients requiring combined laparotomy and thoracotomy	41 %	59 %	19 %

CPR cardiopulmonary resuscitation, *RTS* Revised Trauma Score, *ISS* Injury Severity Score, *EBL* estimated blood loss
Dash in the cells mean that data is not provided
Constructed from data provided in:
Hirshberg A, Wall Jr MJ, Allen MK, Mattox KL. Double jeopardy: thoracoabdominal injuries requiring surgical intervention in both chest and abdomen. J Trauma 1995;39:225–9
Asensio JA, Arroyo Jr H, Veloz W et al. Penetrating thoracoabdominal injuries: ongoing dilemma- which cavity and when? World Journal of Surgery 2002;26:539–43
Clarke DL, Gall TMH, Thomson SR. Double jeopardy revisited: clinical decision making in unstable patients with, thoracoabdominal stab wounds and, potential injuries in multiple body cavities. Injury 2011;42:478–81

while in another scenario blood from the abdominal cavity can find its way to the chest via an injured diaphragm [101]. Such occurrences may develop in many interesting ways. For example, penetrating trauma to the bare area of the liver (area not covered by peritoneum) and diaphragm can present with blood draining from the chest tube, suggesting the need for a thoracotomy when the injury is in the abdomen (Fig. 11.15) [101]. Further, when the abdomen is opened in this situation, no hemoperitoneum may be encountered because under negative pressure, blood drains through the injured diaphragm into the pleural cavity and the chest tube. With the use of bedside sonography (EFAST) preoperatively, some of these pitfalls are eliminated. For example, cardiac tamponade, hemothorax, and the absence or presence of intra-abdominal blood can be easily demonstrated with this diagnostic method.

Intraoperatively the anesthesiologist has an important role in directing the surgeon to the correct surgical target. Apart from careful physiologic monitoring, tracking blood loss and chest tube drainage, observing airway pressures, and replacing lost blood with appropriate blood products, TEE monitoring can help in identifying life-threatening cardiac and great vessel injuries [101]. Likewise hemodynamic and oxygenation changes, when communicated with the surgeon,

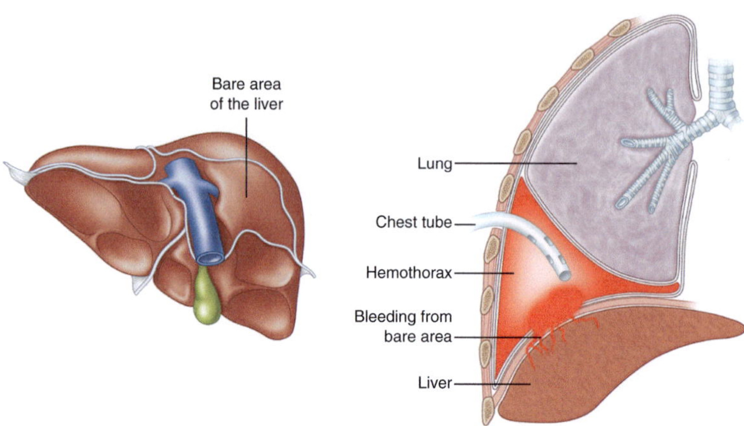

Fig. 11.15 Bare area of the liver (*left panel*), gunshot wound injuring the bare area of the liver, and the diaphragm causing bleeding into the right pleural cavity suctioned by the chest tube (*right panel*)

can help redirect efforts to the alternate cavity in a timely manner. It should be emphasized that in thoracoabdominal injuries, the penetrating object may not only cross the diaphragm but also the midline. Thus the clinician is dealing with three cavities, right chest, left chest, and abdomen, which adds yet more difficulty to preoperative evaluation and intraoperative management.

Management of thoracoabdominal injuries may necessitate several relatively unusual procedures including resuscitative thoracotomy in the emergency department or the operating room, and reoperation to repair missed injuries and to evaluate, irrigate, and debride the abdominal cavity left open as part of the damage control procedure. Resuscitative thoracotomy is performed in 10–20 % of patients with a survival rate of only 10–14 %. Reoperation occurs in about 14 % of these patients. When a wrong cavity is entered, there are several possibilities. For example, after a negative laparotomy, the decision may be to perform a thoracotomy, transabdominal pericardial window, or insertion of a new chest tube for intraoperative diagnosis and intervention. Preservation of the thoracoabdominal barrier is always preferred in order to prevent contamination of the thorax and to preserve diaphragmatic function. Thus an anterolateral thoracotomy may be preferred, at times, over phrenotomy for entry into the thoracic cavity.

Patients with blunt thoracoabdominal injuries often present to the hospital with hypotension, tachycardia, and head injury. Many present without vital signs and require resuscitative thoracotomy in the emergency department, which carries an extremely low rate (1–4 %) of recovery. In one study, age ≥55 years; ISS ≥25; GCS <8; hypotension; massive transfusion; and liver, cardiac, or abdominal vascular trauma were found to be independent risk factors for mortality from these injuries [103].

Although most patients with blunt thoracoabdominal trauma are managed nonoperatively, in some instances operative intervention is indicated. If surgery is contemplated, the abdomen is more likely to be the first cavity to be entered, as the vast majority of organ injuries occur in this cavity [103]. In the thorax, the lung is most commonly damaged, whereas in the abdomen, the spleen and the liver are usually involved. Hollow viscus injuries are not common (2.6 %) and, if present, should be treated expeditiously. The overall mortality from these injuries is about 17–21 % [103]. This rate increases significantly with surgical exploration. Nonoperative management, if possible, is associated with better survival [103].

Pelvic Injuries

Hemorrhage is the most important initial problem and cause of mortality in these injuries: approximately 25 % of these patients present with major bleeding and 1 % with exsanguination. In the vast majority of pelvic fractures bleeding originates from veins injured by bony fragments. Retroperitoneal venous pelvic bleeding is self-limited because of the tamponading effect of the closed pelvic space. In open pelvic fractures, however, venous bleeding will not stop. Pelvic arterial bleeding occurs in about 20 % of patients, usually with severe injuries, and cannot be tamponaded; the retroperitoneal space expands superiorly and anteriorly with continuing bleeding. Occasionally the enlarged retroperitoneal space may reach the anterior abdominal wall, increasing intra-abdominal, intrathoracic, and intracranial pressures. Often pelvic fractures are accompanied by abdominal, thoracic, or cranial injuries with already increased intracavitary pressures. Further compromise of these injured areas results in a substantial increase in morbidity and mortality. Component therapy with blood products should be instituted during this initial period until the bleeding is under control [104].

Shock in these patients is most likely related to hemorrhage, but its source may not necessarily be limited to the pelvis. Associated injuries, especially of the abdomen and the thorax, may be contributing to the hypotension. Rapid evaluation with EFAST, chest radiograph, and laboratory studies may provide some information. The best diagnostic information can be obtained from multidetector CT scanning if the hemodynamic status allows transport of the patient to the radiology unit. Pelvic ring disruption, arterial extravasation (CT blush), and elevated bladder pressure secondary to compression of a hematoma exceeding 500 mL can be detected on CT examination, in addition to the findings of associated injuries. Initially, measures to control pelvic bleeding include use of a pelvic binder, an external fixator, or a C-Clamp that decreases friction between bone fragments. The type and location of arterial bleeding can be diagnosed with pelvic angiography and treated with embolization. If bleeding from associated abdominal, thoracic, and cranial injuries is suspected, their surgical control is usually given priority before

embolization of the pelvic vasculature. The angiography suite must be prepared for anesthesia and resuscitation in advance as soon as angiography and embolization are contemplated.

If embolization must be delayed because of the need for more urgent surgery or for other reasons, control of bleeding in the operating room with extraperitoneal or preperitoneal packing when the pelvic fracture is externally stabilized can aid in reducing blood loss and thus transfusion requirement [105]. Embolization can follow after the patient is stabilized or surgery for associated injuries is completed. Packing is performed by a midline, 6–7 cm long vertical incision starting from the pubic symphysis and continuing superiorly without joining the abdominal incision. The pelvic hematoma is accessed and a few abdominal lap pads are introduced deep into the pelvis.

It has recently been suggested that after external stabilization of the pelvis, extraperitoneal packing under general anesthesia followed by angiography, and, if indicated, arterial embolization may be more beneficial than only external fixation and angiography [105]. Laparotomy for associated abdominal injuries should not be performed indiscriminately; a negative laparotomy in the presence of major pelvic fracture may worsen the overall outcome [106]. Also, during laparotomy every effort should be made to ensure that entry into the retroperitoneal hematoma is avoided in order to prevent uncontrollable bleeding. During preperitoneal packing, the retroperitoneal hematoma is entered outside the peritoneum and bleeding is not likely. Although diagnostic infraumbilical peritoneal lavage, a procedure performed regularly in the past, is seldom utilized now, occasionally it may be used to rule in or rule out an intra-abdominal process. If indicated in the presence of a pelvic fracture, this procedure should be performed above the umbilicus to avoid entry into the retroperitoneal hematoma.

Bladder and urethral injury are also possible in pelvic fractures. A high-riding prostate suggests the presence of this injury. In any case a urethrogram should be performed before insertion of a urinary catheter to avoid further damage to the urethra.

Damage Control Surgery

Trauma to the thorax, abdomen, and pelvis is frequently associated with massive hemorrhage necessitating activation of the massive transfusion protocol. However, administering large quantities of fluids and blood products during a prolonged definitive repair of injuries is likely to result in coagulopathy, hypothermia, and metabolic acidosis, the so-called self-perpetuating vicious cycle which carries a high mortality. In 1983 Stone and colleagues [107] introduced the concept of limiting the extent of surgery in hemorrhaging trauma patients to control of life-threatening bleeding and postponing definitive repair of other injuries, including hollow viscus injuries, to another session. Patients were quickly moved to the postanesthesia care unit (PACU) to be warmed and treated for their metabolic acidosis and coagulopathy. Later, using this strategy Rotondo et al. [108] demonstrated a major improvement in the outcome of patients with abdominal trauma and termed the concept "Damage Control Surgery." Since then this surgical practice has been used extensively in major abdominal trauma and for injuries of other regions including the chest and extremities.

With widespread use of damage control surgery the phenomenon of "Abdominal Compartment Syndrome" surfaced [109]. This results from intra-abdominal hypertension producing multiple organ dysfunction after major abdominal trauma and surgery. The pathophysiology of abdominal compartment syndrome includes a combination of excessive fluid resuscitation, shock-induced inflammatory mediators, surgical manipulation, and closure of the abdominal fascia. The definitive diagnosis is made by measuring urinary bladder pressure through a Foley catheter; this indirectly reflects intra-abdominal pressure. Values exceeding 20–25 mmHg suggest compartment syndrome with the possibility of inadequate organ perfusion and the potential for multiorgan failure and death. Clinical signs include a tense and distended abdomen, elevated airway pressure and $PaCO_2$, and decreased urine output.

This picture is rarely seen at present owing to limited crystalloid infusion, damage control surgery and resuscitation, and an open abdomen strategy. The latter involves leaving the fascia open and covering the abdominal wall with various types of dressings, including a vacuum dressing which permits drainage of exudate formed in the abdominal cavity. These measures have decreased the occurrence of abdominal compartment syndrome and of multiorgan failure. In the majority of patients with open abdomen, fascial closure is performed within a few days. Failure to achieve definitive fascial closure occurs in a small percentage of patients and is related to multiple required reexplorations, development of intra-abdominal abscess, septicemia, acute renal failure, enteric fistula, and ISS >15 [110].

Damage Control Resuscitation

Hypovolemic shock caused by hemorrhage after trauma has both systemic and local consequences, such as development of immunosuppression, systemic inflammatory response, infections, multiple organ failure, and death. The resuscitation technique used until definitive control of blood loss with either direct pressure, tourniquet, suture ligation, or surgery appears to have an influence on the development of these complications. Classically, treatment of hemorrhagic shock involves a bolus infusion of 2 L of warmed crystalloid solution followed by replacement of ongoing fluid or blood loss with isotonic fluids in a 3:1 ratio. Packed red blood cells (PRBCs) are administered only if the patient fails to respond with increased blood pressure to a crystalloid bolus. Although up to 74 % of major trauma patients come to the ER with coagulopathy, generally this complication develops later during classical resuscitation. Consequently, blood components such as fresh frozen plasma (FFP), platelets, and fibrinogen are not part of initial trauma resuscitation. These components are typically given either when coagulopathy is clinically obvious or when laboratory evidence of deficiencies is noted during resuscitation. The classical triggers of component therapy are PT or PTT 1.5–1.8 times normal for FFP, a platelet count <50,000 for platelets, and fibrinogen <0.8 g/L for cryoprecipitate.

The disadvantages of the classical resuscitation strategy are increased bleeding caused by clot dislodgement secondary to blood pressure increase during aggressive fluid resuscitation; the adverse effects of large quantities of fluids, such as hyperchloremic acidosis with large doses of normal saline; a theoretical risk of hyperkalemia with Ringer's Lactate (RL), especially in those with acute kidney injury or chronic renal insufficiency; increased mortality following albumin in severe trauma and burn patients; and the risk of coagulopathy and renal failure with hydroxyethyl starch solutions. Furthermore, it is well known that crystalloids can cause third spacing, which may produce bowel edema, anastomotic leaks, ARDS, and interference with wound healing. Dilutional coagulopathy is another feature of classical resuscitation. Finally, a large amount of fluids can produce hypothermia even when they are warmed.

The so-called bloody vicious cycle is one of the consequences of classical resuscitation in which hemorrhage and acidosis caused by trauma, dilution of coagulation factors and platelets, and hypothermia together produce a clinical scenario which ultimately may lead to death [111]. "Damage control resuscitation," which was introduced during the recent wars, is designed to overcome, at least partly, the problems associated with classical resuscitation. The tenets of damage control resuscitation include selective use of "permissive hypotension," early and aggressive transfusion in a 1:1:1 ratio of PRBCs to FFP to platelets, and selective use of adjuncts. The goals of damage control resuscitation are to minimize bleeding, increase end organ perfusion, prevent coagulopathy, and minimize the risk of multisystem organ failure. During brief periods of permissive hypotension, fluids are withheld or minimized as long as cerebral perfusion is evident and systolic blood pressure remains above a threshold value of 70–80 mmHg. These levels should be maintained until bleeding is controlled. This strategy is thought to decrease both blood loss and transfusion, which are thought to aggravate the inflammatory response and precipitate immunosuppression. Current studies demonstrate some survival benefit with this technique (98 % vs. 83 %) [112].

Early aggressive use of blood transfusion involves the use of whole blood as in the military. In civilian trauma, it is impossible to find whole blood and therefore clinicians have focused on increasing the FFP:PRBC and Platelet:PRBC ratios. The most impressive evidence from the military is Borgman's [113] study, in which he showed a major improvement in survival with transfusion at an equal plasma:PRBC ratio. Subsequent studies by military and civilian investigators showed that an FFP:PRBC ratio between 1:1.3 and 1: 2.0 had a beneficial effect on survival of major trauma patients [112]. The same is also true for Platelets:PRBC ratio [112]. However it should be understood that all of these studies are retrospective in nature and are handicapped by the potential for survival bias.

Recently Lustenberger and colleagues [114] from Germany have tried to compensate for this bias by performing a time-dependent covariate analysis among blunt trauma patients requiring massive transfusion, and demonstrated that even after correcting for survivor bias, an FFP:PRBC ratio of 1:1.5 or greater was associated with improved survival. Studies of platelets:PRBC ratios have shown a similar improvement in mortality although it was not statistically significant.

Bedside thromboelastography (TEG) is being used increasingly during damage control resuscitation to titrate blood component transfusion with favorable results [115]. Previously it was thought that fibrinolysis is unlikely after trauma. It has now been demonstrated by TEG that some major trauma patients develop fibrinolysis requiring administration of cryoprecipitate. Furthermore, TEG has revealed hyperfibrinolysis on admission; this occurs in only 2 % of major trauma patients but is a predictor of a very high mortality [116].

As far as hemostatic adjuncts are concerned, Factor VIIa, once used extensively, is now seldom used, mainly because it does not seem to offer a significant mortality benefit. In addition, it is associated with increased thromboembolic complications, particularly affecting the arterial circulation [117].

Prothrombin complex is composed of a combination of three (II, IX, and X) or four (II, VII, IX, and X) vitamin K-dependent factors. Its major advantage over FFP is its rapid action without the need for large volumes of fluids. It is used primarily in patients with anticoagulant drug-induced coagulopathy [118]. In trauma patients, the use of prothrombin complex may be associated with, decreased transfusion requirement, fewer complications, and shorter length of stay [118]. Tranexamic acid is a promising drug. It works by preventing fibrinolysis. In the CRASH-2 prospective randomized trial, it decreased both all-cause mortality and mortality from bleeding. It should be given within 3 h after injury; otherwise, it is ineffective [117].

References

1. Khandhar SJ, Johnson SB, Calhoon JH. Overview of thoracic trauma in the United States. Thorac Surg Clin. 2007;17:9.
2. Morrison JJ, Rasmussen TE. Noncompressible torso hemorrhage: a review with contemporary definitions and management strategies. Surg Clin North Am. 2012;92:843–58. vii.
3. Ferraris VA, Ferraris SP, Saha SP. The relationship between mortality and preexisting cardiac disease in 5,971 trauma patients. J Trauma. 2010;69:645–52.
4. Council NS. Injury facts. Itasca, IL: National Safety Council; 2012. p. 29
5. Cheynel N, Gentil J, Freitz M, Rat P, Ortega Deballon P, Bonithon Kopp C. Abdominal and pelvic injuries caused by road traffic accidents: characteristics and outcomes in a French cohort of 2,009 casualties. World J Surg. 2011;35:1621–5.
6. Meredith JW, Hoth JJ. Thoracic trauma: when and how to intervene. Surg Clin North Am. 2007;87:95–118. vii.
7. Haynes D, Baumann MH. Management of pneumothorax. Semin Respir Crit Care Med. 2010;31:769–80.
8. Wolfman NT, Myers WS, Glauser SJ, Meredith JW, Chen MY. Validity of CT classification on management of occult pneumothorax: a prospective study. AJR Am J Roentgenol. 1998;171:1317–20.
9. Yadav K, Jalili M, Zehtabchi S. Management of traumatic occult pneumothorax. Resuscitation. 2010;81:1063–8.
10. Enderson BL, Abdalla R, Frame SB, Casey MT, Gould H, Maull KI. Tube thoracostomy for occult pneumothorax: a prospective randomized study of its use. J Trauma. 1993;35:726–9. discussion 729–30.
11. Weissberg D, Refaely Y. Pneumothorax: experience with 1,199 patients. Chest. 2000;117:1279–85.
12. Kulvatunyou N, Vijayasekaran A, Hansen A, Wynne JL, O'Keeffe T, Friese RS, Joseph B, Tang A, Rhee P. Two-year experience of using pigtail catheters to treat traumatic pneumothorax: a changing trend. J Trauma. 2011;71:1104–7. discussion 1107.
13. Bosman A, de Jong MB, Debeij J, van den Broek PJ, Schipper IB. Systematic review and meta-analysis of antibiotic prophylaxis to prevent infections from chest drains in blunt and penetrating thoracic injuries. Br J Surg. 2012;99:506–13.
14. Dominguez KM, Ekeh AP, Tchorz KM, Woods RJ, Walusimbi MS, Saxe JM, McCarthy MC. Is routine tube thoracostomy necessary after prehospital needle decompression for tension pneumothorax? Am J Surg. 2013;205:329–32. discussion 332.
15. Lichtenstein DA, Meziere G, Lascols N, Biderman P, Courret JP, Gepner A, Goldstein I, Tenoudji-Cohen M. Ultrasound diagnosis of occult pneumothorax. Crit Care Med. 2005;33:1231–8.
16. Reissig A, Copetti R, Kroegel C. Current role of emergency ultrasound of the chest. Crit Care Med. 2011;39:839–45.
17. Durham III LA, Richardson RJ, Wall Jr MJ, Pepe PE, Mattox KL. Emergency center thoracotomy: impact of prehospital resuscitation. J Trauma. 1992;32:775–9.
18. Millham FH, Grindlinger GA. Survival determinants in patients undergoing emergency room thoracotomy for penetrating chest injury. J Trauma. 1993;34:332–6.
19. Hopson LR, Hirsh E, Delgado J, Domeier RM, McSwain NE, Krohmer J, National Association of EMSP, American College of Surgeons Committee on Trauma. Guidelines for withholding or termination of resuscitation in prehospital traumatic cardiopulmonary arrest: joint position statement of the National Association of EMS Physicians and the American College of Surgeons Committee on Trauma. J Am Coll Surg. 2003;196:106–12.
20. Moore EE, Knudson MM, Burlew CC, Inaba K, Dicker RA, Biffl WL, Malhotra AK, Schreiber MA, Browder TD, Coimbra R, Gonzalez EA, Meredith JW, Livingston DH, Kaups KL, Group WTAS. Defining the limits of resuscitative emergency department thoracotomy: a contemporary Western

Trauma Association perspective. J Trauma. 2011;70:334–9.

21. Smith CA, Galante JM, Pierce JL, Scherer LA. Laparoscopic transdiaphragmatic pericardial window: getting to the heart of the matter. J Am Coll Surg. 2011;213:736–42.

22. Ho AM, Ling E. Systemic air embolism after lung trauma. Anesthesiology. 1999;90:564–75.

23. Saada M, Goarin JP, Riou B, Rouby JJ, Jacquens Y, Guesde R, Viars P. Systemic gas embolism complicating pulmonary contusion. Diagnosis and management using transesophageal echocardiography. Am J Respir Crit Care Med. 1995;152:812–5.

24. Platz E. Tangential gunshot wound to the chest causing venous air embolism: a case report and review. J Emerg Med. 2011;41:e25–9.

25. Boersma WG, Stigt JA, Smit HJ. Treatment of haemothorax. Respir Med. 2010;104:1583–7.

26. Stewart KC, Urschel JD, Nakai SS, Gelfand ET, Hamilton SM. Pulmonary resection for lung trauma. Ann Thorac Surg. 1997;63:1587–8.

27. Carrillo EH, Block EF, Zeppa R, Sosa JL. Urgent lobectomy and pneumonectomy. Eur J Emerg Med. 1994;1:126–30.

28. Walker JL, Wiersch J, Benson C, Young HA, Dearmond DT, Johnson SB. The successful use of cardiopulmonary support for a transected bronchus. Perfusion. 2012;27:34–8.

29. Brakman M, Buddingh KT, Smit M, Struys MM, Zijlstra JG, van Meurs M. A 28-year-old man with air in the mediastinal space after a car accident. Anesthesiology. 2012;117:878.

30. Singh KE, Baum VC. The anesthetic management of cardiovascular trauma. Curr Opin Anaesthesiol. 2011;24:98–103.

31. Mastroroberto P, Di Mizio G, Colosimo F, Ricci P. Occlusion of left and right coronary arteries and coronary sinus following blunt chest trauma. J Forensic Sci. 2011;56:1349–51.

32. Guo H, Chi J, Yuan M, Qiu Y. Acute myocardial infarction caused by blunt chest trauma: a case report. Int J Cardiol. 2011;149:e80–1.

33. Co SJ, Yong-Hing CJ, Galea-Soler S, Ruzsics B, Schoepf UJ, Ajlan A, Farand P, Nicolaou S. Role of imaging in penetrating and blunt traumatic injury to the heart. Radiographics. 2011;31:E101–15.

34. Teixeira PG, Inaba K, Barmparas G, Georgiou C, Toms C, Noguchi TT, Rogers C, Sathyavagiswaran L, Demetriades D. Blunt thoracic aortic injuries: an autopsy study. J Trauma. 2011;70:197–202.

35. Wong YC, Ng CJ, Wang LJ, Hsu KH, Chen CJ. Left mediastinal width and mediastinal width ratio are better radiographic criteria than general mediastinal width for predicting blunt aortic injury. J Trauma. 2004;57:88–94.

36. Vignon P, Boncoeur MP, Francois B, Rambaud G, Maubon A, Gastinne H. Comparison of multiplane transesophageal echocardiography and contrast-enhanced helical CT in the diagnosis of blunt traumatic cardiovascular injuries. Anesthesiology. 2001;94:615–22. discussion 5A.

37. Lamarche Y, Berger FH, Nicolaou S, Bilawich AM, Louis L, Inacio JR, Janusz MT, Evans D. Vancouver simplified grading system with computed tomographic angiography for blunt aortic injury. J Thorac Cardiovasc Surg. 2012;144:347–54. e1.

38. Azizzadeh A, Keyhani K, Miller III CC, Coogan SM, Safi HJ, Estrera AL. Blunt traumatic aortic injury: initial experience with endovascular repair. J Vasc Surg. 2009;49:1403–8.

39. Gavant ML. Helical CT grading of traumatic aortic injuries. Impact on clinical guidelines for medical and surgical management. Radiol Clin North Am. 1999;37:553–74. vi.

40. Simeone A, Freitas M, Frankel HL. Management options in blunt aortic injury: a case series and literature review. Am Surg. 2006;72:25–30.

41. Goarin JP, Cluzel P, Gosgnach M, Lamine K, Coriat P, Riou B. Evaluation of transesophageal echocardiography for diagnosis of traumatic aortic injury. Anesthesiology. 2000;93:1373–7.

42. Demetriades D, Velmahos GC, Scalea TM, Jurkovich GJ, Karmy-Jones R, Teixeira PG, Hemmila MR, O'Connor JV, McKenney MO, Moore FO, London J, Singh MJ, Spaniolas K, Keel M, Sugrue M, Wahl WL, Hill J, Wall MJ, Moore EE, Lineen E, Margulies D, Malka V, Chan LS. Diagnosis and treatment of blunt thoracic aortic injuries: changing perspectives. J Trauma. 2008;64:1415–8. discussion 1418–9.

43. de Mestral C, Dueck A, Sharma SS, Haas B, Gomez D, Hsiao M, Hill A, Nathens AB. Evolution of the incidence, management, and mortality of blunt thoracic aortic injury: a population-based analysis. J Am Coll Surg. 2013;216:1110–5.

44. Demetriades D. Blunt thoracic aortic injuries: crossing the Rubicon. J Am Coll Surg. 2012;214:247–59.

45. Feezor RJ, Hess Jr PJ, Martin TD, Klodell CT, Beaver TM, Lottenberg L, Martin LC, Lee WA. Endovascular treatment of traumatic thoracic aortic injuries. J Am Coll Surg. 2009;208:510–6.

46. Connolly JE. Hume Memorial lecture. Prevention of spinal cord complications in aortic surgery. Am J Surg. 1998;176:92–101.

47. Demetriades D. Penetrating injuries to the thoracic great vessels. J Card Surg. 1997;12:173–9. discussion 179–80.

48. Wall Jr MJ, Hirshberg A, LeMaire SA, Holcomb J, Mattox K. Thoracic aortic and thoracic vascular injuries. Surg Clin North Am. 2001;81:1375–93.

49. Asensio JA, Chahwan S, Forno W, MacKersie R, Wall M, Lake J, Minard G, Kirton O, Nagy K, Karmy-Jones R, Brundage S, Hoyt D, Winchell R, Kralovich K, Shapiro M, Falcone R, McGuire E, Ivatury R, Stoner M, Yelon J, Ledgerwood A, Luchette F, Schwab CW, Frankel H, Chang B,

Coscia R, Maull K, Wang D, Hirsch E, Cue J, Schmacht D, Dunn E, Miller F, Powell M, Sherck J, Enderson B, Rue III L, Warren R, Rodriquez J, West M, Weireter L, Britt LD, Dries D, Dunham CM, Malangoni M, Fallon W, Simon R, Bell R, Hanpeter D, Gambaro E, Ceballos J, Torcal J, Alo K, Ramicone E, Chan L. American Association for the Surgery of T: penetrating esophageal injuries: multicenter study of the American Association for the Surgery of Trauma. J Trauma. 2001;50:289–96.

50. Ryb GE, Dischinger PC, Ho S. Causation and outcomes of diaphragmatic injuries in vehicular crashes. J Trauma Acute Care Surg. 2013;74:835–8.

51. Morgan BS, Watcyn-Jones T, Garner JP. Traumatic diaphragmatic injury. J R Army Med Corps. 2010;156:139–44.

52. Picetti E, Mergoni M. Images in clinical medicine. Traumatic diaphragmatic hernia. N Engl J Med. 2011;365:e30.

53. DuBose J, Inaba K, Okoye O, Demetriades D, Scalea T, O'Connor J, Menaker J, Morales C, Shiflett T, Brown C, Copwood B, Group ARHS. Development of posttraumatic empyema in patients with retained hemothorax: results of a prospective, observational AAST study. J Trauma Acute Care Surg. 2012;73:752–7.

54. Wall Jr MJ, Soltero E. Damage control for thoracic injuries. Surg Clin North Am. 1997;77:863–78.

55. Kiraly L, Schreiber M. Management of the crushed chest. Crit Care Med. 2010;38:S469–77.

56. Cohn SM, Dubose JJ. Pulmonary contusion: an update on recent advances in clinical management. World J Surg. 2010;34:1959–70.

57. Wu J, Sheng L, Ma Y, Gu J, Zhang M, Gan J, Xu S, Jiang G. The analysis of risk factors of impacting mortality rate in severe multiple trauma patients with posttraumatic acute respiratory distress syndrome. Am J Emerg Med. 2008;26:419–24.

58. Wu JS, Sheng L, Wang SH, Gu J, Ma YF, Zhang M, Gan JX, Xu SW, Zhou W, Xu SX, Li Q, Jiang GY. The impact of clinical risk factors in the conversion from acute lung injury to acute respiratory distress syndrome in severe multiple trauma patients. J Int Med Res. 2008;36:579–86.

59. Battle CE, Hutchings H, Evans PA. Risk factors that predict mortality in patients with blunt chest wall trauma: a systematic review and meta-analysis. Injury. 2012;43:8–17.

60. Miller PR, Croce MA, Bee TK, Qaisi WG, Smith CP, Collins GL, Fabian TC. ARDS after pulmonary contusion: accurate measurement of contusion volume identifies high-risk patients. J Trauma. 2001;51:223–8. discussion 229–30.

61. Becher RD, Colonna AL, Enniss TM, Weaver AA, Crane DK, Martin RS, Mowery NT, Miller PR, Stitzel JD, Hoth JJ. An innovative approach to predict the development of adult respiratory distress syndrome in patients with blunt trauma. J Trauma Acute Care Surg. 2012;73:1229–35.

62. Croce MA, Brasel KJ, Coimbra R, Adams Jr CA, Miller PR, Pasquale MD, McDonald CS, Vuthipadadon S, Fabian TC, Tolley EA. National Trauma Institute prospective evaluation of the ventilator bundle in trauma patients: does it really work? J Trauma Acute Care Surg. 2013;74:354–60. discussion 360–2.

63. Trinkle JK, Furman RW, Hinshaw MA, Bryant LR, Griffen WO. Pulmonary contusion. Pathogenesis and effect of various resuscitative measures. Ann Thorac Surg. 1973;16:568–73.

64. Walkey AJ, Nair S, Papadopoulos S, Agarwal S, Reardon CC. Use of airway pressure release ventilation is associated with a reduced incidence of ventilator-associated pneumonia in patients with pulmonary contusion. J Trauma. 2011;70:E42–7.

65. McCunn M, Habashi NM. Airway pressure release ventilation in the acute respiratory distress syndrome following traumatic injury. Int Anesthesiol Clin. 2002;40:89–102.

66. Maung AA, Luckianow G, Kaplan LJ. Lessons learned from airway pressure release ventilation. J Trauma Acute Care Surg. 2012;72:624–8.

67. Maung AA, Schuster KM, Kaplan LJ, Ditillo MF, Piper GL, Maerz LL, Lui FY, Johnson DC, Davis KA. Compared to conventional ventilation, airway pressure release ventilation may increase ventilator days in trauma patients. J Trauma Acute Care Surg. 2012;73:507–10.

68. Pillow JJ. High-frequency oscillatory ventilation: mechanisms of gas exchange and lung mechanics. Crit Care Med. 2005;33:S135–41.

69. Derdak S, Mehta S, Stewart TE, Smith T, Rogers M, Buchman TG, Carlin B, Lowson S, Granton J. Multicenter Oscillatory Ventilation For Acute Respiratory Distress Syndrome Trial Study I: high-frequency oscillatory ventilation for acute respiratory distress syndrome in adults: a randomized, controlled trial. Am J Respir Crit Care Med. 2002;166:801–8.

70. Slobogean GP, MacPherson CA, Sun T, Pelletier ME, Hameed SM. Surgical fixation vs nonoperative management of flail chest: a meta-analysis. J Am Coll Surg. 2013;216:302–11.

71. Marasco SF, Davies AR, Cooper J, Varma D, Bennett V, Nevill R, Lee G, Bailey M, Fitzgerald M. Prospective randomized controlled trial of operative rib fixation in traumatic flail chest. J Am Coll Surg. 2013;216:924–32.

72. Bhatnagar A, Mayberry J, Nirula R. Rib fracture fixation for flail chest: what is the benefit? J Am Coll Surg. 2012;215:201–5.

73. Paydar S, Mousavi SM, Niakan H, Abbasi HR, Bolandparvaz S. Appropriate management of flail chest needs proper injury classification. J Am Coll Surg. 2012;215:743–4.

74. Simon B, Ebert J, Bokhari F, Capella J, Emhoff T, Hayward III T, Rodriguez A, Smith L. Eastern

Association for the Surgery of T: Management of pulmonary contusion and flail chest: an Eastern Association for the Surgery of Trauma practice management guideline. J Trauma Acute Care Surg. 2012;73:S351–61.

75. Ahn Y, Gorlinger K, Alam HB, Eikermann M. Pain-associated respiratory failure in chest trauma. Anesthesiology. 2013;118:701–8.

76. Ho AM, Karmakar MK, Critchley LA. Acute pain management of patients with multiple fractured ribs: a focus on regional techniques. Curr Opin Crit Care. 2011;17:323–7.

77. Buckley M, Edwards H, Buckenmaier III CC, Plunkett AR. Continuous thoracic paravertebral nerve block in a working anesthesia resident-when opioids are not an option. Mil Med. 2011;176:578–80.

78. Truitt MS, Murry J, Amos J, Lorenzo M, Mangram A, Dunn E, Moore EE. Continuous intercostal nerve blockade for rib fractures: ready for primetime? J Trauma. 2011;71:1548–52. discussion 1552.

79. Leone M, Bregeon F, Antonini F, Chaumoitre K, Charvet A, Ban LH, Jammes Y, Albanese J, Martin C. Long-term outcome in chest trauma. Anesthesiology. 2008;109:864–71.

80. Amital A, Shitrit D, Fox BD, Raviv Y, Fuks L, Terner I, Kramer MR. Long-term pulmonary function after recovery from pulmonary contusion due to blunt chest trauma. Isr Med Assoc J. 2009;11:673–6.

81. Orliaguet G, Ferjani M, Riou B. The heart in blunt trauma. Anesthesiology. 2001;95:544–8.

82. Clancy K, Velopulos C, Bilaniuk JW, Collier B, Crowley W, Kurek S, Lui F, Nayduch D, Sangosanya A, Tucker B, Haut ER. Eastern Association for the Surgery of T: screening for blunt cardiac injury: an Eastern Association for the Surgery of Trauma practice management guideline. J Trauma Acute Care Surg. 2012;73:S301–6.

83. Maron BJ, Estes III NA. Commotio cordis. N Engl J Med. 2010;362:917–27.

84. Isenhour JL, Marx J. Advances in abdominal trauma. Emerg Med Clin North Am. 2007;25:713–33. ix.

85. Farrath S, Parreira JG, Perlingeiro JA, Solda SC, Assef JC. Predictors of abdominal injuries in blunt trauma. Rev Col Bras Cir. 2012;39:295–301.

86. Lima SO, Cabral FL, Pinto Neto AF, Mesquita FN, Feitosa MF, de Santana VR. Epidemiological evaluation of abdominal trauma victims submitted to surgical treatment. Rev Col Bras Cir. 2012;39:302–6.

87. Renz BM, Feliciano DV. Unnecessary laparotomies for trauma: a prospective study of morbidity. J Trauma. 1995;38:350–6.

88. Como JJ, Bokhari F, Chiu WC, Duane TM, Holevar MR, Tandoh MA, Ivatury RR, Scalea TM. Practice management guidelines for selective nonoperative management of penetrating abdominal trauma. J Trauma. 2010;68:721–33.

89. Velmahos GC, Demetriades D, Toutouzas KG, Sarkisyan G, Chan LS, Ishak R, Alo K, Vassiliu P, Murray JA, Salim A, Asensio J, Belzberg H, Katkhouda N, Berne TV. Selective nonoperative management in 1,856 patients with abdominal gunshot wounds: should routine laparotomy still be the standard of care? Ann Surg. 2001;234:395–402. discussion 402–3.

90. Zafar SN, Rushing A, Haut ER, Kisat MT, Villegas CV, Chi A, Stevens K, Efron DT, Zafar H, Haider AH. Outcome of selective non-operative management of penetrating abdominal injuries from the North American National Trauma database. Br J Surg. 2012;99(Suppl 1):155–164.

91. Watson GA, Rosengart MR, Zenati MS, Tsung A, Forsythe RM, Peitzman AB, Harbrecht BG. Nonoperative management of severe blunt splenic injury: are we getting better? J Trauma. 2006;61:1113–8. discussion 1118–9.

92. Nishijima DK, Simel DL, Wisner DH, Holmes JF. Does this adult patient have a blunt intra-abdominal injury? JAMA. 2012;307:1517–27.

93. Gaarder C, Kroepelien CF, Loekke R, Hestnes M, Dormage JB, Naess PA. Ultrasound performed by radiologists-confirming the truth about FAST in trauma. J Trauma. 2009;67:323–7. discussion 328–9.

94. Berardoni NE, Kopelman TR, O'Neill PJ, August DL, Vail SJ, Pieri PG, Singer Pressman MA. Use of computed tomography in the initial evaluation of anterior abdominal stab wounds. Am J Surg. 2011;202:690–5. discussion 695–6.

95. Joseph DK, Kunac A, Kinler RL, Staff I, Butler KL. Diagnosing blunt hollow viscus injury: is computed tomography the answer? Am J Surg. 2013;205:414–8.

96. Petrosoniak A, Engels PT, Hamilton P, Tien HC. Detection of significant bowel and mesenteric injuries in blunt abdominal trauma with 64-slice computed tomography. J Trauma Acute Care Surg. 2013;74:1081–6.

97. Hoff WS, Holevar M, Nagy KK, Patterson L, Young JS, Arrillaga A, Najarian MP, Valenziano CP. Eastern Association for the Surgery of T: practice management guidelines for the evaluation of blunt abdominal trauma: the East practice management guidelines work group. J Trauma. 2002;53:602–15.

98. Johnson JJ, Garwe T, Raines AR, Thurman JB, Carter S, Bender JS, Albrecht RM. The use of laparoscopy in the diagnosis and treatment of blunt and penetrating abdominal injuries: 10-year experience at a level 1 trauma center. Am J Surg. 2013;205:317–20. discussion 321.

99. Villavicencio RT, Aucar JA. Analysis of laparoscopy in trauma. J Am Coll Surg. 1999;189:11–20.

100. Clarke DL, Gall TM, Thomson SR. Double jeopardy revisited: clinical decision making in unstable patients with, thoraco-abdominal stab wounds and, potential injuries in multiple body cavities. Injury. 2011;42:478–81.

101. Hirshberg A, Wall Jr MJ, Allen MK, Mattox KL. Double jeopardy: thoracoabdominal injuries requiring surgical intervention in both chest and abdomen. J Trauma. 1995;39:225–9. discussion 229–31.

102. Asensio JA, Arroyo Jr H, Veloz W, Forno W, Gambaro E, Roldan GA, Murray J, Velmahos G, Demetriades D. Penetrating thoracoabdominal injuries: ongoing dilemma-which cavity and when? World J Surg. 2002;26:539–43.

103. Berg RJ, Okoye O, Teixeira PG, Inaba K, Demetriades D. The double jeopardy of blunt thoracoabdominal trauma. Arch Surg. 2012;147:498–504.

104. White C, Hsu J, Holcomb JB. Hemodynamically unstable pelvic fractures. Injury. 2009;40:7.

105. Cothren CC, Osborn PM, Moore EE, Morgan SJ, Johnson JL, Smith WR. Preperitonal pelvic packing for hemodynamically unstable pelvic fractures: a paradigm shift. J Trauma. 2007;62:834–9. discussion 839–42.

106. Verbeek D, Sugrue M, Balogh Z, Cass D, Civil I, Harris I, Kossmann T, Leibman S, Malka V, Pohl A, Rao S, Richardson M, Schuetz M, Ursic C, Wills V. Acute management of hemodynamically unstable pelvic trauma patients: time for a change? Multicenter review of recent practice. World J Surg. 2008;32:1874–82.

107. Stone HH, Strom PR, Mullins RJ. Management of the major coagulopathy with onset during laparotomy. Ann Surg. 1983;197:532–5.

108. Rotondo MF, Schwab CW, McGonigal MD, Phillips III GR, Fruchterman TM, Kauder DR, Latenser BA, Angood PA. 'Damage control': an approach for improved survival in exsanguinating penetrating abdominal injury. J Trauma. 1993;35:375–82. discussion 382–3.

109. Fabian TC. Damage control in trauma: laparotomy wound management acute to chronic. Surg Clin North Am. 2007;87:73–93. vi.

110. Dubose JJ, Scalea TM, Holcomb JB, Shrestha B, Okoye O, Inaba K, Bee TK, Fabian TC, Whelan J, Ivatury RR, Group AOAS. Open abdominal management after damage-control laparotomy for trauma: a prospective observational American Association for the Surgery of Trauma multicenter study. J Trauma Acute Care Surg. 2013;74:113–20. discussion 1120–2.

111. Cohen MJ. Towards hemostatic resuscitation: the changing understanding of acute traumatic biology, massive bleeding, and damage-control resuscitation. Surg Clin North Am. 2012;92:877–91. viii.

112. Kobayashi L, Costantini TW, Coimbra R. Hypovolemic shock resuscitation. Surg Clin North Am. 2012;92:1403–23.

113. Borgman MA, Spinella PC, Perkins JG, Grathwohl KW, Repine T, Beekley AC, Sebesta J, Jenkins D, Wade CE, Holcomb JB. The ratio of blood products transfused affects mortality in patients receiving massive transfusions at a combat support hospital. J Trauma. 2007;63:805–13.

114. Lustenberger T, Frischknecht A, Bruesch M, Keel MJ. Blood component ratios in massively transfused, blunt trauma patients—a time-dependent covariate analysis. J Trauma. 2011;71:1144–50. discussion 1150–1.

115. Tapia NM, Chang A, Norman M, Welsh F, Scott B, Wall Jr MJ, Mattox KL, Suliburk J. TEG-guided resuscitation is superior to standardized MTP resuscitation in massively transfused penetrating trauma patients. J Trauma Acute Care Surg. 2013;74:378–85. discussion 385–6.

116. Cotton BA, Harvin JA, Kostousouv V, Minei KM, Radwan ZA, Schochl H, Wade CE, Holcomb JB, Matijevic N. Hyperfibrinolysis at admission is an uncommon but highly lethal event associated with shock and prehospital fluid administration. J Trauma Acute Care Surg. 2012;73:365–70. discussion 370.

117. Tobin JM, Varon AJ. Review article: update in trauma anesthesiology: perioperative resuscitation management. Anesth Analg. 2012;115:1326–33.

118. Bolliger D, Gorlinger K, Tanaka KA. Pathophysiology and treatment of coagulopathy in massive hemorrhage and hemodilution. Anesthesiology. 2010;113:1205–19.

Musculoskeletal Injuries and Microvascular Surgery

David W. Boldt and Zarah D. Antongiorgi

Musculoskeletal Injuries

Musculoskeletal injuries are a major source of disability and represent a significant proportion of the global disease burden. According to the World Health Organization, non-fatal musculoskeletal injuries comprised of open wounds and fractures are cited as the most common reason for hospital admission worldwide [1, 2]. The extremities suffer the majority of the musculoskeletal insults, primarily as a consequence of blunt trauma from falls and traffic collisions. In high-income countries, rates of extremity injuries are 500/100,000 per year, while rates in low-middle income countries are two to five times greater at 1,000 to 2,600/100,000 per year [1]. According to the 2012 National Trauma Data Bank which collects admission data from 744 trauma centers in the USA and Canada, a total of 278,100 lower extremity and 223,650 upper extremity injuries were treated in 2011, accounting for 65 % of all injuries treated [3]. Around 30 % of trauma patients admitted to the hospital will have sustained serious limb threatening injuries [4]. Injury severity is often dependent on the energy level of the injuring forces. Open comminuted fractures with significant soft-tissue loss affecting nerve and vascular supply can result after high-energy impact. Low-energy injuries are characterized by compression and shear forces resulting in simple fractures with crush and avulsion injuries. Machinery-related accidents are also responsible for a significant number of civilian extremity injuries. Rotational and shear forces on extremities can cause degloving injuries in which the skin and subcutaneous fat are avulsed off of the underlying tissue. Electrical injury due to electrocution is another source of musculoskeletal injury, most often involving the upper extremity. High-voltage injuries, defined as exposure to electrical energy >1,000 V, cause extensive soft-tissue damage leading to thrombosis and tissue necrosis, resulting in a relatively high amputation rate. Traumatic amputation is the loss of a limb or limb component at the time of traumatic injury. Traumatic amputation represents a special category of extremity injury in which upper or lower limb replantation may be possible if the amputated limb is relatively intact.

Mortality after trauma in civilians is well described and follows a bimodal distribution with peaks in incidence among men aged 16–40 and again in females older than 65 years of age [4]. A survey of the specific demographics of orthopedic trauma at Level I trauma centers in Australia also demonstrated a bimodal

D.W. Boldt, M.D., M.S. (✉)
Department of Anesthesiology and Critical Care, UCLA
David Geffen School of Medicine, Ronald Reagan UCLA
Medical Center, 757 Westwood Plaza, Suite 3325,
Los Angeles, CA 90095, USA
e-mail: dboldt@mednet.ucla.edu

Z.D. Antongiorgi, M.D.
Department of Anesthesiology, UCLA David Geffen
School of Medicine, Ronald Reagan UCLA Medical
Center, 757 Westwood Plaza, Suite 3325, Los Angeles,
CA 90095, USA

C.S. Scher (ed.), *Anesthesia for Trauma*, DOI 10.1007/978-1-4939-0909-4_12,
© Springer Science+Business Media New York 2014

distribution of age with a major peak among 21–30 year olds and a minor peak in patients 81 years and older [5]. Of the patients who were under 65 years of age, which accounted for 70 % of all trauma patients, 71 % were male, while men over 65 years of age only accounted for 30 % of orthopedic traumas. The nature of the extremity injury was also distributed according to age; older patients suffered significantly more femoral fractures while tibia, pelvic, and spine fractures were more prevalent among younger patients [5].

Among military personnel, blast and penetrating injuries are the major causes of musculoskeletal injury and are associated with open fractures and vascular damage more often when compared to civilians. The nature of combat has changed dramatically since World War I and so too have the musculoskeletal injuries of war. In reviewing registry data over a 5-year period of the Iraq and Afghanistan conflicts, the incidence of musculoskeletal combat casualties was 3.06 per 1,000 deployed personnel per year, with fractures occurring in 3.41 per 1,000 deployed personnel a year [6]. Explosive blasts accounted for 82 % of the injuries while only 14 % were due to gunshot wounds. Soft-tissue injuries comprised the bulk of the injuries while fractures were the second most prevalent type of injury. Tibia and fibula fractures were most common, of which 20 % were open, followed by hand and forearm fractures. Prompted by the increasing incidence of bombings and attacks outside of war zones, such as the bombing incident at the 2013 Boston Marathon, blast and explosive injury is a topic of new concern for civilian trauma physicians. Primary blast injury often damages lungs, eardrums, and hollow viscera via propagation of a blast wave through air-fluid filled cavities of the body. Secondary blast injury is characterized by the tissue penetration of explosive shrapnel while a tertiary blast injury is the blunt trauma that results from being thrown down or being buried by structural collapse. In an attempt to better understand how terrorist-related musculoskeletal injuries compare with more common motor-vehicle injuries data from the

Israeli National Trauma Registry was evaluated during a year of increasing suicide bombings and gunman attacks. Data analysis revealed that motor-vehicle victims were more likely to have closed fractures and crush injuries while terrorist-related victims had a significantly higher incidence of open fractures and soft-tissue injury with neurovascular compromise. Additionally, terrorist-related victims were more likely to need an operative intervention and had an overall 4 % mortality compared to 2.9 % mortality for the motor-vehicle victims [7].

Assessment of Injury

Whatever the etiology, the severity of extremity injury should be categorized based on involvement of the bones, blood vessels, nerves, and soft tissue. A "mangled" extremity is one where three of the four components are damaged often leaving the limb unrecognizable [8]. Determining whether an injured limb requires primary amputation or is potentially salvageable is not always straightforward and depends not only on the extent of extremity injury, but also on the presence of other life threatening injuries. When a bony fracture and soft-tissue laceration are in communication with one another, the fracture is considered an open fracture. The annual incidence of open long bone fracture is estimated at 11.5 per 100,000 and the tibia is the most commonly affected long bone [9]. The presence of an open fracture significantly increases the risk of amputation and is most often the result of high-energy motor-vehicle collisions. In 1976, Gustilo and Anderson developed a grading system for the classification of open fractures [10]. The system classifies open fractures into three categories, types I–III, with grading based on wound size, extent of soft-tissue damage and contamination, adequacy of soft-tissue coverage, and associated arterial injury. Higher grades are associated with higher rates of infection. An update to the Gustilo system in 1984 subdivided type III injuries into three subcategories, (A, B, and C) to help further delineate the extent of soft-tissue injury,

Table 12.1 Gustilo open fracture classification system

Gustilo grade	Open fracture definition
I	Wound <1 cm, minimal contamination, simple fracture
II	Wound >1 cm, moderate soft-tissue damage with adequate bone coverage
IIIA	High-energy trauma with extensive soft-tissue laceration with gross contamination but adequate soft-tissue coverage of fractured bone
IIIB	Extensive soft-tissue injury loss with periosteal stripping and bone exposure
IIIC	Open fracture associated with arterial injury requiring repair

contamination, and bone coverage (Table 12.1). Injuries classified as IIIB or higher often require some form of flap coverage. Type IIIC fractures are characterized by vascular injury requiring repair. Bony injuries, especially comminuted fractures, increase the chance of concomitant vascular injury. Suspicion for vascular injury should be high when patients present with fractures of the proximal humerus, humeral shaft, distal radius or ulna, mid-femur and mid- or distal tibia-fibula. When overt signs of a vascular injury are present such as pulsatile bleeding, bruit over the wound, expanding hematoma, loss of pulses or signs of distal ischemia patients should be taken to the operating room for immediate intervention. If the patient has stable skeletal injuries with a minimally contaminated wound and stable hemodynamics a direct repair is safe to pursue. Otherwise, a temporary intraluminal shunt should be considered. In the setting of limb injury, the threshold to perform a fasciotomy should be low, as the risk of compartment syndrome with complex extremity injuries is high.

Although interobserver variability is a cited drawback of the Gustilo system, it provides a reasonably efficient and universal manner of conveying the extent of injury among care providers. Attempts to further expand Injury Severity Score (ISS) classification systems such as the Mangled Extremity Score (MESS); Limb Salvage Index (LSI); and Nerve Injury, Ischemia, Soft-Tissue Injury, Skeletal Injury and Age of Patient Score (NISSSA) to help guide decision making regarding limb salvage or amputation have not been widely accepted [11]. Whichever scoring system is used, it is recommended that the classification of the injury takes place in the operating room where the full extent of soft-tissue and bony damage can be appreciated [12]. It is especially important to note that many of these classification systems were formulated in the 1990s, and surgical technique has progressed significantly since then. Many injuries that might have been designated for amputation 20 years ago are now able to be successfully salvaged.

Microsurgery: A History

Trauma management follows the "life before limb" adage, but once the patient is stabilized the ultimate goal of surgery in musculoskeletal injury is tissue and limb preservation. The ability to salvage tissues has progressed dramatically with the development and rapid expansion in the field of microsurgery. In 1902 Alexis Carrel developed the fundamental technique for anastomosing blood vessels, a feat which earned him the Nobel Prize in Medicine in 1912 [13]. In 1916, heparin was discovered and allowed vascular repair without complication of thrombosis. In 1960, Jacobson and Suarez created the concept of microvascular surgery by introducing the use of a microscope to suture vessels between 0.5 and 3 mm in diameter. During the early 1960s, the American plastic surgeon Harry Buncke earned the title of the "father of microsurgery" through his work with rabbit ear replantation and monkey toe transfers. In 1962, Malt and MaKhann performed the first arm replantation on a 12-year-old boy in Boston. At the same time, orthopedic surgeons in Japan were actively researching the field of microsurgery in traumatology and in 1968 Tamai and Komatsu were the first to apply the principles of microsurgery for the first successful thumb replantation. The 1970s saw advancements in tissue transfers including skin, muscle, and bone to fill defects and reconstruct damaged tissue. First came pedicle flaps where tissues were transferred to the recipient site while remaining attached to a vascular pedicle at the donor site. In 1973, Daniel and Taylor performed the first groin free flap in which the vascular supply is cut and reconnected microsurgically to recipient site vessels [13]. In 1989 the first perforator free flap was described by Koshima and Soeda, which used smaller perforator vessels from the graft site, obviating the need to sacrifice larger blood vessels and muscle groups [14–16]. With the more recent development of the free-style perforator flap, the surgeon has the ability to create custom fit grafts from any anatomic region where a Doppler signal is present. Continued advancements in surgical methods and equipment have improved flap survival rates to over 95 % at most microsurgical centers [14].

Microsurgery in Trauma

As mentioned earlier, basic trauma management principles dictate prioritizing immediate threats to life before dealing with musculoskeletal injuries. Basic tenets to musculoskeletal injury include starting with hemorrhage control. Once stabilized, a thorough assessment of the injured extremity is necessary to determine a plan of action, including wound size and extent of damage to soft-tissue, nerves, vessels, and bone. If there is vascular injury and a flap is a treatment option, angiography or ultrasonography should be considered to evaluate adequacy of vascular targets [17]. Skeletal components need to be stabilized, usually via external fixation, and early and aggressive debridement of necrotic tissue under tourniquet control is paramount before embarking on any reconstruction [15, 18]. In 1986, Godina revolutionized the concept of emergency microsurgical reconstruction in traumatic extremity injury [19]. He published a report of 532 patients with complex lower extremity injuries who were divided into three groups based on timing of free flap reconstruction. Patients who had reconstructive surgery after 72 h of injury had significantly worse outcomes with regards to bone healing time, flap failure rate, infection rate, length of hospital stay, and need for multiple surgical interventions. Based on his findings, recommendations were to perform flap reconstruction of traumatic injuries within 72 h of the insult under the hypothesis that early wound coverage would prevent microbial seeding, protect the wound from dessication, optimize blood flow to promote healing and provide a better revascularization environment before onset of edema or fibrosis thereby increasing the chance of earlier mobility. Since Godina's publication, controversy has existed regarding the optimal timing for flap reconstruction. In light of newer irrigation and wound management (VAC) systems, better wound care is possible and delay of reconstruction may need further investigation [20]. One of the problems with early flap reconstruction is the lack of uniformity in the definition of timing. In 1995, Ninkovic et al. introduced terminology akin to wound healing nomenclature to help compare and contrast institutional practices of timing for free flap closure [18]. According to Ninkovic, primary free flap closure is one that occurs within 12–24 h of injury. Delayed primary closure occurs within 2–7 days, and secondary closure occurs after 7 days. Early reconstruction is contraindicated in unstable patients incapable of tolerating long operations or for patients who would have superior functional outcomes with amputation and prosthesis. Delayed reconstruction is often better tolerated in lower extremity injuries compared to upper extremity injuries where immobilization leads to earlier contractures from tendon adhesions and stiffening of joints. To avoid this complication, joints must be actively or passively moved to maintain range of motion [15].

Significant soft-tissue defects with exposed vital tissues such as bones, tendons, nerves, and vessels require flap coverage and reconstruction. The use of free flap tissue transfer for traumatic injuries is usually preferred over pedicle flap since donor-site burden is minimal and further surgical trauma to the already compromised limb can be avoided. Most free flaps are composite flaps, containing multiple tissue types such as bone, muscle, skin, adipose, fascia, or nerves. Free flaps may be contraindicated in patients with significant comorbidities that may impair flap success, such as diabetes, tobacco use, or use of immunosuppressants and steroids [15]. When considering free flap selection, consideration must be given to the size of the defect, tissues needing to be repaired, level of contamination, available vessels, the aesthetics of both the donor and recipient sites, and the impact on patient's mobility and need for sensation. Myocutaneous flaps are excellent for filling large defects and provide excellent blood flow, which is ideal for highly contaminated or chronically infected wounds. Fasciocutaneous flaps are less bulky and provide well-contoured coverage for more shallow wounds. Additionally, they are ideal for staged reconstructive procedures since they are amenable to elevation with minimal fibrotic scarring [16]. Examples of fasciocutaneous flaps include the parascapular/scapular flap, anterolateral thigh flap, radial forearm flap, and lateral arm flap. Vascularized bone from the humerus can be included in the lateral arm flap. The radial forearm flap can be utilized for composite reconstruction by incorporating vascularized bone from the radius, palmaris tendon, antebrachial cutaneous nerve, and flexor radialis muscle [15]. Commonly used musculocutaneous flaps include the lastissimus dorsi, serratus, rectus abdominis and the gracilis. The latissumus dorsi is a workhorse flap that provides a long pedicle with many options for reconstructing large defects and options to combine with the scapular/parascapular flaps. In terms of bone reconstruction and transfer, the fibula provides an excellent source of free vascularized bone for long bony defects and mandibular replacement.

Anesthesia for Microvascular Surgery

Optimizing the Anesthetic for Flap Success

The success rate of microvascular free tissue transfer has improved greatly over the last few decades, and currently has been reported to be 91–99 % [21]. Accounting for this broad difference in success are a variety of medical, surgical,

and anesthetic variables. Careful preoperative assessment, treatment, and optimization of comorbid disease can minimize the medical risk factors contributing to graft failure. Preexisting hypertension, coronary artery disease, alcohol abuse, smoking, and uncontrolled diabetes have all been shown to correlate with graft failure and/or increased complication rates [21]. Surgical variables affecting graft success have been studied extensively, and techniques have improved significantly in the past few decades. These improvements are most responsible for the observed increase in the success rate of these surgeries. Among anesthetic variables that can be manipulated and optimized in order to increase the success of the surgery and the survival of the transplanted tissue, there are some that are generally agreed upon to have real, observable effects on outcomes while others remain heavily debated. The goal of this chapter is to discuss the effects of these anesthetic variables on microvascular perfusion, to differentiate what is known and agreed upon from what is still debated, and to define areas in which further research is needed prior to drawing more conclusions.

There are several stages associated with a typical microvascular free flap procedure, and the events that occur during each stage of surgery should be taken into consideration when administering an anesthetic. The first step is induction of general anesthesia, which results in peripheral vasodilation resulting in relative hypovolemia and loss of thermoregulation leading to heat loss. The first surgical stage involves the preparation of tissue at the recipient site, which leads to blood loss and insensible fluid loss. The next stage involves harvesting of the flap, which is characterized by tissue denervation leading to sympathectomy and vasodilation of the tissue's vascular bed. It is during this stage following clamping of the vessels that primary ischemia begins. Anaerobic metabolism within the flap results in the accumulation of lactate, calcium, and proinflammatory mediators, decreasing intracellular pH [22]. The severity of these changes is proportional to the duration of ischemia. Furthermore, handling of the flap by the surgeons, as well as the aforementioned release of local inflammatory mediators due to tissue ischemia and anaerobic metabolism, both lead to vasoconstriction within the flap [21]. Subsequent reperfusion of the flap, although restoring normal cellular metabolism, results in a degree of ischemia-reperfusion injury that is dependent on the length of ischemia time and the accumulation of inflammatory mediators [21]. In addition, the restoration of blood flow exposes the new flap to circulating catecholamines. The new flap is also at risk for significant tissue edema due to a compromised vascular endothelial barrier and the absence of lymphatic drainage. Tissue edema results in an increase in extravascular pressure, which reduces the vascular transmural pressure and ultimately leads to decreased blood flow [23]. Furthermore, it is important to note that although denervated free flaps have lost their intrinsic sympathetic tone, the artery and vein maintain innervation and therefore respond to local, physical, and chemical stimuli, such as cold, manipulation, and medications [22]. These factors all combine to influence the perfusion of the newly vascularized free flap. Hypoperfusion of the flap following reperfusion is considered secondary ischemia, and it is this period of ischemia that can be minimized with the appropriate anesthetic technique [22].

Of the anesthetic variables that can be manipulated, intraoperative temperature control and the maintenance of normothermia are among the most important. Intraoperative hypothermia can result in a number of complications, including coagulopathy leading to increased blood loss, higher rate of wound infections, and delayed wound healing [21, 22]. Even mild degrees of hypothermia result in vasoconstriction in peripheral vascular beds and decreased tissue perfusion. In addition, hypothermia increases blood viscosity, further worsening tissue perfusion. Active warming of the patient should begin prior to induction with the use of blankets or forced air warmers, and continued intraoperatively by warming IV fluids and blood products. A patient under anesthesia begins to cool rapidly following induction due in part to widespread vasodilation and anesthetic-related disruption of the body's normal thermoregulatory response [21]. It is therefore recommended that active warming measures be initiated as soon as possible prior to or immediately following induction. In addition, warming measures should be continued into the postoperative period for at least 24 to 48 h to ensure optimal flap perfusion [22].

Another intraoperative variable shown to have effects on outcomes is the restrictive use of blood transfusions. Although increasing hemoglobin levels results in increased oxygen delivery to the tissues, increased hematocrit levels lead to increased blood viscosity, which decreases blood flow and tissue perfusion. Despite this, the ideal hematocrit at which the balance between oxygen content and decreased viscosity results in the optimal oxygen delivery to the tissue remains in question. Current literature does not support a higher transfusion threshold for patients undergoing microvascular surgery as compared to other types of major surgery, especially when the hazards and increased morbidity and mortality of the transfusion of even a single unit of blood is considered [24]. In determining the transfusion threshold, patient-specific factors such as a history of active cardiac disease, rather than surgical factors should dictate a higher target hematocrit, and this should be determined on a patient-by-patient basis. In fact, normovolemic hemodilution in these patients has been shown to be beneficial, as it increases tissue perfusion and improves skin flap survival through decreased blood viscosity [25]. In an animal model using hamsters, Erni et al. measured the oxygen tension and blood flow in the microcirculation of ischemic skin flaps following the induction of normovolemic hemodilution by isovolemic exchange of 50 % of their total blood volume with colloid solution [25]. He demonstrated that normovolemic hemodilution resulted in improved blood flow as well as increased tissue oxygenation in the ischemic flap tissue. This supports the role for a restrictive transfusion strategy in the management of patients undergoing microvascular surgery and suggests the need for future studies to confirm these results in humans to delineate the optimal hematocrit goal below which the detrimental effects of decreased oxygen content outweigh the beneficial effects of improved blood flow through decreased viscosity.

The ideal anesthestic technique for microvascular surgery remains unclear. Given the lengthy surgical time of most of these operations, general anesthesia, either by itself or in combination with regional anesthesia, is commonly chosen. Awake patients under regional anesthesia are often unable to tolerate laying flat for many hours and therefore require some degree of sedation, which may lead to hypercarbia, hypoxia, and respiratory acidosis, all of which may compromise flap perfusion. In addition to these concerns, there is evidence that the vasodilation and decreased systemic blood pressure that accompanies epidural anesthesia can lead to a vascular "steal" phenomenon, reducing blood flow to the free flap. Twisk et al. used measured laser Doppler flow to demonstrate that an epidural infusion decreased flap blood flow by about 30 % [26]. The presumed mechanism is that the sympathectomy induced by the epidural results in vasodilation of the skin leading to a reduction of perfusion to the deeper tissues. They also noted an increased rate of bleeding, making it difficult to perform the vascular anastomoses. Similarly, Erni et al. found that epidural anesthesia resulted in a 20–30 % decrease in blood flow to the free flap [27], while causing no change in the blood flow to intact tissue. Based on these findings, it is possible to conclude that the vasodilation produced by an epidural anesthetic is greater in the intact, normally innervated tissue than in the denervated tissue of the free flap, effectively resulting in a redistribution of blood flow away from the free flap in a vascular "steal" phenomenon.

On the other hand, in many major surgeries, the use of epidural anesthesia results in a reduced incidence of deep venous thrombosis, decreased intraoperative blood loss, and faster postoperative recovery [23]. Within the field of microvascular surgery, a few studies have demonstrated promising results. Strecker et al. in 1988 published a paper on 20 successful cases of lower extremity free tissue transfer under epidural anesthesia [28]. They reported better maintenance of normothermia and decreased

risk of thrombosis at the vascular anastomosis site, which they attributed to the increased postoperative lower limb blood flow induced by the epidural sympathectomy. Similarly, in a retrospective cohort study 5 years later, Scott et al. found a lower rate of both microvascular and major complications in 35 patients who had free flap surgery to the lower extremity under combined epidural and general anesthesia versus general anesthesia alone [29]. There were no flap losses in the epidural group, compared with one flap loss in the non-epidural group, and four more major complications in the nonepidural group, three of which were microvascular complications.

Despite these reports, concern still exists for a circulatory steal phenomenon leading to decreased flap perfusion when using epidural anesthesia. Animal studies analyzing the effects of epidural anesthesia in the setting of microvascular surgery have produced mixed results. Some have demonstrated a reduction in blood flow to the transplanted tissue, while others seem to show no difference [30, 31]. One of these studies [30], which also looked at the volume status of the animals at the time of epidural anesthesia, demonstrated two important points. First, in the animals who were slightly hypovolemic, the reduction in mean arterial blood pressure, cardiac output, and microcirculatory blood flow were all greater when compared to the animals who were euvolemic, emphasizing the importance of maintenance of euvolemia in patients in whom epidural anesthesia is chosen as a technique. Second, following the initiation of a phenylephrine infusion in these same animals, the cardiac output remained unchanged and, although a significant increase in the mean arterial pressure was noted, this resulted in only a minor increase in microcirculatory blood flow, suggesting that the use of phenylephrine to offset the epidural-induced sympathectomy does not completely restore flap tissue perfusion. Until more human studies are performed with reliably reproducible results, it is unlikely that the use of epidural anesthesia in these surgeries will become routine.

Although there seems to be no consensus regarding the benefit of epidural anesthesia in microvascular surgery for free tissue transfer, it appears that these surgeries can be performed safely with epidural anesthetics, despite the demonstrated reduction in flap blood flow that occurs following sympathectomy. Thus, epidural anesthesia cannot be ruled out, particularly in patients whose comorbid conditions make general anesthesia too risky. It is well known that when compared to general anesthesia alone, epidural anesthesia results in a lower risk of respiratory complications and lower pain scores following major surgery. In a large randomized trial of 915 high-risk patients undergoing major abdominal surgery with or without epidural anesthesia, the epidural group had a statistically significant lower incidence of postoperative respiratory failure [32]. In addition, this group had lower pain scores in the first three postoperative days. However, no statistically significant differences were observed in the rates of postoperative 30-day mortality, cardiovascular events, sepsis, gastrointestinal complications, hepatic failure, or renal failure. There were no major adverse consequences of epidural catheterization. Alam et al. [33] reported three successful cases of gracilis-free muscle transfer under epidural anesthesia in two patients deemed too high risk for general anesthesia (two of the flaps were done on the same patient). One of the patients was suffering from respiratory failure due to recent acute respiratory distress syndrome (ARDS) secondary to severe community acquired pneumonia, precluding the use of general anesthesia. The other patient had symptomatic right heart failure secondary to ischemic cardiomyopathy due to long-standing diabetes mellitus. These cases emphasize the important role for epidural anesthesia in selected patients undergoing free tissue transfer to the lower extremity whose comorbid conditions make the risks of general anesthesia prohibitively high.

If general anesthesia is chosen as the preferred anesthetic technique for microvascular surgery, there are several other variables that may affect surgical outcomes. The effect of volatile anesthetics on systemic macrohemodynamics has been well studied, with all of the agents having similar effects [34]. Recently, their effects on regional blood flow and microcirculation have been further investigated. In healthy patients exposed to the usual concentrations of inhaled or intravenous anesthetics, vital organ perfusion remains intact and regional blood flow is adequate [34]. Within microvascular beds, it has been demonstrated that general anesthesia results in increased tissue blood volume and decreased microvascular resistance [35]. This effect was the same whether general anesthesia was conducted with sevoflurane plus remifentanil or propofol plus remifentanil, suggesting that microvascular changes are not significantly different between the two methods [35]. Although microvascular hemodynamic changes appear to be no different between inhaled and intravenous agents, other studies have suggested the potential of other benefits of one agent over the other. Bruegger et al. used a method called venous congestion plethysmography to measure the capillary filtration coefficient (CFC), an index of microvascular permeability, in twenty patients undergoing elective breast surgery [36]. They found that general anesthesia with sevoflurane resulted in a significant decrease in the CFC, while propofol caused no change in CFC. Theoretically, the authors explain, this decreased CFC should result in less extravasation of fluids into the interstitial space. Interestingly, and in support of their theory, they found a significant positive correlation between the decrease in CFC and the perioperative fluid requirements, which were decreased in the sevoflurane group. The lowering of CFC, the authors conclude, resulted in less leakage of fluid into the interstitial space, and in turn less hypovolemia and a lower need for fluid replacement. In addition, this reduction in CFC should result in less interstitial edema formation that may lead to impaired tissue perfusion. Though these results are interesting, further studies are needed to confirm these findings and establish their clinical relevance. Another beneficial effect of volatile anesthetic agents is that it has been demonstrated that the halogenated anesthetic agents isoflurane, sevoflurane, and desflurane result in ischemic preconditioning of the myocardium, conferring a cardioprotective effect [34].

This should be considered when choosing the ideal anesthetic agent, particularly in patients with known cardiovascular disease or those at high risk for such disease.

In regard to the intravenous anesthetic agent propofol, several studies have demonstrated its free radical scavenging properties and its ability to attenuate neutrophil activity [37–39]. In microvascular surgery in particular, neutrophil activity within the flap leads to free radical production, which may contribute to flap failure. Therefore, propofol may be able to improve flap survival. This theory was tested by Tyner et al. who studied propofol-mediated reduction in neutrophil activity in a rat model of skin flaps [40]. To assess for neutrophil activity, flap biopsies were taken at regular intervals and analyzed for myeloperoxidase enzyme content. They found that flap survival was significantly increased with the use of propofol, and this correlated well with the observed reduction in myeloperoxidase activity associated with its use. This implicates a possible important role for propofol use during microvascular surgery, either as the sole general anesthetic in a TIVA technique, or as part of a combined regimen along with an inhaled volatile anesthetic. Further studies are needed to confirm this data and determine the optimal dose needed to observe this beneficial effect of propofol on flap survival.

During emergence from anesthesia, every effort should be taken to avoid coughing and straining due to endotracheal tube irritation, which increases venous pressure within the flap and leads to decreased perfusion and worsened congestion. Many techniques can be employed to achieve this, such as ensuring adequate pain control prior to emergence, the administration of endotracheal lidocaine, deep extubation, or switching from an endotracheal tube to a laryngeal mask airway prior to emergence.

Hemodynamic Support

Despite marked improvements in the success of microvascular free flap surgery in the past few decades, perioperative hypoperfusion and subsequent ischemia remains a continued threat to flap survival. Maintaining adequate perfusion to the flap both intraoperatively and in the early postoperative period continues to be a challenge in these patients due to the many factors that influence microvascular blood flow. Patient comorbidities, anesthetic technique, intravascular volume status, body temperature, and the degree of edema in the flap are several of the factors that can alter perfusion to the newly reanastomosed flap. Maintenance of perfusion to the surgical site may dictate the need for vasoconstrictors, vasodilators, and inotropic agents in order to optimize perfusion pressure, vascular resistance, or cardiac output. In the past two decades, multiple studies have been performed with various agents, some with mixed results and others with fairly conclusive evidence, all suggesting that a singular and superior agent to achieve these goals does not exist. When conceptualizing the factors that determine microvascular blood flow and considering the known effects of specific pharmacologic agents on these factors, it is easy to hypothesize that certain agents may have overall benefit to the success of flap surgery through increased perfusion. The evidence, however, does not always agree with our theories. Milrinone, for example, is a phosphodiesterase III (PDE-III) inhibitor, an enzyme found in cardiac and peripheral vascular muscle. Inhibition of PDE-III leads to a decreased breakdown of cyclic adenosine monophosphate (cAMP), resulting in increased intracellular ionized calcium levels and the subsequent dual effect of improved cardiac contractility and arterial vasodilation via the induction of contractile protein phosphorylation and relaxation in vascular smooth muscle. Arterial vasospasm has been identified as an element in flap failure. In theory, milrinone might augment the cardiac output and promote peripheral arterial vasodilation, improving graft survival via increased perfusion and prevention of arterial vasospasm. Jones et al. tested this theory in a double-blinded randomized controlled clinical trial [41]. Eighty-eight patients undergoing elective microvascular free flap surgery were randomized to receive either a milrinone infusion or placebo with normal saline throughout surgery. The use of milrinone did not result in improved graft survival or prevent arterial vasospasm. It did, however, result in the increased need for vasopressor support.

Nevertheless, inotropes may result in improved graft function by increasing cardiac output and tissue perfusion. Scholz et al. studied the use of dobutamine, another inotropic agent with systemic vasodilatory effects, in twenty patients undergoing elective free tissue transfer surgery [42]. After completion of the microvascular anastomoses, dobutamine infusions of 2, 4, and 6 mcg/kg/min were initiated in a randomized order and both mean and maximum blood flow in the anastomosed recipient artery were measured with an ultrasonic flowmeter by an investigator who was blinded to the infusion rates. At 4 and 6 mcg/kg/min, investigators noticed a significant increase in both mean and maximum blood flow in the recipient anastomosed artery as well as an increased cardiac output. However, overall surgical outcomes were not investigated in this study. It is unclear if the investigators used vasopressors in their study cohort due to the arterial vasodilation that accompanies the use of dobutamine. They did note, though, that as the infusion rate of dobutamine increased, so did the heart rate and systemic mean arterial blood pressure of the study patients. This is in contrast to the study by Jones, in which milrinone resulted in decreasing mean arterial pressure, necessitating the use of vasopressors. The difference in these observations may be attributable to the differing mechanism of action of dobutamine. Like milrinone, dobutamine results in increased inotropy and cardiac output while causing systemic vasodilation, but this effect is achieved through direct stimulation of beta-1 and beta-2- receptors. Beta-1 stimulation results not only in inotropy, but also in chronotropy, thereby increasing heart rate. It has been hypothesized that this increase in chronotropy maintains mean arterial pressure minimizes the need for vasopressor support. These conclusions have been confirmed by other studies. Suominen et al. studied microvascular blood flow during transversus

rectus abdominus muscle (TRAM) flap surgery and compared the effects of dopamine and dobutamine infusions [43]. Dobutamine at 8 mcg/kg/min resulted in increased CO, decreased SVR, but increased flap blood flow. Dopamine at the same infusion rate resulted in an increased CO but unchanged SVR and flap blood flow. Comparing the same two agents in a swine model, Cordeiro et al. [44] demonstrated that blood flow in musculocutaneous flaps is primarily determined by CO and SVR. Similarly, in this study, dobutamine resulted in increased CO and flap blood flow, while dopamine resulted in no change in flap blood flow despite an increase in CO. Phenylephrine, a direct acting alpha-agonist, results in decreased flap blood flow at doses from 1.5–3 mcg/kg/min [44]. Decreasing the resistance to blood flow, as measured by a fall in SVR, while increasing CO and maintaining a reasonable mean arterial perfusion pressure appears to strike the ideal balance of hemodynamics for microvascular procedures.

The use of vasoconstrictors in an attempt to maintain adequate perfusion pressure may prove to be particularly contentious in the realm of microvascular surgery. In normal peripheral tissue with an intact sympathetically innervated microcirculation, it is well known that the use of vasopressors such as phenylephrine results in decreased blood flow. Maier et al. studied the effects of phenylephrine on the sublingual microcirculation of fifteen patients during cardiopulmonary bypass (CPB) for coronary artery bypass graft surgery and found that the increased perfusion pressure induced by phenylephrine at a constant CPB flow rate resulted in decreased microcirculatory blood flow in the sublingual mucosa [45]. This finding can be explained by microvascular shunting, as the phenylephrine-induced decrease in blood flow was observed only in the capillary vessels and not in medium-sized vessels. Of note, despite a significant reduction of perfusion pressure following the initiation of CPB (from 73 to 47 mmHg), no changes in microcirculatory blood flow were observed in the absence of phenylephrine. It was not until phenylephrine infusion was initiated, raising the perfusion pressure from 47 to

68 mmHg, that the reduction in microcirculatory blood flow was seen.

These observations of the effects of phenylephrine, however, were in microvascular blood flow in normal tissue. Investigators have looked into whether sympathetically denervated tissue, such as that in a surgical flap, responds in the same way to these agents. In a porcine model of free latissimus dorsi flaps to the lower extremity, Banic and colleagues studied the effects of both phenylephrine and nitroprusside on systemic cardiac output and microcirculatory blood flow using laser Doppler flowmetry (LDF) while infusing the agents either systemically or locally through the peripheral artery feeding the flap [46]. Systemic nitroprusside resulting in a decrease of mean arterial pressure by 30 % did not affect CO but decreased the flap blood flow by 40 %. Locally infused nitroprusside at a dose proportionate to the systemic dose based on the fraction of global CO present in the feeding artery of the flap resulted in an increase of flap blood flow by 20 %. Of further interest is the fact that systemic phenylephrine at a dose resulting in a 30 % increase in MAP did not result in any significant changes in CO or flap blood flow. Locally infused phenylephrine, on the other hand, decreased total flap blood flow by 30 %. The finding that systemic nitroprusside decreases flap blood flow confirms that a vascular steal phenomenon occurs as a result of widespread systemic vasodilation, similar to that which occurs during general anesthesia or due to neuraxial anesthesia-induced sympathectomy. It is not surprising that locally infused vasodilators or vasoconstrictors result in increased or decreased flap blood flow, respectively. Interestingly, however, systemic phenylephrine seemed to have no effect of flap blood flow, contrary to the findings of other studies. It should be kept in mind, however, that the dose of systemic phenylephrine used in this study was only 1 mcg/kg/min. It is conceivable that with higher doses of phenylephrine, the effects of decreased flap perfusion demonstrated in other studies may become more pronounced. In another porcine model of vertical rectus abdominus muscle rotational flaps, Massey et al. studied the effects of systemic phenylephrine and epinephrine on both the pedicle artery blood flow and microvascular perfusion [47]. Phenylephrine infusions at doses of 20, 40, and 80 mcg/min resulted in decreases in both the pedicle artery blood flow and the microvascular perfusion of the flap. Epinephrine, on the other hand, at doses of 0.5, 1, and 2 mcg/kg/min increased the flows in both the pedicle artery and in the microvascular circulation. The epinephrine-induced increases in perfusion paralleled the increases in systemic MAP and CO that were observed with increasing doses. Of note, a key difference between the Banic and Massey studies lies in the types of flaps studied. The Banic group studied free flaps, while the Massey group studied rotational or pedicled flaps. The vascular hemodynamics of these two types of flaps are significantly different. In free flaps, the combination of the total sympathectomy of the vessels within the tissue and the damage of ischemia-reperfusion injury result in microvasculature that does not respond in the usual manner to systemically administered vasoactive agents. In rotational or pedicled flaps, the flap is released and twisted around the neurovascular bundle without interrupting blood flow. This results in intact sympathetic innervation of the pedicle artery and the avoidance of significant ischemia-reperfusion injury, leading to flap blood flow that responds more readily to these systemic agents [22]. In regard to the findings in the Massey study with systemic epinephrine infusions, the observed increases in flap perfusion are likely related to the increased CO, similar to the effect of dobutamine as previously discussed. In addition to the increased CO due to epinephrine's beta-adrenergic effects, the alpha-adrenergic stimulation led to an increased MAP. Unlike the isolated alpha-agonist effects of phenylephrine, the presence of alpha agonism in conjunction with beta agonist activity may confer some benefit.

Norepinephrine, another mixed alpha and beta-adrenergic agent, was studied by Hiltunen et al. [48]. Using a pig model of microvascular and pedicled rectus abdominus myocutaneous flaps, the technique of microdialysis was used to detect metabolic changes as an early marker for decreased tissue perfusion and ischemia. Two significant findings resulted. First, sevoflurane-induced hypotension to a MAP of 50 mmHg resulted in no changes in flap perfusion as assessed by microdialysis. In addition, correction of the hypotension with norepinephrine to a MAP of 80–90 mmHg with a mean dosage of 2.84 mcg/kg/min also resulted in no changes in microvascular perfusion. These findings emphasize that pressure does not always correlate with flow and highlight our lack of understanding of the hemodynamic principles governing these complex vascular networks. In spite of these findings, norepinephrine remains a poorly studied agent, and further studies are needed before its routine use in microvascular surgery can be recommended.

The blood flow in a microvascular flap is very complex, influenced by multiple factors, many of which are unable to be practically measured or predicted in modern anesthetic and surgical practice. Systemic arterial pressure is the major determinant of the pressure gradient across the transplanted flap, but flow can also decrease due to an increase in venous pressure or an increase in resistance due to vasoconstriction or vasospasm. Although transplanted tissue is sympathetically denervated, the blood vessels can still vasospasm due to cold, manipulation, systemic catecholamines, and metabolites generated by ischemia [42]. The impact of vasoactive medications on the flap is also influenced by the method of administration (i.e., local vs. systemic, as demonstrated by Banic et al.), the flap model itself (pedicled vs. free flaps), and other factors, which are currently unknown or unable to be measured. It is important to take into account that in clinical practice, a patient's systemic circulatory response to these medications can exhibit significant individual variability and is often unpredictable. Without question, the realm of microcirculatory hemodynamics is full of unanswered questions, and its future is wide open for further research and clinical experimentation to improve our understanding and management of these complex situations.

Intravascular Volume Status and Blood Viscosity

The goal of fluid management in microvascular surgery is to maintain intravascular fluid volume at a level that is optimal for tissue blood flow and oxygenation, while avoiding fluid overload, which leads to worsening of flap edema and congestion. Flaps have a tendency to develop edema due to a lack of lymphatic drainage and a reduced ability to reabsorb interstitial fluid. Ideally, the replacement fluid should not be able to pass freely through the damaged endothelium. In theory, colloids might be a better choice versus crystalloids in this patient population. However, recent data does not support the use of colloid solutions over crystalloids [23]. Despite this, many experts recommend colloids, specifically synthetic colloids, as the preferred replacement fluid in microvascular surgery [49]. The superiority of synthetic colloids over albumin, however, has not been demonstrated, and concerns regarding their negative effects on coagulation have limited their use in microvascular surgery. A more pertinent dilemma is not the type of fluid that is administered, but the amount. Multiple studies have demonstrated the beneficial effects and improved outcomes resulting from a restrictive fluid management strategy in major surgery. Zhong and colleagues performed a retrospective review of 354 cases of microsurgical free flap breast reconstruction performed at a single institution over a period of 8 years and discovered that the IV fluid infusion rate over the first 24 h, when standardized for weight and after adjusting for the effects of other covariables, significantly predicted postoperative complications, especially at the extremes of crystalloid infusion rates [50]. Similar findings on the negative effects and complications associated with increased fluid administration in free flap surgery have been demonstrated in other studies, making a restrictive fluid management strategy in microvascular surgery a topic that is generally agreed upon [50]. It is unclear, however, how practitioners are to manage intraoperative fluid administration, avoiding the hypotension and increased vasopressor needs associated with hypovolemia, while preventing the postoperative complications and tissue edema associated with overzealous fluid replacement. Conventional methods used to monitor the intravascular volume status, such as central venous pressure (CVP) monitoring, have been shown to be inaccurate in guiding fluid replacement [51–55]. This is not surprising, considering the limitations of CVP monitoring in determining fluid balance and predicting the hemodynamic response to fluid administration. One has to make a series of assumptions when using CVP values to assess volume status, including the equality of the pressure–volume relationship between the right and left atrium and the preservation of the Frank–Starling mechanism in relation to volume loading and cardiac contractility. Further, following fluid administration, changes in CVP are delayed when compared to changes in measured stroke volume. In fact, the CVP will not appreciably increase until the venous capacitance system is full, making its measurement much less sensitive to minute-by-minute hemodynamic changes that might be affected by volume administration. With these limitations in mind, it is easy to explain why flow monitoring, rather than pressure monitoring, with the use of devices that measure cardiac output is more accurate and is associated with less complications than the use of CVP to guide fluid replacement [53, 54]. Traditionally, the pulmonary arterial Swan-Ganz catheter has been used to measure cardiac output via the principle of thermodilution. The complications associated with its placement, however, have limited its widespread use in non-cardiac surgery. Recently, esophageal Doppler (ED) has been used intraoperatively to assess for volume status with more promising results [52–54]. By the placement of an esophageal probe, stroke volume, cardiac output, and fluid responsiveness are measured by using the principle of Doppler shift in the descending thoracic aorta. This method has been proven in several studies to be superior to the use of CVP in guiding fluid replacement and has even been shown to be comparable to the determination of cardiac output by pulmonary

arterial catheter thermodilution technique [56]. The use of ED for hemodynamic monitoring has been successfully described in major cardiothoracic, orthopedic, vascular, laparoscopic, and open abdominopelvic surgeries. In a study by Figus and colleagues, ED was compared to CVP monitoring to guide intraoperative fluid replacement in 104 patients undergoing free perforator flap surgery [56]. They found that the use of ED resulted in less intraoperative positive fluid balance, less monitoring and flap complications, and a shorter hospital stay. In addition, there were no complications related to ED monitoring. Additionally, the relatively short time it takes to place the device when compared with a central venous catheter led to statistically significant shorter anesthetic times. The only limitation to the use of ED is that its accuracy is dependent on correct positioning within the esophagus, typically 30–40 cm from the lips of the patient, and the probe may need to be repositioned multiple times intraoperatively.

Other devices are available that use analysis of the arterial pressure waveform rather than Doppler to measure stroke volume and predict the response to fluid administration. These devices require the presence of an arterial catheter but are not subject to the same positioning variables as esophageal probes. The usefulness of these devices in major surgery, particularly in high-risk patients, has been demonstrated [57]. Although the use of cardiac output monitoring to guide fluid therapy is rapidly expanding in multiple surgical specialties, its use in microvascular surgery is still not widespread. In a survey conducted in the United Kingdom and published in 2011 by Chalmers et al. the anesthesiology departments of 40 major head and neck surgery centers performing free flap surgery were surveyed on their use of intraoperative cardiac output monitoring. Of the 40 departments surveyed, only three reported the routine use of intraoperative CO monitoring to guide fluid replacement [58]. These three centers all used arterial pressure waveform monitoring devices. In other surgical specialties, use of these devices have resulted in shorter hospital stays and reduced morbidity related to fluid balance [51, 53–55,

57]. The cost of these devices, as well as the reluctance to trust the data gathered from them, have been cited as reasons why their use is not increasing as rapidly as would be expected. As costs decrease over time and further studies are done to validate the accuracy of measurements taken from these devices, it is likely that their use will increase. In addition, data demonstrating reduced hospital stays and decreased morbidity with these devices may prompt closer cost-benefit analyses, resulting in increased use of these devices in spite of their cost. Until that time, and at centers where these capabilities are not available, the careful use of intraoperative fluids guided by traditional methods such as CVP monitoring, arterial blood gas analysis, and urine output remain an important part of the intraoperative and perioperative care of these patients.

Intraoperative Hemodynamic Monitoring

As previously discussed, the routine use of intraoperative cardiac output monitoring is not common. However, the presence of moderate to severe cardiac disease in some patients makes monitoring of CO necessary to guide therapy in the form of inotropic support. This can be achieved with a Swan-Ganz pulmonary arterial catheter, intraoperative transesophageal echocardiography, esophageal Doppler, or arterial pressure waveform analysis. The use and interpretation of transesophageal echocardiography requires specialized training in order to accurately and safely guide care, and this generally limits its use by the non-cardiac anesthesiologist. The use of the Swan-Ganz catheter for measurement of CO via thermodilution is still considered by many to be the standard of care. For some anesthesiologists and surgeons, the decreased risk of major complications of less invasive CO monitors, such as esophageal Doppler and arterial pressure waveform analyzers, might make their use preferable provided they are available. The decision of which monitor to use is less relevant than managing a low CO in the setting

of cardiomyopathy. The previous discussion and evidence presented comparing the major inotropic agents milrinone and dobutamine, and the mixed vasopressor and inotropic agents epinephrine and dopamine, should help determine the appropriate agent for a particular patient. For example, in a patient with known existing coronary artery disease in whom tachycardia should be avoided, milrinone might be preferred over dobutamine, given the chronotropic effects of dobutamine.

Non-pharmacologic means of supporting CO should also be considered. Jennings et al. describe the case of a patient who presented for elective maxillofacial free flap reconstructive surgery with an ejection fraction of 15 % secondary to alcohol use and chemotherapy toxicity [59]. An intra-aortic balloon pump was placed prior to induction in order to aid with perioperative augmentation of CO and flap perfusion. In addition to IABP support at 1:1 augmentation, dobutamine and norepinephrine infusions were used to maintain hemodynamics. The surgery was successful, and the patient was admitted to the ICU postoperatively for continued IABP support and discharged to the ward on the sixth postoperative day. Although dobutamine and norepinephrine were required intraoperatively to maintain hemodynamics, the authors concluded that the placement of the IABP helped to minimize the use of vasopressor agents, which can unfavorably affect graft perfusion in a dose-dependent manner.

Techniques in Microcirculation Perfusion Monitoring

As mentioned above, patient comorbidities, anesthetic technique, intravascular volume status, body temperature, and the use of vasoactive medications can all alter perfusion to the newly reanastomosed tissue. Decreasing any one or more of these variables to a critical threshold could result in inadequate perfusion to the anastomotic site for even a brief, albeit crucial, time period, resulting in graft ischemia and failure. Most flap failures occur within the first 3 days following surgery [21]. Postoperative flap perfusion monitoring is a largely clinical assessment, based on skin color, turgor, capillary refill, surface temperature, bleeding with pinprick, and bedside Doppler ultrasound signal monitoring of the feeding artery. While these techniques are easy to perform, they require experience to interpret and have a number of limitations. Recently, noninvasive techniques to monitor the perfusion of the newly vascularized tissue have improved and been introduced into clinical and experimental research. Some of these techniques include orthogonal polarization spectral (OPS) imaging, side stream dark-field (SDF) imaging, and LDF. OPS and SDF imaging noninvasively visualize and quantify blood flow within the microcirculation via erythrocyte movement detection [34]. LDF, on the other hand, measures microvascular blood flow through the detection of frequency shifts that occur when low-energy laser light encounters erythrocytes [34]. The probes used in these techniques have been implemented into handheld, needle, and endoscopic devices, resulting in broader applicability and further ease of use in clinical settings. Over time, these techniques may become part of routine intraoperative and even postoperative monitoring to ensure adequate microcirculatory perfusion.

Postoperative Considerations

It has been demonstrated that the blood flow in a free tissue flap decreases to about half of its pre-transfer rate during the first 6–12 h after surgery [23]. Therefore, vigilant postoperative management is paramount in maintaining perfusion to the graft. Postoperative care of patients following flap surgery involves the maintenance of many of the same parameters as were discussed intraoperatively, such as normothermia, normovolemia, and moderate hemodilution. Judicious administration of IV fluids is important to avoid hypervolemia, which leads to worsening flap edema, and hypovolemia, both resulting in decreased flap perfusion. Postoperative shivering should be avoided, as it increases oxygen

consumption and causes peripheral vasoconstriction. Pain should be adequately controlled in order to avoid catecholamine release and subsequent vasoconstriction, but over sedation should also be avoided as hypoventilation leads to hypercarbia, hypoxemia, and acidosis, all of which can also result in catecholamine release and vasoconstriction. NSAIDs should be avoided given the risk of perioperative hematoma formation.

In summary, despite the recent advances and research in the area of microvascular surgery and the anesthetic variables affecting its outcomes, flap ischemia and failure remain problematic. Although much is known about the effects of certain variables on flap perfusion, data is either lacking or conflicting in many other areas, indicating the need for further research to determine their influence on flap outcomes.

References

1. World Health Organization. The burden of musculoskeletal conditions at the start of the new millennium, Report of a WHO Scientific Group, WHO Technical Report Series 919. Geneva: WHO; 2003.
2. Mock C, Cherian MN. The global burden of musculoskeletal injuries challenges and solutions. Clin Orthop Relat Res. 2008;466:2306–16.
3. Nance ML. National Trauma Data Bank Annual Report 2012. American College of Surgeons.
4. Esposito TJ, Brasel KJ. Epidemiology. In: Mattox KL, Moore EE, Feliciano DV, editors. Trauma. 7th ed. New York: MGraw-Hill Medical; 2013.
5. Urquhart DM, Edwards ER, Graves SE, Williamson OD, McNeil JJ, Kossman T, et al. Characterisation of orthopedic trauma admitted to adult level I trauma centres. Injury Int J Care Injured. 2006;37:120–7.
6. Belmont PJ, McCriskin BJ, Hsiao M, Burks R, Nelson KJ, Schoenfeld AJ. The nature and incidence of musculoskeletal combat wounds in Iraq and Afghanistan (2005–2009). J Orthop Trauma. 2013;27:e107–13.
7. Weil YA, Peleg K, Givon A, Mosheiff R. Musculoskeletal injuries in terrorist attacks—a comparison between the injuries sustained and those related to motor vehicle accidents, based on a national registry database. Injury Int J Care Injured. 2008;39:1359–64.
8. Bumbasirevic M. Current management of the mangled upper extremity. Int Orthop. 2012;36:2189–95.
9. Court-Brown CM, Rimmer S, Prakash U, McQueen MM. The epidemiology of open long bone fractures. Injury. 1998;29:529–34.

10. Gustilo R, Anderson J. Prevention of infection in the treatment of one thousand and twenty five open fractures of the long bones: retrospective and prospective analysis. J Bone Joint Surg Am. 1976;58:453–8.

11. Durrant CAT, Mackey SP. Orthoplastic classification systems: the good, the bad, and the ungainly. Ann Plast Surg. 2011;66:9–12.

12. Okike B, Bhattacharyya T. Current concepts review: trends in the management of open fractures. J Bone Joint Surg. 2006;88:2739–48.

13. Tamai S. History of microsurgery. Plast Reconstr Surg. 2009;124:282e–94e.

14. Spyropopulou A, Jeng SF. Microsurgical coverage reconstruction in upper and lower extremities. Seminars Plast Surg. 2002;20:24–42.

15. Saint-Cyr M, Wong C, Buchel EW, Colohan S, Pederson WC. Free tissue transfers and replantation. Plast Reconstr Surg. 2012;130:858e–78e.

16. Tintle SM, Levin LS. The reconstructive microsurgery ladder in orthopedics. Injury Int J Care Injured. 2013;44:376–85.

17. Management of Complex Extremity Trauma. American College of Surgeons Committee on Trauma Ad Hoc Committee on Outcomes. 2005.

18. Ninkovic M, Voight S, Dornseifer U, Lorenz S, Ninkovic M. Microsurgical advances in extremity salvage. Clin Plast Surg. 2012;39:491–505.

19. Godina M. Early microsurgical reconstruction of complex trauma of the extremities. Plast Reconstr Surg. 1986;78:285–92.

20. Hill JB, Vogel JE, Sexton KW, Guillamondegui OD, Del Corral GA, Shack RB. Re-evaluating the paradigm of early free flap coverage in lower extremity trauma. Microsurgery. 2013;33(1):9–13.

21. Gardiner MD, Nanchahal J. Strategies to ensure success of microvascular free tissue transfer. J Plast Reconstr Aesthet Surg. 2010;63(9):e665–73.

22. Pereira CMB, et al. Anesthesia and surgical microvascular flaps. Rev Bras Anesthesiol. 2012;62(4):563–79.

23. Hagau N, Longrois D. Anesthesia for free vascularized tissue transfer. Microsurgery. 2009;29(2):161–7.

24. Hajjar LA, et al. Transfusion requirements after cardiac surgery: the TRACS randomized controlled trial. JAMA. 2010;304(14):1559–67.

25. Erni D, et al. Haemodynamics and oxygen tension in the microcirculation of ischaemic skin flaps after neural blockade and haemodilution. Br J Plast Surg. 1999;52(7):565–72.

26. van Twisk R, et al. Is additional epidural sympathetic block in microvascular surgery contraindicated? A preliminary report. Br J Plast Surg. 1988;41(1):37–40.

27. Erni D, et al. Effects of epidural anaesthesia on microcirculatory blood flow in free flap patients under general anaesthesia. Eur J Anaesthesiol. 1999;16(10):692–8.

28. Strecker WB, et al. Epidural anaesthesia during lower extremity free tissue transfer. J Reconstr Microsurg. 1988;4(4):327–9.

29. Scott GR, et al. Efficacy of epidural anaesthesia in free flaps to the lower extremity. Plast Reconstr Surg. 1993;91(4):673–7.

30. Banic A, et al. Effects of extradural anesthesia on microcirculatory blood flow in free latissimus dorsi musculocutaneous flaps in pigs. Plast Reconstr Surg. 1997;100(4):945–55. discussion 956.

31. Lanz OI, et al. Effects of epidural anesthesia on microcirculatory blood flow in free medial saphenous fasciocutaneous flaps in dogs. Vet Surg. 2001;30(4):374–9.

32. Rigg JRA, et al. Epidural anaesthesia and analgesia and outcome of major surgery: a randomized trial, for MASTER Anaesthesia Trial Study Group. Lancet. 2002;359:1276–82.

33. Alam NH, et al. Three episodes of gracilis free muscle transfer under epidural anesthesia. J Plast Reconstr Aesthet Surg. 2006;59(12):1463–6.

34. Turek Z, et al. Anesthesia and the microcirculation. Semin Cardiothorac Vasc Anesth. 2009;13(4):249–58.

35. De Blasi RA, et al. Effects of remifentanil-based general anaesthesia with propofol or sevoflurane on muscle microcirculation as assessed by near-infrared spectroscopy. Br J Anaesth. 2008;101(2):171–7.

36. Bruegger D, et al. Microvascular changes during anesthesia: sevoflurane compared with propofol. Acta Anaesthesiol Scand. 2002;46(5):481–7.

37. Murphy PG, et al. Effect of propofol and thiopentone on free radical mediated oxidative stress on the erythrocyte. Br J Anaesth. 1996;76:536–43.

38. Kokita N, Hara A. Propofol attenuates hydrogen peroxide-induced mechanical and metabolic derangements in the isolated rat heart. Anesthesiology. 1996;84:117–27.

39. Young Y, et al. Propofol neuroprotection in a rat model of ischaemia reperfusion injury. Eur J Anaesthesiol. 1997;14:320–6.

40. Tyner TR, et al. Propofol improves skin flap survival in a rat model: correlating reduction in flap-induced neutrophil activity. Ann Plast Surg. 2004;53(3):273–7.

41. Jones SJ, et al. Milrinone does not improve free flap survival in microvascular surgery. Anaesth Intensive Care. 2007;35(5):720–5.

42. Scholz A, et al. The effect of dobutamine on blood flow of free tissue transfer flaps during head and neck reconstructive surgery. Anaesthesia. 2009;64(10):1089–93.

43. Suominen S, et al. The effect of intravenous dopamine and dobutamine on blood circulation during a microvascular TRAM flap operation. Ann Plast Surg. 2004;53(5):425–31.

44. Cordeiro PG, et al. Effects of vasoactive medications on the blood flow of island musculocutaneous flaps in swine. Ann Plast Surg. 1997;39(5):524–31.

45. Maier S, et al. Effects of phenylephrine on the sublingual microcirculation during cardiopulmonary bypass. Br J Anaesth. 2009;102(4):485–91.

46. Banic A, et al. Effects of sodium nitroprusside and phenylephrine on blood flow in free musculo-cutaneous flaps during general anesthesia. Anesthesiology. 1999;90(1):147–55.
47. Massey MF, Gupta DK. The effects of systemic phenylephrine and epinephrine on pedicle artery and microvascular perfusion in a pig model of myoadipo-cutaneous rotational flaps. Plast Reconstr Surg. 2007;120(5):1289–99.
48. Hiltunen P, et al. The effects of hypotension and norepinephrine on microvascular flap perfusion. J Reconstr Microsurg. 2011;27(7):419–26.
49. Sigurdsson GH. Perioperative fluid management in microvascular surgery. J Reconstr Microsurg. 1995;11:57–65.
50. Zhong T, et al. Intravenous fluid infusion rate in microsurgical breast reconstruction: Important lessons learned from 354 free flaps. Plast Reconstr Surg. 2011;128(6):1153–60.
51. Junghans T, et al. Hypovolemia after traditional pre-operative care in patients undergoing colonic surgery is underrepresented in conventional hemodynamic monitoring. Int J Colorectal Dis. 2006;21:693–7.
52. Lee JH, et al. Evaluation of corrected flow time in oesophageal Doppler as a predictor of fluid responsiveness. Br J Anaesth. 2007;99:343–8.
53. Noblett SE, et al. Randomized clinical trial assessing the effect of Doppler-optimized fluid management on outcome after elective colorectal resection. Br J Surg. 2006;93:1069–76.
54. Wakeling HG, et al. Intraoperative oesophageal Doppler guided fluid management shortens postoperative hospital stay after major bowel surgery. Br J Anaesth. 2005;95:634–42.
55. Venn R, et al. Randomized controlled trial to investigate influence of the fluid challenge on duration of hospital stay and perioperative morbidity in patients with hip fractures. Br J Anaesth. 2002;88:65–71.
56. Figus A, et al. Intraoperative esophageal Doppler hemodynamic monitoring in free perforator flap surgery. Ann Plast Surg. 2013;70:301–7.
57. Green D, et al. Latest developments in peri-operative monitoring of the high-risk major surgery patient. Int J Surg. 2010;8:90–9.
58. Chalmers A, et al. Cardiac output monitoring to guide fluid replacement in head and neck microvascular free flap surgery—what is current practice in the UK? Br J Oral Maxillofac Surg. 2012;50(6):500–3.
59. Jennings A, et al. Elective peri-operative intra-aortic balloon counterpulsation during maxillofacial free flap reconstructive surgery in a patient with severe cardiomyopathy. Anaesthesia. 2010;65(2):204–6.

Assessment and Physiology of Burns

13

Cynthia Wang

Epidemiology

Burn injuries rank as some of the most devastating injuries worldwide. Burns are the fourth most common type of trauma worldwide, following traffic accidents, falls, and interpersonal violence [1]. The American Burn Association estimates that last year, there were approximately 450,000 burns that required some form of hospital treatment in the United States. Three thousand five hundred deaths result from burns every year, with 3,000 resulting from residential burns while 500 occur from other sources such as motor vehicle and aircraft crashes, electrical, chemical, and hot liquid burns. Seventy-five percent of these deaths occur either on the scene or during initial transport to a healthcare facility. Nevertheless, for those who make it to a treatment center, the survival rate among patients admitted to a burn center from 2001 to 2010 was just over 96 %. Within the same 10-year period, the mortality rate for burns decreased from 4.5 to 3 % for males, and from 6.8 to 3.6 % for females. Though overall mortality decreased, deaths from burns are noticeably higher with advanced age, increased burn size, and the presence of inhalation injury.

Sixty-eight percent of burn injuries occur at home, with those at extremes of age more prevalently represented in this statistic. Children under the age of 5 years accounted for 18 % of all cases, while those aged 60 years or older accounted for 12 % of all cases. Those with preexisting conditions, such as alcoholism or epilepsy, as well as those with psychiatric illnesses are also more prone to burn injury [2]. For children under the age of 5 years, scald injuries are the most prevalent cause of burns. For all other age categories, fire and flame injuries dominate the list of causes [3]. It has been reported that certain socioeconomic factors are associated with a higher incidence of burn injury. These include:

- Non-white ethnicity
- Low household income
- Crowded household living conditions
- Low maternal education
- Unemployment [4]

Worldwide, burns are far more common in underdeveloped or developing countries. In low to middle income countries, the incidence of burns is 1.3 occurrences per 100,000 people, while in high income countries, the incidence drops to 0.14 occurrences per 100,000 people [5]. Often, these burns occur in the winter, particularly in lower income countries where cooking, heating, and lighting is accomplished via open flames and other non-electrical apparatuses. The risk of fire is even higher in light of the fact that often, homes and facilities lack exits for escape in case of fire.

C. Wang, M.D. (⊠)
Department of Anesthesiology, Ronald Reagan UCLA Medical Center, 757 Westwood Plaza, Los Angeles, CA 90095, USA
e-mail: cynthiawang@mednet.ucla.edu

C.S. Scher (ed.), *Anesthesia for Trauma*, DOI 10.1007/978-1-4939-0909-4_13,
© Springer Science+Business Media New York 2014

Poor storage of flammable fuels, and the presence of flammable clothing and building materials further increase the risk [6–13]. Overall, worldwide mortality from burns is estimated at approximately 300,000 a year [1].

Despite these statistics, the mortality from burns has decreased over the years. This is largely in part due to an increased awareness that specialized care for burn patients can drastically improve outcomes in patients suffering from burn injuries. Burn injuries present a very unique set of clinical challenges that require knowledgeable and vigilant care from all members of an organized care team.

Classification of Burns

Thermal burns: The severity of thermal burns is dependent on the contact temperature, duration of contact to the heat source, and the thickness of the skin. Most commonly, thermal burns result from exposure to flames, hot liquids or solids, and steam. The majority of these burns involve the epidermis and at least part of the dermis. Thermal burns may be further classified as scalds, flame burns, or contact burns. Scalds most often occur in children or the elderly and tend to be superficial or superficial partial-thickness burns. Flame burns account for 50 % of all adult burns. They often present with inhalational injury or other types of trauma and are often deep partial-thickness burns or full thickness burns. Contact burns result from direct or prolonged contact with objects that are extremely hot. This often occurs in a setting in which the patient is altered or unconscious, such as in the case of epilepsy or drug or alcohol abuse. They are also most commonly deep partial-thickness or full thickness burns [14, 15].

Cold exposure: Tissue damage from frostbite occurs when ice crystals form both inside and outside of cells. The fluid and electrolyte shifts that ensue cause lysis of cell membranes and, eventually, cellular necrosis. Vasoconstriction and hemoconcentration also ensue, resulting in thrombosis, decreased tissue perfusion and tissue hypoxia [16, 17].

Chemical Burns

Both acidic and alkaline burns can cause significant tissue damage. These can be difficult to assess at times because burns that appear to only be superficial can be associated with severe injury to deeper tissues. Furthermore, the corrosive effect of the chemical agent often continues to deepen the burn until the agent is fully removed. Acidic agents denature skin proteins, ultimately causing coagulation necrosis. Alkaline agents dissolve protein and collagen in the skin, creating soluble protein complexes that allow the agent to penetrate deeper into the skin, thereby causing greater damage than acidic agents. Depending on the offending agent, simple irrigation with water may not be sufficient or may be inappropriate [15, 18].

Electrical Burns

Electricity causes injury via several mechanisms. These include its direct effect on tissues, the conversion of electrical energy to thermal energy resulting in superficial and deep burns, or by blunt mechanical injury from a muscular convulsion or a fall as a result of the electrical shock. The severity of injury is primarily determined by the amount of current flowing through the body. Usually, the electrical current creates an entry and exit point as it travels through the body, subjecting any tissue in its trajectory to injury. The degree of injury is most highly correlated to the voltage, as expressed by the formula $0.24 \times V^2 \times R$, where V represents the voltage and R represents the resistance.

Domestic electricity tends to have low voltages and thus produces small, deep contact burns at the entry and exit sites. If the current is an alternating current, it may also interfere with cardiac conduction, causing arrhythmias. High tension injuries occur when the patient has come into contact with currents of 1,000 V or greater. In these types of injuries, extensive tissue damage occurs and can result in rhabdomyolysis and renal failure. High tension injuries that involve currents greater than 70,000 V are almost always fatal. Flash burns may also occur with electrical injuries. These occur when no actual current passes through the patient. However, the arc of current from a high tension voltage source can cause superficial flash burns to exposed body parts or set fire to clothing [15, 19].

Though rare, lightning injuries do occur and often result in long-term disability, if not death. Approximately 30 % of lightning injuries result in death, while 70 % of lighting strike victims suffer some sort of permanent or long-term disability. Two-thirds of deaths occur within the first hour after the injury and are due to arrhythmia or respiratory failure [20–22].

Inhalational Burns

While thermal injuries are often limited to the supraglottic airways, resulting in upper airway edema and/or blistering, hot steam can cause injury to lower areas of the respiratory tract. Additionally, patients may suffer from the systemic toxicity of inhaled products of combustion. Inhalational injury to the airways can take up to hours after the initial injury to manifest. Thus, caregivers must consistently monitor patients with burn injuries for the development of respiratory complications [23].

Characterizing the Burn

The severity of a burn is generally classified by the body surface area (BSA) involved and the depth of the injury. The terms first degree, second degree, third degree, and fourth degree in describing the depth of burns have been replaced by terminology that better correlates with and reflects the need for surgical intervention: superficial, superficial partial-thickness, deep partial-thickness, and full thickness [24].

Superficial burns only involve the epidermal layer of skin and are most commonly seen with sunburns. These burns are painful, dry, red, and blanch when pressure is applied. There is no blistering in superficial burns. Usually, by the fourth day following the initial injury, the epithelium peels away, revealing fresh, healed epidermis.

Superficial partial-thickness burns are those that extend to the area between the epidermis

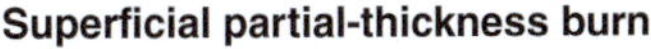

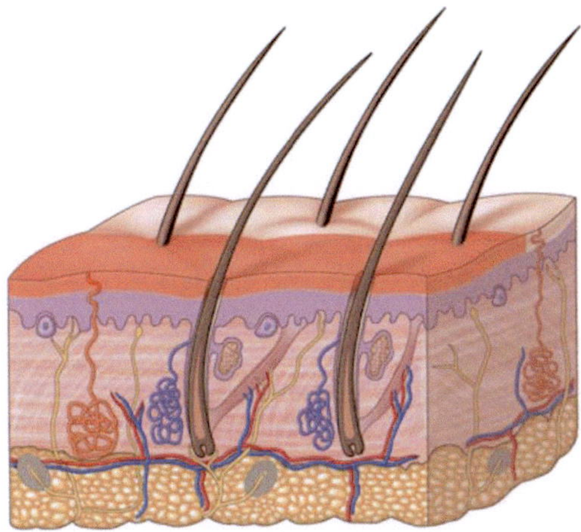

Fig. 13.1 Superficial partial-thickness burn. Reprinted from Ref. [75] with permission

and the dermis. In these types of injuries, blisters form between the epidermal and dermal layers within 24 h of injury. They are painful, red, and also blanch when pressure is applied, but unlike purely superficial burns, they weep. Scar formation and functional impairment usually do not occur; however, skin pigmentation may change. Healing is usually complete within 7–21 days, as long as the healing process is not complicated by bacterial infection. Deep partial-thickness burns are those that extend deeper into the dermis. Glandular tissue and hair follicles can sustain significant damage from deep partial-thickness burns. These injuries always blister, are painful only when pressure is applied, can be wet or waxy dry, and have variable coloring that can be patchy white or red. These burns, unlike superficial and superficial partial-thickness burns, do not blanch when pressure is applied. As they heal over the course of 3–9 weeks, the skin hypertrophies and scars, which can cause limitations in movement, especially if the injury has occurred over a joint. At times, deep partial-thickness burns can be difficult to distinguish from full thickness burns (Figs. 13.1 and 13.2).

Full thickness burns involve all layers of the dermis and often injure the underlying subcutaneous tissue layers. These burns leave an eschar, or dead, but intact, layer of dermis. Sensation is decreased, leaving the skin over these areas

Deep partial-thickness burn

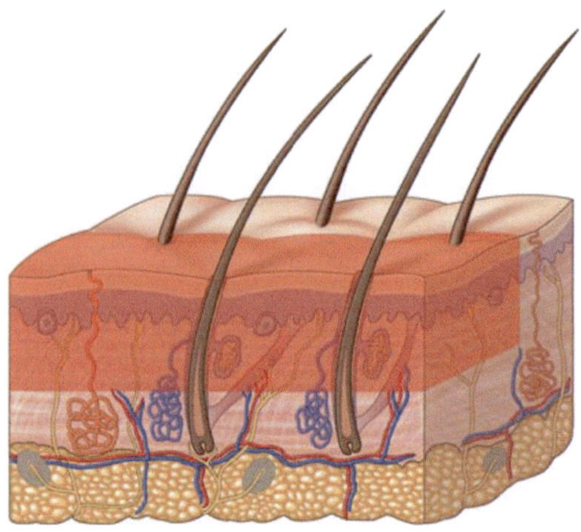

Fig. 13.2 Deep partial-thickness burn. Reprinted from Ref. [75] with permission

completely anesthetized or hypoesthetic. The skin is dry, stiff, and the coloration can vary from waxy and white, to gray, to charred and black. Regardless of color, it does not blanch with pressure. No blisters are formed. Because hair follicles are completely destroyed in full thickness burns, hair can be pulled easily and painlessly from follicles. Over time, the eschar contracts and separates from underlying viable tissue. Because of the degree of contracture, if the eschar spans the circumference of a limb, it can jeopardize perfusion to and survival of the limb. Complete spontaneous healing in full thickness burns in not possible. A summary of the characteristics associated with burns of various depths can be found in Table 13.1.

Although the terminology used to describe most burns has evolved to describe the layers of epidermis and dermis involved, the term fourth degree burn is still used to describe burns that extend through the skin into underlying tissue such as fascia, muscle, and bone. These burns are life-threatening, and if the patient survives the initial injury, surgical intervention is always required [25].

In addition to classifying burn depth, tissue injury following a burn can be classified into several zones. The zone of necrosis, also known as the zone of coagulation, refers to the tissue that is nonviable and that needs to be debrided in order to decrease the incidence of infection and promote healing. In the zone of stasis, tissue is salvageable but hypoxic and at risk of dying. If prolonged hypotension, edema, or infection occurs, it can transition to becoming a zone of necrosis. The zone of hyperemia is an area of tissue in which cytokine release and inflammatory mediators result in leaky capillaries, resulting in extravasation of fluid and tissue edema. In cases where the burn injury exceeds 30 % of BSA, the effects of these inflammatory mediators manifest systemically, affecting other organ systems such as the cardiovascular, respiratory, and gastrointestinal systems.

Accurate estimation of the BSA affected is crucial to appropriate assessment and treatment of the patient. Underestimation of the BSA involved may result in under-resuscitation of the patient and poor outcomes. Furthermore, accurate classification of burns may help triage patients to major burn centers for appropriate care. The extent of burns is expressed as a percentage of the total BSA. When estimating burn surface area, superficial burns are not taken into consideration. Burns that appear to be either deep partial-thickness or full thickness burns are assumed to be full thickness until proven otherwise. There are several methods for estimating TBSA involved in burns. These include the Lund-Browder method, the rule of nines, and the palm method [26, 27].

Lund-Browder Chart

The Lund-Browder (LB) chart consists of two drawings of the patient: one of the anterior aspect and one of the posterior aspect (Fig. 13.3). The BSA assigned to corresponding parts of the body appear on the drawing or on a table that accompanies the drawing. The table also indicates BSA differences in age, accounting for variations attributed to growth. Although the Lund Brower method is useful in that it provides an illustrated record of precisely where the burn injuries are located, there can also be several problems associated with LB charts. Studies have suggested that BSA estimates produced by LB charts can be

Table 13.1 Characteristics of burns at varying depths

Assessment of burn depth

| | Burn type | | | |
	Superficial	Superficial dermal	Deep dermal	Full thickness
Bleeding on pin prick	Brisk	Brisk	Delayed	None
Sensation	Painful	Painful	Dull	None
Appearance	Red, glistening	Dry, whiter	Cherry red	Dry, white, leathery
Blanching to pressure	Yes, brisk return	Yes, slow return	No	No

Reprinted from British Medical Journal, Ref. [74], copyright 2004 with permission from BMJ Publishing Group Ltd

inconsistent when performed by different operators or even by the same operators in different settings. Furthermore, anatomical variations among the patient population also produce inconsistencies in BSA estimates. For instance, large-breasted patients, pregnant women, or patients who are obese are inadequately represented in LB charts. In fact, it has been shown that large-chested women have significantly more BSA in the anterior chest region than men (16 % vs. 11 %), and with every increase in cup size, the BSA increases by a factor of 0.1 when compared to the posterior trunk. Lateral body parts and areas between fingers and toes are also difficult to delineate on such charts. Despite these shortcomings, LB charts remain one of the more commonly used methods to estimate BSA [28–30].

Rule of Nines

In using the Rule of Nines, a percentage that is a multiple of 9 % is assigned to each body region. Each leg represents 18 % of total BSA, each arm is 9 %, the anterior trunk and posterior trunk each represent 18 % of total BSA, and the head represents 9 %. The Rule of Nines method is perhaps one of the easiest and quickest ways of estimating BSA. However, it is probably also the least accurate, often overestimating the size of the burn area. One study estimates that the discrepancy in BSA estimates is 3 % higher when using the Rule of Nines versus LB charts. Estimates derived from the Rule of Nines method have also been shown to be less reproducible and therefore less precise [31, 32].

Palm Method

The palm method is one by which the area of burns is approximated by using the surface area of the patient's palm as a standard measurement. The surface area of the patient's palm (excluding fingers) is generally estimated to be 0.5 % of the total BSA. The surface area of the palmar surface of the hand including the fingers is estimated to be 1 % of the total BSA. This method tends to be more useful in cases in which the burn areas are patchy and incoherent. As with other methods of estimating BSA, however, the palm method has also been shown to exhibit inaccuracies. One particular study that obtained hand tracings of approximately 800 volunteers ranging in age from 2 years to 89 years found that the palmar surface of an adult hand accounted for approximately 0.78 % of the total BSA on average. In children, this was found to be slighter higher at 0.86 %. Thus, the standard 1 % BSA-palmar surface correlation probably results in gross overestimates in most cases. The palm method has also been shown to be inconsistent in patients who are obese, particularly when the BMI exceeds 31. Some have suggested that using only the palm (excluding the fingers) is perhaps the best way to estimate BSA with the palm method, since the palm more consistently correlates with the 0.5 % BSA estimate [33–36].

Given that all three methods of estimating BSA have been shown to be inaccurate under certain circumstances, some have postulated that there might be other, more effective ways of estimating BSA. One group in Japan has proposed that using the number of pieces of

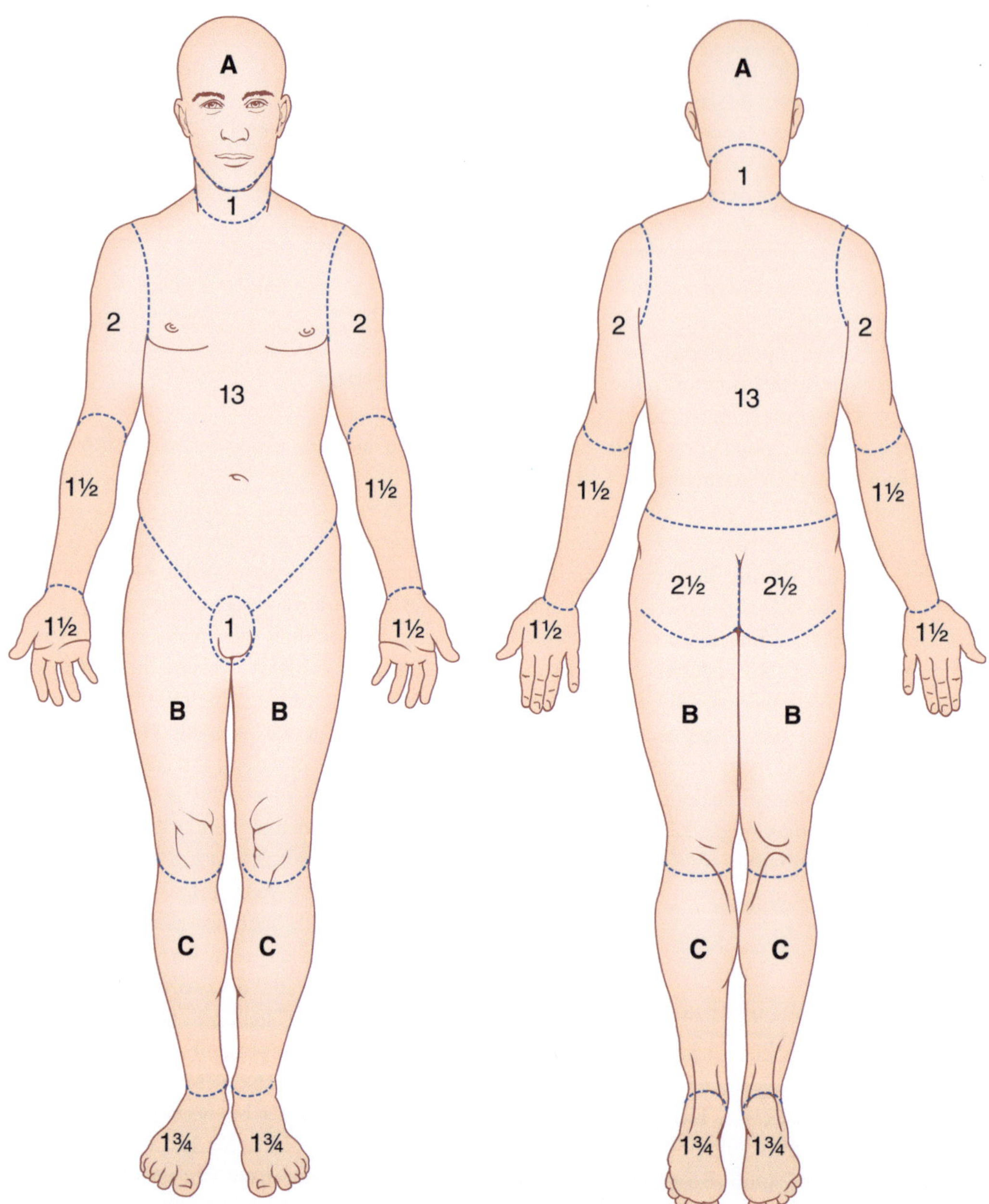

Relative percentage of areas affected by growth

Age in years	0	1	5	10	15	Adult
A – ½ of head	9½	8½	6½	5½	4½	3½
B – ½ of one thigh	2¾	3¼	4	4¼	4½	4¾
C – ½ of one leg	2½	2½	2¾	3	3¼	3½

Fig. 13.3 Example of Lund-Browder chart. Reprinted from Ref. [28] with permission

Table 13.2 American Burn Association injury grading system

Minor burn	Moderate burn	Major burn
• 15 % TBSA or less in adults • 10 % TBSA or less in children and the elderly • 2 % or less full thickness burns in children and adults without cosmetic or functional risk to eyes, ears, face, hands, feet, and perineum	• 15–25 % TBSA in adults with less than 10 % full thickness burn • 10–20 % partial-thickness burn in children under 10 and adults over 40 years of age with less than 10 % full thickness burn • 10 % TBSA or less full thickness burn in children or adults without cosmetic or functional risk to eyes, ears, face, hands, feet, and perineum	• 25 % TBSA or greater • 20 % TBSA or greater in children under 10 and adults over 40 years of age • 10 % TBSA or greater full thickness burn • All burns involving eyes, ears, face, hands, feet, and perineum that are likely to result in cosmetic or functional impairment • All high voltage electrical burns • All burn injury complicated by major trauma or inhalation injury • All poor risk patients with burn injury

Intertulle gauze that is required to cover the burned areas is more accurate than traditional methods of estimating BSA. Since the size of each piece of gauze is known, the group argues that the burn area can be more precisely estimated [37]. This method, however, is still subjective and operator dependent. In the years to come, computer aided two-dimensional and three-dimensional scanners may prove to be the most accurate in estimating burn areas [38].

Combining information about the burn surface area and the depth of involvement, burns are further classified as minor, moderate, or major burns. Burns are categorized as designated in Table 13.2. This level of classification is important because different categories of burns are associated with varying degrees of inflammation and systemic involvement that may dictate a need for higher levels of care, care at a specialized burn center, or both. Inflammatory mediators are released within minutes to hours after the initial burn injury and can begin to exhibit systemic effects quickly, particularly following major burns. Timely recognition of the severity of the burn and the category in which it falls is crucial to the patient receiving adequate and appropriate therapy [31, 39].

It is important, however, to remember not to take these classifications in isolation. The many factors contributing to morbidity and mortality in burn patients are complex. For instance, a burn involving 20 % TBSA carries a 30 % mortality in a 70-year-old patient but is generally very survivable for an otherwise healthy 20-year-old patient.

Thus, when classifying and risk stratifying burn injuries, all patient characteristics, the mechanism of burn injury, comorbidities, and severity of the burn must all be weighed with equal importance.

The inflammatory response to a burn injury is extremely complex, and in cases of major burns, can affect almost every organ system in the body (Fig. 13.4). Although this response is immediate after the initial insult, noticeable systemic effects may take as long as 5–7 days to manifest. Ultimately, successful management of the adverse effects of these inflammatory mediators determines the overall survival of compromised tissue as well as recovery of the patient.

Cardiovascular and Hemodynamic Changes

The cardiovascular response following a burn injury is comprised of two phases: the acute, or resuscitative phase, and the hypermetabolic phase. The acute phase, which usually lasts for approximately 48 h, is characterized by hypovolemia, resulting in decreased tissue perfusion and, if not addressed aggressively, tissue ischemia, metabolic acidosis, and renal failure. Hypovolemia results from the release of inflammatory mediators from the injured area that increase capillary permeability and fluid and protein loss into the extravascular space. Mediators involved in the vascular response to burn injury include histamine, prostaglandins PGE2 and PGI2, leukotrienes LB4 and LD2, thromboxane

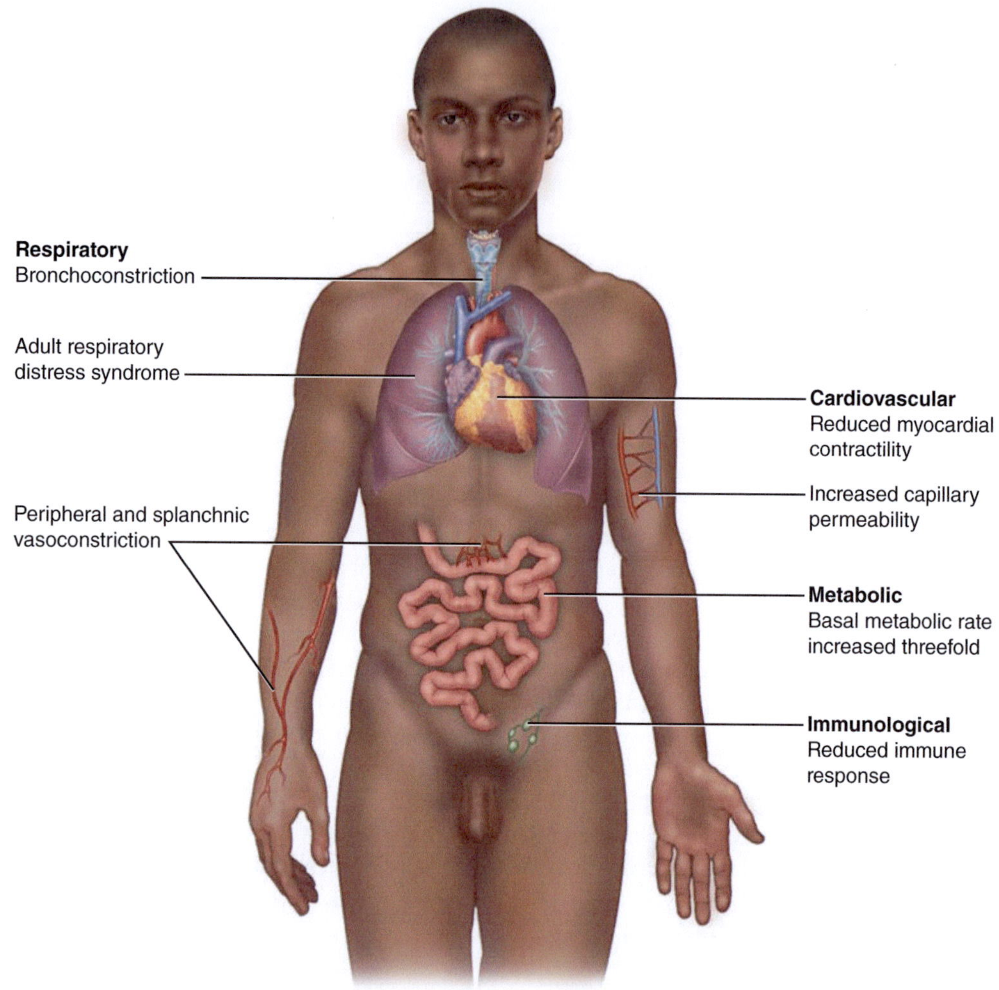

Fig. 13.4 Systemic changes that occur after burn injury. Reproduced from British Medical Journal, Ref. [15], copyright 2004 with permission from BMJ Publishing Group Ltd

A2, interleukin-6, catecholamines, oxygen free radicals, platelet aggregation factor, angiotensin II, and vasopressin. It is also prudent to note that inhalational injury, hypoalbuminemia, and sepsis can exacerbate the increase in vascular permeability, contributing to extravascular fluid sequestration. Evaporative losses from the burn area are also a major contributor to hypovolemia and hypotension. Fluid loss from evaporation occurs at approximately 1.2 mL/kg/% BSA/24 h in patients with greater than 40 % BSA involved [40].

Cardiac output decreases as a result of decreased preload and from the direct myocardial depressant effects of burn toxins, and the magnitude of this decrease is proportional to the size of the burn area. Impaired contractility may also be attributed in some cases to the apoptotic destruction of cardiac myocytes, which has been demonstrated to occur in the left ventricle 24 h after the burn injury. Myocardial depression in burn injury is characterized by a low left ventricular contractility in the presence of adequate or elevated filling pressures. Right ventricular function may also be impaired due to an increase in pulmonary arterial pressures as a result of inhalational injury [41]. In severe cases, myocardial dysfunction and heart failure may persist for long periods of time after the initial injury. Circulating myocardial depressants as well as myocardial edema may also lead to clinically significant diastolic dysfunction, which has been shown to be an independent marker for mortality in patients who are critically ill. In cases in which myocyte apoptosis is suspected to be the primary cause of heart failure, inotropic support is preferred over flooding the failing heart with large volumes of fluid. However, inotropes may produce vasoconstriction at the wound site, further compromising wound healing. Therefore, inotropic medications should not be administered unless the patient has been as adequately fluid resuscitated as can be tolerated. If inotropic support is required despite adequate fluid resuscitation, it is prudent to select medications such as dobutamine that do not result in vasoconstriction in order to maximize wound viability, as long as hypotension is not significant. The overall volume status of the patient is often assessed using filling pressures measured with a pulmonary artery catheter or through echocardiography. Additional methods of assessing the adequacy of fluid resuscitation, such as the use of transcardiopulmonary thermodilution, have been shown to be successful in guiding fluid therapy and decreasing overall morbidity. Although base deficit and lactate levels are good indicators of cellular perfusion, fluid resuscitation is rarely guided by following trends in base deficit and serum lactate levels [42–47].

The hypermetabolic phase that follows is characterized by a dramatic increase in blood flow to tissues resulting in significant edema formation, which can be exacerbated by hypoproteinemia. This physiological process is triggered by an adrenergic response to the burn injury, increasing catecholamine production and release. During this time, the risk of myocardial infarction and cardiac arrhythmias is increased. Furthermore, for those patients with an underlying history of coronary artery disease, the hypercoagulability that accompanies burn injury increases the risk for acute coronary syndrome. Other hematologic changes that occur with burn injuries will be discussed in more detail at a later stage [48–51].

Pulmonary Changes

Although there have been drastic advances in the treatment of cutaneous burn injuries, mortality rates for patients with inhalational injuries have shown little improvement in the last couple of decades. There are three ways in which smoke inhalation injury affects the airway: thermal injury to the upper airway as well as to the pulmonary system as a whole, chemical irritation of the respiratory tract, and systemic effects of toxic gases. Smoke inhalational injury can affect the upper airway, the tracheobronchial tree, the lung parenchyma, or a combination of the three. The response to inhalational injury occurs within hours, producing an inflammatory reaction within the lungs that can persist for up to 5 days after the initial insult. Changes that occur within 24–72 h after an inhalational injury include pulmonary arterial hypertension, bronchial constriction, increased airway resistance, reduced pulmonary compliance, atelectasis, and increased pulmonary shunt fraction. Interestingly, if inhalational injury occurs in conjunction with cutaneous burns, the incidence of respiratory complications increases significantly. In fact, respiratory failure is one of the major causes of death after a burn; the mortality rate of patients who develop pulmonary complications is as high as 80 %. Among burn patients who are hospitalized, pneumonia is the most common clinical complication.

The primary source of injury to the upper airway during smoke inhalation is thermal injury. Normally, the nasopharynx clears inspired gases of particulate matter larger than 5 μm in size. During a fire, however, victims breathe through the mouth due to nasopharyngeal irritation, increasing the deposition of toxic, particulate, foreign matter into the airway. The heat also damages the epithelial layer, denaturing proteins and leading to activation of the complement cascade and the release of histamine. Histamine release also stimulates the formation of nitric oxide, which in turn forms reactive nitrogen species. Xanthine oxidase is formed from the heat damage, catalyzing the formation of reactive oxygen species. The presence of both reactive oxygen species and reactive nitrogen species increases endothelial permeability, thereby resulting in edema. Acutely, thermal injury leads to progressive swelling of the upper airway, leading to potential airway obstruction. Clinical findings such as stridor and increased work of breathing may not be evident until the edema has progressed to the point of obstruction. The swelling may persist for several days and may be further complicated by scarring and contractures, especially if the burn injury involves the head and neck region. Edema may also be exacerbated by fluid resuscitation requirements dictated by the extent of cutaneous burns. Ciliary function is also impaired, increasing the risk of infection in the lungs. The formation of viscous secretions and the inability to clear these secretions contribute to airway obstruction and atelectasis.

The tracheobronchial tree is less likely to suffer from thermal injury unless the patient has inhaled very high specific heat capacity particles, such as superheated steam. Usually, injury to the tracheobronchial tree is due to chemicals in smoke, which can cause inflammation, mucosal sloughing, airway irritability, and activation of the systemic inflammatory response. The tracheobronchial tree is heavily populated with vasomotor and sensory nerve endings. Stimulation of these nerve endings by smoke inhalation causes the release of neuropeptides, which result in intense bronchoconstriction. Neuropeptides also enhance the production of nitric oxide, which can react with reactive oxygen species to form harmful reactive nitrogen species. High NO production can also result in the loss of hypoxic pulmonary vasoconstriction, which, along with a dramatic increase in bronchial blood flow, can worsen pulmonary edema. Studies have suggested that bronchial blood flow increases by up to tenfold within 20 min after the injury. Histologically, damage to the bronchial endothelium results in a profuse transudate of protein solution. Early after the inhalational injury, this transudate forms foamy secretions. Later on, however, the transudate solidifies and potentially obstructs the lower airways. The obstructive material forms a cast that consists of mucous secretions, denuded epithelial cells, inflammatory cells, and fibrin. In a patient who is mechanically ventilated, these casts may obstruct the airway enough to cause barotrauma to ventilated areas. In severe cases, the bronchoconstriction and edema can progress to acute respiratory distress syndrome (ARDS).

Damage to the lung parenchyma in inhalational injury is often delayed. The time it takes to develop changes to the lung parenchyma after the initial insult can be indicative of the severity of injury. Increased transvascular fluid displacement results in alveolar damage and atelectasis. Fibrin, an inhibitor of surfactant and a pro-inflammatory substance, deposits in the airway, further worsening the effects of atelectasis and ventilation defects. Activated neutrophils in the airway cause damage by adhering to the alveolar wall, causing the release of proteases and reactive oxygen species. Damaged cell membranes within the lungs release arachidonic acid, which is converted by cyclooxygenase to thromboxane A2 and prostacyclin PGI2. An increase in the levels of these mediators can worsen ventilation and perfusion defects by causing pulmonary hypertension, adversely affecting gas exchange and oxygenation. More often than not, however, the increase in pulmonary pressures is offset by the release of nitric oxide, which in its own right can also contribute to ventilation/perfusion defects.

Depending on the composition of inhaled toxins, the degree of airway injury may vary. Household components such as PVC, Teflon, and polyurethane, when combusted, produce particularly toxic substances such as hydrogen chloride, phosgene, hydrogen cyanide (HCN), and isocyanate. These toxins have adverse effects on the cellular respiratory chain, exacerbating hypoxemia. Even after patient has recovered from the acute effects of the inhalational injury, these toxins may result in increased airway reactivity that persists for several months after the injury due to their corrosive effects on the airway. Table 13.3 lists some of these toxic compounds and their effects on the body [48, 50–52].

Carbon monoxide (CO) poisoning is common in burn injuries, as the concentration of CO in smoke rapidly rises in a fire. In fact, it is one of

Table 13.3 Toxic compounds and their effects [52]

Toxic compound	Material	Source	Pathophysiology
Arolein/ propenal	Acrylics Cellulose Polypropylene	Aircraft windows, textiles, wall coverings Cotton, jute, paper, wood Carpet, upholstery	Severe irritation of upper respiratory tract, mucosa necrosis, and death within 10 min with concentrations over 50 ppm
Aldehydes	Acrylics Cellulose Polyamine resins	Aircraft windows, textiles, wall coverings Cotton, jute, paper, wood Household, kitchen goods	Corrosive, denatures proteins; formaldehyde: denatures ribonucleic acid
Ammonia	Polyamide Polyamide resins Polyurethane Silk, wool	Carpet, clothing Household, kitchen goods Insulation, upholstery Blankets, clothing, fabric, furniture	Airway irritant leading to cough, increasing secretions and bronchoconstriction; ammonium hydroxide: tissue necrosis
Carbon monoxide	All materials	All combustible products	Tissue hypoxia, organ failure, death within 1 h with concentrations of 80–90 %
Hydrogen chloride	Polyester Polyvinyl chloride	Clothing, fabrics Floor, furniture, upholstery, wall, wire/ pipe coating	Mucosal necrosis and acute bronchitis
Hydrogen cyanide	Fire retardants Polyacrylonitrile Polyamide Polyamide resins Polyurethane Silk, wool	Polymeric material Appliances, engineering, plastics Carpet, clothing Household, kitchen goods Insulation, upholstery Blankets, clothing, fabric, furniture	Tissue hypoxia, organ failure, death; death possible with concentrations over 1 µg/mL
Hydrogen sulfide	Rubber Silk, wool	Tires Blankets, clothing, fabric, furniture	Airway irritant, corrosive
Phosgene	Polyvinyl chloride	Floor, furniture, upholstery, wall, wire/ pipe coating	Mucosal necrosis, primarily in small airways and alveoli
Sulfur dioxide	Rubber	Tires	Strong irritation to eyes and airway, lower airway injury, and pulmonary edema

the most frequent causes of immediate death following smoke inhalation injury. Carbon monoxide is odorless and colorless. It binds to hemoglobin with a 200 % greater affinity than oxygen, reducing oxygen carrying capacity and shifting the oxyhemoglobin dissociation curve to the left, making it more difficult for oxygen to be released from the hemoglobin to the tissues. Although very high concentrations of CO are required to produce lethal carboxyhemoglobin (COHb) levels of 50 or 60 %, inhalation of even 0.1 % carbon monoxide can result in lethal levels because it so readily displaces oxygen, especially if the exposure is prolonged. Carbon monoxide also combines with myoglobin, inhibiting the diffusion of oxygen to cardiac and skeletal muscles. Furthermore, it interferes with mitochondrial function, uncoupling oxidative phosphorylation and therefore decreasing ATP production. The results of its effects at the mitochondrial level are metabolic acidosis and direct myocardial toxicity. COHb levels of 90 % or greater result in immediate cardiac arrest. Patients who have suffered from cardiac arrest as a result of carbon monoxide poisoning may be unresponsive to resuscitation and hyperbaric oxygen due to the direct toxic effects of carbon monoxide on the mitochondria of cardiac

Table 13.4 Symptoms of carbon monoxide toxicity [53]

Blood level of COHgb (%)	Symptoms
<15–20	Headache, dizziness, confusion
20–40	Nausea, vomiting, disorientation, visual impairment
40–60	Agitation, combativeness, hallucinations, coma, shock
>60	Death

myocytes. At lower COHb levels of 30 % or higher, the patient experiences weakness and altered mental status (Table 13.4). Neurological symptoms worsen up to COHb levels of 60 %, at which point the effects are fatal.

Pulse oximetry may reveal a normal saturation even in the presence of carbon monoxide toxicity. However, cooximetry can reveal the presence of abnormal hemoglobin species. Tachypnea in patients with isolated carbon monoxide poisoning without concomitant lung injury is often absent, as the carotid bodies are sensitive to arterial O_2 tension, not the overall O_2 content. Patients with COHb levels of 40 % or greater may exhibit the classic cherry red coloring of blood; however, if the patient is hypoxic and cyanotic, this finding may be obscured [54–56].

If the burning material contains nitrogen, such as wool or nylon, the smoke will also contain HCN. HCN is much quicker acting and much more potent than carbon monoxide; in fact, it is one of the most lethal toxins known to mankind. Inhalational injury is the foremost cause of cyanide poisoning in the world, which is found to be present in 35 % of all fire victims. HCN is a colorless gas with the smell of bitter almonds that binds to cytochrome oxidase in the mitochondria, preventing oxidative phosphorylation. In order to produce ATP, cells must resort to anaerobic metabolism, thus producing more lactic acid and worsening metabolic acidosis. Cyanide is also a nonspecific inhibitor of antioxidants, increasing levels of oxygen free radicals. Additionally, cyanide inhibits the enzyme responsible for the formation of gamma amino-butyric acid (GABA), thereby decreasing the seizure threshold in patients with cyanide toxicity. Symptomatically, HCN inhalation initially causes a brief episode of tachypnea followed by respiratory depression and, eventually, apnea. In some cases, patients may experience pulmonary edema. Oxygen utilization is low, resulting in high venous oxyhemoglobin content, and cyanosis is not seen until very late stages of cyanide poisoning. Because of the complicated distribution and metabolism of HCN, it is difficult to pinpoint a blood cyanide level that can be classified as lethal. The release of various toxic gases during a fire does not usually occur simultaneously; rather, peak concentrations of these gases occur at varying points of time, and isolated measurements of COHb, cyanide, or other toxins may not reflect maximum exposure. The degree of damage due to inhalational injury is correlated with the synergistic effects of CO and HCN levels, O_2 depletion, and the effects of any other inhaled products of combustion, making it difficult to attribute the severity of injury to any one factor [57–60].

Renal and Electrolyte Changes

The incidence of acute renal failure in burn patients ranges anywhere from 1.3 to 38 %, and the presence of renal failure is associated with high mortality rates, as high as 73 to 100 %. During the acute phase following a burn injury, renal blood flow (RBF) and glomerular filtration rate (GFR) are both decreased due to the decrease in cardiac output. A decrease in RBF activates the renin-angiotensin-aldosterone system and stimulates the release of antidiuretic hormone. The overall effect is sodium and water retention accompanied by dramatic losses of potassium, calcium, and magnesium. As the patient transitions into the hypermetabolic phase, RBF and GFR are increased; however, tubular function at this time is often impaired. Two different mechanisms of renal failure have been described in burn patients. The first occurs within a few days after the injury and is primarily due to hypovolemia, low cardiac output, and systemic vasoconstriction. These changes, in conjunction with some degree of myoglobinuria, can destroy tubular cells. This results in an oliguric acute tubular necrosis. Elevated levels of catecholamines, angiotensin, aldosterone, and vasopressin have been associated with this type of renal failure. This early onset renal failure due to early acute tubular necrosis can be avoided with aggressive, early fluid resuscitation; however, in patients with deep, extensive burns or burns due to electrical trauma, it may be difficult to avoid. The other type of renal failure that prevails in this patient population has a more complex etiology and is thought to arise as a result of sepsis, multiorgan failure, or both. The exact pathophysiology of how this later occurring renal failure develops is still unclear. Statistically, it is more common in patients with concurrent inhalational injury or who arrive to the hospital intubated. This late developing renal failure more frequently leads to the need for hemodialysis than early onset renal failure due to oliguric acute tubular necrosis. Identification of patients that are prone to developing late onset renal failure may be crucial to determining the need for early intervention, which may decrease mortality in this patient population [48, 61–63].

Renal failure, particularly when associated with sepsis and multiorgan failure in the burn population, is associated with an extremely high mortality rate. In one particular review of burn patients who died of multiorgan failure, renal failure was present in every patient. A decrease in urine output as well as an eventual rise in urea concentrations and serum creatinine should be clues to the development of early renal insufficiency or failure. Early initiation of renal replacement therapy is the best strategy in order to prevent electrolyte imbalances and in order to complement early, aggressive fluid resuscitation and nutritional supplementation. Some have argued that continuous veno-venous hemodialysis (CVVHD) may be more appropriate in the burn patient than intermittent single pass dialysis. Continuous filtration allows the patient to maintain stable levels of electrolytes and a consistent intravascular volume status while avoiding large hemodynamic shifts that occur with intermittent hemodialysis, therefore decreasing the risk of compromising perfusion to wound areas [42, 64].

Increased serum potassium concentrations are often seen in burn patients within the first 2 days after the initial injury. After the first 2 days, marked hypokalemia is the more common finding due to exaggerated renal losses. The loss of potassium can be exacerbated by diarrhea or by frequent suctioning of gastric fluids. The hypokalemia that ensues can be severe enough to result in cardiac dysrhythmias, especially if it is worsened by drugs that promote the intracellular transfer of potassium such as insulin, glucose, and sodium bicarbonate, or if drugs that counter the myocardial effects of potassium are administered (such as calcium). Patients with hypokalemia are particularly sensitive to the dysrhythic effects of digitalis, which should be avoided. Calcium levels are also depressed in post-burn patients, primarily due to renal losses. Pediatric patients are particularly sensitive to hypocalcemia and should receive calcium replacement therapy, particularly if blood is being transfused [63].

Gastrointestinal Changes

Patients who suffer from burn injuries experience a number of changes to the gastrointestinal system. Decreased mesenteric and splanchnic blood flow result in intestinal ischemia, which in turn activates neutrophils and tissue bound enzymes such as xanthine oxidase, which destroy the gut's mucosal barrier. This leads to increased intestinal permeability and bacterial translocation, promoting the development of endotoxemia. Bacterial translocation can begin as early as 1 h after thermal injury, and peak plasma levels of endotoxin occur at 12 h and peak again at 4 days after the burn. Endotoxins activate macrophages and neutrophils, leading to further release of oxidants, arachidonic acid metabolites, and proteases, all of which exacerbate local and systemic inflammatory processes. Burn patients also experience a higher incidence of gastric ulcer formation (also known as Curling's ulcers) and gastrointestinal hemorrhage. Up to 86 % of burn patients demonstrate erosion of the stomach lining within 72 h of the injury. In fact, Curling's ulcer formation is the most frequent life-threatening gastrointestinal complication associated with burns. Duodenal ulcers occur twice as frequently in children than in adults. Ulcer prophylaxis is achieved by the administration of antacids or H_2-antagonist drugs. In severe cases, however, gastric ulcers resulting from burn injuries may require a vagotomy or partial gastrectomy. Gastrointestinal bleeding, another common complication, occurs in up to 40 % of burn patients. Given all of these changes in the gastrointestinal tract, nutrient absorption through the gut is often found to be impaired following a burn injury. Burn injury combined with the use of narcotic medications leads to impaired gastrointestinal motility in this patient population, resulting in delayed gastric emptying and ileus. Adynamic ileus is almost always present in patients who have suffered from burns involving 20 % or greater TBSA. Severe gastrointestinal dysfunction can be minimized or, in mild cases, prevented with adequate and early fluid resuscitation, early excision of necrotic tissue, staged feeding, and administration of supplemental nutrients [48, 63, 65]. Hepatic blood flow is also decreased, even the patient has been adequately volume resuscitated, which can result in hepatic ischemia and dysfunction. An increase in lipolysis in the post-burn period can produce an increase in liver size, which can be enlarged up to twice its size.

Metabolic and Endocrine Changes

After a burn injury, the patient experiences a dramatic increase in metabolic rate, which is generally proportional to the size of the burn. For instance, if more than 50 % BSA is involved in the burn, the metabolic rate can be more than doubled. Due to altered hypothalamic function, the metabolic thermostat is reset upward, increasing skin and core temperatures to levels above normal. Many of the thermoregulatory activities of the skin are destroyed or diminished as a result of the burn injury, impairing skin vasoactivity, sweating, piloerection, and insulation. The skin loses its function as a water vapor barrier, resulting in loss of free water. Evaporative water loss has been estimated at 4 L/m^2 of burn surface in children while in adults, it is estimated at 2.5 L/m^2 of burn surface. For every milliliter of water loss, calories are also lost. The estimated energy loss is estimated to be 0.58 cal for every milliliter of water that is lost. For instance, if 4 L of water is lost, the corresponding calorie loss would amount to 2,400 cal. Other contributors to the hypermetabolic state after burns include wound-generated mediators, hormonal mediators, and endotoxemia.

During the post-burn hypermetabolic response, the patient experiences an increase in glycogenolysis, gluconeogenesis, and levels of glucogenic precursors, which result in hyperglycemia and impaired insulin responsiveness. Although glucose delivery is dramatically increased, glucose oxidation is severely impaired, leading to elevated fasting glucose levels. Glycosuria is a common finding in these patients. Burn patients may also be susceptible to developing non-ketotic hyperosmolar coma, especially if total parenteral nutrition is being administered. Another component of the hypermetabolic post-burn response is a dramatic increase in serum catecholamine levels, which peak 3–4 days after the burn. Peak serum catecholamine levels can be up to 26 times normal levels and result in intense vasoconstriction throughout the body. This immense increase in systemic catecholamines has been associated with many adverse outcomes in burn patients, including ischemia of the gastrointestinal tract, liver dysfunction, Curling's ulcers, oliguria, disseminated intravascular coagulation, cardiac dysfunction, and hypertensive crises.

The catabolic state in the post-burn period leads to degradation of muscle protein at a rate that is much faster than it can be synthesized. Over time, continued catabolism of muscle protein leads to severe muscle wasting and a dramatic decrease in lean body mass. This elevated metabolic state can persist for as long as 24 months after the initial burn injury. In children who have suffered from burns, this prolonged period of catabolism can lead to growth retardation. Nitrogen loss has been estimated to be 20–25 g/m^2 TBSA/day. This means that if nutritional needs are not addressed early in the treatment period, lethal cachexia can occur in less than 30 days. Thus, early and aggressive alimentation of burn patients, ideally within 24 h after the initial burn injury, is essential in meeting the incredible metabolic requirements in this patient population. Some have championed the initiation of enteral feeds as soon as 1–2 h after the burn in order to offset the effects of hypermetabolism, hypercatabolism, and systemic inflammation. However, in reality, this is often not feasible due to the risk of aspiration and difficulties with proper feeding tube placement during the acute resuscitation phase. Furthermore, within the first 2 h after burn injury, intestinal ischemia due to hypovolemia and hypotension cannot be ruled yet, making the decision to initiate early feeds difficult. Nevertheless, early feeding is known to have definitive benefits in burn patients. Studies in patients receiving enteral nutrition within 24 h after a burn injury show a decrease in overall levels of catecholamines, cortisol, and glucagon, thereby achieving an early attenuation of the hypermetabolic response. Early enteral feeding is also thought to maintain intestinal integrity and slow the translocation of bacteria, therefore decreasing the risk of endotoxemia. In severe cases, however, enteral nutrition may not be possible for a protracted period of time. In these cases, total parenteral nutrition may be necessary in order to meet nutritional needs and prevent lethal nutritional deficiencies [63, 66–68].

Hematologic and Immunologic Changes

The hematological system is affected on several levels from burn injuries. Hemoconcentration, resulting from the loss of circulating plasma volume, is one of the earliest findings. However, after the initial resuscitation, patients are more often anemic due to hemodilution from fluid administration. Over time, suppression of erythropoietin production, blood loss from frequent debridements and other surgical procedures, and hemolysis of heat-damaged red blood cells contribute to long-standing anemia in this patient population. Heat-damaged red blood cells also have a decreased half-life of 7 days versus 21 days for normal red blood cells. Autoimmune hemolytic anemia may also develop. Within the first week, platelet sequestration can lead to clinically significant thrombocytopenia. After the first week, platelet levels return to normal or above normal values. If thrombocytopenia persists, sepsis must be ruled out. Also within the early stages after burn injury, prothrombin time (PT) and partial thromboplastin time (PTT) may be elevated due to liver dysfunction but generally return to normal after a few

weeks. For the first several days after the burn, fibrinogen is decreased and fibrin split products are increased, suggesting fibrinolysis, but subsequently return to normal levels after a few days. In fact, fibrinogen levels, along with factor V and VIII levels can be above normal after the first few days following the injury, reflecting the hypercoagulable state that is often present after the acute period in burn injuries. The burn injury itself along with the hypercoagulability that ensues may predispose the patient to disseminated intravascular coagulation and/or episodes of vascular occlusion. White blood cell counts are usually elevated following burn injuries; however, severe sepsis and silver sulfadiazine in wound dressings may cause leukopenia, therefore offsetting the leukocytosis. Leukocyte function tends to be low after burn injury, and levels of immunoglobulins G and M are depressed. Burn patients are extremely susceptible to bacteremia and sepsis from pneumonia, suppurative thrombophlebitis, and bacterial invasion of the burned areas. However, in half of burn patients, an offending bacterial agent cannot be isolated. This suggests that systemic inflammatory changes are often due to a mediator driven response initiated by the injured tissue rather than an infectious agent. Pro-inflammatory cytokines such as TNF-α, IL-1, and IL-6 trigger a number of primary and secondary responses that result in a shock-like state. Several other changes in the immune system also increase the susceptibility to developing sepsis in burn victims. For instance, phagocytosis is impaired, as is neutrophil chemotaxis. Similar changes occur in macrophages, especially in alveolar macrophages. Lymphocytes also exhibit a faulty response to mitogen stimulation. After a burn injury, the number of T suppressor lymphocytes, which inhibit normal T cell stimulation of antibody production, increases. In fact, the number of circulating T suppressor lymphocytes has been correlated with the risk for developing sepsis. The best way to minimize these adverse immunologic changes is early wound care. Studies have suggested that early excision of burned tissue and wound closure reverses many of the immunologic changes that occur, thereby reducing the severity of the inflammatory response to burn injury and decreasing the risk of developing disseminated infection [48, 69–72].

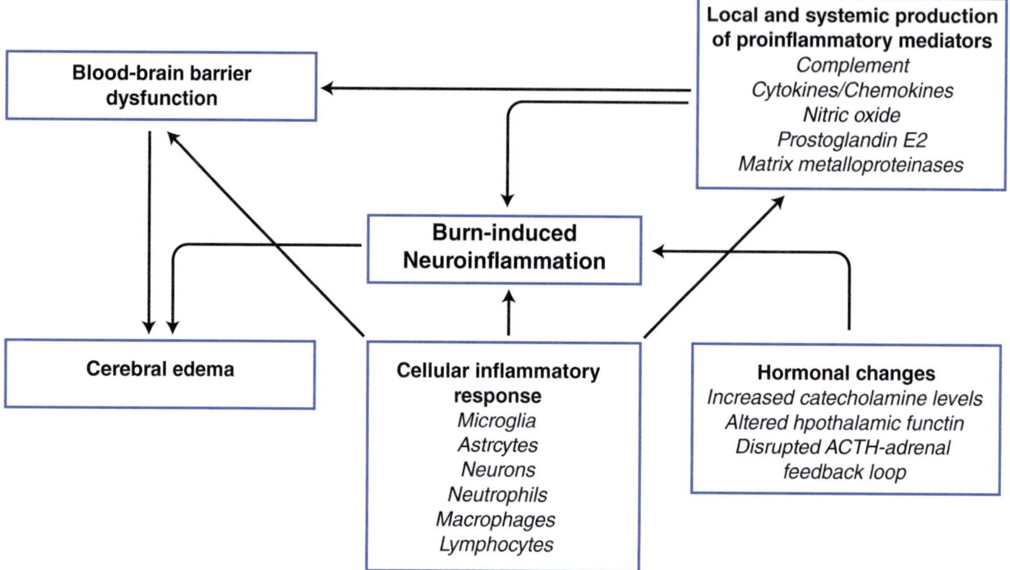

Fig. 13.5 Pathophysiology of blood brain barrier breakdown and development of cerebral edema. From Ref. [73]

Neurologic Changes

The neurologic system is not immune to injury in patients with burn injuries. Cerebral complications are highly correlated with mortality in burn patients, but they are often overlooked. Hypoxic cerebral injury is often seen among this patient population and is the cause of death in up to 10 % of patients with severe burn injury. Furthermore, liberal fluid administration in conjunction with the neuronal damage caused by the inflammatory process may lead to the development of potentially dangerous cerebral edema. Under normal conditions, the blood brain barrier tightly regulates molecules that enter the brain tissue. However, during the inflammatory process, the integrity of this barrier can be seriously compromised, and cerebral microvascular permeability is increased. Reactive oxygen species, reactive nitrogen species, proteases, cytokines, chemokines, and complement proteins all contribute to the compromise of the barrier as well as direct neuronal damage. If increased intracranial pressure is suspected, consultation with neurologist and neurosurgical colleagues is imperative, and external decompression of intracranial pressures must be considered (Fig. 13.5).

The hypothalamic-pituitary axis, which is implicated in the hypermetabolic response after injury, is also impaired in patients after a burn. Elevated serum prolactin levels have also been positively correlated with the severity of the burn. Additionally, burn victims commonly exhibit transient adrenal insufficiency, which has been associated with an increase in mortality rates following a burn [42, 73].

References

1. World Health Organization. The Global Burden of Disease: 2004 Update. Geneva 2008. http://www.who.int/healthinfo/global_burden_disease/GBD_report_2004update_full.pdf.
2. Langley K, Sim K. Anaesthesia for patients with burns injuries. Curr Anaesth Crit Care. 2002;13 (2):70–5.
3. National Burn Repository. 2011 Report of National Data from 2001–2010. 2011. http://www.ameriburn.org/2011NBRAnnualReport.pdf.
4. Edelman LS. Social and economic factors associated with the risk of burn injury. Burns. 2007;33 (8):958–65. PubMed PMID: 17869003. Epub 2007/09/18. eng.
5. WHO. Global Burden of Disease 2004 Summary Tables. Geneva2008. http://www.who.int/healthinfo/global_burden_disease/estimates_regional/en/index.htm.

6. Peck MD, Kruger GE, van der Merwe AE, Godakumbura W, Ahuja RB. Burns and fires from non-electric domestic appliances in low and middle income countries Part I. The scope of the problem. Burns. 2008;34(3):303–11. PubMed PMID: 18206314. Epub 2008/01/22. eng.

7. Sawhney CP. Flame burns involving kerosene pressure stoves in India. Burns. 1989;15(6):362–4. PubMed PMID: 2624690. Epub 1989/12/01. eng.

8. Barss P, Baker S, Mohan D. Injury prevention: an international perspective: epidemiology, surveillance, and policy. New York: Oxford University Press; 1998.

9. Grange AO, Akinsulie AO, Sowemimo GO. Flame burns disasters from kerosene appliance explosions in Lagos, Nigeria. Burns. 1988;14(2):147–50. PubMed PMID: 3390735. Epub 1988/04/01. eng.

10. Gupta M, Bansal M, Gupta A, Goil P. The kerosene tragedy of 1994, an unusual epidemic of burns: epidemiological aspects and management of patients. Burns. 1996;22(1):3–9. PubMed PMID: 8719308. Epub 1996/02/01. eng.

11. Marsh D, Sheikh A, Khalil A, Kamil S, Jaffer Z, Qureshi I, et al. Epidemiology of adults hospitalized with burns in Karachi, Pakistan. Burns. 1996;22(3):225–9.

12. El-Badawy A, Mabrouk AR. Epidemiology of childhood burns in the burn unit of Ain Shams University in Cairo, Egypt. Burns. 1998;24(8):728–32. PubMed PMID: 9915673. Epub 1999/01/23. eng.

13. Mabrouk A, El Badawy A, Sherif M. Kerosene stove as a cause of burns admitted to the Ain Shams burn unit. Burns. 2000;26(5):474–7. PubMed PMID: 10812271. Epub 2000/05/17. eng.

14. Orgill DP, Solari MG, Barlow MS, O'Connor NE. A finite-element model predicts thermal damage in cutaneous contact burns. J Burn Care Rehabil. 1998;19 (3):203–9. PubMed PMID: 9622462. Epub 1998/06/11. eng.

15. Hettiaratchy S, Dziewulski P. ABC of burns: pathophysiology and types of burns. BMJ. 2004;328 (7453):1427–9. PubMed PMID: 15191982. Pubmed Central PMCID: PMC421790. Epub 2004/06/12. eng.

16. Petrone P, Kuncir EJ, Asensio JA. Surgical management and strategies in the treatment of hypothermia and cold injury. Emerg Med Clin North Am. 2003;21 (4):1165–78. PubMed PMID: 14708823. Epub 2004/01/08. eng.

17. Murphy JV, Banwell PE, Roberts AH, McGrouther DA. Frostbite: pathogenesis and treatment. J Trauma. 2000;48(1):171–8. PubMed PMID: 10647591. Epub 2000/01/27. eng.

18. Cartotto RC, Peters WJ, Neligan PC, Douglas LG, Beeston J. Chemical burns. Can J Surg. 1996;39 (3):205–11. PubMed PMID: 8640619. Epub 1996/06/01. eng.

19. Cooper MA. Electrical and lightning injuries. Emerg Med Clin North Am. 1984;2(3):489–501. PubMed PMID: 6534739. Epub 1984/08/01. eng.

20. Browne BJ, Gaasch WR. Electrical injuries and lightning. Emerg Med Clin North Am. 1992;10(2):211–29. PubMed PMID: 1559466. Epub 1992/05/01. eng.

21. Ritenour AE, Morton MJ, McManus JG, Barillo DJ, Cancio LC. Lightning injury: a review. Burns. 2008;34(5):585–94. PubMed PMID: 18395987. Epub 2008/04/09. eng.

22. Duclos PJ, Sanderson LM. An epidemiological description of lightning-related deaths in the United States. Int J Epidemiol. 1990;19(3):673–9. PubMed PMID: 2262263. Epub 1990/09/01. eng.

23. Weiss SM, Lakshminarayan S. Acute inhalation injury. Clin Chest Med. 1994;15(1):103–16. PubMed PMID: 8200187. Epub 1994/03/01. eng.

24. Mertens DM, Jenkins ME, Warden GD. Outpatient burn management. Nurs Clin North Am. 1997;32 (2):343–64. PubMed PMID: 9115481. Epub 1997/06/01. eng.

25. Paper ABAW. Surgical management of the burn wound and use of skin substitutes 2009. http://www.ameriburn.org.

26. Collis N, Smith G, Fenton OM. Accuracy of burn size estimation and subsequent fluid resuscitation prior to arrival at the Yorkshire Regional Burns Unit. A three year retrospective study. Burns. 1999;25(4):345–51. PubMed PMID: 10431984. Epub 1999/08/04. eng.

27. Freiburg C, Igneri P, Sartorelli K, Rogers F. Effects of differences in percent total body surface area estimation on fluid resuscitation of transferred burn patients. J Burn Care Res. 2007;28(1):42–8. PubMed PMID: 17211199. Epub 2007/01/11. eng.

28. Minimas D. A critical evaluation of the Lund-Browder chart. Wounds UK. 2007;3(3):58–68.

29. Hidvegi N, Nduka C, Myers S, Dziewulski P. Estimation of breast burn size. Plast Reconstr Surg. 2004;113 (6):1591–7. PubMed PMID: 15114118. Epub 2004/04/29. eng.

30. Lund C, Browder N. The estimation of areas of burns. Surg Gynecol Obstet. 1944;79:352–8.

31. Monafo WW. Initial management of burns. N Engl J Med. 1996;335(21):1581–6. PubMed PMID: 8900093. Epub 1996/11/21. eng.

32. Wachtel TL, Berry CC, Wachtel EE, Frank HA. The inter-rater reliability of estimating the size of burns from various burn area chart drawings. Burns. 2000;26(2):156–70. PubMed PMID: 10716359. Epub 2000/03/15. eng.

33. Amirsheybani HR, Crecelius GM, Timothy NH, Pfeiffer M, Saggers GC, Manders EK. The natural history of the growth of the hand: I. Hand area as a percentage of body surface area. Plast Reconstr Surg. 2001;107(3):726–33. PubMed PMID: 11304598. Epub 2001/04/17. eng.

34. Jose RM, Roy DK, Vidyadharan R, Erdmann M. Burns area estimation-an error perpetuated. Burns. 2004;30(5):481–2. PubMed PMID: 15225916. Epub 2004/07/01. eng.

35. Perry RJ, Moore CA, Morgan BD, Plummer DL. Determining the approximate area of a burn: an inconsistency investigated and re-evaluated. BMJ. 1996;312(7042):1338. PubMed PMID: 8646048. Pubmed Central PMCID: PMC2350999. Epub 1996/05/25. eng.

36. Sheridan RL, Petras L, Basha G, Salvo P, Cifrino C, Hinson M, et al. Planimetry study of the percent of body surface represented by the hand and palm: sizing irregular burns is more accurately done with the palm. J Burn Care Rehabil. 1995;16(6):605–6. PubMed PMID: 8582938. Epub 1995/11/01. eng.

37. Ichiki Y, Kato Y, Kitajima Y. Assessment of burn area: most objective method. Burns. 2008;34 (3):425–6. PubMed PMID: 17920774. Epub 2007/ 10/09. eng.

38. Neuwalder JM, Sampson C, Breuing KH, Orgill DP. A review of computer-aided body surface area determination: SAGE II and EPRI's 3D Burn Vision. J Burn Care Rehabil. 2002;23(1):55–9. PubMed PMID: 11803314. discussion 4; Epub 2002/01/23. eng.

39. Hartford CE. Care of outpatient burns. 3rd ed. Philadelphia, PA: Elsevier; 2007.

40. Harrison HN, Moncrief JA, Duckett Jr JW, Mason Jr AD. The relationship between energy metabolism and water loss from vaporization in severely burned patients. Surgery. 1964;56:203–11. PubMed PMID: 14174738. Epub 1964/07/01. eng.

41. Schultz AM, Werba A, Wolrab C. Early cardiorespiratory patterns in severely burned patients with concomitant inhalation injury. Burns. 1997;23(5):421–5. PubMed PMID: 9426912. Epub 1997/08/01. eng.

42. Ansermino M, Hemsley C. Intensive care management and control of infection. BMJ. 2004;329 (7459):220–3. PubMed PMID: 15271835. Pubmed Central PMCID: PMC487741. Epub 2004/07/24. eng.

43. Sheridan RL, Ryan CM, Yin LM, Hurley J, Tompkins RG. Death in the burn unit: sterile multiple organ failure. Burns. 1998;24(4):307–11. PubMed PMID: 9688194. Epub 1998/08/04. eng.

44. Kraft R, Herndon DN, Branski LK, Finnerty CC, Leonard KR, Jeschke MG. Optimized fluid management improves outcomes of pediatric burn patients. J Surg Res. 2013;181(1):121–8. PubMed PMID: 22703982. Pubmed Central PMCID: PMC3465500. Epub 2012/06/19. eng.

45. Lin CY, Wu CK, Yeong EK, Lin HH, Huang YT, Lee JK, et al. Prognostic significance of left ventricular diastolic function in burn patients. Shock. 2012;37 (5):457–62. PubMed PMID: 22508290. Epub 2012/ 04/18. eng.

46. Kallinen O, Maisniemi K, Bohling T, Tukiainen E, Koljonen V. Multiple organ failure as a cause of death in patients with severe burns. J Burn Care Res. 2012;33(2):206–11. PubMed PMID: 21979843. Epub 2011/10/08. eng.

47. Abu-Sittah GS, Sarhane KA, Dibo SA, Ibrahim A. Cardiovascular dysfunction in burns: review of the literature. Ann Burns Fire disasters. 2012;25 (1):26–37. PubMed PMID: 23012613. Pubmed Central PMCID: PMC3431724. Epub 2012/09/27. eng.

48. Cakir B, Yegen BC. Systemic responses to burn injury. Turk J Med Sci. 2004;34:215–26.

49. Porter JM, Shakespeare PG. Cardiac output after burn injury. Ann R Coll Surg Engl. 1984;66(1):33–5. PubMed PMID: 6691694. Pubmed Central PMCID: PMC2493656. Epub 1984/01/01. eng.

50. de Campo T, Aldrete JA. The anesthetic management of the severely burned patient. Intensive Care Med. 1981;7(2):55–62. PubMed PMID: 7009689. Epub 1981/01/01. eng.

51. Black R, Kinsella J. Anaesthetic management for burns patients. Br J Anaesth. 2001;1(6):177–80.

52. Rehberg S, Maybauer MO, Enkhbaatar P, Maybauer DM, Yamamoto Y, Traber DL. Pathophysiology, management and treatment of smoke inhalation injury. Exp Rev Resp Med. 2009;3(3):283–97. PubMed PMID: 20161170. Pubmed Central PMCID: PMC2722076. Epub 2010/02/18. Eng.

53. Barasch P, Cullen BF, Stoelting RK. Clinical anesthesia. 5th ed. Philadelphia, PA: Lippincott Williams and Wilkins; 2006.

54. Hampson NB, Zmaeff JL. Outcome of patients experiencing cardiac arrest with carbon monoxide poisoning treated with hyperbaric oxygen. Ann Emerg Med. 2001;38(1):36–41. PubMed PMID: 11423810. Epub 2001/06/26. eng.

55. Vegfors M, Lennmarken C. Carboxyhaemoglobinaemia and pulse oximetry. Br J Anaesth. 1991;66(5):625–6. PubMed PMID: 2031826. Epub 1991/05/01. eng.

56. Haney M, Tait AR, Tremper KK. Effect of carboxyhemoglobin on the accuracy of mixed venous oximetry monitors in dogs. Crit Care Med. 1994;22(7):1181–5. PubMed PMID: 8026210. Epub 1994/07/01. eng.

57. Alarie Y. Toxicity of fire smoke. Crit Rev Toxicol. 2002;32(4):259–89. PubMed PMID: 12184505. Epub 2002/08/20. eng.

58. Mizock BA. Lactic acidosis. Disease-a-month: DM. 1989;35(4):233–300. PubMed PMID: 2656163. Epub 1989/04/01. eng.

59. Tursky T, Sajter V. The influence of potassium cyanide poisoning on the gamma-aminobutyric acid level in rat brain. J Neurochem. 1962;9:519–23. PubMed PMID: 13994947. Epub 1962/09/01. eng.

60. Morocco AP. Cyanides is the. Crit Care Clin. 2005;21 (4):691–705. vi. PubMed PMID: 16168309. Epub 2005/09/20. eng.

61. Planas M, Wachtel T, Frank H, Henderson LW. Characterization of acute renal failure in the burned patient. Archiv Intern Med. 1982;142(12):2087–91. PubMed PMID: 7138158. Epub 1982/11/01. eng.

62. Schneider DF, Dobrowolsky A, Shakir IA, Sinacore JM, Mosier MJ, Gamelli RL. Predicting acute kidney injury among burn patients in the 21st century: a classification and regression tree analysis. J Burn Care Res. 2012;33 (2):242–351. PubMed PMID: 22370901. Pubmed Central PMCID: PMC3310938. Epub 2012/03/01. eng.

63. Stoelting R, Dierdorf SF. Anesthesia and co-existing disease. 4th ed. Philadelphia, PA: Churchill Livingstone; 2002.

64. Davies MP, Evans J, McGonigle RJ. The dialysis debate: acute renal failure in burns patients. Burns. 1994;20(1):71–3. PubMed PMID: 8148082. Epub 1994/02/01. eng.

65. Xiao SC, Zhu SH, Xia ZF, Lu W, Wang GQ, Ben DF, et al. Prevention and treatment of gastrointestinal dysfunction following severe burns: a summary of recent 30-year clinical experience. World J Gastroenterol. 2008;14(20):3231–5. PubMed PMID: 18506931. Pubmed Central PMCID: PMC2712858. Epub 2008/05/29. eng.

66. Deitch EA. The management of burns. N Engl J Med. 1990;323(18):1249–53. PubMed PMID: 2120587. Epub 1990/11/01. eng.

67. Rodriguez NA, Jeschke MG, Williams FN, Kamolz LP, Herndon DN. Nutrition in burns: Galveston contributions. J Parenter Enteral Nutr. 2011;35 (6):704–14. PubMed PMID: 21975669. Epub 2011/ 10/07. eng.

68. Kasten KR, Makley AT, Kagan RJ. Update on the critical care management of severe burns. J Intens Care Med. 2011;26(4):223–336. PubMed PMID: 21764766. Epub 2011/07/19. eng.

69. Gregory G. Gregory's pediatric anesthesia. 5th ed. Oxford: Blackwell Publishing; 2012.

70. Demling RH. Burns. N Engl J Med. 1985;313 (22):1389–98. PubMed PMID: 3903505. Epub 1985/ 11/28. eng.

71. Alexander JW, Ogle CK, Stinnett JD, Macmillan BG. A sequential, prospective analysis of immunologic abnormalities and infection following severe thermal injury. Ann Surg. 1978;188(6):809–16. PubMed PMID: 736659. Pubmed Central PMCID: PMC1397007. Epub 1978/12/01. eng.

72. Davis JM, Dineen P, Gallin JI. Neutrophil degranulation and abnormal chemotaxis after thermal injury. J Immunol. 1980;124(3):1467–71. PubMed PMID: 7358988. Epub 1980/03/01. eng.

73. Flierl MA, Stahel PF, Touban BM, Beauchamp KM, Morgan SJ, Smith WR, et al. Bench-to-bedside review: burn-induced cerebral inflammation—a neglected entity? Crit Care. 2009;13(3):215. PubMed PMID: 19638180. Pubmed Central PMCID: PMC2717412. Epub 2009/07/30. eng.

74. Hettiaratchy S, Papini R. Initial management of a major burn: II—assessment and resuscitation. BMJ. 2004;329(7457):101–3. PubMed PMID: 15242917. Pubmed Central PMCID: PMC449823. Epub 2004/ 07/10. eng.

75. DeSanti L. Pathophysiology and current management of burn injury. Adv Skin Wound Care. 2005;18 (6):333–4.

Management of Burns and Anesthetic Implications

14

Cynthia Wang

Initial Management of Burns

All patients who present with burn injuries should be thoroughly evaluated using the Advanced Trauma Life Support (ATLS) protocol. Approximately 10 % of patients with burn injuries also present with concomitant traumatic injuries, so a head to toe evaluation is imperative. An ABCDEF primary survey should be performed: airway, breathing, circulation, disability, exposure, and fluid resuscitation. If the heat source is not yet removed at initial point of contact, it must be immediately removed. Even after flames have been extinguished, clothing can still retain heat and must be removed as quickly as possible. The exception to this is material that is adherent to the skin such as tar or nylon, which should be left in place to prevent further skin injury. The burn area should first be irrigated with tepid water (approximately 15 °C). Ice water should be avoided due to its vasoconstrictive effects and because of the risk of hypothermia in patients with extensive burns who lose copious amounts of heat due to evaporative losses from disrupted skin barrier. Tepid irrigation for at least 20 min cools the burned area, removes any noxious agents, and also helps to stabilize mast cells and temper histamine release [1–3].

If the patient has not yet arrived to a care facility, the burned area should be covered after generous irrigation in order to prevent heat loss and to serve as a barrier against further evaporative losses and pathogens. Polyvinyl chloride film, otherwise known as common household plastic wrap, is ideal as it is non-adherent, transparent so that the burn area can be visually inspected, and impermeable. This should be gently laid onto the wound rather than wrapped so that in case the area swells, a tight wrap does not create ischemia or compartment syndrome. If plastic wrap is not available, a clean cotton sheet may be used instead, though it is less ideal. Wet dressings should be avoided due to the risk of rapid heat loss. Any topical creams should be avoided at this stage.

Chemical burns must be irrigated with particular care, as the deleterious effects of the offending agent only subside upon complete removal of the agent. If a chemical burn is suspected, a prompt search for the causative agent must be conducted, as simply irrigating with tepid water may not be adequate (Table 14.1). After rinsing with water and removing all contaminated clothing, the agent can be tested with litmus paper to determine whether it was acidic or alkaline. Certain chemical agents are neutralized with specific treatments. Hydrofluoric acid, for instance, which is commonly used for glass etching and can cause industrial burns, must be neutralized with topical calcium gluconate. Any eye injuries must also be irrigated copiously and examined promptly by an ophthalmologist.

C. Wang, M.D. (✉)
Department of Anesthesiology, Ronald Reagan UCLA Medical Center, 757 Westwood Plaza, Los Angeles, CA 90095, USA
e-mail: cynthiawang@mednet.ucla.edu

C.S. Scher (ed.), *Anesthesia for Trauma*, DOI 10.1007/978-1-4939-0909-4_14,
© Springer Science+Business Media New York 2014

Table 14.1 Specific chemical burns and treatments

Specific chemical burns and treatments
Chromic acid—Rinse with dilute sodium hyposulphite
Dichromate salts—Rinse with dilute sodium hyposulphite
Hydrofluoric acid—10 % calcium gluconate applied topically as a gel or injected

Reprinted from British Medical Journal, Ref. [4], copyright 2004 with permission from BMJ Publishing Group Ltd

Approximately 60–70 % of burns seen in the emergency department are minor. If the burn is minor, it may be suitable for treatment in an outpatient setting. Generally, these are small (less than 10 % BSA), superficial burns that do not affect critical areas. The victim of the burn should also be relatively healthy with few or no significant comorbidities. If treated in an outpatient setting, maintenance of sterility is of utmost importance. The wound may be washed with soap and water or cleaned with a very dilute chlorhexidine solution. There is some controversy over how to manage blisters from burns in the outpatient setting; however, if the blister is large, it should be unroofed and the dead skin should be removed in a sterile fashion. The burned area should be securely dressed with sterile gauze and covered with a cotton wool dressing. The area should be inspected every 24 h. After the first 48 h, the dressing should be changed. After the first dressing change, subsequent dressing changes should be done every 3–5 days. If a minor burn has not healed within 2 weeks, it should be referred to a specialist. As the burn area heals, the skin becomes dry, scaly, and may itch. Changes in pigmentation may also occur as healing progresses. Sun exposure to the burned area should be minimized for 6–12 months after the initial injury [4, 5].

Burns that involve more than 10 % BSA or extend beyond the superficial layer of skin merit further evaluation and treatment, possibly in an inpatient setting. Patients who have evidence of electrical burns mandate a detailed evaluation given their tendencies to develop compartment syndrome, cardiac dysrhythmias, and muscle necrosis. Those who fail outpatient therapy or require supplemental nutritional support may also require continuing treatment at an inpatient facility. Patients at extremes of age, with large burns, or with burns involving critical areas should be transferred to a specialized burn center [6, 7].

Management of Airway and Inhalational Injuries

While the treatment for cutaneous burns has improved dramatically in the last few decades, mortality rates for patients with inhalational injuries have not changed significantly. Airway assessment is extremely important after a burn injury as inhalational injury can be present even in the absence of cutaneous burn injuries. Any closed space burn injuries involving steam, hot gases, combustibles, or explosions should raise suspicion for airway involvement and/or inhalational injuries. The oropharynx should be inspected carefully for soot. Carbonaceous sputum, singed facial or nasal hairs, or any burn injuries to the face or neck region may also be clues to inhalation injury. The patient should be observed over time for any signs of respiratory distress such as wheezing, stridor, tachypnea, or hoarseness, which may not be immediately apparent. These symptoms can develop as the airway becomes more edematous over the course of many hours (up to 18 h or more). Confusion, agitation, obtundation, or altered mental status may be indicators of carbon monoxide or cyanide poisoning. Pulse oximetry can often be deceptively normal in patients with burn injury, as it does not reflect abnormal hemoglobin species, nor does it reflect the metabolic ramifications of toxic gaseous byproducts. Arterial blood gas may be a somewhat better indicator for the presence of inhalational injury. A $PaO_2:FiO_2$ ratio of <300 has been shown to be an indicator of poor outcomes in patients with burn injuries. Chest radiographs and computed tomography are generally not useful. Fiberoptic bronchoscopy, however, can be used to directly inspect the supra- and infra-glottic airway for edema and for carbonaceous material. Fiberoptic bronchoscopy also aides in safely placing endotracheal tubes as well as in removing mucous plugs, exudate, and foreign irritants [6, 8].

All patients who are suspected to have suffered from inhalational injuries should receive 100 % O_2 as soon as possible. As was previously discussed, carbon monoxide poisoning is common in patients with burn and/or inhalational injuries. The half-life of carbon monoxide is normally 240–320 min. However, with the administration of normobaric 100 % O_2, this half-life decreases to 40–80 min. One hundred percent O_2 should be administered for as long as it is necessary, or at least until the carbon monoxide concentration reaches 10 % or below. Hyperbaric oxygen therapy may also be considered for carbon monoxide poisoning. However, there is little evidence to suggest that it improves outcomes, and there is no consensus regarding the duration and intensity of treatment. Hyperbaric oxygen therapy also increases the risk of barotrauma in this patient population.

Obstruction, critical hypoxia, and death can quickly ensue after inhalational injuries, even if the airway is patent upon initial assessment, so establishment of a secure airway in a timely manner is crucial. Delay can result in a difficult intubation. Patients with facial trauma or burns may also be difficult to mask ventilate. Even if intubation is performed promptly, administration of an induction agent can result in obstruction due to relaxation of the upper airways, especially in the presence of upper respiratory tract injuries. Patients with inhalational injuries may also have very swollen tongues, making visualization of the airway cumbersome. Depending on the degree of airway involvement in the burn injury, an awake intubation with a fiberoptic bronchoscope may be the most suitable method of establishing an airway. If the patient is intubated, the endotracheal tube must be very carefully secured as accidental dislodgment of the tube can be fatal. If there is evidence or suspicion of vocal cord damage, a tracheostomy may be the preferred method of establishing an airway in order to prevent any exacerbation of vocal cord injury from an endotracheal tube. However, whether or not an airway is established with an endotracheal tube or a tracheostomy, resources and personnel able to establish a surgical airway should always be available given the dynamic changes to the airway in burn patients over time. Following intubation, the head of the bed should be kept elevated in order to minimize facial and airway edema. Over the long term, as the patient heals, scars and contractures in the head and neck area can limit mouth opening and neck mobility, creating difficulties in establishing an airway for subsequent surgical procedures [6, 9–13].

Patients with inhalational injury may require unconventional ventilation modes in the intensive care unit. Volumetric diffusive respiratory mode (VDR) is a ventilation mode in which high frequency, sub-tidal volume breaths are progressively accumulated until a certain airway pressure is met. At this point, passive exhalation is permitted to occur. The goal of VDR is to reduce mean airway pressures and increase overall PaO_2 and PaO_2:FiO_2 ratios without adversely affecting hemodynamics. It has also been shown to help mobilize secretions more effectively than conventional modes of ventilation. Additionally, studies have suggested that the incidence of pneumonia is decreased in patients who are ventilated with VDR modes versus conventional ventilation modes. Airway pressure release ventilation mode (APRV) is another alternative mode of ventilation that may be beneficial in patients with burn injuries. APRV uses high and low PEEP in order to recruit closed alveoli and therefore improve oxygenation. Essentially, it is a continuous positive airway pressure mode that is interrupted by an intermittent release phase. This mode of ventilation results in improved oxygenation due to improved V:Q matching, and decreased sedation and paralysis requirements. It has also been shown to improve blood flow not only to the lung and muscles of respiration, but also the gastrointestinal system and the kidneys [14–16].

Adjunctive therapies such as the use of bronchodilators, nitric oxide, nebulized heparin, N-acetylcysteine, and aggressive pulmonary toilet are also important in decreasing the incidence of respiratory morbidity and mortality. When inhaled, nitric oxide selectively dilates capillaries that supply ventilated lung regions, improving V:

Q ratios. Although some patients exhibit dramatic improvement in $PaO_2:FiO_2$ ratios with the use of nitric oxide, studies have suggested that if there is no response to nitric oxide within 60 min of therapy using concentrations between 5 and 20 ppm, nitric oxide is unlikely to be of benefit, and it should be abandoned as a therapeutic option. In patients who are responders to inhaled nitric oxide, however, the drug has been shown to have an overall survival benefit. Nebulized heparin and TPA have also been shown to be of benefit in some studies. These agents are thought to improve ventilation by breaking down fibrin deposits that form as a result of inhalational injury. This in turn improves alveolar oxygenation and ventilation by reducing obstruction. *N*-acetylcysteine, otherwise known as Mucomyst, has not been shown to confer any survival benefit on patients with burn injuries. However, it has been shown to decrease leukocyte numbers in bronchoalveolar lavage. One particular study that reviewed the benefits of inhaled heparin and *N*-acetylcysteine in patients with inhalational injury revealed that the combination of the two agents resulted in a statistically significant survival benefit by attenuating the progression of acute respiratory distress syndrome. Inhaled β-agonist agents can also produce bronchodilation and reduce lung inflammation without systemic hemodynamic effects. Aerosolized corticosteroids, though often used to treat chronic pulmonary diseases, have not been shown to be of benefit in patients with inhalational injury. Though some have suggested that corticosteroids confer a limited benefit in patients with late stage ARDS, this conclusion is not definitive [17–21].

In patients in whom conventional or unconventional ventilation modes fail to provide adequate oxygenation and ventilation, veno-venous extracorporeal membrane oxygenation (ECMO) may be considered. ECMO may help to maintain oxygenation while minimizing barotrauma to already injured lung parenchyma. There have been isolated case reports of patients who have successfully survived severe respiratory failure due to the use of extracorporeal life support. However, one retrospective study of patients who failed conventional ventilation and were placed on ECMO revealed low survival rates amongst trauma and burn victims. Other predictors of poor survival on ECMO included older age, prolonged mechanical ventilation prior to initiation of ECMO, multiple organ failure, and long ECMO runs [22, 23].

Burn Resuscitation

Patients with burn injuries must be resuscitated promptly; any delay can significantly increase mortality. The greatest fluid loss in patients who have suffered from burns occurs within the first 24 h. For those with small burns, peripheral intravenous access is generally adequate. However, for patients with burns involving more than 20 % BSA, central line placement for intravenous access is more appropriate.

Several formulas have been developed in order to help guide fluid resuscitation. Generally, these formulas provide guidelines for aggressive but steady fluid resuscitation. Boluses of fluid typically are ineffective and sometimes even deleterious for burn patients, as the rapid rise in intravascular hydrostatic pressure simply drives more fluid out of the circulation. One of the most popular formulas for guiding resuscitation is the Parkland formula, otherwise known as the Baxter formula. It was developed in 1970 by Dr. Charles R. Baxter at Parkland Memorial Hospital who discovered that more aggressive volume resuscitation within the first 8 h after an injury improved cardiac output. The Parkland formula calls for the administration of 4 mL/kg/% TBSA burned for the first 24 h. The Parkland formula does not apply to superficial burn areas. One-half of the calculated fluid need is administered within the first 8 h, and the remaining half is given over the next 16 h. The modified Brooke formula calls for 2 mL/kg for each percentage of TBSA burned over 24 h. Some have suggested that using the Parkland formula more frequently results in over-resuscitation, which can be a risk factor for increased mortality. However, other studies have shown no differences in mortality between the two formulas. Children require maintenance fluid in addition to the calculated resuscitation volumes. The Galveston formula has been used to determine appropriate resuscitation and maintenance volumes for children with burn injuries. It calls for 5 L/m^2 burned for resuscitation with an additional 2 L/m^2 per day for maintenance. Like both the Parkland and Brooke formulas, half of the resuscitation and maintenance is administered over the first 8 h, and the remaining half is given over the next 16 h. Of note, high tension electrical injuries require more fluid, up to 9 mL/kg/%TBSA in the first 24 h. Patients with concomitant inhalational injuries may also have higher fluid requirements [24–30].

Despite the formulas and guidelines for fluid resuscitation, there is no consensus on a standardized formula or protocol for burn patients. In fact, empiric experience suggests that these formulas often underestimate the fluid requirements in burn patients. Because of these observations, some have advocated that resuscitation be tailored to clinical endpoints. These include urine output of 0.5 mL to 1 mL/kg/h in adults and children with guidance from hemodynamic parameters. Hemodynamic monitoring not only includes the use of invasive or non-invasive blood pressure monitoring, but also cardiac output monitoring. Swan-Ganz catheters are used less and less in burn patients and replaced by monitoring devices that measure the cardiac output using non-invasive methods, such as the end-tidal carbon dioxide tracing, esophageal Doppler and pulse contour cardiac output, which uses the shape of the arterial pulse tracing to determine the stroke volume and cardiac output [6, 24, 31–33].

Usually, for initial resuscitation, crystalloid solution is preferred. There is no consensus on the ideal solution, but generally, 0.9 % normal saline is avoided due to the risk of developing hyperchloremic metabolic acidosis with large resuscitation volumes. Isotonic solutions such as lactated Ringer's, Plasmalyte, or Hartmann's solution that contain more physiologic concentrations of electrolytes are preferred. Historically, albumin was routinely administered as part of the initial resuscitation within the first 24 h. In theory, colloid administration should be beneficial since serum protein levels decrease after burn injuries. Some have shown that those receiving colloid receive less crystalloid and less fluid overall during the resuscitative period. However, recent evidence has suggested that colloid resuscitation does not reduce mortality and adds to the overall cost of care. For children weighing less than 20 kg, 5 % dextrose should be added to the resuscitation fluid in order to prevent hypoglycemia. After the first 24 h, some centers begin administering colloid at 0.5 mL/kg/%TBSA along with crystalloid at 1.5 mL/kg/%TBSA, titrating resuscitation to urine output [6, 30, 34–36].

Although delayed resuscitation can result in poor perfusion to both vital organs and otherwise viable tissue, over-resuscitation is also risky and can lead to its own set of complications. Compartment syndrome has been reported in cases involving circumferential, deep, full-thickness burns and has been linked to the amount of fluid infused. In addition, the systemic inflammatory response results in microvascular leak, vasodilation, and decreased cardiac output and contractility, all of which can confound fluid management goals in burn patients while contributing to the development of compartment syndrome. The development of abdominal compartment syndrome may be suspected if the patient develops abdominal distension, oliguria, and if he or she becomes increasingly difficult to mechanically ventilate. Abdominal compartment syndrome is particularly concerning as it decreases perfusion to many vital organs, including the bowel, liver, and kidneys, and leads to multiorgan compromise or failure. Serial bladder pressure measurements may provide insight into the development of abdominal compartment syndrome and help determine whether a decompressive laparotomy is necessary in order to prevent organ damage. Another treatment option is percutaneous drainage of fluid with a peritoneal dialysis catheter. For suspected compartment syndrome in other parts of the body, such as the extremities, compartment pressures may be measured by inserting an 18G needle under the eschar into the subfascial tissue and transducing pressure measurements. Pressures greater than 30 mmHg are considered to be diagnostic of compartment syndrome, and measures should be taken to decompress the area. This is usually accomplished by performing an escharotomy or fasciotomy. An escharotomy can be performed at bedside with light sedation and involves making an incision along the entire length of the eschar with extension of the incision to viable tissue. Only burnt tissue is divided, sparing the fascia.

A fasciotomy must be performed in the operating room as it involves opening the full length of fascial compartments. The pressure within the affected area can be monitored after decompression with a bedside manometry device [6, 37–39].

Wound Management

Wounds must be carefully managed, as inadequately treated wound sites may convert to deeper wounds that mandate surgical intervention. The wound can be cleaned with simply soap and water or chlorhexidine and normal saline washes. Most recommend that blisters greater than 0.5 cm in size be debrided in order to reduce the risk of bacterial colonization. Wounds should be cultured upon admission and recultured at intervals in order to monitor for colonization. Most often, wounds are colonized within a few hours with gram-positive organisms such as *Staphylococcus aureus* and *Staphylococcus epidermis*, or with intestinal flora within a few days such as *Pseudomonas aeruginosa*, *Enterobacter cloacae*, and *Escherichia coli*. Bacterial colonization does not always dictate the need for systemic antibiotics; however, early debridement and topical and/or biological dressings may prevent further spread of infection. Furthermore, healthcare workers must be vigilant in maintaining hand hygiene and a clean environment in order to minimize the chances of cross contamination. Following cleaning of the wound, a topical antimicrobial agent is applied and the wound should be covered with several layers of absorptive gauze and Kerlix in order to minimize evaporative fluid losses [6, 40].

Several types of topical agents can be used, including silver sulfadiazine (Silvadene), mafenide acetate (Sulfamylon), and silver nitrate. Silver sulfadiazine has proven over time to be inexpensive, easy to apply, and to effectively control wound colonization. However, eschar penetration

with Silvadene is minimal, and some have linked leukopenia and hemolysis with Silvadene use. Furthermore, it has been shown to have a direct toxic effect on keratinocytes, which in turn delays wound healing. Mafenide acetate, or Sulfamylon cream, is easy to apply but can be painful when applied to superficial partial thickness burns. Nevertheless, Sulfamylon provides good eschar penetration and is therefore useful in cases when eschar excision is not expected to be performed immediately or when control of *Pseudomonas aeruginosa* infection is needed. Sulfamylon is also a carbonic anhydrase inhibitor, and its use can lead to the development of metabolic acidosis. Silver nitrate solution has become less popular over time due to its poor tissue penetration and association with electrolyte abnormalities. However, it is still a good agent for the prevention or treatment of gram-negative bacterial colonization or fungal infection. In other parts of the world, Granulflex, a hydrocolloid dressing with a thin polyurethane foam sheet bonded onto a semipermeable film that is adhesive and waterproof, is sometimes used. Granulflex is particularly useful in areas that are difficult to cover with normal dressings. Another option is Mepitel, a nonadhesive dressing that consists of a flexible polyamide net coated with soft silicone [5, 6, 41, 42].

Generally, purely epidermal burns, though painful, only require supportive therapy and heal in about a week via regeneration of undamaged keratinocytes within skin adnexae. Burns that involve layers beyond just the epidermis, however, require more attention. Superficial partial thickness burns must be treated in order to prevent wound progression. These wounds rarely progress to deeper burns, but this can happen if the wound becomes dry or if the patient is hypotensive for prolonged periods of time. This is accomplished with antimicrobial creams and occlusive dressings, creating a moist environment that promotes epithelialization. Healing occurs usually within 2 weeks as the epidermis regenerates from keratinocytes within sweat glands and hair follicles. Because of the source of epithelialization, regeneration depends heavily on the density of skin adnexae. In other words, thin, hairless skin tends to heal more slowly than thick, hairy skin. Deep partial thickness burns are perhaps some of the most difficult to address, primarily because they may be unrecognized as deep burns at initial assessment. There are fewer skin adnexae at deeper levels, and therefore, healing occurs at a much slower rate and is more frequently associated with contraction. There are few deep partial thickness burns that can heal without surgical excision by keeping the wound area warm, moist, and free of infection. However, most deep partial thickness burns are best managed by excising the burnt tissue and grafting skin. In full-thickness burns, all regenerative elements of skin are lost, and healing only occurs from the edges of skin. Significant contraction occurs. All full-thickness burns should be excised and grafted unless they involve an area of less than 1 cm in a part of the body that does not affect function (Fig. 14.1) [43].

Grafts used following surgical excision include xenograft, allograft, autograft, or cultured skin substitute. Most burn surgeons recommend that surgical wound excision occur within the first 1–7 days after injury in order to attenuate the systemic inflammatory response to burns and to reduce the risk of sepsis. Aggressive early excision, however, has not been universally supported. One particular study involving adults over 30 years of age with more than 30 % TBSA injured suggests that there is no difference in outcomes between those who are treated conservatively versus those who receive surgical attention within 72 h after the burn. The same study, however, also suggested that in pediatric patients and those between the ages of 17 and 30, early excision led to decreased mortality rates when compared to patients who were managed conservatively. On the whole, many factors including the patient's age, comorbidities, and extent of injury should be taken into account when deciding when the wound should be excised. For the most part, deep burn wounds must be excised early, before it triggers the development of multiple organ failure or becomes infected. When the decision to proceed with surgery is made, some centers stage the excision and grafting process, performing the excision on one day and grafting skin the next in order to shorten operating times, optimize hemostasis, and minimize hypothermia. Post surgical topical antibiotic treatment of the

grafted area is crucial for graft survival and prevention of wound infection [6, 44–47].

The ideal graft material is split thickness skin autograft from neighboring, unburnt areas. The depth of excision of the burnt areas determines the thickness of the skin harvested. It is important to note when grafting skin that thinner grafts generally contract more. Usually, the donor harvest site is adjacent to the burned area, as this improves color matching. Sometimes, if donor sites are sparse, the graft can be perforated with a mesher to allow for expansion. This, however, produces cosmetically undesirable results as the mesh pattern is permanent. Because of this, meshed graft is rarely used on the face and hands.

Other options to consider when donor sites are sparse is to rotate donor sites and use grafts from several areas of unburned skin in sequence, or to wait until donor sites have regenerated and may be reharvested. In either case, the wound can be covered in antimicrobial creams or covered with a temporary covering until skin can be harvested. Examples of temporary coverings include cadaveric allograft, synthetic products, xenograft (such as pigskin), or cultured epithelial autograft. Cultured epithelial autografts help to extend available donor sites. It can be cultured into sheets, which take three weeks to develop, or in suspension, which are available after just 1 week [43].

Nutritional Supplementation in Burn Patients

After a burn injury, patients enter a hypermetabolic state that can persist for up to 12 months. Because of the hypercatabolism and loss of lean body mass in the immediate post-burn phase, a negative nitrogen balance is seen during the first 1 to 2 weeks post injury. Although indirect calorimetry remains the gold standard for measuring resting energy expenditure (REE), the energy requirements of patients are usually overestimated. It is also important to keep in mind that indirect calorimetry measurements only provide insight into energy expenditures during a discreet moment in the post-injury period. Energy expenditure and requirements may vary

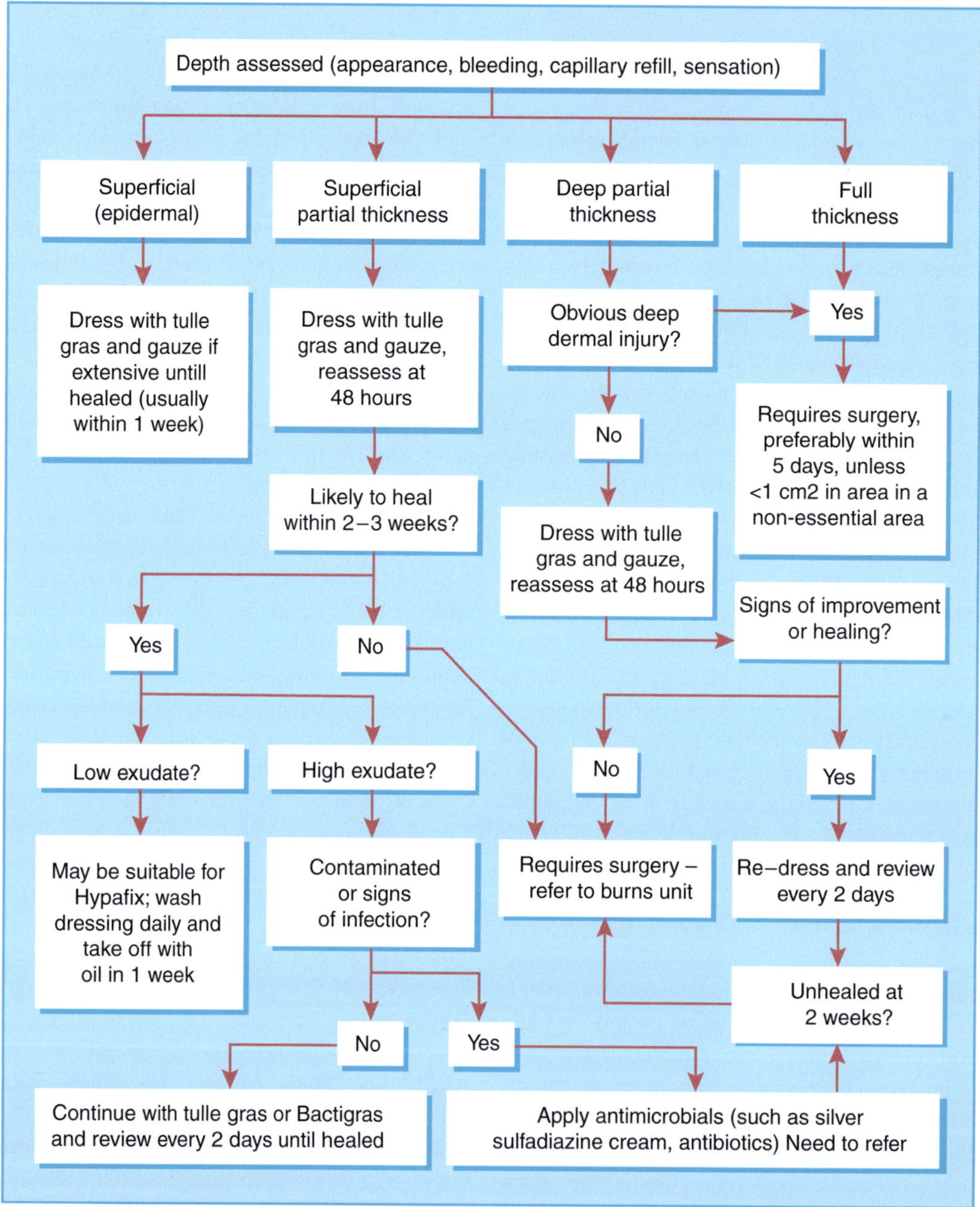

Fig. 14.1 Algorithm for approach to wound assessment and care. Reproduced from British Medical Journal, Ref. [43], copyright 2004 with permission from BMJ Publishing Group Ltd

substantially over the course of the healing process. Care providers must also keep in mind that clinically controlled variables and environmental factors, such as management of heat loss, sedation, and mechanical ventilation may alter energy needs, making nutritional requirements a dynamic issue (Table 14.2). Therefore, performing indirect calorimetry measurements at several points in time in the post-burn period may provide more accurate insight into actual energy requirements.

Overestimating energy requirements can be just as deleterious as underestimating energy

Table 14.2 Factors affecting energy expenditure in burn patients

	Increase	Decrease	No effect
Physiologic effects			
Age		√	
Malnutrition		√	
Wound size	√		
Sepsis			√
Protein catabolism	√		
Pancreatitis	√		
Pain	√		
Fever	√		
Treatment effects			
Mechanical ventilation	√		
Wound closure			√
Warm environment		√	
Surgical procedure			√
Initiation of nutrition support			√
Physical therapy	√		
Medication effects			
Growth hormone			√
Corticosteroids	√		
Vasoactive agents	√		
Neuromuscular blockade			√

Reprinted from Burns: Journal of the International Society for Burn Injuries, Ref. [56], Copyright 2007, with permission from Elsevier

needs, as overfeeding can be detrimental to burn patients. Excess carbohydrate intake increases CO_2 production, fat stores, hepatic dysfunction, hyperglycemia, and prolongs the wound healing process. Severe burns result in the efflux of amino acids from skeletal muscle, presumably in order to accommodate for the amino acid needs mandated by tissue injury and repair. Furthermore, increased cortisol levels result in increased proteolysis, protein breakdown, and protein oxidation. Inadequate protein intake after burn injury compromises wound healing, muscle function, and the immune system. However, excess protein supplementation may also exacerbate the catabolic process. The goal for protein supplementation should be to slow the efflux of amino acids from skeletal muscle and to maximize protein synthesis needed for maintenance of immune function and wound healing. For adults, protein intake of 1.5 g/kg/day

is associated with a net balance between protein synthesis and breakdown. Lipolysis also occurs in burn patients. However, supplementing with exogenous fat usually exacerbates this process or contributes to increased storage of fatty tissue, making it unnecessary and ineffective. Underfeeding has been demonstrated by some to have positive results in critically ill patients who have not suffered from burns. However, it can be dangerous in the patient with burn injuries. An appropriate nutritional strategy is essential for adequate wound healing, mediation of the inflammatory response, control of the hypermetabolic response, and reduction of sepsis-related morbidity and mortality. Although serum albumin levels are often used to assess the nutritional status in critically ill patients, albumin levels in burn patients are poorly reflective of overall nutritional status since albumin levels fall rapidly after the initial burn injury. Replacement or resuscitation with albumin has not been shown to produce positive clinical outcomes. Other nutritional markers, such as transferrin, carotene, iron, and calcium are also unreliable as markers for nutritional status. Over the long term care of burn patients, prealbumin levels may be an indicator of nutritional status, as it is a marker of protein synthesis. In the acute phase, however, prealbumin levels have less of a role [6, 48–56].

Glucose monitoring is perhaps the most central chemical marker for nutritional status in the burn patient. Hyperglycemia occurs in most patients with burn injury regardless of the degree of injury due to increased glucose production and impaired glucose extraction by tissue. The liver and peripheral tissue are also much less responsive to insulin, making it difficult to achieve normoglycemia, even with very high doses of insulin supplementation. Tight glucose control along with modulation of the inflammatory response has been shown to increase survival, improve wound healing, and decrease the incidence of sepsis. Interestingly, beta blockers have been used to modulate glucose levels, enhance the immune response to sepsis, and mediate catecholamine release after severe injury. Some have shown that burn patients who were taking beta blockers prior to the injury exhibited decreased mortality and improved healing times when compared to those who were administered beta blockade therapy in the hospital after the injury. Others have observed that patients who are administered beta blocker therapy benefit from decreased hospital stays. In children, beta blocker therapy has been shown to be associated with decreased cardiac work, attenuation of the inflammatory response without an increase in the incidence or severity of sepsis, and reversal of catabolism [6, 57–67].

In patients who have suffered from a burn injury, enteral feeding is the preferred route for nutritional supplementation. Maintaining gut integrity is thought to decrease the chances of bacterial translocation and reduce the incidence of sepsis. If it is anticipated that oral nutritional intake will be inadequate within 5–7 days after the injury, a feeding tube should be placed. Timing of enteral nutrition is not universally agreed upon, though many advocate initiating feeds within hours after the burn injury. This, however, may be logistically very difficult to manage and potentially dangerous. There is a risk of developing complications, including misplacement of the feeding tube, aspiration, and intestinal necrosis. In fact, some have demonstrated that the incidence of intestinal necrosis was much higher in those who received early feedings. This may be related to altered intestinal perfusion and hypotension during the early burn resuscitation phase in conjunction with the need for increased blood flow to the gut during feeding. It is unclear whether or not initiation of feeding within several hours of injury confers any noticeable benefit when compared to initiation of feeding at a later stage (i.e., 72 h or more following the injury). There is also debate regarding the route of enteral feeding and whether there is a significant difference between small bowel and gastric feeds. Those who are in favor of small bowel feeds maintain that burn patients exhibit delayed gastric emptying, and that, as a result, small bowel feeds decrease the risk of aspiration. Post-pyloric feeds also enable patients to continue feeds throughout surgery. However, placement of small bowel feeding tubes in post-burn injury patients can be tricky and is not without complications. Small bowel feeds are also associated with a high incidence of diarrhea.

Gastric tube feeds not only prevent gastric ulcer formation, but also are associated with a much lower rate of diarrhea. Gastric feeds are also much more simple to administer. For patients who require repeated trips to the operating room, however, gastric tube feeds must be stopped prior to going to the OR in order to prevent aspiration. Frequent interruptions to gastric feeds may necessitate alternatives for providing nutrition, such as supplemental parenteral nutrition. Parenteral nutrition is mainly reserved for those patients who are absolutely unable to tolerate enteral feeds due to gastrointestinal diseases or complications. It remains the second line method of feeding and carries with it an increased risk of sepsis due to central line infection. It is important to note that problems with gut barrier failure and infection are associated with the lack of enteral feeding rather than the provision of parenteral feeding. Thus, in cases in which patients are unable to tolerate enteral feeds, parenteral nutrition must be initiated without delay in order to ensure that nutritional needs are adequately met. In many cases, a combination of enteral and parenteral feeding may be used to achieve this. Intravenous lipids are generally avoided unless parenteral nutrition is required in excess of 3 weeks. This is due to the association of lipid supplementation with platelet dysfunction, poor immune function, and worsened lung function [6, 51, 54, 56, 68, 69].

Vitamin supplementation is also a crucial part of the nutritional regimen in the post-burn patient. Vitamin A has been shown to help in wound healing, and supplementation with vitamin A is recommended in patients with greater than 20 % TBSA burn involvement. Vitamin C should also be administered, as it plays a significant role in collagen synthesis and wound healing. Trace elements are often lost through wound exudates. This, in conjunction with decreased gastrointestinal absorption, increased urinary losses, and altered distribution of nutrients, necessitates more careful assessment and supplementation than in critically ill patients who are not victims of burn injury. Zinc, for instance, is crucial in the wound healing process. Studies have suggested that zinc deficiencies in septic patients are associated with poor outcomes. Despite this, it is consistently difficult to accurately measure levels of micronutrients, partly because trace elements exist in pools that are in a constant state of flux. Many of these micronutrients are bound to protein carriers, and concomitant hypoproteinemia can impair the nutrient's ability to be transported from its storage form to tissues. Thus, isolated measurements of micronutrient concentrations of micronutrients may not reflect actual functional deficiencies. Given the highly catabolic physiology following a burn injury, some have suggested that anabolic steroids may confer some benefit. However, the administration of anabolic steroids in burn patients remains controversial, and there have not been any clear indication that it confers any clinically significant benefit. Other anabolic agents, such as oxandrolone, have also been used in order to restore lean body mass, improve wound healing, and improve overall nutritional status. However, as is the case with steroids, the benefit is observational and supported with little evidence [6, 56, 70–73].

Anesthetic Management for the Burn Patient

Anesthetic management for patients with burn injuries can be challenging. In addition to the airway and resuscitation challenges described above, these patients present unique considerations in the operating room that often require some degree of creativity on the anesthesiologist's part. For one, monitoring can be extremely difficult in these patients for whom access to the chest (for ECG monitoring), arms (blood pressure monitoring), and digits (pulse oximetry) may be limited. For ECG monitoring, skin staples or subcutaneous needles attached to crocodile clips can be used if the thorax has suffered from extensive burns. Even if digits are available for pulse oximetry monitoring, values may be inaccurate due to hypothermia, hypoperfusion, or both. Alternative sites for pulse oximetry such as the nose, lip, or tongue may be necessary. If there is no suitable location for placement of a non-invasive blood pressure cuff, an arterial line may be necessary. Invasive central venous monitoring and monitoring of urine output may also be helpful, but information may be limited if the patient is exhibiting signs of renal insufficiency or failure or if the patient has developed intra-abdominal compartment syndrome. The hypermetabolic state that ensues post-burn injury along with physiology consistent with a systemic inflammatory response may make hemodynamic parameters difficult to interpret.

Induction may be achieved via intravenous or inhalational technique. Maintenance of anesthesia can also be done via inhalational, nitrous-narcotic, intravenous technique, or a combination of techniques. There is no evidence to suggest that one method is superior to the other. Ketamine may be used to augment the anesthetic while adding analgesic effects, particularly in patients who may not be hemodynamically stable. Regional blocks may be considered as a supplement to the anesthetic or, in rare cases, as the primary anesthetic. However, its use is limited by the risk of infection and the area of injury, which may not be isolated to a specific nerve distribution. Extra junctional nicotinic acetylcholine receptors are upregulated 24–48 h after the initial injury. Therefore, succinylcholine must be avoided, as it may result in fatal hyperkalemia. If needed, it may only be used within the first 24 h after injury. The risk of hyperkalemia may persist up to years after the burn injury. A general rule regarding the use of succinylcholine is that once wounds are healed and the patient is mobile, the patient should no longer be susceptible to fatal hyperkalemia from succinylcholine administration. The upregulation of receptors, increased volume of distribution, and increase in metabolic rate also render the patient relatively resistant to the effects of non-depolarizing neuromuscular blockers, mandating much higher doses than usual. Higher doses of induction agents such as thiopental are also required. These physiological changes in addition to increased tolerance with multiple administration also mandate higher doses of opioids. Blood loss can be significant and at times, insidious. Though average predicted blood loss can be variable from center to center, the anesthesiologist should be prepared for at least 50–100 mL of blood loss per percent of body surface area excised. This amount can also vary depending on the age of the wound and the presence of infection. As the wound becomes more hyperemic with time, bleeding during excision can worsen. Infection also exacerbates bleeding. Achieving hemostasis can also be complicated by the presence of thrombocytopenia and by abnormal levels of clotting factors. The best way to manage blood loss is to frequently check hemoglobin and hematocrit levels. In efforts to conserve blood and reduce blood loss, surgeons may employ measures such as infiltration with vasoconstrictors, limb tourniquets, compressive dressings, and performing excisions as early as possible. Blood loss can be minimized by performing excisions within 24 h of injury or after 16 days from the time of initial injury. Infiltration with vasoconstrictors may reduce blood loss; however, there is potential for systemic absorption of tumescent solution, resulting in hemodynamic fluctuations and fluid overload.

Depending on the area being operated on, careful consideration must be given to patient positioning. Pressure points must be carefully padded and excessive pressure should be avoided on burned areas. Due to the physiological changes and areas of burned, exposed, tissue, temperature monitoring is mandatory, as are measures to prevent hypothermia, including administering warmed fluids, maintaining higher ambient temperatures, and forced air warming. Other measures that may be taken include using heat lamps, placing reflective barriers over the patient, and humidifying anesthetic gases. Given that these patients often require multiple anesthetics, the best approach is to carefully review prior anesthetic encounters while keeping in mind that analgesic requirements will likely be increased. Anxiolysis is usually mandatory for these patients. Over time, if face or neck contractures are present, airway anatomy may become distorted due to flexion abnormalities or limited mouth opening. In extreme cases, surgical neck release may be required prior to induction of anesthesia. Alternatively, in the presence of dramatic craniofacial deformities, ECMO has been used in some cases as a bridge to securing the airway until neck release can be performed. This however, should be reserved as a last resort and rescue strategy. As more time progresses and wounds heal, heat loss becomes less of a concern.

Procedures later in the healing process are generally superficial and should require less aggressive pain control [74, 75].

Sepsis and Multiorgan Failure in the Burn Patient

Although great strides have been made in burn resuscitation, thereby reducing the morbidity and mortality from burn shock, the risk of infection and sepsis remains high. Protective skin barriers are compromised in burn injury, and this is the primary point of entry for life threatening infections. Necrotic tissue and serosanguinous exudate from wound beds is an ideal medium for pathogenesis. A depressed immune system following burn injury further increases the risk of infection. Wound care is especially important, as is frequent culturing of open wound beds. This may help in detecting infection in early stages before it has spread into the blood stream. It is important to remember, however, that extensive microbial colonization of the wound surface can make wound cultures very difficult to interpret and treat. Wound biopsy with histological examination and quantitative culture is perhaps the most definitive way of diagnosing infection in the wound bed. This process, however, is time consuming and expensive, making it impractical. Gram-positive bacteria populate the wound within 48 h of injury. Gram-negative organisms appear anywhere from 3 to 21 days after the injury. Fungal infection is seen even later. The most common infectious agents tend to vary from center to center, but in general, the source of infection in many centers has shifted away from β-hemolytic *Streptococci* to resistant gram-negative organisms such as *Pseudomonas*, resistant gram-positive organisms, and fungi (Table 14.3). It is prudent to note that the longer the wound stays open, the greater the risk of fatal infection, particularly in the case of fungal infections, which are also prone to spreading to the lung. Viral infections, most commonly from CMV or HSV, are less likely to spread systemically and appear to have less of an effect than bacteria on overall morbidity and mortality. However, the diagnosis of viral infections can

Table 14.3 Causative agents of wound infection [76]

Pathogen	Examples	Clinical manifestations
β-hemolytic streptococci	*Strepotococcus pyogenes*	Acute cellulitis, occasionally toxic shock syndrome
Staphylococci	Methicillin-resistant *Staphylococcus aureus*	Abcesses, subeschar pus
Gram-negative bacteria	*Pseudomonas aeruginosa* *Acinetobacter baumanii* *Proteus* species	Common in specialized burn units
Fungi	*Candida*	Most common fungal infection; colonizes the surface but has low potential for disseminated invasion
Filamentous fungi	*Aspergillus* *Fusarium* Phycomycetes	Can aggressively invade subcutaneous tissue; must be treated with surgical debridement
Virus	*Herpes simplex*	Causes vesicular lesions

be challenging in the burn patient; therefore, the true effect of viral infections on morbidity and mortality may be underestimated.

Pneumonia is also a leading cause of sepsis in patients who have suffered from burn injury, though it is not nearly as common as wound infection. Patients who are intubated and on mechanical ventilation are at higher risk, as are patients who have suffered inhalational injuries, those with circumferential chest wall burns, and those who remain immobile for long periods of time after injury. For patients in whom early pneumonia is suspected, aggressive bronchoscopy and bronchoalveolar lavage may prevent dissemination of infection, help tailor antibiotic therapy, and decrease needs for mechanical ventilation and length of overall hospital stays. Catheter based infections from indwelling lines are also a significant source of infection. Prompt removal of unnecessary catheters is perhaps one of the best preventative strategies. For lines and catheters that still remain clinically relevant, frequent evaluation and maintenance of the line, followed by catheter exchange (when possible) may help decrease the incidence of line-related infections. Some have advocated the use of silver impregnated, chlorhexidine/silver sulfadiazine coated, or antibiotic coated catheters to reduce the incidence of line-related infections. However, there is little evidence to suggest that the use of these catheters results in outcomes that are any better than vigilant maintenance and routine line care. Urinary tract infections are seen not only in patients with indwelling urinary catheters, but also in those who have suffered burns to the perineum. Sinus and middle ear infections may arise in patients who are fed through nasogastric tubes for prolonged periods of time. Corneal burns may result in secondary infections in the eye. Other less common sites of infection include infective endocarditis—most commonly a result of disseminated bloodstream infections from wound beds or indwelling catheters—as well as intra-abdominal infections, which are quite rare [76–80].

Sepsis is an independent predictor of mortality following a burn injury, particularly in the presence of multiorgan failure. After the initial resuscitation, up to 75 % of mortality in burn patients can be attributed to infection. Often the diagnosis of sepsis may be delayed, as its symptoms of tachycardia, tachypnea, fever, and leukocytosis may be attributed to the burn injury itself rather than to a brewing infection. Although laboratory markers may be used to predict the development of infection, white blood cell counts, neutrophil percentages, and body temperature are poor predictors of bloodstream infection in the burn patient. Some have advocated the use of other markers, such as procalcitonin and C-reactive protein; however, the correlation of these markers with the development of sepsis is poorly agreed upon and inconclusive. The American Burn Association has developed a consensus criteria for the definition of sepsis in patients who have suffered from burns. It includes at least three of the following parameters:

- Temperature >102.2 °F (39 °C) or <97.7 °F (36.5 °C)
- Progressive tachycardia (adults >90 bpm; children >2 standard deviations above age specific normal values)
- Progressive tachypnea (adults >30 breathes per minute; children >2 standard deviations above age specific normal values)
- Refractory hypotension (adults SBP <90 mmHg or a decrease of >40 mmHg or mean arterial BP <70 mmHg; children <2 SD below normal)
- Leukocytosis (adults WBC >12,000/μL; children >2SD above normal) or leukocytopenia (<4,000/μL)
- Thrombocytopenia that occurs 3 days after resuscitation (adults plt <100,000/μL; children <2 SD below age specific normal values)
- Hyperglycemia >110 mg/dL in the absence of pre-existing diabetes mellitus
- Inability to tolerate enteral feeds for more than 24 h based upon:
  - Abdominal distension
  - Residual volumes (two times the feeding rate in adults and >150 mL/h in children)
  - Uncontrollable diarrhea (>2,500 mL/day for adults and >400 mL/day for children)

Additionally, the ABA definition requires that the infection be documented by one of the following modalities:

- Infection is confirmed on culture (wound, blood, urine) OR
- Pathologic tissue source is identified (<10^5 bacteria on quantitative wound biopsy or microbial invasion on biopsy) OR
- A clinical response to antimicrobial administration is documented.

Signs of burn wound infection include conversion of a previously partial thickness wound to full-thickness wound and/or infection that develops at a site that was previously epithelialized. Invasive burn wound characteristics include the following:

- Rapid change in appearance of the wound

- Appearance of focal, multifocal, or generalized dark brown, black, or violaceous discoloration of the wound
- Separation or discoloration of the eschar
- Hemorrhagic discoloration of subeschar tissue
- Presence of green pigment (pyocyanin) in subcutaneous fat (i.e., *Pseudomonas* infection)
- Erythema, edema, pain, warmth of surrounding skin
- Edema and/or violaceous discoloration at the margin between burned and unburned skin
- Presence of initially erythematous and later black necrotic nodular lesions (ecthyma gangrenosa) in adjacent unburned skin
- Exophthalmos may be the first sign of mucormycosis in midface burns (retrobulbar space involvement)

The approach to treatment of infection in burn patients can also be tricky. Excessive and overly aggressive administration of antibiotics may only perpetuate colonization with resistant microorganisms. Because of this, prophylactic systemic antibiotics are generally not recommended. Broad-spectrum antibiotics in order to cover wound manipulation are also not recommended unless the burn involves greater than 40 % of TBSA. A better strategy might involve using shorter courses of narrow spectrum antibiotics in an attempt to deliver more targeted therapy. Careful wound care, including the use of topical antibiotic agents, is an important retardant to wound and bloodstream infections. Early surgical closure of the burn wound also helps to minimize entry points for infection [6, 76, 81–84].

The American Burn Association's registry of causes of burn mortalities reveals that nearly 50 % of patients who did not survive burn injuries died as a result of organ failure. Both multiorgan failure and sepsis in burn patients are associated with burn size, age, male gender, length of stay in intensive care, and duration of mechanical ventilation. The gut hypothesis behind multiple organ failure has gone through many changes over time. Initially, it was thought that loss of gut barrier integrity led to bacterial translocation, bloodstream infection, and systemic inflammation that subsequently resulted in multiorgan failure. This has evolved to the idea that loss of gut barrier function leads to the production of endogenous pro-inflammatory factors and tissue factors that lead to organ injury and eventually, failure. In fact, some have noted that multiple organ failure occurs in burn patients despite the clinical absence of uncontrolled infection, suggesting that the etiology of organ failure is multifactorial and complex in this patient population and may not be solely attributable to sepsis. In fact, in one particular review of burn patients in a specialized facility over the course of 6 years, researchers observed that in most cases of multiorgan failure, patients were actually clinically uninfected at the time of death, even if they had suffered from multiple isolated infectious events over the course of their care. The theory behind this phenomenon is that although the infections and soft tissue injuries that incite the inflammatory process are successfully treated, the systemic inflammatory process persists [85, 86].

It is much more effective to prevent the development of multiorgan failure rather than to treat it after it has begun its course. Minimizing the incidence of sepsis and inflammation through early wound excision and closure, hemodynamic support in order to ensure adequate oxygen delivery to tissues, and early enteral nutrition in order to support the gut and minimize bacterial translocation across the bowel wall are measures that should be taken to prevent the onset of organ failure. Attenuation of the hypermetabolic response—therefore dampening the acute rise in catecholamine, glucagon, and cortisol levels—can also decrease the incidence of multiorgan failure and overall morbidity and mortality. Although there are cases in which multiorgan failure develops in the absence of sepsis, disseminated infection is still a leading cause of multiorgan failure. This is particularly true now with the abundance of multi-drug resistant organisms. Between 1989 and 1999, only 42 % of patients died from sepsis from multi-drug resistant organisms. Twenty-five percent of those patients who died were infected with *Pseudomonas*. Other common offending organisms include *Staphylococcus aureus*,

Escherichia coli, and *Klebsiella pneumonia*. Between 1999 and 2009, the number of patients who died from sepsis and multiorgan failure as a result of infection with multi-drug resistant organisms increased to 86 %, with *Pseudomonas* being present in 64 % of those patients. The incidence of *Acinetobacter* has also risen precipitously over the last few years, whereas prior to 2000, it was seldom in burn patients with sepsis and multiorgan failure. Colistin has emerged as an effective treatment for multi-drug resistant *Pseudomonas* and *Acinetobacter* infections; however, some studies have suggested that there is no difference in mortality between patients who receive colistin versus piperacillin/ tazobactam and vancomycin. Clindamycin and vancomycin are perhaps the most popular and effective treatments for methicillin-resistant *Staphylococcus aureus* infection. Although advancements in fungal treatments have improved dramatically over the last two decades, there are still drug-resistant fungi that may not respond to traditional therapies. *Aspergillus terreus*, for instance, is innately resistant to amphotericin B. Alternative, newer, agents, such as azoles (voriconazole, posaconazole) and echinocandins (caspofungin, micofungin) may be used to treat resistant fungi, but each agent's limitations and side effect profile must be carefully considered prior to selecting a drug. Ultimately, given the complex etiology of wound infection and sepsis in this patient population, infectious disease specialist consultation is often helpful [79, 85, 87, 88].

Rehabilitation After Burns

Even with aggressive fluid resuscitation, wound and infection management, and surgical rehabilitation, burn patients are at extremely high risk of developing long-term limitations to mobility. They must be engaged early and aggressively in physical activity to help maintain range of motion. Immobilization should only be allowed if it is medically necessary. Generally, immobilization is only mandated if there is concomitant injury to tendon and/or bone, or after tissue repair such as skin reconstruction. It was once thought that immobilization time after a grafting procedure should be about 5–7 days. However, the trend has been to decrease the immobilization time after grafting to 3–5 days, promoting passive range of motion exercises as soon as the graft takes and advancing to monitored active range of motion exercises. If a body part must be immobilized, it should be splinted or fixed in an anti-deformity position for as little time as possible. Otherwise, studies have suggested that range of motion exercises be performed anywhere from 2 to 4 times a day with independent activity by the patient in between therapy sessions. Overall, there has been a trend in burn centers toward early ambulation, preferably by postoperative day 5. However, the ability to ambulate by postoperative day 5 is at times limited by the location of the injury and may be more difficult in patients whose injuries involved the lower extremities, particularly below the knees. Patients who are able to ambulate within 24 h after surgery have been shown in some studies to have shorter lengths of stay. Early ambulation also decreases the risk of deep vein thrombosis and pulmonary emboli.

Splinting, though sometimes used to intentionally limit mobility, has also been used to prevent loss of range of motion. There are generally two schools of thought when it comes to splinting: it can be instituted early and used as a preventative measure or initiated therapeutically when the patient begins to show signs of contracture. Generally, the frequency with which this modality is employed is dependent on the depth of burn. Patients with full-thickness burns are more frequently placed in splints than those with more superficial burns. Early splinting is most commonly performed when the injury involves the hand, followed by the ankle, elbow, and axilla. Delayed splinting most often occurs when the injury involves the neck, elbow, perioral region, and knee. Tendon exposure may also mandate splinting in order to preserve range of motion. If the burn involves the hand, particular attention should be paid to rehabilitation efforts as hand function has been found to be a strong predictor of physical quality of life. If the burn has involved the extensor mechanism in the

hand, flexion at the proximal interphalangeal joint can result in the development of a boutonniere deformity, in which the proximal interphalangeal joint is permanently flexed while the distal interphalangeal joint is extended. Early splinting is encouraged in hand burns to prevent boutonniere deformities. Exposed tendons are splinted in the slack position to prevent tendon rupture. Alternatives to splinting the hand in the case of exposed tendons include the use of Kirschner wires or direct contact casts. Others have resorted to pinning the joint in a straightened position. If pinned, care must be taken to remove the pins early unless the intention is to fuse the joint. If the joint becomes fused, the patient may lose his ability to grip, a function which remains preserved in patients with boutonniere deformities. Achilles tendon injury and exposure is another type of injury in which splinting is employed. Some have advocated splinting the foot and ankle in the neutral position, while others support splinting in slight plantar flexion. Exercise and motion of the foot and ankle must be done very gingerly in order to minimize the risk of rupturing the Achilles tendon [89, 90].

Scar formation can be one of the factors that contribute to loss of range of motion. Scarring can vary depending on a number of external factors, such as fluid resuscitation, positioning in the hospital, surgical intervention, and wound dressing and management. However, it can also be influenced by patient specific factors such as age, pregnancy, skin pigmentation, and degree of motivation and compliance with rehabilitation programs. There are two primary types of scars that can develop. Hypertrophic scarring results from the buildup of excess collagen fibers during wound healing and the reorientation of fibers in non-uniform patterns. Keloid scarring extends beyond the boundary of the initial injury and tends to be more common in patients with pigmented skin. Scar formation can be minimized if the wound is well managed from an early stage. Pressure garments are the primary intervention in scar management and should be used immediately after the skin has healed. Pressure is thought to reduce scarring by potentiating scar maturation and encouraging collagen fibers to reorient into uniform, parallel patterns as opposed to the whorled pattern that is seen in untreated scars. Pressure garments need to be tailored to each individual patient, and it is best if they are reassessed and refitted every few months to accommodate the changing contours of the healing wound. For patients with burns that involve the face and/or neck area, an acrylic mask that helps provide conforming pressure over the burned areas may be worn. Masks made of fabric may also be made for patients to wear overnight while sleeping.

Alternatives to pressure garments include pressure devices or non-custom wraps. Although they may not conform to the wound as well as customized garments, they still help to minimize trauma to fragile, healing wound grafts. For areas of scar tissue that have not responded well to pressure garments, other techniques such as massage, creams, and contact media may be considered. Massage helps to soften restrictive bands of scar tissue, making the scar area more pliable. Moisturizing creams prevent the skin from drying and cracking, creating ports of entry for secondary wound infection and skin breakdown. Moisturizing is beneficial to burn patients even if the scar has healed well. There are several different types of contact media that have been used to promote healthy scar formation. Silicone gel sheets are thought to limit the degree of scar contraction through hydration and occlusion. In areas of the body where it is logistically difficult to place silicone sheets such as digits or the web spaces between digits, elastomer molds can be used to help flatten the scar. Hydrocolloid sheets can also be used in lieu of silicone gel sheets. They are also thought to limit scar contraction. Unlike silicone gel sheets, they can be left on the skin for up to 7 days and are very thin, so massage can be given through the thin sheets. Another tool thought to aide in healthy scar formation is ultrasound, which is postulated to help the inflammatory process progress more quickly. Adequate sun protection is mandatory in patients who have suffered from burn injuries for up to 2 years after the initial injury [91, 92].

Heterotopic ossification (HO), which is the extra-articular formation of lamellar bone in connective tissue, is not frequently seen in burn injury, but when it is present, it can lead to serious functional limitations. When HO does occur, the elbow joint tends to be the most common site. The incidence of heterotopic ossification is increased when 25 % or more TBSA is involved in the burn injury. If it develops, it can result in significant pain, loss of range of motion, and even nerve injury for patients. There is little known about what can be done to prevent the development of HO, though early wound closure may play a role. The treatment of HO remains unclear. Active assistive range of motion exercises, gentle terminal stretch, and terminal resistance training are recommended to minimize the development of heterotopic ossification. However, it is probably best to limit the extent of stretching and exercise. Animal models have suggested that aggressive stretching exercises may in fact contribute to the formation of HO and some have suggested that aggressive stretching after development of HO can exacerbate the condition. One particular study demonstrated that forced manipulation during a time of immobilization provoked the development of HO, and remobilization actually increased the density in areas of calcification. Another group showed that passive stretching beyond the pain free range of motion led to progression of HO to complete ankylosis. Thus, once HO has developed, some recommend that exercise should be limited to active range of motion exercises within a pain free range. This issue is particularly tricky in burn patients since stretching plays a critical role in preventing soft tissue contracture in the wound healing process. In severe cases of heterotopic ossification, surgical intervention may be required, followed by a period of aggressive physical therapy. If surgical excision is required to treat HO, it is typically performed a year or more after the initial injury. Local radiation therapy has also produced positive results in some patients. Other treatments, such as the use of non-steroidal anti-inflammatory agents and bisphosphonates, have also been described, but the outcomes have been inconsistent at best. Furthermore, the use of these medications in burn patients may be limited due to concerns for renal toxicity and coagulopathy [93–95].

Another practice that was once common but has become less popular over time is burn hydrotherapy. Hydrotherapy is thought to promote healing by softening and removing dead tissue, therefore enabling new tissue to form. Other theoretical benefits include preventing excessive loss of moisture through burned tissue, removing pus, minimizing scar tissue formation, providing comfort, and in some cases, aiding in physical therapy. There are several different modes of hydrotherapy. Immersion hydrotherapy occurs when the patient is completely submerged in a disinfected pool of sterile water, regardless of the location of the burn. Shower hydrotherapy is directed toward a specific area of injury and is thought to be just as effective as immersion hydrotherapy. The primary risk with either type of hydrotherapy, however, is infection. Hydrotherapy equipment has been shown in some centers to be contaminated with *Pseudomonas* despite meticulous sterilization procedures. In the early 1990s, as many as 90 % of burn centers in North America reported regularly employing hydrotherapy as an integral part of rehabilitation for burn patients. However, due to the risk of infection, only 10 % of burn centers now report regular use of hydrotherapy [96, 97].

Pain Control in Burn Patients

Pain control in burn patients is a particularly challenging issue. Despite efforts to improve the quality of pain management in burn victims, patients continue to report unrelieved moderate to severe levels of pain. There are many reasons that burn pain remains a challenge for caregivers. For one, burn pain can vary drastically from patient to patient, and it can also fluctuate significantly over the course of the recovery period. As the wound heals and scar tissue forms, pain often begins to de-escalate, though this is not to say that burn patients do not experience pain at all once healing has completed. Even after healing, burn patients may have to return frequently to the operating room for reconstructive procedures

that may become a significant source of anxiety and pain. Over time, chronic neuropathic pain and neuropathies may ensue as damaged neurons regenerate. The inflammatory response from nerve and tissue injury can often result in allodynia and primary hyperalgesia in the injured area and secondary hyperalgesia in the surrounding area. Repetitive painful stimuli can cause neuroplastic adaptations throughout the central nervous system whereby afferent pain sensory impulses undergo facilitation and amplification to a given stimulus, contributing to the generation of chronic pain. Associated pathologies such as depression, anxiety, and posttraumatic stress disorder also exacerbate pain symptoms. The degree and nature of pain can also vary depending on the depth of the burn. Superficial burns generally result in hyperalgesia and mild to moderate levels of pain. Superficial partial thickness burns are associated with marked hyperalgesia and moderate to severe pain as sensory receptors at the level of the dermis are damaged. Deep partial thickness to full-thickness burns are often associated with the absence of pain, and hyperalgesia tends to be uncommon. This is primarily due to the fact that the dermis, along with its sensory and vascular structures, is completely destroyed. Acute pain from dressing changes and surgery can be minimal, though there is usually pain in the transition zone between burned and unburned layers of skin. However, this does not mean that patients with deep burns do not experience pain. These patients often describe a deep aching pain that is likely related to the inflammatory response. There are also a number of psychosocial issues and comorbidities that may affect the patient's experience of pain (Fig. 14.2) [98–100].

There are three types of pain that must be addressed in burn patients. Not only do burn patients have a chronic, underlying background pain for which there is no end in sight, patients must deal with the acute pain associated with bedside and surgical procedures (procedural pain). Furthermore, burn patients can also experience significant breakthrough pain that is frequently associated with movement. This mechanical hyperalgesia is especially common

Fig. 14.2 Factors affecting patient's perception of burn pain. Reprinted from Burns: Journal of the International Society for Burn Injuries, Ref. [100], Copyright 2009, with permission from Elsevier

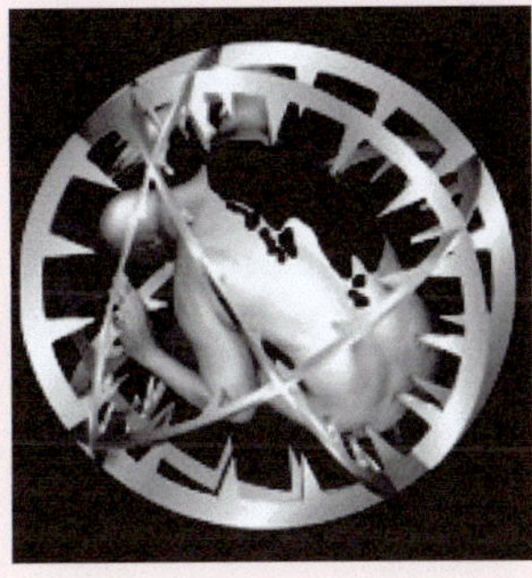

in patients who remain immobilized for extended periods of time. At times, however, breakthrough pain may also occur spontaneously with no apparent inciting event. Background pain, though generally less intense than procedural or breakthrough pain, can worsen significantly before epithelialization is complete.

Adequate assessment of pain levels is extremely important. Assessment tools must be practical and reliable and must address the three facets of pain: pain intensity, behavioral reactions, and physiologic reactions. Although there is no single assessment technique that is universally agreed upon, it is important to select an approach and use it consistently. For adults, assessment of pain is done with adjective scales, such as "none, mild, moderate, and severe." Alternatively, some prefer the numeric scale, using 0 as an indicator of no pain and 10 to reflect the worst, most excruciating pain a patient has ever experienced. The caveat to using these methods is that it may be impossible to elicit a meaningful response in a patient who is sedated and on mechanical ventilation, or in a patient

who is demented. The assessment of pain in children can be much more difficult than it is in adults, particularly for children who are pre-verbal. Physiological indicators such as heart rate, blood pressure, and respiratory rate, which are often used to assess pain in children, are unreliable indicators as they are affected by processes related to the burn injury itself. Instead, scales that assess pain based on behaviors are thought to be more specific. For instance, facial expressions and length of cry have been used to assess pain in children. The FLACC scale (Faces Legs Activity Cry Consolability scale) is perhaps one of the most widely employed observer based pain scales used in children. For children that are pre-school age and older, self-reported verbal scales may be used instead. The Wong-Baker FACES pain scale is designed for children 3 years or older and uses a pictogram of faces displaying varying degrees of pain and discomfort. The child is then asked to choose the face that most closely corresponds with their own level of pain. The OUCHER scale uses a picture scale for very young children and a numerical scale for children 5 years or older [99, 101–105].

The approach to pain management in burn patients must be multimodal, using a combination of pharmacological and non-pharmacological treatment modalities. Pharmacologic agents used for treating pain include opioids, non-opioids, anxiolytics, and anesthetics. Opioid agonists are amongst the more popular pharmacologic analgesics. However, high dose opioids can be associated with short-term adverse side effects such as respiratory depression and constipation, as well as the development of long-term consequences such as tolerance and, in severe cases, addiction. As pain subsides, opioid analgesics cannot simply be abruptly discontinued. For patients who have been on high dose opioids for extended periods of time, abrupt discontinuation may lead to severe withdrawal symptoms. Thus, just as it is important to have a protocol for administering and escalating pain medications, it is important to systematically wean patients who have been on opioids in order to avoid withdrawal symptoms. Of note, there is no evidence that the use of opioids during the management of acute burn pain increases the likelihood of opioid dependency, so opioid analgesics should not be withheld for fear of its adverse side effects. Generally, long-acting opioids such as oral morphine are used to treat chronic, background pain while shorter acting opioids such as fentanyl are given for brief, painful stimuli such as wound care and surgical procedures. When addressing background pain, medication must be administered regularly in order to ensure a steady state of analgesic. Establishing a protocol for medication escalation and administration is crucial to ensure that doses of pain medication are not missed, creating an iatrogenic episode of breakthrough pain. Though opioids can be administered intravenously or orally, the optimal route of administration is intravenous due to its rapid onset of action and titratability. Patient controlled analgesia (PCA) with IV opioids gives patients the flexibility to titrate medication based on patient needs. Oral and gastrointestinal administration of opioids through a feeding tube is also an option and provides equally good pain relief. Though this route of administration is less titratable, it requires minimal monitoring as the risk of fatal overdose is somewhat less.

Oral transmucosal administration of opioids is also useful, particularly in the pediatric population. Intramuscular administration of opioids is not recommended for burn patients. The injections need to be administered frequently, they are painful, and the drug absorption can be extremely variable due to compartment shifts.

Morphine is the standard analgesic against which other analgesics are compared. Morphine tends to be somewhat less effective for short, acute episodes of pain given that its onset and peak effect are somewhat more delayed than other opioids. It is generally reserved for the treatment of chronic, background pain. Oxycodone is an effective alternative to morphine, and some patients exhibit a better response to one versus the other. However, there is no evidence that oxycodone is superior to morphine or vice versa. Fentanyl has a quicker onset and time to peak effect, making it suitable for use in acute pain settings. It is easy to administer intravenously, transmucosally through the buccal or nasal mucosa, and transdermally. Remifentanil is an ultra-short acting opioid that is useful for acute, procedural pain. Given its short half-life and easy titratability, it achieves maximum analgesic effect with a lower risk of delayed side effects. It is, however, extremely potent and should only be administered by trained personnel since it can cause sudden respiratory depression and apnea during administration. Alfentanil is also a short-acting opioid but has a longer half-life than remifentanil. It is also used primarily to treat procedural pain, but given its pharmacokinetics, it provides a greater degree of post-procedural pain relief than remifentanil. Tramadol acts on mu receptors and enhances the reuptake of norepinephrine as well as the release of serotonin. It is generally well tolerated and has an analgesic effect similar to that of morphine. When considering analgesic options for chronic pain, methadone is often used to treat or prevent chronic hyperalgesia related to central sensitization and neuropathic pain [100, 106].

Non-opioid analgesics are also an integral part of the treatment regimen in the burn patient. Dexmedetomidine, a central alpha-2 agonist, provides sedation, anxiolysis, and analgesia with minimal risk for respiratory depression, particularly in children. It is useful for limited stimuli from debridements and dressing changes. Clonidine, like dexmedetomidine, is also a central alpha-2 agonist that augments descending inhibitory spinal cord pathways. It can be effective as an adjunctive analgesic when administered in doses of 1–3 µg/kg/day in adults and children alike. Ketamine is frequently used for the treatment of acute procedural pain. Case reports have suggested that ketamine, when used in conjunction with clonidine, is an extremely effective analgesic and sedative in children who experience severe burn pain, especially during dressing changes. The NMDA antagonizing effects of ketamine also make it useful in treating chronic pain, since it is thought that NMDA receptors play a role in central sensitization after burn injury. Acetaminophen and non-steroidal anti-inflammatory medications (NSAIDs) can also be added to the pharmacological regimen for pain control in burn patients. Both acetaminophen and NSAIDs exhibit a ceiling effect in their dose response relationship. Therefore, their use is usually limited to treating minor burn pain in the outpatient setting. If used for treating severe burn pain, they are usually used as adjuncts to other agents. For procedures and dressing changes, topical analgesics such as lidocaine may also help augment pain control. The data for topical local anesthetics, however, does not show that it produces a significant reduction in procedural pain. There have been some studies that suggest there may be a role for intravenous lidocaine, particularly for acute increases in painful stimuli caused by dressing changes and surgical procedures. Intravenous lidocaine may help improve analgesic efficiency, alleviate some of the deleterious effects of opioid administration, and minimize the necessity of escalating opioid doses in patients with burn injuries. Systemic lidocaine is thought to achieve this by depressing conduction in afferent nerves, inhibiting dorsal horn neural transmission and modifying the cerebral perception of pain. Lidocaine is also thought to possess anti-inflammatory properties that may play a significant role in the suppression of pain in burns, which stem in part from inflammatory processes. However, many studies have failed to demonstrate a decrease in opioid requirements when intravenous lidocaine was used as an adjunctive analgesic. Consultation with pain specialists may be helpful in achieving satisfactory pain control by helping to develop and adhere to protocols as well as for monitoring the evolution and improvement of pain [107–112].

Anxiolytics play an important role in pain control in the burn patient, whose anxiety levels can contribute significantly to their perception of pain. Anxiety is prevalent in the post-burn population given the needs for aggressive surgical treatment and frequent wound debridements, and patients who report high levels of background pain tend to also exhibit higher anxiety levels. Anxiolytics are a particularly effective premedication prior to wound care in order to address the anticipatory anxiety experienced by patients. In fact, benzodiazepines have been shown to improve post-procedure pain scores in patients. Antipsychotic medications are another option for the treatment of anxiety and agitation associated with burn treatments. First generation antipsychotics such as haloperidol are often used for the treatment or even prevention of delirium in critically ill patients. Second generation antipsychotics, such as quetiapine, are used for the treatment of anxiety disorders and are often administered in conjunction with benzodiazepines in burn patients in order to help with sleep. Other centrally acting agents such as antidepressants (amitriptyline) and anticonvulsants (gabapentin) may help to modulate central neuropathic pain. Amitriptyline modulates pain by inhibiting descending spinal cord pain pathways. It can cause sedation, which may be beneficial in helping the patient sleep at night. Patients on amitriptyline may also experience anticholinergic side effects such as dry mouth and blurred vision. Gabapentin binds to presynaptic calcium channel receptors that are involved in pain hypersensitivity and indirectly inhibits NMDA receptors [99, 100, 113–115].

Anesthetics, whether general, neuraxial, targeted non-neuraxial, or regional, are also useful in managing burn pain. General anesthesia or deep sedation is reserved for the relatively brief, intense pain associated with procedures. For moderately painful procedures, inhaled nitrous oxide can be administered to provide analgesia without loss of consciousness. Usually, this is delivered through a face mask in a mixture of 50 % nitrous oxide and 50 % oxygen. Regional anesthesia can be useful for procedures, particularly when the burned area involves extremities. The most common nerve groups involved include the brachial plexus (interscalene block, infraclavicular and supraclavicular blocks, and axillary block), the sciatic nerve, and the femoral nerve. Interestingly, patients who undergo skin grafting procedures often experience more pain at the donor graft site than the grafted area. Thus, regional anesthetic blocks are often used to treat donor graft site pain. Most commonly, bupivacaine and lidocaine are used for these blocks, though other local anesthetics may be selected depending on the nature and length of stimulus. Neuraxial techniques, which involve the administration of local anesthetic into the intrathecal or epidural space have also been used. Prior to catheter placement, coagulation studies must be done to ensure that the risk of hematoma formation is minimal. Care must be taken in the case of indwelling epidural or spinal catheters to monitor for infection, as burn patients may be at higher risk of developing infectious complications such as meningitis and epidural abscess. Targeted non-neuraxial blocks are another option for pain control. For example, a fascia iliaca compartment block can be performed to provide analgesia to the lower extremity following skin graft harvesting. The risks associated with these blocks are minimal as long as the procedures are performed by experienced practitioners [116–118].

Non-pharmacological pain control techniques should complement pharmacologic agents. Choosing a technique should be based on how the patient has responded to the stress of the burn injury. Some patients exhibit signs of avoidance in which they give up control of all medical decision making to health care professionals. These patients typically respond well to distraction techniques that help them avoid focusing on painful stimuli. Avoidance techniques are those that are designed to psychologically distract or distance the patient from the painful stimulus. Diverting attention toward a nonpainful stimulus may lessen the intensity of perceived pain. Avoidance interventions include distraction, guided imagery, hypnosis, and virtual reality. Distraction is perhaps the most effective in children, whose attention is easily diverted with activities such as story-telling, singing songs, or counting. In adults, distraction might require somewhat more creativity and effort. Guided imagery involves the use of imagined pictures, sounds, or sensations to draw attention away from the stimulus. The imagery in this technique is simply one that the patient creates in his mind and can revisit anytime. Hypnosis is an altered state of consciousness characterized by an increased receptivity to suggestion, the ability to alter perceptions, and an increased capacity for dissociation. The dramatic shift in consciousness that occurs with hypnosis is thought to be the mechanism by which attention is shifted away from the perception of pain. Hypnosis is a very involved process and depends heavily on the clinician–patient relationship. It also involves several stages, including deep breathing, suggestions for enhancing the hypnotic state, narrowing the patient's attention, providing posthypnotic suggestions, and finally, reaching the alert stage. If planned well, hypnosis sessions can be scheduled prior to scheduled surgical procedures. Hypnosis is particularly powerful in burn patients because patients with burn injuries often experience a dissociative response that may render them more hypnotizable. Furthermore, many burn patients demonstrate behavioral regression, making them more willing to be taken care of by others and to relinquish control. Studies have suggested that patients with higher baseline pain levels experience a greater decrease in pain after hypnosis than those with lower baseline pain levels. It is important to realize, however, that many of these studies only involve very small cohorts of burn patients and use inconsistent methodologies to assess pain and the effectiveness of treatment with hypnosis. Virtual reality is another method that has been utilized to treat pain. Since attentional focus is limited and the person cannot attend to more than one stimulus at a time, virtual reality creates an environment in which patients can be absorbed by a controlled, alternative stimulus during painful procedures, thus taking the focus away from the procedure being performed. Hypnosis and virtual reality, often used concomitantly, are perhaps the most effective distraction techniques. They have been shown to significantly reduce pain for patients undergoing procedures or dressing changes when used in conjunction with pharmacologic agents. Another subset of patients tend to seek information, actively participate in care, and are reluctant to relinquish control throughout the treatment process. These patients may find distraction techniques stressful as they feel a sense of loss of control in the situation. For patients who demonstrate a desire to be deeply involved in care, the best approach is to keep the patient as informed as possible. Helping the patient understand each issue, alternative, and solution puts the patient at ease by building a sense of trust and mutual understanding.

Other techniques include relaxation techniques that help to lower arousal, thus shifting focus away from the source of pain. Deep breathing, otherwise known as diaphragmatic breathing, is a simple and effective measure that can help the patient relax. Often, pain or anxiety lead to rapid, shallow breathing, also known as thoracic breathing, which can exacerbate muscle tension and contribute to a heightened sense of pain. Deep breathing techniques help the patient avert this phenomenon. Cognitive behavioral techniques (CBT) are also popular non-pharmacologic tools used for addressing pain and anxiety in burn patients. CBT helps to change the way patients think and respond to pain and the anticipation of pain. With cognitive behavioral therapy, patients are given the tools to recognize that certain stimuli will cause pain, mentally block the anticipation of pain, and distract themselves from the pain by diverting their thoughts toward something else. Other non-pharmacological techniques such as massage, progressive muscle relaxation, and acupressure/acupuncture can also be considered in patients who continue to experience severe pain despite best efforts [99, 114, 119–124].

In addition to the treatment of burn pain, burn associated pruritus is also an important symptom that affects patient rehabilitation. The pathophysiology of itching in burn patients is not completely understood. Although histamine is thought to be a contributing factor, the central nervous system has also been implicated in the development and maintenance of these symptoms (Fig. 14.3). It appears that after a burn injury, factors such as female sex, number of surgical procedures, and the presence of posttraumatic stress disorder are associated with a higher incidence of pruritus. Although pruritus can be pervasive throughout the healing process, it is thought that pruritus in the "acute" phase (i.e., within 3 months of injury) is related to the transition from wound closure to early remodeling. Chronic pruritus, or itching that persists 12–24 months after injury, tends to be more commonly seen in patients with deep burns who require multiple surgical procedures and who suffer from psychological sequelae from the burn and its aftermath.

Burn pruritus is a multifactorial phenomenon and can be classified into several different categories:

1. Pruritoceptive, originating in the skin as exemplified in urticarial conditions
2. Neuropathic, arising from anatomical dysfunction in the afferent pathway (e.g., postherpetic pruritus and brain tumors)
3. Neurogenic, resulting from CNS dysfunction without evidence of anatomical pathology, indicating abnormal neurochemical activity (e.g., the action of opioid peptides in liver disease)
4. Psychogenic, associated with psychiatric conditions

Antihistamines have been the mainstay therapy for burn pruritus. When given in the early stages after burn injury, they can be effective. However, studies have suggested that the use of a central agent such as gabapentin in conjunction with two antihistamines achieves superior relief than when using three antihistamines. When antihistamines are administered for the treatment of itching in the late proliferative and remodeling stages of the burn, significantly fewer patients report achieving good symptomatic relief. For patients in the later stages of healing, gabapentin in addition to antihistamine therapy again achieved better symptomatic relief than antihistamines alone. Ondansetron, a 5HT3 receptor antagonist, has been used to treat cholestatic pruritus. The ability of serotonin antagonists to inhibit the excitatory CNS pathways that contribute to itching may make ondansetron a useful agent in treating burn pruritus. Transcutaneous electrical nerve stimulation (TENS) is a therapeutic modality that involves the use of controlled,

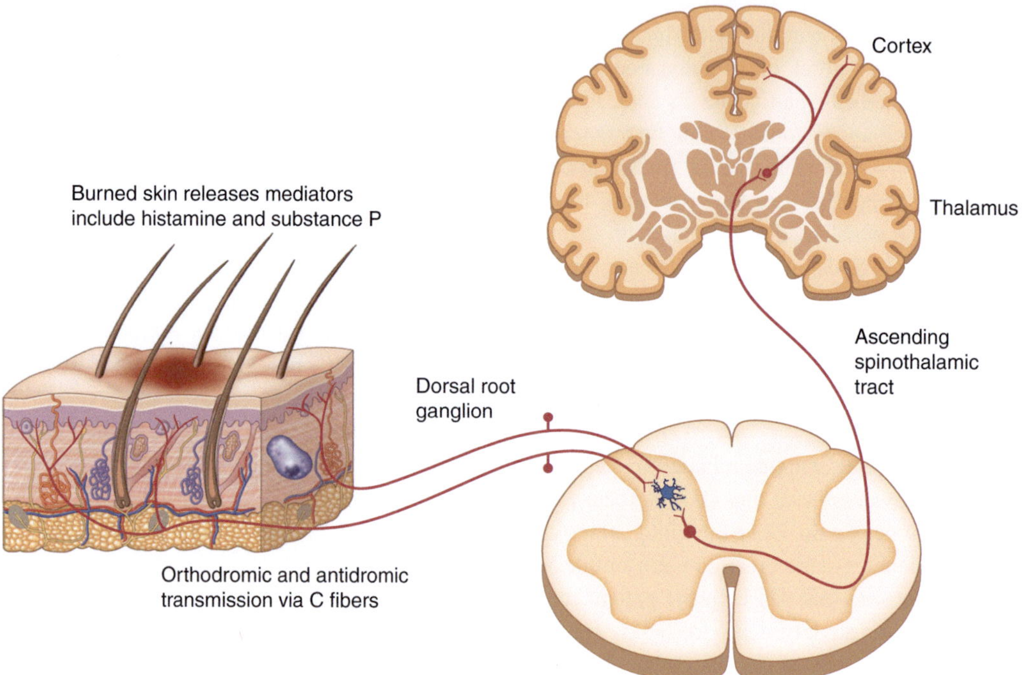

Fig. 14.3 Schematic diagram of the pruritic pathway. Healing/healed burned skin releases a wide variety of pruritic mediators including histamine and neuroinflammatory transmitters like substance P (SP). A subset of C fibers transmits impulses in an orthodromic manner to the spinal cord via the dorsal root ganglion. In addition, impulses spread from afferents in the injured area to neighboring nerve fibers via the antidromic axon reflex (*arrow*); this involves the release of SP from neurons and mast cells (depicted in the skin), which enhances the input to the CNS. Impulses are carried via the ascending spinothalamic tract and the thalamus to higher CNS areas (including the contralateral somatosensory cortex, ipsilateral, contralateral motor areas, and the prefrontal cortex and cingulated gyrus) for sensory registration. Reprinted from Ref. [125], with permission

low-voltage electrical impulses to the nervous system via electrodes that are placed on the skin. This is thought to trigger a release of endogenous opioids that inhibit descending excitatory CNS pathways, thereby alleviating the sensation of pruritus [125].

Conclusion

The effective treatment of burns involves a coordinated, multidisciplinary team. Knowledge of the pathophysiology of burns and management of the multitude of complex physiological changes associated with burns is the key to the successful management of a potentially very complicated injury.

References

1. Cuttle L, Pearn J, McMillan JR, Kimble RM. A review of first aid treatments for burn injuries. Burns. 2009;35(6):768–75. PubMed PMID: 19269746. Epub 2009/03/10. eng.
2. Sawada Y, Urushidate S, Yotsuyanagi T, Ishita K. Is prolonged and excessive cooling of a scalded wound effective? Burns. 1997;23(1):55–8. PubMed PMID: 9115611. Epub 1997/02/01. eng.
3. Ofeigsson OJ, Mitchell R, Patrick RS. Observations on the cold water treatment of cutaneous burns. J Pathol. 1972;108(2):145–50. PubMed PMID: 4647507. Epub 1972/10/01. eng.
4. Hettiaratchy S, Dziewulski P. ABC of burns: pathophysiology and types of burns. BMJ. 2004;328

(7453):1427–9. PubMed PMID: 15191982. Pubmed Central PMCID: PMC421790. Epub 2004/06/12. eng.

5. Hudspith J, Rayatt S. First aid and treatment of minor burns. BMJ. 2004;328(7454):1487–9. PubMed PMID: 15205294. Pubmed Central PMCID: PMC428524. Epub 2004/06/19. eng.

6. Kasten KR, Makley AT, Kagan RJ. Update on the critical care management of severe burns. J Intensive Care Med. 2011;26(4):223–36. PubMed PMID: 21764766. Epub 2011/07/19. eng.

7. Latenser BA. Critical care of the burn patient: the first 48 hours. Crit Care Med. 2009;37(10):2819–26. PubMed PMID: 19707133. Epub 2009/08/27. eng.

8. Rehberg S, Maybauer MO, Enkhbaatar P, Maybauer DM, Yamamoto Y, Traber DL. Pathophysiology, management and treatment of smoke inhalation injury. Expert Rev Respir Med. 2009;3(3):283–97. PubMed PMID: 20161170. Pubmed Central PMCID: PMC2722076. Epub 2010/02/18. Eng.

9. Krafft P, Fridrich P, Pernerstorfer T, Fitzgerald RD, Koc D, Schneider B, et al. The acute respiratory distress syndrome: definitions, severity and clinical outcome. An analysis of 101 clinical investigations. Intensive Care Med. 1996;22(6):519–29.

10. Yilmaz M, Iscimen R, Keegan MT, Vlahakis NE, Afessa B, Hubmayr RD, et al. Six-month survival of patients with acute lung injury: prospective cohort study. Crit Care Med. 2007;35(10):2303–7. PubMed PMID: 17944018. Epub 2007/10/19. eng.

11. Weaver LK, Howe S, Hopkins R, Chan KJ. Carboxyhemoglobin half-life in carbon monoxide-poisoned patients treated with 100 % oxygen at atmospheric pressure. Chest. 2000;117(3):801–8. PubMed PMID: 10713010. Epub 2000/03/14. eng.

12. de Campo T, Aldrete JA. The anesthetic management of the severely burned patient. Intensive Care Med. 1981;7(2):55–62. PubMed PMID: 7009689. Epub 1981/01/01. eng.

13. Demling RH. Smoke inhalation lung injury: an update. Eplasty. 2008;8:e27. PubMed PMID: 18552974. Pubmed Central PMCID: PMC2396464. Epub 2008/06/17. eng.

14. Rodeberg DA, Housinger TA, Greenhalgh DG, Maschinot NE, Warden GD. Improved ventilatory function in burn patients using volumetric diffusive respiration. J Am Coll Surg. 1994;179(5):518–22. PubMed PMID: 7952452. Epub 1994/11/01. eng.

15. Carman B, Cahill T, Warden G, McCall J. A prospective, randomized comparison of the volume diffusive respirator vs conventional ventilation for ventilation of burned children. 2001 ABA paper. J Burn Care Rehabil. 2002;23(6):444–8. PubMed PMID: 12432322. Epub 2002/11/15. eng.

16. Daoud EG. Airway pressure release ventilation. Ann Thorac Med. 2007;2(4):176–9. PubMed PMID: 19727373. Pubmed Central PMCID: PMC2732103. Epub 2007/10/01. eng.

17. Sheridan RL, Hess D. Inhaled nitric oxide in inhalation injury. J Burn Care Res. 2009;30(1):162–4. PubMed PMID: 19060730. Epub 2008/12/09. eng.

18. Enkhbaatar P, Murakami K, Cox R, Westphal M, Morita N, Brantley K, et al. Aerosolized tissue plasminogen inhibitor improves pulmonary function in sheep with burn and smoke inhalation. Shock. 2004;22(1):70–5. PubMed PMID: 15201705. Epub 2004/06/18. eng.

19. Miller AC, Rivero A, Ziad S, Smith DJ, Elamin EM. Influence of nebulized unfractionated heparin and N-acetylcysteine in acute lung injury after smoke inhalation injury. J Burn Care Res. 2009;30(2):249–56. PubMed PMID: 19165116. Epub 2009/01/24. eng.

20. Adhikari N, Burns KE, Meade MO. Pharmacologic treatments for acute respiratory distress syndrome and acute lung injury: systematic review and meta-analysis. Treat Respir Med. 2004;3(5):307–28. PubMed PMID: 15606221. Epub 2004/12/21. eng.

21. Palmieri TL. Use of beta-agonists in inhalation injury. J Burn Care Res. 2009;30(1):156–9. PubMed PMID: 19060734. Epub 2008/12/09. eng.

22. Thompson JT, Molnar JA, Hines MH, Chang MC, Pranikoff T. Successful management of adult smoke inhalation with extracorporeal membrane oxygenation. J Burn Care Rehabil. 2005;26(1):62–6. PubMed PMID: 15640737. Epub 2005/01/11. eng.

23. Nehra D, Goldstein AM, Doody DP, Ryan DP, Chang Y, Masiakos PT. Extracorporeal membrane oxygenation for nonneonatal acute respiratory failure: the Massachusetts General Hospital experience from 1990 to 2008. Arch Surg. 2009;144(5):427–32. PubMed PMID: 19451484. discussion 32; Epub 2009/05/20. eng.

24. Pruitt Jr BA. Fluid and electrolyte replacement in the burned patient. Surg Clin North Am. 1978;58(6):1291–312. PubMed PMID: 734610. Epub 1978/12/01. eng.

25. Gueugniaud PY, Carsin H, Bertin-Maghit M, Petit P. Current advances in the initial management of major thermal burns. Intensive Care Med. 2000;26(7):848–56. PubMed PMID: 10990098. Epub 2000/09/16. eng.

26. Chung KK, Wolf SE, Cancio LC, Alvarado R, Jones JA, McCorcle J, et al. Resuscitation of severely burned military casualties: fluid begets more fluid. J Trauma. 2009;67(2):231–7. PubMed PMID: 19667873. discussion 7; Epub 2009/08/12. eng.

27. Cancio LC, Chavez S, Alvarado-Ortega M, Barillo DJ, Walker SC, McManus AT, et al. Predicting increased fluid requirements during the resuscitation of thermally injured patients. J Trauma. 2004;56(2):404–13. PubMed PMID: 14960986. discussion 13–4; Epub 2004/02/13. eng.

28. Barrow RE, Jeschke MG, Herndon DN. Early fluid resuscitation improves outcomes in severely burned children. Resuscitation. 2000;45(2):91–6. PubMed PMID: 10950316. Epub 2000/08/19. eng.

29. Graves TA, Cioffi WG, McManus WF, Mason Jr AD, Pruitt Jr BA. Fluid resuscitation of infants and children with massive thermal injury. J Trauma. 1988;28(12):1656–9. PubMed PMID: 3199467. Epub 1988/12/01. eng.

30. Hettiaratchy S, Papini R. Initial management of a major burn: II—assessment and resuscitation. BMJ. 2004;329(7457):101–3. PubMed PMID: 15242917. Pubmed Central PMCID: PMC449823. Epub 2004/07/10. eng.

31. Reid RD, Jayamaha J. The use of a cardiac output monitor to guide the initial fluid resuscitation in a patient with burns. Emerg Med J. 2007;24(5):e32. PubMed PMID: 17452692. Pubmed Central PMCID: PMC2658516. Epub 2007/04/25. eng.

32. Jaffe MB. Partial CO2 rebreathing cardiac output—operating principles of the NICO system. J Clin Monit Comput. 1999;15(6):387–401. PubMed PMID: 12578034. Epub 2003/02/13. eng.

33. Berton C, Cholley B. Equipment review: new techniques for cardiac output measurement—oesophageal Doppler, Fick principle using carbon dioxide, and pulse contour analysis. Crit Care. 2002;6(3):216–21. PubMed PMID: 12133181. Pubmed Central PMCID: PMC137448. Epub 2002/07/23. eng.

34. Perel P, Roberts I. Colloids versus crystalloids for fluid resuscitation in critically ill patients. Cochrane database of systematic reviews (Online). 2012;6: CD000567. PubMed PMID: 22696320. Epub 2012/06/15. eng.

35. Warden GD. Burn shock resuscitation. World J Surg. 1992;16(1):16–23. PubMed PMID: 1290260. Epub 1992/01/01. eng.

36. Alderson P, Bunn F, Lefebvre C, Li WP, Li L, Roberts I, et al. Human albumin solution for resuscitation and volume expansion in critically ill patients. Cochrane database of systematic reviews (Online). 2004 (4):CD001208. PubMed PMID: 15495011. Epub 2004/10/21. eng.

37. Ivy ME, Atweh NA, Palmer J, Possenti PP, Pineau M, D'Aiuto M. Intra-abdominal hypertension and abdominal compartment syndrome in burn patients. J Trauma. 2000;49(3):387–91. PubMed PMID: 11003313. Epub 2000/09/26. eng.

38. Hershberger RC, Hunt JL, Arnoldo BD, Purdue GF. Abdominal compartment syndrome in the severely burned patient. J Burn Care Res. 2007;28(5):708–14. PubMed PMID: 17667839. Epub 2007/08/02. eng.

39. Brown RL, Greenhalgh DG, Kagan RJ, Warden GD. The adequacy of limb escharotomies-fasciotomies after referral to a major burn center. J Trauma. 1994;37(6):916–20. PubMed PMID: 7996604. Epub 1994/12/01. eng.

40. Caldwell Jr FT, Bowser BH, Crabtree JH. The effect of occlusive dressings on the energy metabolism of severely burned children. Ann Surg. 1981;193 (5):579–91. PubMed PMID: 7235763. Pubmed Central PMCID: PMC1345123. Epub 1981/05/01. eng.

41. Thomson PD, Moore NP, Rice TL, Prasad JK. Leukopenia in acute thermal injury: evidence against topical silver sulfadiazine as the causative agent. J Burn Care Rehabil. 1989;10(5):418–20. PubMed PMID: 2793919. Epub 1989/09/01. eng.

42. Wasiak J, Cleland H. Burns (minor thermal). Clin Evid. 2005;14:2388–96. PubMed PMID: 16620494. Epub 2006/04/20. eng.

43. Papini R. Management of burn injuries of various depths. BMJ. 2004;329(7458):158–60. PubMed PMID: 15258073. Pubmed Central PMCID: PMC478230. Epub 2004/07/20. eng.

44. Hart DW, Wolf SE, Chinkes DL, Beauford RB, Mlcak RP, Heggers JP, et al. Effects of early excision and aggressive enteral feeding on hypermetabolism, catabolism, and sepsis after severe burn. J Trauma. 2003;54(4):755–61. PubMed PMID: 12707540. discussion 61–4; Epub 2003/04/23. eng.

45. Barret JP, Herndon DN. Modulation of inflammatory and catabolic responses in severely burned children by early burn wound excision in the first 24 hours. Arch Surg. 2003;138(2):127–32. PubMed PMID: 12578404. Epub 2003/02/13. eng.

46. Barret JP, Herndon DN. Effects of burn wound excision on bacterial colonization and invasion. Plast Reconstr Surg. 2003;111(2):744–50. PubMed PMID: 12560695. discussion 51–2; Epub 2003/02/01. eng.

47. Herndon DN, Barrow RE, Rutan RL, Rutan TC, Desai MH, Abston S. A comparison of conservative versus early excision. Therapies in severely burned patients. Ann Surg. 1989;209(5):547–52. PubMed PMID: 2650643. Pubmed Central PMCID: PMC1494069. discussion 52–3; Epub 1989/05/01. eng.

48. Curreri PW. Nutritional support of burn patients. World J Surg. 1978;2(2):215–22. PubMed PMID: 97867. Epub 1978/03/01. eng.

49. Herndon DN, Curreri PW. Metabolic response to thermal injury and its nutritional support. Cutis. 1978;22(4):501–6. PubMed PMID: 699632. Epub 1978/10/01. eng.

50. Ireton-Jones C, Jones JD. Improved equations for predicting energy expenditure in patients: the Ireton-Jones Equations. Nutr Clin Pract. 2002;17 (1):29–31. PubMed PMID: 16214963. Epub 2005/10/11. eng.

51. Schulman CI, Ivascu FA. Nutritional and metabolic consequences in the pediatric burn patient. J Craniofac Surg. 2008;19(4):891–4. PubMed PMID: 18650706. Epub 2008/07/25. eng.

52. Joffe A, Anton N, Lequier L, Vandermeer B, Tjosvold L, Larsen B, et al. Nutritional support for critically ill children. Cochrane database of systematic reviews (Online). 2009 (2):CD005144. PubMed PMID: 19370617. Epub 2009/04/17. eng.

53. Chan MM, Chan GM. Nutritional therapy for burns in children and adults. Nutrition. 2009;25 (3):261–9. PubMed PMID: 19097858. Epub 2008/12/23. eng.

54. Gottschlich MM, Jenkins ME, Mayes T, Khoury J, Kagan RJ, Warden GD. The 2002 Clinical Research Award. An evaluation of the safety of early vs delayed enteral support and effects on clinical, nutritional, and endocrine outcomes after severe burns. J Burn Care Rehabil. 2002;23(6):401–15. PubMed PMID: 12432317. Epub 2002/11/15. eng.

55. Rettmer RL, Williamson JC, Labbe RF, Heimbach DM. Laboratory monitoring of nutritional status in burn patients. Clin Chem. 1992;38(3):334–7. PubMed PMID: 1547547. Epub 1992/03/01. eng.

56. Prelack K, Dylewski M, Sheridan RL. Practical guidelines for nutritional management of burn injury and recovery. Burns. 2007;33(1):14–24. PubMed PMID: 17116370. Epub 2006/11/23. eng.

57. Gore DC, Ferrando A, Barnett J, Wolf SE, Desai M, Herndon DN, et al. Influence of glucose kinetics on plasma lactate concentration and energy expenditure in severely burned patients. J Trauma. 2000;49(4):673–7. PubMed PMID: 11038085. discussion 7–8; Epub 2000/10/19. eng.

58. Wolfe RR, Miller HI, Spitzer JJ. Glucose and lactate kinetics in burn shock. Am J Physiol. 1977;232(4):E415–8. PubMed PMID: 15459. Epub 1977/04/01. eng.

59. Jeschke MG, Boehning DF, Finnerty CC, Herndon DN. Effect of insulin on the inflammatory and acute phase response after burn injury. Crit Care Med. 2007;35(9 Suppl):S519–23. PubMed PMID: 17713402. Epub 2007/09/22. eng.

60. Holm C, Horbrand F, Mayr M, von Donnersmarck GH, Muhlbauer W. Acute hyperglycaemia following thermal injury: friend or foe? Resuscitation. 2004;60(1):71–7. PubMed PMID: 14987787. Epub 2004/02/28. eng.

61. Ellger B, Westphal M, Stubbe HD, Van den Heuvel I, Van Aken H, Van den Berghe G. Glycemic control in sepsis and septic shock: friend or foe? Anaesthesist. 2008;57(1):43–8. PubMed PMID: 18034219. Epub 2007/11/24. Blutzuckerkontrolle bei Patienten mit Sepsis und septischem Schock: Freund oder Feind? ger.

62. Norbury WB, Jeschke MG, Herndon DN. Metabolism modulators in sepsis: propranolol. Crit Care Med. 2007;35(9 Suppl):S616–20. PubMed PMID: 17713418. Epub 2007/09/22. eng.

63. Arbabi S, Ahrns KS, Wahl WL, Hemmila MR, Wang SC, Brandt MM, et al. Beta-blocker use is associated with improved outcomes in adult burn patients. J Trauma. 2004;56(2):265–9. PubMed PMID: 14960966. discussion 9–71; Epub 2004/02/13. eng.

64. Mohammadi AA, Bakhshaeekia A, Alibeigi P, Hasheminasab MJ, Tolide-ei HR, Tavakkolian AR, et al. Efficacy of propranolol in wound healing for hospitalized burn patients. J Burn Care Res. 2009;30(6):1013–7. PubMed PMID: 19826272. Epub 2009/10/15. eng.

65. Baron PW, Barrow RE, Pierre EJ, Herndon DN. Prolonged use of propranolol safely decreases cardiac work in burned children. J Burn Care Rehabil. 1997;18(3):223–7. PubMed PMID: 9169945. Epub 1997/05/01. eng.

66. Herndon DN, Hart DW, Wolf SE, Chinkes DL, Wolfe RR. Reversal of catabolism by beta-blockade after severe burns. N Engl J Med. 2001;345(17):1223–9. PubMed PMID: 11680441. Epub 2001/10/30. eng.

67. Jeschke MG, Norbury WB, Finnerty CC, Branski LK, Herndon DN. Propranolol does not increase inflammation, sepsis, or infectious episodes in severely burned children. J Trauma. 2007;62(3):676–81. PubMed PMID: 17414346. Epub 2007/04/07. eng.

68. Peng X, Yan H, You Z, Wang P, Wang S. Effects of enteral supplementation with glutamine granules on intestinal mucosal barrier function in severe burned patients. Burns. 2004;30(2):135–9. PubMed PMID: 15019120. Epub 2004/03/17. eng.

69. Alexander JW. Nutritional pharmacology in surgical patients. Am J Surg. 2002;183(4):349–52. PubMed PMID: 11975921. Epub 2002/04/27. eng.

70. Aida T, Murata J, Asano G, Kanda Y, Yoshino Y. Effects of polyprenoic acid on thermal injury. Br J Exp Pathol. 1987;68(3):351–8. PubMed PMID: 3620330. Pubmed Central PMCID: PMC2013252. Epub 1987/06/01. eng.

71. Voruganti VS, Klein GL, Lu HX, Thomas S, Freeland-Graves JH, Herndon DN. Impaired zinc and copper status in children with burn injuries: need to reassess nutritional requirements. Burns. 2005;31(6):711–6. PubMed PMID: 16006043. Epub 2005/07/12. eng.

72. Berger MM, Rothen C, Cavadini C, Chiolero RL. Exudative mineral losses after serious burns: a clue to the alterations of magnesium and phosphate metabolism. Am J Clin Nutr. 1997;65(5):1473–81. PubMed PMID: 9129479. Epub 1997/05/01. eng.

73. Cunningham JJ, Leffell M, Harmatz P. Burn severity, copper dose, and plasma ceruloplasmin in burned children during total parenteral nutrition. Nutrition. 1993;9(4):329–32. PubMed PMID: 8400588. Epub 1993/07/01. eng.

74. Bishop S, Maguire S. Anaesthesia and intensive care for major burns 2012. Available from: http://ceaccp.oxfordjournals.org/content/early/2012/02/23/bjaceaccp.mks001.full.

75. Fuzaylov G, Fidkowski CW. Anesthetic considerations for major burn injury in pediatric patients. Paediatr Anaesth. 2009;19(3):202–11. PubMed PMID: 19187044. Epub 2009/02/04. eng.

76. Ansermino M, Hemsley C. Intensive care management and control of infection. BMJ. 2004;329(7459):220–3. PubMed PMID: 15271835. Pubmed Central PMCID: PMC487741. Epub 2004/07/24. eng.

77. Wahl WL, Taddonio MA, Arbabi S, Hemmila MR. Duration of antibiotic therapy for ventilator-associated pneumonia in burn patients. J Burn Care Res. 2009;30(5):801–6. PubMed PMID: 19734728. Epub 2009/09/08. eng.

78. Schuerer DJ, Zack JE, Thomas J, Borecki IB, Sona CS, Schallom ME, et al. Effect of chlorhexidine/silver sulfadiazine-impregnated central venous catheters in an intensive care unit with a low blood stream infection rate after implementation of an educational program: a before-after trial. Surg Infect (Larchmt). 2007;8(4):445–54. PubMed PMID: 17883361. Epub 2007/09/22. eng.

79. Murray CK, Loo FL, Hospenthal DR, Cancio LC, Jones JA, Kim SH, et al. Incidence of systemic fungal infection and related mortality following severe burns. Burns. 2008;34(8):1108–12. PubMed PMID: 18691821. Epub 2008/08/12. eng.

80. D'Avignon LC, Hogan BK, Murray CK, Loo FL, Hospenthal DR, Cancio LC, et al. Contribution of bacterial and viral infections to attributable mortality in patients with severe burns: an autopsy series. Burns. 2010;36(6):773–9. PubMed PMID: 20074860. Epub 2010/01/16. eng.

81. Nguyen LN, Nguyen TG. Characteristics and outcomes of multiple organ dysfunction syndrome among severe-burn patients. Burns. 2009;35(7): 937–41. PubMed PMID: 19553020. Epub 2009/06/26. eng.

82. Greenhalgh DG, Saffle JR, Holmes JH, Gamelli RL, Palmieri TL, Horton JW, et al. American Burn Association consensus conference to define sepsis and infection in burns. J Burn Care Res. 2007;28(6):776–90. PubMed PMID: 17925660. Epub 2007/10/11. eng.

83. Church D, Elsayed S, Reid O, Winston B, Lindsay R. Burn wound infections. Clin Microbiol Rev. 2006;19(2):403–34. PubMed PMID: 16614255. Pubmed Central PMCID: PMC1471990. Epub 2006/04/15. eng.

84. Pruitt Jr BA. The diagnosis and treatment of infection in the burn patient. Burns. 1984;11(2):79–91. PubMed PMID: 6525539. Epub 1984/12/01. eng.

85. Sheridan RL, Ryan CM, Yin LM, Hurley J, Tompkins RG. Death in the burn unit: sterile multiple organ failure. Burns. 1998;24(4):307–11. PubMed PMID: 9688194. Epub 1998/08/04. eng.

86. Magnotti LJ, Deitch EA. Burns, bacterial translocation, gut barrier function, and failure. J Burn Care Rehabil. 2005;26(5):383–91. PubMed PMID: 16151282. Epub 2005/09/10. eng.

87. Williams FN, Herndon DN, Hawkins HK, Lee JO, Cox RA, Kulp GA, et al. The leading causes of death after burn injury in a single pediatric burn center. Crit Care. 2009;13(6):R183. PubMed PMID: 19919684. Pubmed Central PMCID: PMC2811947. Epub 2009/11/19. eng.

88. Branski LK, Al-Mousawi A, Rivero H, Jeschke MG, Sanford AP, Herndon DN. Emerging infections in burns. Surg Infect (Larchmt). 2009;10(5):389–97. PubMed PMID: 19810827. Pubmed Central PMCID: PMC2956561. Epub 2009/10/09. eng.

89. Smith MA, Munster AM, Spence RJ. Burns of the hand and upper limb—a review. Burns. 1998;24(6): 493–505. PubMed PMID: 9776087. Epub 1998/10/17. eng.

90. Kamolz LP, Kitzinger HB, Karle B, Frey M. The treatment of hand burns. Burns. 2009;35(3):327–37. PubMed PMID: 18952379. Epub 2008/10/28. eng.

91. Edgar D, Brereton M. Rehabilitation after burn injury. BMJ. 2004;329(7461):343–5. PubMed PMID: 15297346. Pubmed Central PMCID: PMC506862. Epub 2004/08/07. eng.

92. Holavanahalli RK, Helm PA, Parry IS, Dolezal CA, Greenhalgh DG. Select practices in management and rehabilitation of burns: a survey report. J Burn Care Res. 2011;32(2):210–23. PubMed PMID: 21240002. Epub 2011/01/18. eng.

93. Coons D, Godleski M. Range of motion exercises in the setting of burn-associated heterotopic ossification at the elbow: case series and discussion. Burns. 2012 Nov 15. PubMed PMID: 23159702. Epub 2012/11/20. Eng.

94. Michelsson JE, Granroth G, Andersson LC. Myositis ossificans following forcible manipulation of the leg. A rabbit model for the study of heterotopic bone formation. J Bone Joint Surg. 1980;62(5):811–5. PubMed PMID: 7391105. Epub 1980/07/01. eng.

95. Crawford CM, Varghese G, Mani MM, Neff JR. Heterotopic ossification: are range of motion exercises contraindicated? J Burn Care Rehabil. 1986;7(4):323–7. PubMed PMID: 3117800. Epub 1986/07/01. eng.

96. Thomson PD, Bowden ML, McDonald K, Smith Jr DJ, Prasad JK. A survey of burn hydrotherapy in the United States. J Burn Care Rehabil. 1990;11(2):151–5. PubMed PMID: 2335554. Epub 1990/03/01. eng.

97. Shankowsky HA, Callioux LS, Tredget EE. North American survey of hydrotherapy in modern burn care. J Burn Care Rehabil. 1994;15(2):143–6. PubMed PMID: 8195254. Epub 1994/03/01. eng.

98. Choiniere M, Melzack R, Rondeau J, Girard N, Paquin MJ. The pain of burns: characteristics and correlates. J Trauma. 1989;29(11):1531–9. PubMed PMID: 2585565. Epub 1989/11/01. eng.

99. Summer GJ, Puntillo KA, Miaskowski C, Green PG, Levine JD. Burn injury pain: the continuing challenge. J Pain. 2007;8(7):533–48. PubMed PMID: 17434800. Epub 2007/04/17. eng.

100. Richardson P, Mustard L. The management of pain in the burns unit. Burns. 2009;35(7):921–36. PubMed PMID: 19505764. Epub 2009/06/10. eng.

101. Wibbenmeyer L, Sevier A, Liao J, Williams I, Latenser B, Lewis II R, et al. Evaluation of the usefulness of two established pain assessment tools in a burn population. J Burn Care Res. 2011;32(1): 52–60. PubMed PMID: 21116190. Epub 2010/12/01. eng.

102. Gaston-Johansson F, Albert M, Fagan E, Zimmerman L. Similarities in pain descriptions of four different ethnic-culture groups. J Pain Symptom Manage. 1990;5(2):94–100. PubMed PMID: 2348093. Epub 1990/04/01. eng.

103. Merkel SI, Voepel-Lewis T, Shayevitz JR, Malviya S. The FLACC: a behavioral scale for scoring postoperative pain in young children. Pediatr Nurs. 1997;23(3):293–7. PubMed PMID: 9220806. Epub 1997/05/01. eng.

104. Wong DL, Hockenbery M, Wilson D, et al. Wong's essentials of pediatric nursing. 6th ed. St. Louis, MO: Elsevier Mosby; 2001.

105. Johnston CC, Strada ME. Acute pain response in infants: a multidimensional description. Pain. 1986;24(3):373–82. PubMed PMID: 3960577. Epub 1986/03/01. eng.

106. Hanafiah Z, Potparic O, Fernandez T. Addressing pain in burn injury. Curr Anaesthesia Crit Care. 2008;19(5–6):287–92.

107. Yang HT, Hur G, Kwak IS, Yim H, Cho YS, Kim D, et al. Improvement of burn pain management through routine pain monitoring and pain management protocol. Burns. 2012 Nov 22. PubMed PMID: 23182650. Epub 2012/11/28. Eng.

108. Wasiak J, Mahar P, McGuinness SK, Spinks A, Danilla S, Cleland H. Intravenous lidocaine for the treatment of background or procedural burn pain. Cochrane database of systematic reviews (Online). 2012;6:CD005622. PubMed PMID: 22696353. Epub 2012/06/15. eng.

109. Lin H, Faraklas I, Sampson C, Saffle JR, Cochran A. Use of dexmedetomidine for sedation in critically ill mechanically ventilated pediatric burn patients. J Burn Care Res. 2011;32(1):98–103. PubMed PMID: 21088616. Epub 2010/11/23. eng.

110. Walker J, Maccallum M, Fischer C, Kopcha R, Saylors R, McCall J. Sedation using dexmedetomidine in pediatric burn patients. J Burn Care Res. 2006;27(2):206–10. PubMed PMID: 16566567. Epub 2006/03/29. eng.

111. Kariya N, Shindoh M, Nishi S, Yukioka H, Asada A. Oral clonidine for sedation and analgesia in a burn patient. J Clin Anesth. 1998;10(6):514–7. PubMed PMID: 9793819. Epub 1998/10/30. eng.

112. Lyons B, Casey W, Doherty P, McHugh M, Moore KP. Pain relief with low-dose intravenous clonidine in a child with severe burns. Intensive Care Med. 1996;22(3):249–51. PubMed PMID: 8727440. Epub 1996/03/01. eng.

113. Vulink NC, Figee M, Denys D. Review of atypical antipsychotics in anxiety. Eur Neuropsychopharmacol. 2011;21(6):429–49. PubMed PMID: 21345655. Epub 2011/02/25. eng.

114. Patterson DR, Ptacek JT. Baseline pain as a moderator of hypnotic analgesia for burn injury treatment. J Consult Clin Psychol. 1997;65(1):60–7. PubMed PMID: 9103735. Epub 1997/02/01. eng.

115. Patterson DR, Ptacek JT, Carrougher GJ, Sharar SR. Lorazepam as an adjunct to opioid analgesics in the treatment of burn pain. Pain. 1997;72(3):367–74. PubMed PMID: 9313277. Epub 1997/10/06. eng.

116. MacLennan N, Heimbach DM, Cullen BF. Anesthesia for major thermal injury. Anesthesiology. 1998;89(3):749–70. PubMed PMID: 9743414. Epub 1998/09/22. eng.

117. Still JM, Abramson R, Law EJ. Development of an epidural abscess following staphylococcal septicemia in an acutely burned patient: case report. J Trauma. 1995;38(6):958–9. PubMed PMID: 7602646. Epub 1995/06/01. eng.

118. Cuignet O, Mbuyamba J, Pirson J. The long-term analgesic efficacy of a single-shot fascia iliaca compartment block in burn patients undergoing skin-grafting procedures. J Burn Care Rehabil. 2005;26(5):409–15. PubMed PMID: 16151286. Epub 2005/09/10. eng.

119. Wiechman SA, Patterson DR. ABC of burns. Psychosocial aspects of burn injuries. BMJ. 2004;329(7462):391–3. PubMed PMID: 15310609. Pubmed Central PMCID: PMC509350. Epub 2004/08/18. eng.

120. Landolt MA, Marti D, Widmer J, Meuli M. Does cartoon movie distraction decrease burned children's pain behavior? J Burn Care Rehabil. 2002;23(1):61–5. PubMed PMID: 11803316. Epub 2002/01/23. eng.

121. Eller LS. Guided imagery interventions for symptom management. Annu Rev Nurs Res. 1999;17:57–84. PubMed PMID: 10418653. Epub 1999/07/27. eng.

122. Patterson DR, Everett JJ, Burns GL, Marvin JA. Hypnosis for the treatment of burn pain. J Consult Clin Psychol. 1992;60(5):713–7. PubMed PMID: 1383302. Epub 1992/10/01. eng.

123. Sharar SR, Miller W, Teeley A, Soltani M, Hoffman HG, Jensen MP, et al. Applications of virtual reality for pain management in burn-injured patients. Expert Rev Neurother. 2008;8(11):1667–74. PubMed PMID: 18986237. Pubmed Central PMCID: PMC2634811. Epub 2008/11/07. eng.

124. Thurber CA, Martin-Herz SP, Patterson DR. Psychological principles of burn wound pain in children. I: theoretical framework. J Burn Care Rehabil. 2000;21(4):376–87. PubMed PMID: 10935822. discussion 5; Epub 2000/08/10. eng.

125. Goutos I. Neuropathic mechanisms in the pathophysiology of burns pruritus: redefining directions for therapy and research. J Burn Care Res. 2013;34(1):82–93. doi:10.1097/BCR.0b013e3182644c44.

Perioperative Pediatric Anesthesia Trauma Considerations

Charles J. Fox, Alan David Kaye, Jacob C. Hummel, and Moises Sidransky

Introduction

Trauma is the leading cause of death among children older than 1 year of age in the United States. Each year approximately 15,000 children die as a result of trauma. Additionally, over 100,000 pediatric patients suffer significant morbidity and disability from trauma. Unfortunately, despite dramatic increases in the number of educational programs and advances in injury prevention technology, this number remains consistent. In school aged children, motor vehicle and bicycle accidents are the most common causes of traumatic injury.

C.J. Fox, M.D. (✉)
Department of Anesthesiology, LSU–Health–Shreveport, 1501 Kings Highway, Shreveport, LA 71102, USA
e-mail: cfox1@LSUhsc.edu

A.D. Kaye, M.D., Ph.D., D.A.B.A., D.A.B.P.M., D.A.B.I.P.P.
Department of Anesthesiology, LSU School of Medicine, Room 656, 1542 Tulane Avenue, New Orleans, LA 70112, USA
e-mail: Alankaye44@hotmail.com

J.C. Hummel, M.D., M.S.B.S.
Department of Anesthesiology, Tulane Hospital, 1415 Tulane Avenue, SL 4, New Orleans, LA 70112, USA
e-mail: Jhummel1@tulane.edu

M. Sidransky, M.D.
Department of Anesthesiology, LSU HSC New Orleans, 1542 Tulane Avenue, 6th Floor, New Orleans, LA 70112, USA
e-mail: msidra@lsuhsc.edu

The most common lethal injuries from blunt trauma are head trauma and severe intrathoracic injuries. Head injuries make up 80 % of isolated injuries and cause 70 % of all pediatric trauma deaths. Due to the compliant and non-calcified chest wall of pediatric patients, those with intrathoracic injuries may present without obvious rib fractures.

The complications from pediatric trauma impact anesthesiologists worldwide. Anesthesiologists are involved in many facets of pediatric trauma. Frequently, care of these patients takes place in adult emergency rooms or trauma centers, outside of the operating rooms. Unfortunately, very few anesthesiology residency programs teach about common traumatic injuries incurred by the pediatric population. It is vital to understand the subtle physiologic and anatomical differences and issues of this population, as compared to adults [1, 2].

Special Pediatric Anatomical and Physiologic Characteristics

Airway

Infants have large heads (prominent occiputs) relative to body size. This results in flexion of both the head relative to the neck, and the neck relative to the chest, when placed supine. Care must be taken to properly position these patients for intubation. Some practitioners place a roll or towel under the shoulders of these patients to

C.S. Scher (ed.), *Anesthesia for Trauma*, DOI 10.1007/978-1-4939-0909-4_15,
© Springer Science+Business Media New York 2014

maximize the "sniffing position" for mask ventilation and intubation. The need for neck stabilization may further complicate management of these patients. The narrowest part of the airway in children is located at the subglottic area, whereas in the adult airway it is at the glottis. The larynx is located at C_2–C_5 in the pediatric population compared with a C_6 location in adults. The large tongue, short and U-shaped epiglottis, and anteriorly placed vocal cords can make airway management challenging, especially for the non-pediatric specialist [1].

When selecting an endotracheal tube, with or without a cuff, one must be cognizant of the delicate vocal cords, which may be easily damaged. Unfortunately, many pediatric patients do not conform to the many tables or formulas used when calculating the correct endotracheal tube size. This may result in large "leaks" when performing positive pressure ventilation. To achieve adequate positive pressure ventilation, some studies have shown a 30 % reintubation rate in patients under the age of 2. This, coupled with recent studies showing no increase in laryngeal injuries in pediatric patients ventilated with a cuffed endotracheal tube, has led to some advocating the use of "cuffed" endotracheal tubes in this group. One must remember that tracheal mucosal damage from increased cuff pressure or oversized endotracheal tubes is increased in hypotensive patients. Meticulous endotracheal cuff pressure monitoring may be required [1–3].

Circulation

Pediatric trauma patients may sustain significant blood loss (25 % of circulating blood volume) before a loss in central arterial pressure is seen. Therefore blood pressure can be an inaccurate measure of hypovolemia in this age group. Other measures such as heart rate, peripheral temperature, and capillary refill are more accurate measures of hypovolemia. Pediatric patients with cool extremities, delayed capillary refill (over 2 s), or tachycardia out of proportion for their age group provide a more accurate

Table 15.1 Hemodynamic parameters

Age	Systolic blood pressure (mmHg)	Heart rate (beats/min)
1 year	80	150
4 years	80	120
6 years	80–100	100
10 years	80–100	90

Table 15.2 Blood volume

Age	Blood volume (mL/kg)
3 months–1 year	70–80
1 year	70

diagnosis of hypovolemia. Tables 15.1 and 15.2 list the normal systolic blood pressures, heart rate, and blood volumes of pediatric patients based on age [3].

Temperature Regulation

Pediatric patients have a larger surface area to body size ratio, less subcutaneous fat, thinner skin, and a higher metabolic rate than adults. In light of these differences, temperature should be monitored with vigilance. Ambient temperature should be adjusted to prevent hypothermia. Forced air convective warming devices and/or warm blankets can be applied to prevent or treat hypothermia after the initial trauma survey is completed. Although hypothermia can be beneficial in neurotrauma patients, it may precipitate decreases in cardiac and renal function. Hypothermia may also increase oxygen demand, cause hemostasis, acidosis, and increase the incidence of arrhythmias [1, 6].

Initial Resuscitation and Primary Survey

The initial survey requires quick identification of life-threatening injuries and prioritizing the delivery of treatment. The initial survey for pediatric trauma patients involves immediate assessment of the "ABCDEs" which is the protocol for Advanced Trauma Life Support. This enables efficient resuscitation and quick restoration of hemodynamic stability. The first hour, commonly referred to as the "Golden Hour," is critical. The following should be achieved within the initial hour to maximize outcome: primary survey, resuscitation, secondary survey, and definitive care.

A = Airway, B = Breathing

On arrival, the patient should be monitored with pulse oximetry and receive supplemental oxygen via nasal cannula or facemask while the initial survey is completed. Airway examination for signs of obstruction or compromise should take priority. This includes an inspection of the face, mouth, mandible, teeth, nose, and neck. It is imperative that one establishes, secures, and maintains a patent airway. Airway obstruction can result in hypoxemia, hypercarbia, and cardiac arrest.

Signs of blood, broken teeth, or edema when inspecting the airway may necessitate immediate airway intervention. In all patients with a closed head injury, it is assumed there is a cervical injury until proven otherwise. All trauma patients are considered to have "full stomachs." Measures should be taken to maintain C-spine precautions and minimize the risk of pulmonary aspiration.

The clinician should look, listen, and feel when assessing breathing and ventilation. Observation can reveal chest rise, an abnormal respiratory rate or pattern, nasal flaring, subcostal or intercostal retractions, and use of accessory muscles. Listening can identify stridor, grunting, or the presence or absence of breath sounds with auscultation. Lastly, one must feel to assess tracheal midline position or the presence of crepitus. A chin lift or jaw thrust can improve airway patency in patients with complete or partial airway obstruction. When executing these maneuvers, special care should be taken not to hyperextend the neck. Oral airway placement may be beneficial, but can lead to gagging and vomiting. This may precipitate pulmonary aspiration in the conscious patient.

The decision to intubate should be made as early as possible. One should not wait until a ventilation crisis occurs. Early intubation is advised in the following scenarios: (1) Patients with impending respiratory failure experiencing hypoventilation, apnea, or hypoxemia necessitating oral airway placement, or a flail chest. (2) Patients who have an initial Glasgow Coma Scale (GCS) score below 9. (3) Patients in shock who have not responded to appropriate fluid resuscitation. (4) Patients with significant burns or airway injury. Before intubation is attempted, airway equipment, drugs, suction, and personnel should be identified. Most emergency departments have an airway cart that contains emergency airway devices such as a fiberoptic bronchoscope, laryngeal mask airway, jet ventilation equipment, a light wand, and various laryngoscope blades and endotracheal tubes. If a difficult intubation is anticipated, a cricothyrotomy and tracheostomy kit and surgical personnel should be identified before proceeding with airway management.

C = Circulation

As previously mentioned, the most common cause of thoracic trauma is blunt trauma. Rib fractures are a poor predictor of major thoracic injury. The ribs are primarily cartilaginous structures and are extremely compliant, usually protecting against fractures. Commonly, pediatric trauma patients who have sustained multiple injuries present in hypovolemic shock. The pediatric patient is able to maintain a normal blood pressure despite a 25–40 % reduction in circulating blood volume. This compensation occurs through vasoconstriction and an increase in heart rate to sustain cardiac output. Therefore mental status, capillary refill, skin mottling, tachycardia, and peripheral skin temperature are more accurate indicators of circulatory status. A narrow pulse pressure and sustained tachycardia may indicate impending circulatory collapse.

Immediate restoration of systemic blood pressure is critical to maintain normal organ perfusion and function. Initial resuscitative efforts should involve administration of a warmed isotonic crystalloid solution. Many clinicians use warmed lactated ringers and initially infuse 20 mL/kg. This may be repeated once or twice. After this, if no increase in blood pressure is noted, then colloid and blood product administration should be considered. The first choice of blood products should be type-specific and fully cross-matched blood, given in 10–20 mL/kg boluses. If type-specific, fully cross-matched blood is not available, then type-specific, partially cross-matched, or type-specific uncross-matched blood is preferred. O Rh-negative blood is the next choice until type-specific blood is available. If the patient remains hemodynamically unstable after the above measures, then vasopressors (epinephrine) and/or inotropes (dopamine and dobutamine) may be indicated. After vasopressors and/or inotropes are used and there is still hemodynamic instability, tension pneumothorax, pericardial tamponade, myocardial contusion, or unrecognized internal bleeding should be considered.

Vascular access can be extremely challenging in the pediatric trauma patient presenting with hemodynamic instability. Peripheral access with a 24 gauge angiocatheter may be an adequate way to start resuscitation. When peripheral access is not possible, central access should be attempted. Cannulation of the external or internal jugular vein via direct venipuncture or Seldinger technique is acceptable. If there is no suspicion of intra-abdominal trauma or disruption of the inferior vena cava, femoral vein cannulation can be attempted. A central venous catheter should not be placed in the internal jugular vein if cerebral perfusion is in question. In the pediatric population subclavian venous catheter placement is associated with a higher incidence of pneumothorax and subclavian artery injury than in adults. The increasing use of ultrasound technology has made visualization and placement of central venous and arterial catheters easier in the pediatric population.

If intravenous access is not obtained after 2–3 min, one should place an intraosseous catheter. An intraosseous needle should be used; however, most large bore needles will suffice. Any nontraumatized long bone can be used for access, but the most common entry point is the tibia. The advised area of entry is the anteromedial aspect of the tibia 2 cm below the tibial tuberosity. Emissary veins that traverse the bony cortex may affect the

Table 15.3 Glasgow Coma Scale in children

Score	Variable
	Best motor response
6	Obeys commands
5	Localizes pain
4	Withdraws from pain
3	Abnormal flexion
2	Abnormal extension
1	Flaccidity
Score	Variable
	Best response
5	Appropriate words or social smiles, fixes, and follows
4	Cries but consolable
3	Persistently irritable
2	Restless agitated (moans only)
1	None
Score	Variable
	Eye opening responses
4	Spontaneous
3	Opens to voices
2	Opens to pain
1	None

Modified from Emerg Med Clin North Am, 16, Cantor RM, Leaming JM, Evaluation and management of pediatric major trauma, pp. 229–56, Copyright 1998, with permission from Elsevier

flow rate. Intraosseous access should only be used temporarily, until venous access can be obtained.

D = Disability

Head trauma is the major cause of death for pediatric trauma patients. The initial examination should include the mnemonic "AVPU" (awareness, response to verbal or pain stimuli, and unresponsiveness to stimuli), or the modified GCS (see Table 15.3) for assessment. The GCS can be unreliable in some pediatric patients. The GCS verbal responses have been modified for children in the hopes of improving predictability. However, in the absence of hypoxic-ischemic injury, the condition of most pediatric patients will improve despite a low GCS score [1].

An initial neurologic assessment sets a baseline for the patient so that trends in neurological function can be observed. Pediatric trauma patients may present with an unaltered mental status, no headaches and no vomiting. A CT scan should be performed despite the lack of these symptoms. Patients under the age of 18 months are able to accommodate an expanding intracranial mass because their fontanelles have not closed. However, if a fontanelle is bulging, immediate action should be undertaken. The large head to body size ratio in pediatric trauma patients predisposes them to flexion-extension injuries of the cervical spine between the second and third vertebrae. In half of patients with spinal cord injury, no radiologic abnormalities are noted. The patient with cervical spine injury may present with profound hypotension. Care to preserve neck stability and spinal cord perfusion should be taken [1, 2].

E = Exposure/Environmental Control

The pediatric trauma patient is frequently undressed to facilitate complete assessment. Patients can quickly become hypothermic due to their lack of subcutaneous tissue and their large surface area relative to body size. Clinicians should prepare to prevent hypothermia by increasing ambient temperature and using warm blankets to cover the patient after examination [7].

Preoperative Evaluation and Intraoperative Management

Secondary Survey

A secondary survey involves a thorough inspection of the patient and each organ system, with careful regard to the patient's hemodynamic status. Usually the anesthesiologist performs this preoperatively, with a thorough history and physical examination. However, pediatric trauma patients often present with urgent or emergent surgical needs. With limited time, a brief history

outlined by the mnemonic "AMPLE" may be obtained for safe delivery of anesthesia. The anesthetist should talk with the patient (if he or she is capable of providing information), or others (family, paramedics, nurses, ED physicians) to determine the following:

A—allergies: Is the patient allergic to any medications, foods, and materials such as latex? If they do have allergies, what happened and how was it treated?

M—medications: What medications are they taking, both prescription and over the counter? If they are taking medications, how often, what dosage, what route, and the when was the last time the medication was taken?

P—past medical and surgical history: What medical conditions do they have? What surgeries have they had? What was their anesthetic experience? Any family history of anesthesia complications?

L—last oral intake: When was the last time they had anything to eat or drink? What did they eat or drink?

E—events related to the injury: What led up to or occurred just prior to the injury? [17]

Other information pertinent to patient care may include: What was the course of events and treatment given at the scene of the accident and in the emergency department? What crystalloid, colloid, or blood products have been given since the event? What are the laboratory, radiologic, and ancillary test results? [1]

Equipment

Having an operating room prepared and available for trauma is essential for taking care of severely injured children. The anesthesia machine should be checked daily. Pressure transducer lines should be set up and zeroed. Ventilators capable of volume control and pressure control ventilation should be available, as well as rapid infusers, warming devices, a cell saver machine, forced air warmers, a difficult airway cart with fiberoptic bronchoscopes, airway equipment of different sizes, an echocardiographic machine and probes, an ultrasound machine for vascular access, a direct telephone line to the clinical lab and blood bank, an emergency resuscitation cart with defibrillator and pacer, an arterial blood gas machine, a glucometer, crystalloid and colloid solutions, and emergency type O-negative blood. Additionally, the operating room ambient temperature should be raised to more than 28 °C for infants and small children [9].

Monitors and Monitoring

In the world of anesthesia there is no better monitor than a focused and vigilant pediatric anesthesiologist. Monitors provide clinically useful information that can aid the timely application of therapeutic interventions. The ASA standard monitors include the electrocardiogram (ECG), noninvasive blood pressure (at least every 5 min), pulse oximetry, temperature probe, capnography, and an oxygen analyzer with a low oxygen concentration limit alarm in use. These monitors should be used for every pediatric patient. Additionally, a nerve stimulator is recommended to assess neuromuscular blockade, as well as an esophageal or precordial stethoscope to continuously monitor breath sounds. The pulse oximeter measures arterial oxygen saturation and gauges the adequacy of oxygenation and tissue perfusion. It may become unreliable when there is vasoconstriction due to hypovolemia, hypothermia, or shock. Other factors that influence the accuracy of pulse oximetry are patient movement, ambient light, dysfunctional hemoglobin (carboxyhemoglobin), and an altered relationship between $PaCO_2$ and SaO_2 (shift in the oxyhemoglobin dissociation curve) [4].

Capnography, or exhaled CO_2 monitoring, is helpful with: (1) determining endotracheal tube placement, (2) assessing ventilation, (3) estimating the $PaCO_2$ (the concentration of expired CO_2 is normally within 2–3 mmHg of that in the arterial blood), (4) gauging the adequacy of ventilation and the effectiveness of CPR, and (5) evaluating dead space [5].

In the mechanically ventilated neonate or young infant, the dead space volume between the breathing circuit and the ETT may be relatively more significant than in an adult, resulting in higher dead space to tidal volume ratio and less accurate, lower, $ETCO_2$ value. Decreases in the $ETCO_2$ value can be due to hyperventilation, hypothermia, low cardiac output, pulmonary embolism, accidental disconnection of the circuit, mainstem tracheal intubation, or cardiac arrest. Therefore, monitoring the trend of $ETCO_2$ as well as the actual $ETCO_2$ value is very important in infants and young children.

Temperature monitoring is mandatory in all children due to their immature thermoregulation, disproportionately greater body surface area to body mass ratio, and fluid and heat loss from exposed surgical sites. Hypothermia in children is associated with many adverse effects, such as increased oxygen consumption, a left shift of the oxyhemoglobin dissociation curve, coagulopathy with prolonged bleeding, metabolic and lactic acidosis, hypoglycemia, apnea, depressed myocardial contractility, arrhythmias, impaired drug metabolism, delayed emergence from anesthesia, and increased mortality. For these reasons, continuous temperature monitoring is mandatory in the care of an injured child [6].

Other monitors to consider include an arterial line, a central venous catheter, a urinary catheter, and an ICP monitoring device. In addition, continuous hemoglobin analysis and near-infrared spectroscopy are being increasingly used in pediatric anesthesia, and may soon have an important role in the care of the pediatric trauma patients. Invasive arterial blood pressure measurement is very useful, but urgent surgery should not be delayed if attempts to place an arterial line are unsuccessful. An arterial line provides access to obtain blood samples for analysis. It also provides continuous and accurate blood pressure measurement, useful when large changes in blood pressure are expected intraoperatively.

The most common reason for emergent or urgent surgery in the pediatric trauma patient is hemodynamic instability, often due to penetrating chest injury or acute bleeding in the head [16]. When transporting an unstable trauma patient, extra care should be placed in securing airways, lines, and monitors. An inventory of lines and monitors should be done immediately upon arrival to the OR. When transferring the patient to the OR table, cervical spine precautions should be maintained. The continuation of resuscitation fluids is imperative during placement of invasive monitors or establishment of additional IV access.

As with any trauma case, the pediatric anesthesiologist's primary responsibility is to focus first on the airway, breathing, and circulation. If the patient is already intubated, correct placement of the ET tube should be confirmed by equal and bilateral breath sounds, symmetrical chest expansion, and a normal $ETCO_2$ waveform on the capnogram, or a color change on the portable $ETCO_2$ detector. Once these are confirmed, mechanical ventilation can be safely initiated to ensure adequate ventilation and oxygenation.

Many infants and children who suffer trauma come to the OR conscious or semiconscious, receiving supplemental oxygen through a face mask or nasal cannula. For most of these patients, endotracheal intubation is often a necessity, so a reasonable and safe plan to secure the airway should be formulated. Before intubation, one should always have an emergency airway tray (including fiberoptic bronchoscope, laryngeal mask airway, light wand, jet ventilation, and appropriate blades and tubes). In addition, familiarity and knowledge of the American Society of Anesthesiologists (ASA) difficult airway algorithm is a necessity.

Anesthesiologists should presume that all trauma patients have full stomachs and a high likelihood of cervical spine injuries. Rapid sequence IV induction and intubation with manual in line cervical spine stabilization is usually indicated. By performing a rapid sequence induction then intubation, the time between loss of airway reflexes and intubation is minimized [10]. Preoxygenation of the patient with 100 % oxygen for four maximal breaths or 3–5 min of normal breathing, followed by intravenous injection of an anesthetic induction agent and a muscle relaxant while cricoid pressure is applied, reduces the risk of aspiration of gastric contents. As soon as the neuromuscular blocking agent takes effect, direct laryngoscopy is performed while in line cervical spine stabilization is maintained. Endotracheal tube placement is confirmed by the presence of continuous $ETCO_2$ capnography waves, auscultation of bilateral equal breath sounds, and the

absence of gastric sounds in the stomach. Cricoid pressure is only discontinued when ETT placement is confirmed and its cuff is inflated. A modified rapid sequence induction is an option when dealing with a combative or uncooperative child. With a combative child, another option is to perform an inhalational induction and apply cricoid pressure as the child loses consciousness. Before choosing a particular induction technique, the risk and benefits of each should be considered, specifically regarding aspiration and exacerbation of injuries due to excessive movement. During induction and intubation, the oxygen saturation of pediatric patients will decrease more quickly than in adults. This is related to their higher metabolic rate and low oxygen reserves (decreased functional residual capacity). Therefore, preoxygenation is very important [11, 12].

The modified rapid sequence induction and intubation has three defining features: (1) oxygen administration before induction, (2) the use of cricoid pressure, and (3) an attempt to ventilate the patient before securing the airway. Inflation pressures should be kept between 15 and 20 cm H_2O to minimize the possibility of gastric distention, regurgitation, and aspiration. Suction should be immediately available in the event of passive regurgitation or vomiting. Oxygenation should be attempted after each failed intubation attempt [10].

When dealing with a difficult airway, particularly when direct laryngoscopy appears to be difficult, the anesthesiologist should have several options for airway maintenance and protection. Spontaneous ventilation may be maintained while an inhalational agent is used to deepen the level of anesthesia in preparation for a fiberoptic intubation. In a non-emergent situation, for children with a limited mouth opening, limited neck movement (common in trauma victims in a cervical collar), or a congenital syndrome associated with a difficult airway, the fiberoptic bronchoscope is a powerful tool. Another helpful adjunct with these patients can be a video-assisted laryngoscope. It may allow for good visualization of the airway with less neck movement. In emergency situations, blind placement of a supraglottic device such as a laryngeal mask airway (LMA) is common. The LMA does not protect the airway from aspiration, but it can be used as a conduit to facilitate either blind or fiberoptic intubation of the trachea. The "Fastrach LMA" is another supraglottic device that is useful when direct visualization of the laryngeal inlet is not possible. However, this device is not yet available for use in small children. Additionally, the lightwand or light-assisted device can be very helpful. This is a rigid stylet with a light at its tip. It uses the technique of transtracheal illumination for blind intubation of the trachea in older children. Advantages to using this in the trauma patient are ease of learning how to use the device, and minimizing neck movement in a patient with a potential cervical spine injury [11, 12].

Induction Agents

When initiating induction of a trauma patient several factors have to be considered. The hemodynamic status is a major concern. Other concerns include the potential side effects of induction agents. A hypovolemic child is particularly sensitive to the vasodepressor and negative inotropic effects of volatile anesthetics, some induction agents, and drugs that promote histamine release. A safe induction technique may include providing small incremental doses of the selected agents. The reduced doses of induction agents are effective because the hypovolemic child has a decreased volume of distribution, while blood flow to the heart and brain are maintained. Also, fluid resuscitation can cause hemodilution resulting in a reduction of drug binding serum proteins. Almost any induction agent can be used in pediatric trauma as long as the agents are titrated carefully to minimize potential deleterious effects.

Sodium thiopental (at this time not commercially available) can be given in the dose of 3–6 mg/kg intravenously. Its dose should be titrated carefully as its side effects include venodilation and myocardial depression. Additionally, thiopental is rapid acting, lowers intraocular pressure (IOP), and does not cause pain on injection. It is a good choice for induction of pediatric patients with head injury and increased

intracranial pressure (ICP) as it causes a dose-dependent decrease in ICP, cerebral oxygen consumption, cerebral blood flow (CBF), and reduces epileptiform activity.

Propofol can be given in a dose of 2–3 mg/kg IV. One of its major side effects is more pronounced hypotension than thiopenthal, especially in hypovolemic patients. Propofol also causes pain on injection, especially when given in smaller caliber vessels. To decrease the pain on injection, lidocaine 0.5–1 mg/kg IV can be given prior to propofol. Propofol decreases ICP and CBF, and has antiemetic, anticonvulsant, and antipruritic properties.

Ketamine can be given in a dose of 1–3 mg/kg IV. Due to its high lipid solubility, it can also be given intramuscularly in trauma patients. It has some very favorable effects during induction of a hypovolemic, hypotensive, hemorrhaging child who needs emergent surgery. As an induction agent, ketamine can elevate blood pressure while providing analgesia and amnesia. It can provide complete anesthesia given as an infusion after induction. Ketamine can produce significant but transient increases in systemic blood pressure, heart rate, and cardiac output via centrally mediated sympathetic stimulation. However, ketamine is a direct myocardial depressant. This effect is usually masked by its stimulation of the sympathetic nervous system. Doses of ketamine used for induction minimally affect the central ventilatory drive, and do not depress upper airway reflexes. Ketamine causes increased salivation that can be attenuated by giving anticholinergic premedication such as glycopyrrolate 0.01 mg/kg IV, or atropine 0.1–0.2 mg/kg IV. Ketamine can cause dose-dependent increases in ICP, CBF, and cerebral oxygen consumption. Therefore it is usually avoided in patients with intracranial pathology, especially those with increased ICP [1, 3].

Etomidate can be given in a dose of 0.2–0.3 mg/kg IV. Advantages of using etomidate are that it is a short acting, potent, non-barbiturate sedative hypnotic, providing hemodynamic stability due to its minimal effects on the cardiovascular system. Etomidate is a potent cerebral vasoconstrictor, decreasing ICP and CBF. Other side effects of etomidate include spontaneous movements (characterized as myoclonus), and it has both anticonvulsant and proconvulsant properties. It can cause adrenocortical suppression, especially after a prolonged continuous infusion [13].

Neuromuscular Blockers

For muscle relaxation, either a depolarizing or a nondepolarizing muscle relaxant can be used. Succinylcholine can be given in a dose of 1.5–2 mg/kg IV. It is a depolarizing muscle relaxant, and may be the best choice for rapid sequence induction and intubation due to its rapid onset of 30–60 s and its short duration of 5–10 min. Its short duration makes it a valuable tool in the event that endotracheal intubation is unexpectedly difficult and bag mask ventilation becomes inadequate. This can allow for the return of potentially life-saving spontaneous respiratory efforts quickly. Infants require larger doses of succinylcholine, typically 2–3 mg/kg IV. This is due to their large volume of distribution. Caution must be taken when administering succinylcholine, especially when given repeatedly, because children are more susceptible than adults to cardiac arrhythmias, hyperkalemia, rhabdomyolysis, myoglobinuria, malignant hyperthermia, and even sinus arrest from succinylcholine. Thus, atropine 0.01–0.02 mg/kg IV (0.1 mg minimum) is often given to children prior to succinylcholine. Other side effects of succinylcholine include increased IOP and ICP, and elevated intragastric and esophageal sphincter pressures. Hyperkalemic cardiac arrest after succinylcholine administration has occurred in children with undiagnosed neuromuscular disorders. Succinylcholine is therefore *contraindicated* in patients with muscular dystrophies, and also in pediatric patients with burns more than 24 h old, denervation injuries, hyperkalemia, disuse atrophy, neuromuscular disorders, prolonged immobility, and a history of malignant hyperthermia.

Nondepolarizing muscle relaxants, such as rocuronium, may also be used for induction. At higher doses of 0.9–1.2 mg/kg IV, rocuronium provides rapid onset of neuromuscular blockade for intubation within 45–90 s. However, larger doses of rocuronium usually prolong its duration of action (up to 90 min). Rocuronium does not cause histamine release. If being given with thiopental, the intravenous line should be flushed before giving rocuronium, as rocuronium precipitates with thiopental. Another nondepolarizing muscle relaxant is vecuronium, which also does not cause histamine release or adverse hemodynamic effects. When given in a dose of 0.25 mg/kg IV, it provides good intubating conditions in 60–90 s. Vecuronium is an acidic compound that can be inactivated by alkaline solutions such as thiopental. Therefore thiopental should be flushed from the intravenous line before administering vecuronium.

Fluids and Blood Replacement

Large amounts of intravenous fluids may be required. They serve one of four purposes in trauma patients: (a) maintenance, (b) to balance ongoing losses, (c) to treat hypovolemia, and (d) to serve as replacement for volume deficits. In general, the non-glucose containing, isotonic crystalloid solutions are the fluids of choice for replacement of fluid losses associated with major surgery, hemorrhagic shock, and trauma. These solutions can rapidly restore circulating blood volume and preserve vital organ perfusion.

Calculating the preoperative deficit may be difficult in pediatric trauma patients. Patients undergoing emergency surgery may have larger fluid deficits related to fever, vomiting, third space loss, or blood loss. Often intraoperatively large deficits must be replaced; therefore fluid warmers should be used. This helps avoid hypothermia. An accurate estimate of fluid loss is often impossible; therefore fluid replacement should be guided by cardiovascular response and urine output.

Maintenance fluids for pediatric patients should be calculated using the 4-2-1 formula. For example, the required maintenance fluid for a 26 kg child would be 4 mL/kg/h for the first 10 kg, plus an additional 2 mL/kg/h for the next 10–20 kg, plus 1 mL/kg/h for weight greater than 20 kg, for a total of 66 mL/h (40 + 20 + 6). Again, non-glucose containing, isotonic crystalloid solutions are the fluids of choice for maintenance. Glucose containing solutions may be necessary in cases of hypoglycemia, or if the patient is at risk for hypoglycemia, such as a neonate with limited glycogen reserves.

Preoperative and intraoperative fluid losses are mostly isotonic, and are commonly replaced by lactated ringers or 0.9 % normal saline solution. Lactated ringers solution is slightly hypotonic (273 mOsm/L, sodium 130 mEq/L, chloride 108 mEq/L) and contains electrolytes. It is thought to be the most physiologic solution, especially when given in large amounts. Normal saline (308 mOsm/L, sodium 154 mEq/L, chloride 154 mEq/L) may also be used, but can lead to hyperchloremic metabolic acidosis when given in large amounts. Albumin 5 % is the most common colloid used in pediatric patients, but disagreement exists as to the efficacy of this therapy versus isotonic crystalloid administration.

Blood loss should be replaced with 3 mL of crystalloid for every 1 mL of blood loss, in combination with 1 mL colloid given for every 1 mL of blood loss, to maintain normovolemia. The hematocrit should be monitored in cases with moderate (4–6 mL/kg/h) or greater blood loss. When a predetermined lower limit of hematocrit has been reached, blood products should be given. Acceptable low hematocrit values vary with age. Premature infants normally have a hematocrit of 40–45 %, with an acceptable low level of 35–40 %. A normal hematocrit for a newborn is 45–65 %, and an acceptable low hematocrit is 35–40 % for this age. A normal hematocrit for a 3-month-old is 30–42 %, and an acceptable low hematocrit is 25 %. A normal hematocrit for a 1-year-old is 34–42 %, with an acceptable low hematocrit of 20–25 %. Children 6 years old or older have a normal hematocrit between 35 and 43 %, and an acceptable low hematocrit of 20–25 %. Red blood cell transfusion is indicated to increase the intravascular oxygen carrying capacity, as well as volume. The use of other blood products such as platelets, fresh frozen plasma (FFP), cryoprecipitate, or other factors should be guided by coagulation studies and clinical signs of coagulopathy. Other factors that influence the decision to transfuse include preoperative hematocrit, estimated blood volume, comorbidities, rate of ongoing blood loss, and the clinical response of the patient to volume resuscitation.

The formula to calculate maximum allowable blood loss is: MABL = EBV X (initial hematocrit-target hematocrit)/initial hematocrit. To calculate the amount of PRBCs needed to reach the target hematocrit value, the following formula can be used: Volume of PRBCs (mL) = EBV X (desired hematocrit-present hematocrit)/ hematocrit of PRBC (typically 60 %). Transfusion of 10–15 mL/kg of PRBCs should increase the hemoglobin concentration by 2–3 g/dL.

Platelets and FFP should be given when blood loss is greater than one to two blood volumes, or when the results of coagulation studies are abnormal. Administration of 5–10 mL/kg of platelet concentrate should increase platelets by 50,000–100,000 per dL. FFP is typically given to correct coagulopathy due to insufficient coagulation factors. Administration of 10–15 mL/kg of FFP will increase factor levels by 15–20 %. Cryoprecipitate is most commonly used as a source of fibrinogen, factor VIII, and factor XIII. Administration of 1 unit of cryoprecipitate for every 5 kg to a maximum of 4 units is typically adequate for correcting coagulopathy due to low levels of fibrinogen.

Recombinant factor VIIa is approved by the FDA for the treatment and prevention of bleeding in patients with factor VII deficiency, and for hemophiliacs with inhibitors to factors VIII and IX. Over the last decade, there have been multiple reports of recombinant factor VIIa being used effectively in controlling life-threatening traumatic and intraoperative bleeding unresponsive to conventional intervention. However, concern remains about potential thromboembolic complications [14].

Postoperative Care of Pediatric Trauma Patients

The percentage of injured children that go on to have surgery is considered low, as one study reported fewer than 15 % of pediatric trauma patients require surgery. Despite this, it is important to realize that those pediatric patients requiring surgery are often critically injured. One study cited that 86 % of pediatric trauma patients at risk for mortality had at least one surgical diagnosis, and that surgical pediatric trauma patients required longer ICU stays (2). Even though pediatric and adult trauma patients undergo similar surgeries to treat their injuries, there are considerable differences in physiology (especially in regards to cardiac and pulmonary physiology) that make postoperative care of pediatric trauma patients much different than in adults.

The challenge of caring for pediatric trauma patients in the postoperative period begins with transport. As stated previously, pediatric trauma patients who require surgery have a higher mortality risk and will often require recovery in an intensive care unit. The transport of pediatric trauma patients to intensive care units is often challenging. The pediatric intensive care units (PICU) are sometimes located a considerable distance from the operating rooms in the hospital. The clinician transporting the patient should focus on airway management, breathing, and the cardiovascular status of the patient. Due to the patient's critical condition, monitors, resuscitative drugs, and airway equipment, as well as other medical equipment, should be on hand during transport to ensure proper care and stability.

Regarding airway management and maintenance of ventilation, the anesthesiologist must decide whether to keep the patient intubated, or to extubate in the operating room. If the patient is extubated in the OR, then supplies for laryngoscopy and intubation should accompany the patient to the PICU in case intervention is needed during transport. In addition to airway supplies, an oxygen source, properly fitting face mask, and a self-inflating bag with reservoir should be transported with the patient should ventilation become inadequate. It is not ideal to intubate a patient during transport from the OR. Bag-mask ventilation is an acceptable method for ventilation, and is frequently used by clinicians when transporting patients to the PICU. If respiratory difficulty occurs during transport, it is advisable to provide bag-mask ventilation until arrival in the PICU. The PICU provides a better setting for intubation if needed.

Maintaining adequate circulation should begin with ensuring that the patient has adequate intravascular access before transport. Supplies such as intravascular catheters of appropriate gauge, intraosseous needles, and isotonic fluids with proper pediatric drip chambers and tubing should be transported with the patient in case intravascular access is lost and emergency medications need to be administered. Key drugs for the management of a pediatric trauma patient include etomidate, ketamine, succinylcholine, vecuronium, cisatracurium, lorazepam, midazolam, fentanyl, morphine, dopamine, dobutamine, epinephrine, atropine, albuterol, and racemic epinephrine.

Portable monitors used to transport patients to the ICU should be able to measure blood pressure, pulse oximetry, and provide a 5-lead EKG tracing. Some monitors may be equipped with defibrillation pads or devices to measure blood glucose. Ultimately it is at the discretion of the anesthesiologist as to which supplies, monitors, and medications are needed for patient transport. It may not be practical to travel with all of the drugs and supplies previously listed [9].

Hemodynamic monitoring in pediatric patients may be more challenging than in adults. One must realize hemodynamic values vary based on the age of the pediatric patient (see Table 15.1). Even more challenging is determining whether pediatric trauma patients are experiencing bleeding related to their injury or surgery, or, more importantly, are in hypovolemic shock. In adults, blood pressure and heart rate are more sensitive values used for diagnosing hypovolemic shock. On the other hand, as previously mentioned, children can maintain normal, age-specific blood pressures despite significant blood loss. For this reason, it is advisable to place an arterial line in all pediatric trauma patients for close blood pressure monitoring. An arterial line also allows for arterial blood gases and other labs to be easily obtained in the postoperative setting. A quick way to determine the normal systolic blood pressure of a child is to multiply the patient's age in years by

2 and then add 80. For newborns, the normal systolic blood pressure is approximately equal to their age in gestational weeks (i.e., 40 mmHg for a term infant). If hypovolemic shock is suspected in the postoperative setting, then a protocol for resuscitation should be followed, especially if the patient has become hypotensive. A bolus of 20 mL/kg of crystalloid should be given twice before initiating transfusion of type-specific, cross-matched PRBCs or O-negative type blood. If there is no improvement, then FFP and platelets should immediately follow the transfusion of blood [19].

Postoperatively, pediatric trauma patients may need to remain intubated with ventilator support. Thoracic trauma is common in pediatric trauma patients. The lung is often injured, even in the absence of rib fractures, due to the very compliant chest wall that allows direct transfer of energy to the lungs. Oxygenation may be compromised, and pediatric patients may present like adult patients present with acute lung injury (ALI) or acute respiratory distress syndrome (ARDS). Pediatric patients presenting with an ARDS-like picture should be treated with the treatment strategy of low tidal volumes (6 mL/kg) [15]. In addition to the lung protective strategy of low tidal volumes, specialized modes of ventilation have been used to help patients recover. High frequency (or oscillator) ventilation allows for continuous airway pressure and low tidal volumes with very high respiratory rates to help maximize the patient's oxygenation. The inspiration to expiration ratio can also be inversed, giving the patient more time in the inspiration phase, allowing permissive hypercapnia [18, 21–23]. When all ventilation modes fail, a trial of extracorporeal membrane oxygenation (ECMO) may allow the heart and lungs time to recover [8].

Postoperatively, we may find that not all of the injuries suffered during trauma were necessarily corrected with surgery. Other injuries may have been stabilized before surgery and require ongoing monitoring and care. The most notable of these injuries are possible cervical spine fractures. Several protocols have been suggested for cervical spine clearance, but there are no procedural or diagnostic standards. The care of patients with possible cervical spine fracture focuses on keeping the head in a neutral position. However, pediatric patients have larger heads than adults, and when lying supine a child's head is often slightly flexed. Extra padding behind the back, or specialized backboards, along with a cervical collar, can help keep the head in a neutral position. Other anatomic differences between children and adults include more flexible interspinous ligaments and joint capsules, vertebral bodies that will slide forward with flexion, flat facet joints, and a different head to neck ratio. Due to a disproportionately larger head, the greater laxity of interspinous ligaments, and flatter facet joints, cervical spine injuries in children are most likely to occur in the first three cervical vertebrae.

As we have continual postoperative hemodynamic monitoring for pediatric trauma patients who may have ongoing internal bleeding, the patient should also be continually observed to identify any undiagnosed fractures. Some pediatric patients may have difficulty communicating effectively due to age. This, coupled with the possibility of distracting injuries, may allow for an undiagnosed fracture to appear postoperatively. Children are at risk for multiple injuries based on their smaller body size. When caring for the pediatric trauma patient postoperatively, it should not be assumed that all of their injuries have been addressed. Bony fractures can also be more difficult to diagnose in pediatric patients due to the presence of growth plates. Given the previous statements, one should pay close attention to the patient's complaints of pain and their ability to move extremities or ambulate [1, 3].

References

1. Loy J. Chapter 24, Pediatric trauma and anesthesia. In: Smith C, editor. Trauma and anesthesia. Cambridge: Cambridge University Press; 2008. p. 367–90.
2. Miller RD, Pardo M. Basics of anesthesia. 6th ed. Philadelphia: Lippincott Williams & Wilkins; 2011. p. 327–686.
3. Varon AJ, Smith CE, editors. Essentials of trauma anesthesia. Cambridge: Cambridge University Press; 2012.

4. Severinghaus JW, Kehheher JF. Recent developments in pulse oximetry. Anesthesiology. 1992;76:1018–38.
5. Marino PL. Oximetry and capnography. The ICU book, vol. 20. 3rd ed. Philadelphia: Lippincott Williams & Wilkins; 2007. p. 395–8.
6. Schubert A. Side effects of mild hypothermia. J Neurosurg Anesthesiol. 1995;7(2):139–45.
7. Bernardo LM, Henker R. Thermoregulation in pediatric trauma: an overview. Int J Trauma Nurs. 1999;5:101–5.
8. Lerman J. Special techniques: acute normovolemic hemodilution, controlled hypotension and hypothermia, ECMO. In: Gregory GA, editor. Pediatric anesthesia. 3rd ed. New York: Churchill Livingstone; 1994.
9. Campbell S, Wilson G, Engelhardt T. Equipment and monitoring—What is in the future to improve safety? Paediatr Anaesth. 2011;21:815–24.
10. Morris J, Cook TM. Rapid sequence induction: a national survey of practice. Anaesthesia. 2001;56:1090–7.
11. Barch B, Rastatter J, Jagannathan N. N Int J Pediatr Otorhinolaryngol. 2012;76(11):1579–82. doi:10.1016/j.ijporl.2012.07.016. Epub 2012 Aug 11.
12. Jain S, Bhadani U. J Anesth. 2011;25(2):291–3. doi:10.1007/s00540-010-1091-2. Epub. 2011 Jan 20.
13. Fragen RJ, Shanks CA, Moteni A, et al. Effects of etomidate on hormonal responses to surgical stress. Anesthesiology. 1984;61:652–6.
14. Alten JA, Benner K, Green K, et al. Pediatric off label use of recombinant factor VIIa. Pediatrics. 2009;123:1066–72.
15. Cullen ML. Pulmonary and respiratory complications of pediatric trauma. Respir Care Clin N Am. 2001;7(1):59–77.
16. Teppas III JJ, et al. Pediatric trauma is very much a surgical disease. Ann Surg. 2003;237(6):775–81.
17. Wathen J, Cooper L, Crossman K, Bastidas MA. Pediatric trauma: module 4. Denver: UC. Accessed in 2013.
18. Baird JS, et al. Noninvasive ventilation during pediatric interhospital ground transport. Prehosp Emerg Care. 2009;13(2):198–202.
19. Feliciano DF, Mattox KL, Moore EE. Trauma. 6th ed. New York: McGraw-Hill; 2008. p. 987–1000.
20. Holmes JE, Lee DE. Pediatric trauma. In: Wilson WC, Grande CM, Hoyt DB, editors. Trauma: emergency resuscitation, periopertive anesthesia and surgical management, vol. 1. New York: Informa Healthcare; 2007.
21. Tovar J. The lung and pediatric trauma. Semin Pediatr Surg. 2008;17(1):53–9.
22. Arnold JH. Prospective randomized comparison of high frequency oscillatory ventilation and conventional mechanical ventilation in pediatric respiratory failure. Crit Care Med. 1994;22(10):1530–9.
23. Walls R, Ratey JJ, Simon RI. Rosen's emergency medicine: expert consult premium edition—enhanced online features and print (Rosen's emergency medicine: concepts & clinical practice (2v.)). St. Louis: Mosby; 2009. p. 262–80.

Trauma in the Pregnant Patient

16

Anjali K. Fedson Hack

Introduction

Trauma is the leading cause of death for women in the United States ages 34 years of age and younger. It is the primary cause of deaths not attributable to medical causes in pregnancy, complicating 6–8 % of pregnancies, and results in emergency surgery in up to 20 % of pregnant women with traumatic injuries [1–7]. Trauma-related deaths are often not included in maternal mortality reviews and the precise contribution of trauma to mortality rates is probably underestimated [8, 9]. Nevertheless, trauma accounts for up to 46 % of pregnancy-associated deaths, or greater than one million deaths annually worldwide [6, 10–12]. While pregnancy-related maternal deaths (those due to medical events during pregnancy) have declined, those due to injury have increased [1]. Causes include active-employment while pregnant, greater number of miles traveled in an automobile, and growing incidence of intimate partner violence.

Maternal injury can have serious consequences, including fetal loss, preterm rupture of membranes, preterm delivery, placental abruption, cesarean delivery, and stillbirth (see Fig. 16.1) [13–18]. One study estimated that as many as one-third of pregnant women hospitalized for trauma will deliver during their hospitalizations [19]. Actual fetal injury and loss

rates may be undercounted due to a lack of standardized reporting methods; for example, medical care for the initial episode of maternal trauma and subsequent fetal loss may occur at different medical centers; the fetal loss may occur after unreported maternal trauma; or the fetal loss may not be recorded because it occurred at less than 20 weeks gestation [20].

Trauma in pregnancy has been associated with younger age, less education, being unmarried, and it is more common among those who have used tobacco, alcohol, or illicit substances while pregnant [21, 22]. Data from the American College of Surgeons National Trauma Data bank indicate that alcohol and illicit substances are implicated in pregnancy-associated trauma in 12.9 % and 19.6 % of cases, respectively [3]. While pregnancy itself does not increase morbidity or mortality due to injury, it has been identified as an independent risk factor for trauma. This includes violent assaults aimed at causing fetal injury [23, 24].

Fetal outcomes after maternal trauma are poor, with mortality reported as high as 40–50 % [25]. Importantly, fetal morbidity and mortality can occur in the setting of insignificant maternal injury [25, 26], and severity scores for maternal injury do not accurately predict placental abruption or fetal death [27–29]. Consequently, it is essential that all women of childbearing age who experience trauma be evaluated for pregnancy, and if pregnant undergo fetal evaluation, even in the setting of minor injury.

A.K.F. Hack, M.D., Ph.D. (✉)
New York, New York 10025, USA
e-mail: fedsonhack@gmail.com

C.S. Scher (ed.), *Anesthesia for Trauma*, DOI 10.1007/978-1-4939-0909-4_16,
© Springer Science+Business Media New York 2014

- Maternal death
- Maternal loss of consciousness
- Injury Severity Score > 15
- Pelvic fracture
- Failure to use seat belts
- Early gestational age
- Vaginal bleeding
- Severe hemorrhage
- Coagulopathy
- Serum lactate > 2 mEq/L

Fig. 16.1 Factors associated with trauma-associated fetal loss

Types of Trauma

Patterns of Injury

The risk for trauma increases as pregnancy progresses, with 10–15 % of injuries occurring in the first trimester and 50–54 % in the third trimester [30], and parturients are more likely to have abdominal rather than head injuries [31]. The uterus is protected within the bony pelvis until 12 weeks gestation, so chances of fetal injury are limited during the first trimester. The American College of Obstetricians and Gynecologists (ACOG) categorizes trauma into three categories: blunt abdominal injury, penetrating trauma, and pelvic fractures [32]. Maternal and fetal mortality may result from the injury itself or from indirect causes, such as maternal shock, disseminated intravascular coagulation, or acute respiratory distress syndrome.

Blunt Injury to the Abdomen

Blunt abdominal injury accounts for two-thirds of trauma cases in pregnancy. The force of the impact directly correlates with degree of maternal and fetal injury. As pregnancy progresses, the gravid uterus pushes abdominal contents upward, thus decreasing the risk of maternal bowel injury from a direct abdominal blow, although the risk of hepatic or splenic rupture and retroperitoneal hemorrhage remains.

With increasing gestational age, the uterus is at greater risk in abdominal injury. While the amniotic fluid absorbs collision energy and prevents its direct transmission to the fetus, premature rupture of membranes can occur because the portion of membranes lying over the internal cervical os is unsupported by the uterine wall and this creates a potential site for tears. Placental abruption is common and it may occur within hours of injury or later.

Forceful direct impact and contrecoup injuries can contribute to traumatic rupture of the uterus itself. Clinical presentation of uterine rupture ranges from hemorrhagic shock with maternal collapse, to nonspecific abdominal discomfort. Fetal injuries following abdominal trauma are most commonly reported during the third trimester and while maternal mortality may be less than 10 %, fetal death rates approach 100 % [33].

Penetrating Trauma

There are few data on outcomes of penetrating injury during pregnancy. A retrospective study of abdominal injuries seen in a level 1 trauma center from 1996 to 2008 reported that blunt injuries occurred in 91 % whereas penetrating injuries accounted for only 9 % of patients [34]. Among penetrating injuries, 73 % were caused by gunshots. Maternal mortality did not differ between the two groups, but fetal mortality was 73 % following penetrating injuries, but only 10 % following blunt trauma. Overall, gunshot wounds are reported to cause fetal injury in 60–70 % and lead to death in 40–65 % of cases [4, 34, 35]. While gunshot wounds require a laparotomy to determine the full scope of injury, stab wounds do so only if the blade appears to have penetrated the peritoneum.

Pelvic Fracture

Pelvic fractures contribute to high maternal and fetal mortality. Medical treatment is complicated by pregnancy and there are increased risks of obstetrical complications. A literature review of 101 case reports of pelvic or acetabular fractures in pregnancy found that maternal and fetal deaths did not correlate with the type of fracture (simple or complex), its location, or trimester of pregnancy [36]. Overall, fetal morality was 35 % and maternal mortality 9 %. However, an institutional study of 148 motor vehicle accident (MVA)-related injuries at a level 1 trauma center, in which there were no maternal deaths, noted that mothers of five of the seven cases of fetal demise had sustained pelvic fractures [37]. The odds of fetal loss were 48 times higher if their mothers sustained a pelvic fracture, versus those who did not, and ten times more likely if the mother lost consciousness on impact [37]. Among the seven fetal deaths, only one was due to direct uterine trauma; the other six were the result of spontaneous abortion.

Pelvic fractures may lead to placental abruption in as many as 30 % of cases [38]. In one retrospective study of maternal fractures, patients who delivered during hospitalization had 15-fold increase in placental abruption and 20-fold increases in transfusions and stillbirths [39]. Those who were discharged and delivered subsequently had a 47 % increase in abruptions and 18 % increase in rate of preterm deliveries. In this study, women with pelvic fractures were the only group in which there was long-term increased risk of fetal death.

Causes of Maternal Trauma

Motor Vehicle Accidents

The overall incidence of motor vehicle accidents (MVA) has been estimated at 2.8 % [21], and MVAs may account for 34–70 % of all traumatic injuries during pregnancy [3, 16, 40, 41]. Maternal mortality following MVAs has been estimated at 1.4 and fetal mortality at 3.7 per 100,000 pregnancies, respectively [42]. Both maternal morbidity and mortality are substantially increased when seat belts are not used or placed incorrectly, and adverse outcomes have been reported in 100 % of women injured in MVAs who were not wearing seatbelts [43]. The use of alcohol and other intoxicants has

been implicated as a risk factor for MVAs during pregnancy, with up to 45 % of collisions involving maternal alcohol use [22, 44].

Seat belts can prevent maternal impact with the steering wheel in both front and rear collisions [45]. Many pregnant women fail to use or correctly place seatbelts [46], and one study reported that only half of patients indicated they received counseling about seatbelt use from their physicians [47]. Fear of injuring their fetus and belt discomfort have been reported as reasons for avoiding their use [43], and when used improperly, seatbelts can cause severe uterine and fetal injury. Yet, fetal deaths are three times more likely in MVAs when the mother is not wearing a seat belt [21]. Recommendations for their correct use, with or without airbag activation during MVAs, have been associated with improved fetal outcomes [48, 49]. Current guidelines recommend using seatbelts throughout pregnancy, with the lap belt portion placed under the abdomen and over the anterior superior iliac spines and pubic symphysis. The shoulder portion of the belt should be between the breasts with the belt as snug as comfort permits [32].

In high-speed automobile crashes, airbags and three-point seatbelts can be life saving, and one study reported they were protective only when vehicle speeds exceed 32–38 mph. There have been case reports of uterine rupture and placental abruption with airbag deployment [50, 51], however, a population-based study of airbag deployment during MVAs in pregnancy failed to find a statistically increased risk of poor fetal outcomes [52]. Another study of 42 pregnant women who were wearing three-point seat belts when they were involved in MVAs found that deployment of airbags further reduced the risk of adverse fetal outcomes [48].

Despite the absence of data regarding airbag injury risk, new manufacturing criteria for "advanced air bags" require supplemental restraint systems that are designed to accommodate children and women as well as standard-sized men. According to the National Highway Traffic and Safety Association, pregnant women should be at least 10 in. away from an airbag in the dashboard or steering wheel and the seat should be pushed back or reclined as the abdomen grows during pregnancy.

During collisions, substantial mechanical forces are placed on the uterus. Both shear force failure (or strain) and tensile failure (by a contrecoup mechanism) have been implicated in uterine injury. The displacement of the uterus forward during a collision can generate negative forces and injure the opposite side of the uterus. In addition, upon impact the mother's torso folds over the abdomen, markedly increasing abdominal pressure. The combination of these two movements can cause placental abruption in additional to maternal injuries [53].

Falls

Falls are estimated to complicate 48.9 of 100,000 pregnancies, and they account for 22–52 % of all traumatic injuries in pregnancy [54, 55]. As many as one-in-four women will fall while pregnant [56, 57]. The likelihood of falling increases in the second and third trimesters when gait and balance are altered by shifts in a women's center of balance [58–60] and women are less able to stabilize themselves when their body position changes abruptly [61]. In one study of pregnant women hospitalized for falls, fractures were the most common injuries, followed by contusions and sprains [56]. This study also reported a 4.4-fold increase in preterm labor, an 8-fold increase in placental abruption, and a 2.9-fold increase in fetal hypoxia compared with those who had not fallen.

Assaults, Homicide, and Suicide

Assault during pregnancy is a leading cause of maternal and fetal deaths [62–66]. The prevalence of domestic violence (DV) or intimate partner violence (IPV) varies worldwide. In the United States, it occurs in 22.1 % of the women of childbearing age, although it is higher in specific groups [67, 68]. Pregnancy appears to be an independent risk factor for battery [23, 69].

Women who are abused while pregnant have a threefold risk of becoming homicide victims during the same pregnancy [61]. Among postpartum women 15–19 years old, the risk of homicide was 2.6-fold greater than that of women who had not been pregnant [70]. One study of mortality among pregnant women 15–44 years of age in New York City found that for injury-related deaths, 63 % were homicides and 13 % were suicides [12]. Another review of pregnancy-associated deaths in Maryland found that homicide was the leading cause of all maternal deaths [71].

Data from the multistate National Violent Death Reporting System (NVDRS) for 2003–2007 reveal that pregnancy-associated violent death mortality in women ages 15–54 accounted for a rate of 4.9 per 100,000 live births [62]. The homicide rate was calculated at 2.9 per 100,000 live births. Of the 139 homicides among women of childbearing age, 108 (77 %) occurred during pregnancy and the remainder within the first postpartum year. Women at extremes of age were at higher risk. Younger women were at greatest risk, with those 24 years and younger accounting for more than half (53.9 %) of pregnancy-associated homicides, but only 33.6 % of live births in reporting states. Women 40 years or older were also at elevated risk of homicide. In this sample, 59.1 % of homicides were due to intimate partner violence [62]. Another study, based on records of the New York City Office of the Chief Medical Examiner between 1998 and 2009, revealed that in 19 of 27 homicides among pregnant women, the victim and suspect were known to each other [72].

Violent abuse in pregnancy is associated with a 2.7-fold increase in preterm births and 5.5-fold increase in low birthweight infants [73]. Risk factors for DV/IPV include substance abuse, less education, low socioeconomic status, African-American race, unintended pregnancy, unmarried status, a history of DV/IPV prior to pregnancy, or witnessing violence by mother or intimate partner as a child [74]. Fetal mortality following intimate partner violence has been reported as high as 16 % [34].

Most studies have reported a lower incidence of suicide in pregnant versus non-pregnant women [63]. According to NVDRS data for 2003–2007, maternal suicide accounted for two deaths per 100,000 live births [62]. In this survey, women over 40 years of age accounted for 17.0 % of pregnancy-related suicides but only 2.8 % of the live births. The homicide and suicide rates in this study were both higher than reported maternal death rates reported from common obstetric causes (hemorrhage/placenta previa, ecclampsia/preeclampsia, and amniotic fluid embolism). Fetal or infant death, and substance abuse are maternal risk factors for attempting suicide in during pregnancy and postpartum [75, 76].

Burns and Electrical Injuries

Our understanding of burns in pregnancy is limited, as the reported incidence of burn injuries is low and burn victims are not consistently screened for pregnancy. Worldwide, approximately 7 % of women of reproductive age who are treated for burns are pregnant [77]. A prospective study of pregnant women admitted to a burn center in Iran over 9 years, found that larger total body surface area burned correlated with those that were self-inflected. In this study, 27.45 % of burns were suicide attempts. Total body surface area burned and degree of burn are related to the extent of maternal and fetal injury. As the body surface area of injury approaches 40 %, mortality rates for mother and fetus approach 100 % [77, 78]. Sepsis complicating burn injury is a major contributor to maternal and fetal mortality [79].

A recent observational study used thromboelastography (TEG) to evaluate hypercoagulability in burn patients and noted a hypercoagulable state developing 1 week after the initial injury. Pregnant patients with burns should receive routine thromboprophylaxis as the hypercoagulable state of pregnancy may be exacerbated and deaths from pulmonary embolisms occur in the setting of burn injury [80].

Smoke inhalation during burn injury significantly increases maternal and fetal mortality [81, 82] due to oxygen depletion, carbon monoxide (CO) poisoning [82] and cyanide (CN) poisoning from combustion of synthetic products silk and wool [83]. Fetal hemoglobin has greater affinity than maternal hemoglobin for CO, and fetal carboxyhemoglobin levels can reach as high as 15 %. The fetal effect of inhaled CO and CN poisoning depends on the gestational age of the fetus and combined exposure exhibits a synergistic effect.

CO poisoning can be treated with normobaric oxygen. Hyperbaric oxygen therapy has been used in pregnancy, but remains controversial. Prompt treatment of CN with intravenous hydroxocobalamin effectively removes CN, raises the threshold for lethal CO poisoning, and is superior to combined treatment with amyl nitrate, sodium nitrate, and sodium thiosulfate, all of which are contraindicated in pregnancy [83].

There are few reports of electrical injuries in pregnancy, and among reported cases there has been wide variance in the degree of injury. In one study of 15 cases of severe electrical injury during pregnancy, fetal mortality was 73 % [84]. A prospective study of minor electrical shocks from household appliances, however, found no difference in birth outcomes compared with controls [85]. The magnitude of the current appears to be related to the degree of fetal injury, as does trajectory through the uterus and conduction of the current to the fetus by amniotic fluid. In cases of severe electric shocks, resulting falls can lead to abdominal injury and placental abruption.

Poisoning

Case reports of poisoning in pregnancy are limited and primarily concern suicide attempts (see above) and inadvertent drug overdoses. One study found that pregnant women accounted for only 0.07 % of calls to a poison control center over 4 years [86]. If all women who sought help had received a pregnancy test, however, the number would likely have been higher [87]. No studies have examined the teratogenic risks of specific poison antidotes, and it is recommended that they not be withheld from pregnant women if there are clear medical indications [88].

Drug overdoses in pregnancy have been reported from both over-the-counter medications such as acetaminophen and prescription drugs.

Lead has been found to contaminate several naturopathic medications. Isolated case reports of accidental overdoses of hospital-delivered medications, such as epidural local anesthetics or misoprostol, have also been noted. Opioid-medications are responsible for the recent dramatic increase in overdose fatalities, with overall mortality rates three times higher in rural compared with metropolitan areas. A study of pregnancy-related deaths in Florida from 1999 to 2005 found that prescription drugs were detected in 54 % of cases, with opioids being the most commonly detected drug, followed by benzodiazapines. Among pregnant women who died, drug toxicity and motor vehicle accidents each accounted for one-third of the total deaths, followed by gunshot wounds in 14 % [89].

Envenomation injuries, caused by snakes, scorpions, spiders, jellyfish, and hymenoptera (bees, wasps, hornets, ants) are rare in pregnancy and treatment has been directed by case reports on non-pregnant subjects. Venom-specific approaches based upon supportive therapy and anti-venom administration is indicated to support the mother [90].

Maternal and Fetal Outcomes Following Trauma

Maternal mortality is directly linked to the severity of the traumatic injury. Traumatic head injuries, internal injuries, and hemorrhagic shock account for the majority of maternal deaths [16, 91, 92]. Pregnant women who are injured and deliver at the time of the initial trauma hospitalization experience worse outcomes. One retrospective analysis of hospital discharge records in California reported that pregnant women who delivered during their hospitalization for trauma had a 9-fold greater risk of placental abruption, a 42-fold greater risk of uterine rupture and 69-fold greater risk of maternal death compared with those who delivered during a subsequent admission [16]. Data are conflicting as to whether being pregnant during traumatic injury is associated with a survival advantage over non-pregnant women of childbearing age [31].

Obstetric complications of trauma include preterm labor and delivery, preterm premature rupture of membranes, placental abruption, feto-maternal hemorrhage, and uterine rupture. After 22–24 weeks gestation, preterm labor occurs in 25 % of trauma cases [4]. Most preterm deliveries occur after discharge from the initial trauma hospitalization. Calcium channel blockers such as nifidipine are widely used off-label for tocolysis for those patients who remain undelivered with preterm labor. Magnesium sulfate can be used for short-term tocolysis (5–7 days), and has been shown to have fetal neuroprotective effects in early preterm deliveries (<32 weeks) for all pregnancies [93, 94].

Abruption of the placenta occurs with 1.7 % of maternal injuries and in up to 40 % of severe injuries [95]. It is more common after blunt trauma [16]. Ultrasound is a relatively insensitive test for placental abruption and due to its delayed occurrence, continuous fetal monitoring is recommended for 6 h, even in the setting of minor trauma [96].

Uterine rupture is a rare consequence of trauma that has grave consequences for the fetus. Rupture occurs most commonly in rapid deceleration or compression injuries, and is typically found in patients with a previous uterine scar. Following uterine rupture, fetal mortality is almost universal and the maternal mortality rate is 10 % [97]. The risk of rupture increases with gestational age and with the severity of trauma. Abdominal pain, uterine tenderness, loss of abdominal shape, cessation of contractions, and maternal hemodynamic instability may be found. The uterus may rupture posteriorly if it is unscarred by previous surgery and typical findings on abdominal examination may be absent. Bladder injury is also associated with posterior ruptures, and blood or meconium may be found in the urine [98].

Of note, uterine rupture and ruptured membranes following blunt abdominal trauma are associated with amniotic fluid embolism (AFE) [99]. Signs and symptoms of AFE vary and include, shock, acute hypertension, seizure, respiratory distress, disseminated intravascular coagulation or cardiac arrest. These clinical findings in the setting of traumatic injury should prompt high suspicion of AFE [100].

Fetomaternal hemorrhage occurs in up to 30 % of pregnant trauma patients and is more common in those who sustain anterior trauma and have an anterior implanted placenta [101]. Hemorrhage can cause fetal anemia, arrhythmias, and exsanguination resulting in fetal death. In addition, mothers are at risk of Rh sensitization: as little as 0.01 mL of Rh-positive blood from the fetus can result in sensitization in Rh-negative women.

In the California study cited above, fetuses delivered during the initial trauma hospitalization had a 2-fold increase in premature delivery, a 4.6-fold increase in fetal death and a 3-fold increase in neonatal death [16]. Because the fetal head is in the pelvis near term, there is a risk of fetal skull fracture and brain injury with pelvic fractures. Even minor trauma during pregnancy can significantly increase the risk of pre-term delivery, despite normal fetal monitoring and observation. Pregnant women who are discharged after hospitalization for trauma should still be considered at risk for the remainder of their pregnancies [26].

The Physiology of Pregnancy and Management of the Trauma Patient

The altered physiology of pregnancy and the fetal response to trauma affect both the severity of trauma and its treatment. Initial management is focused on maternal stabilization. Treatment must be guided by pregnancy-related changes in maternal physiology and how they affect trauma life support protocols. Physiologic changes in pregnancy involve alterations of the airway anatomy, gastrointestinal, respiratory, cardiovascular, and hematologic physiology that are particularly relevant in the trauma patient [102] and can influence the evaluation and treatment of traumatic injury (see Table 16.1). These changes allow for greater clinical compensation to trauma, but this can sometimes delay recognition of the extent of injury and hemorrhagic shock (see Fig. 16.2).

Airway Management

Airway management in normal pregnancy presents additional risks over the non-pregnant patient. Changes in oncotic pressure and increases in circulating blood volume lead to engorgement of the naso- and oropharyngeal mucosa and larynx, resulting in edema and friability of the upper airway and a predisposition to airway obstruction. Smaller endotracheal tubes (6–7 mm internal diameter) may be needed for intubation, and caution is indicated when inserting nasopharyngeal airways or endotracheal tubes. Soft tissue edema, enlargement of the tongue and breast tissue, and generalized weight gain can complicate laryngoscopy. A shorter laryngoscope handle may be needed to facilitate visualization of the airway structures.

Trauma can further complicate airway management. Fluctuating levels of consciousness as a result of intracranial injuries, alcohol or drug ingestion, hypoxia or shock, can lead to loss of airway reflexes. Specific injuries, such as facial fractures, burns, and cervical spine instability pose additional challenges.

In late-trimester pregnancies, difficult airway management should be anticipated and additional equipment made available, such as a stylet, gum elastic bougie, levered-laryngoscope, lightwand, intubating laryngeal mask airway (LMA), and fiberoptic or video laryngoscope. A study of maternal airway grades at 12 and 28 weeks found that the percent of Mallampati Grade IV airways, with only views of the hard palate and no view of soft palate or uvula, increased by 34 % [103].

In obese patients, an airway ramp can be made up of a rolled towel or blanket placed under the patient's upper back and head until horizontal alignment is achieved between the external auditory meatus and sternal notch. This has been found to be superior to the traditional "sniff" position that is created by placing a cushion under the patient's head and raising the occiput [104, 105]. In pregnant trauma patients, once cervical spine instability has been ruled out, ramped positioning may facilitate direct laryngoscopy.

Table 16.1 Physiologic changes of pregnancy

Cardiovascular			Clinical significance
Heart rate	Increased 15–20 bpm	75–95 bpm	Adaption to tolerate blood loss
Cardiac output	Increased 30–50 %	6–8 L/min	
Mean arterial blood pressure	Decreased 10 mmHg	Midtrimester 80 mmHg	
Systemic vascular resistance	Decreased 10–15 %	1,200–1,500 dyn/s/cm^{-5}	
Respiratory			
Tidal volume	Increased 40 %	700 mL	
Minute ventilation	Increased 40 %	10.5 L/min	Respiratory alkalosis
Expiratory reserve volume	Decreased 15–20 %	550 mL	
Functional residual capacity	Decreased 20–25 %	1,350 mL	Rapid desaturation
Blood gas			
pH	Unchanged	7.4–7.45	
pCO_2	Decreased	27–32 mmHg	
pO_2	Increased	100–108 mmHg	
HCO_3	Decreased	18–21 mEq/L	
Hematologic			
Blood volume	Increased 30–50 % 13–18 weeks	4,500 mL	
Erythrocyte volume	Increased 10–15 %		Dilutional anemia
Hemoglobin	Decreased 1–2 g/dL	9–11 g/dL	
Leukocytes	Increased up to 18×10^9 Leukocytes/L 24–40 weeks	5,000–150,000/mm^3	
Coagulation			
Factors I, II, V, VII, IX, X, and XII	Increased		Hypercoagulable state

There are no studies that compare direct and video laryngoscopes in pregnant patients. In cases of neck trauma, there are conflicting data regarding decreased motion of the cervical spine using videolaryngoscopes [106, 107]. One study which randomized non-pregnant trauma patients to intubation with Glidescope® video laryngoscope or direct laryngoscopy with Macintosh blade found that the use of the Glidescope resulted in longer median intubation times without a mortality benefit [108]. Video laryngoscopes may have theoretical benefits in late-term pregnancy or in cases of maternal obesity, but there are no robust supporting data. Once intubation has been achieved, nasogastric decompression should be initiated to minimize the risk of aspiration. If intubation is impossible, a LMA may permit ventilation, although the risk of aspiration remains. Some patients may require cricothyrotomy or tracheostomy.

Gastrointestinal Changes

While all trauma patients are at risk for aspiration, the risk is increased in pregnant patients due to progesterone-mediated relaxation of the lower esophageal sphincter, gastric tone and mobility. One case-controlled study of non-trauma patients reported an aspiration risk as high as 8 % [109]. Prolonged bag/mask ventilation in a trauma setting will increase the risk of aspiration. While pregnancy itself does not prolong gastric emptying, delays occur with obesity, labor, and the presence of pain, or opioid administration. In addition, many pregnant women may resort to

Fig. 16.2 Maternal physiologic changes associated with hemorrhage

Compensated blood loss: 10–15% of blood volume (600 mL–900 mL)
- Heart rate unchanged
- Mean arterial pressure unchanged

Mild blood loss: 20–25% of blood volume (1200 mL–1500mL)
- Tachycardia (95–105 bpm)
- Mean arterial pressure drops 10–15% (70–75 mmHg)
- Vasoconstriction–cold, pale extremities, poor capillary refill

Moderate blood loss: 25–35% of blood volume (1500 mL–2000 mL)
- Tachycardia (105–120 bpm)
- Mean arterial pressure drop 25–30% (50–60 mmHg)
- Tissue hypoxia
- Oliguria
- Restlessness

Severe blood loss: > 35% of blood volume (>2000 mL)
- Tachycardia (>120 bpm)
- Hypotension (mean arterial pressure <50 mmHg)
- Tissue hypoxia
- Oliguria
- Altered consciousness
- Coagulopathy–disseminated intravascular and/or trauma–associated

small frequent meals, increasing the likelihood of a full stomach when presenting with trauma.

Respiratory Changes

Weight gain and enlargement of the uterus during pregnancy cause decreased functional residual capacity (FRC) and can lead to rapid desaturation, further complicating airway management. Oxygen should be provided to all pregnant trauma patients, with early consideration of an oral, nasal, or endotracheal airway. Metabolic needs and oxygen consumption are high in pregnancy, both of which worsen hypoxia. Denitrogenation with 100 % oxygen must be performed prior to intubation. Maternal oxygen saturation should be maintained at $\geq$95 % in order to maintain a $PaO_2 > 70$ mmHg and optimize oxygen diffusion across the placenta. When maternal oxygenation falls below 60–70 mmHg, fetal oxygenation is compromised.

Maternal minute ventilation rate increases as a result of expanded tidal volume and progesterone-mediated stimulation of the medullary respiratory center that controls ventilatory drive. This results in lower carbon dioxide tensions of between 28 and 32 mmHg. There is a compensatory excretion of bicarbonate to maintain an arterial pH of 7.40–7.45. These values need to be taken into account when interpreting blood gases and adjusting ventilator settings.

In trauma patients, ventilatory drive can be reduced following drug overdose, poisoning, alcohol ingestion, head injury, pneumothorax, hemothorax, lung, or chest wall injury. Successful management of these injuries may involve drainage of air or blood. In pregnancy, the thoracic anteriorposterior diameter increases and the diaphragm moves 4 cm cephalad. If a thoracostomy procedure is needed, needle entry should be made one or two intercostal spaces higher than in non-pregnant patients to avoid injuring the diaphragm and abdominal organs.

Cardiovascular Changes

Many of the cardiovascular changes seen in pregnancy can complicate the evaluation and management of pregnant trauma patients. The enlarged uterus causes the heart to shift cephalad and to the left. The electrocardiogram (ECG) can show sinus tachycardia, left-axis deviation, nonspecific ST-T changes, and inverted or flattened

T-waves. Q-waves may also be present in leads III and avF. Premature atrial and ventricular beats are common. As the body adjusts to expanded circulating volume and preload, the heart becomes hypertrophic and dilated with an enlarged left ventricular end-diastolic volume. Afterload, however, is reduced due to decreased peripheral vascular resistance. The heart rate and stroke volume begin to increase early and peak at 28–32 weeks' gestation. Heart murmurs, such as a pulmonary mid-systolic murmur and a supraclavicular murmur, may be present.

As the pregnant patient prepares for the blood loss of delivery, blood volume increases 50 % with a 30 % increase in red cell volume. The greater increase of plasma volume over erythrocyte count leads to a dilutional anemia resulting in hemoglobin values of 9–11 g/dL. Significantly, the pregnant patient can lose 2,000 mL of blood (30–40 % of blood volume) before she reveals changes in heart rate or blood pressure. As blood loss approaches 2,500 mL, rapid deterioration occurs [110]. These normal physiologic changes of pregnancy may provide better organ perfusion and maternal tolerance of "shock" state and may partially contribute to increased survival after traumatic injury [111].

Blood pressure is lower than normal in pregnancy due to the vasodilatory effects of progesterone and the low-resistance placental bed, which causes a decrease in peripheral vascular resistance that reaches its nadir at 28 weeks. Normal mean arterial blood pressures in pregnancy are 80 mmHg. By the second trimester, heart rates are mildly elevated by 15–20 bpm. Vascular remodeling and deterioration of the arterial media during pregnancy can predispose the patient to vascular aneurysms and injury. Spontaneous rupture of the aorta and coronary, vertebral, splenic, hepatic, gastric, and renal arteries has been reported in pregnancy independent of traumatic injury.

Engorgement of the pelvic vasculature during pregnancy increases the risk of retroperitoneal hemorrhage and hematoma following lower abdominal or pelvic trauma. At term, uterine blood flow accounts for approximately 20 % of cardiac output and may be up to 600 mL/min [112]. The placenta is a large and inelastic vascular structure with high blood flow and low vascular resistance, and following trauma these changes can lead to rapid maternal and fetal exsanguination. Uterine perfusion is not autoregulated and is thus dependent on maternal mean arterial blood pressure. Fetal distress, due to inadequate placental perfusion, can be one of the first indicators of maternal hemodynamic deterioration.

By 18–20 weeks gestation, the enlarged uterus exerts pressure on the inferior vena cava which can restrict venous return. In the supine position, this can reduce cardiac output by up to 30 % and cause pallor, diaphoresis, nausea, vomiting, and hypotension. Inferior vena caval compression makes the saphenous and femoral veins less preferable for delivering medication, but lower extremity access is possible in emergencies. In order to release inferior vena caval pressure and promote venous return left uterine displacement with either a hip wedge, tilted backboard, or manual displacement, should be used during resuscitation.

Coagulation

Most procoagulant factors are increased in pregnancy. This adaptive mechanism can be beneficial in achieving hemostasis after delivery and in trauma. Nonetheless, venous stasis, dilation of the pelvic vessels, and endothelial damage accompanying trauma increase the risk of thromboembolism, and prophylaxis is indicated. Fibrinogen levels are normally higher in pregnancy, thus a low fibrinogen level (<100 mg/dL) can be an early indication of massive hemorrhage or disseminated intravascular coagulation. This finding can help guide transfusion therapy.

Field Intervention and Resuscitation

Management of trauma involves a multidisciplinary team of paramedics, nurses, emergency physicians, surgeons, obstetricians, and anesthesiologists. Evaluation and resuscitation should follow the Advanced Trauma Life Support (ATLS) guidelines for rapid assessment and management of injury, which have been shown to decrease deaths during initial stages of resuscitation for all trauma patients [112, 113]. Modification of ATLS protocols for trauma in pregnancy may include supplemental oxygen, upper-extremity intravenous access, and left uterine displacement.

Newer strategies for pre-hospital treatment of trauma patients in the United States have been termed "load and go" or "scoop and run," as opposed to the "stay and play" strategies of Germany and France. The US strategies provide patients with minimal life-saving treatment at the site of injury before rapid transfer to trauma centers. Current guidelines for field trauma indicate that patients at >20 weeks pregnant should be transported to the closest trauma center even if they fail to meet physiologic, anatomic, or mechanistic injury criteria for severe injury [114]. This avoids the under triage of pregnant women that would occur if only physiologic and anatomic triage criteria considerations were applied [115]. Injuries that are not significant to general patients can be serious to pregnant women and even minor injuries can lead to poor fetal outcomes [25, 116, 117]. This has been shown in a retrospective cohort study of approximately 10,000 deliveries that were associated with trauma [16]. Patients with non-severe injury scores had 7.7-fold increased risk of abruption, a 16-fold increase in uterine rupture, a 4.9-fold increase in maternal death, and a 2.7-fold increase in fetal death for non-severe injuries compared with uninjured patients.

Primary Survey

The primary survey summarizes the "ABCs" of resuscitation: immediate attention to "airway, breathing, and circulation." The trauma protocol is completed with "D and E," which refer to disability assessment and exposing the patient for identification of all injuries [6]. In the pregnant patient "D" should also prompt left uterine displacement (see below and Fig. 16.3).

The primary survey is designed to be efficient and begins with airway assessment, maintaining inline cervical immobilization, ascertaining that the airway is free from obstruction and that airway reflexes are intact. Oral or nasal airways, or tracheal intubation may be necessary.

Respiratory effort and rate are determined in the spontaneously breathing patient, and high-flow oxygen can be given via a non-rebreather facemask to insure adequate oxygen delivery to mother and fetus. Hyperventilation is required for treating patients with maternal head injury and suspected increased intracranial pressure, but it may result in decreased uterine blood flow. When possible, carbon dioxide tension should be maintained within normal limits for pregnancy.

Blood pressure and peripheral pulses can be decreased by aortocaval compression. Left uterine displacement can be achieved with tilt of a spine board to 15° angle with a 6-in. diameter rolled towel (or bag of crystalloid fluid) or, once spinal injuries are ruled out, through manual uterine displacement [117].

Early volume replacement must be achieved to maintain placental perfusion and fetal well-being and needs to be adjusted to reflect the increased circulating volume of pregnancy. Sources of bleeding should be identified and controlled and blood pressure parameters kept within values normal for the gestational age of the pregnancy.

Venous access should be obtained with two large bore peripheral intravenous catheters in the upper extremities, particular in the setting of aortocaval compression, but may be difficult to obtain in hypovolemic shock. In pregnancy the internal jugular vein overlies the carotid artery to a greater degree than in non-pregnant patients, making the traditional landmarks technique more risky for carotid puncture [118]. Use of ultrasound and the Seldinger technique can help to guide needle placement. Needle puncture of the internal jugular vein is preferred over the subclavian vein because it is less frequently associated with hemo- or pneumathoraces. Obtaining venous access through the femoral veins can increase the risk of thromboembolism and sepsis and should only be used in emergencies. Direct visualization of the vessel with a cutdown

Airway
- Prepare for difficult intubation with airway edema and friability, aspiration risk, rapid desaturation
- Use smaller endotracheal tube (6–7)

Breathing
- If a chest tube is needed, place in 3rd or 4th intercostal space

Circulation
- Place 2 large bore IVs above diaphragm

Disability
- Consider eclampsia as cause of altered mental status

Displacement
- Displace uterus after 18–20 weeks to avoid aortocaval compression

Exposure
- Locate entry and exit wounds

Fig. 16.3 Primary survey in the pregnant trauma patient

technique can also be employed. Finally, the use of interosseous needles has been reported in a case of massive obstetric hemorrhage [119].

The brief evaluation for disability should focus on the patient's level of consciousness using the Injury Severity Score or the Glasgow Coma Scale. A more detailed evaluation of neurologic injury should also evaluate pupil size and reactivity, lateralizing signs, and level of spinal cord injury. Eclampsia should be considered as a reason for altered mental status or seizures. Injury scales are not useful in prospectively identifying those at risk for adverse fetal outcomes, as even minor injuries are associated with increased risk [14, 25, 26]. Indicators of maternal hypoperfusion and hypoxia, direct uterine injury, and maternal head injury have been repeatedly associated with poor fetal outcomes.

After immobilizing the cervical spine to maintain the airway and providing respiratory support and fluid resuscitation, the patient should be fully exposed and evaluated for any missed injuries. In the case of gunshot injury, it is mandatory to locate entry and exit wounds.

Fluid Resuscitation

In the past 10–15 years there has been a paradigm shift regarding the best strategies to resuscitate trauma patients before achieving definitive surgical control of hemorrhage. Current prehospital trauma life support recommends 1–2 L of fluids be given in the field [120]. The most recent ATLS guidelines advocate aggressive crystalloid resuscitation as 3:1 replacement of estimated blood loss, with administration of fresh frozen plasma (FFP) and platelets (PLT) when one whole blood volume had been replaced or 1 unit FFP for every 5 units packed red blood cells (RBC) administered [113, 121].

The dilutional effects of crystalloid administration can affect coagulation function [122], and large volumes can lead to acidosis, interstitial edema, tissue swelling, dysfunction of the microcirculation, and impaired oxygenation [123]. Normal saline is isotonic with respect to extracellular fluid and large volumes can result in a hyperchloremic metabolic acidosis [124]. Concern about water and sodium overload has led to the notion of "small volume" resuscitation with hypertonic saline [125]. The early use of hypertonic saline for resuscitation, however, has not improved short- or long-term outcomes, and it is not recommended in traumatic brain injury [126]. Balanced salt solutions, such as Hartmann's or Ringer's solutions, are increasingly recommended for resuscitation; they are relatively hypotonic and use lactate, acetate, gluconate, or malate as anions [127]. A recent study has shown that in the setting of hemostatic transfusion, trauma patients who received restricted crystalloid fluids <150 mL rather than standard fluid resuscitation had better survival [128].

Colloids interfere with coagulation more extensively than crystalloids by reducing fibrin polymerization. Albumin, prepared by fractionation and heat-treatment of blood, is the reference colloid solution. A comparison of the use of saline versus albumin (the SAFE Study) showed no significant difference between the two in ICU death rates at 28 days [129]. However, albumin was associated with increased deaths at 2 years in patients with traumatic brain injury due to increased intracranial pressure in the first weeks of treatment [130]. Hemodilution with albumin results in a coagulopathy that is more easily reversed with fibrinogen and factor XIII than that of synthetic colloids [131], but it is unclear whether specific groups of patients benefit more from albumin resuscitation compared with saline. Moreover, albumin is unlikely to be widely used given its cost and problems with storage.

Worldwide, hydroxyethyl starch (HES) solutions are the most commonly used semi-synthetic colloids. HES causes movement of plasma proteins into the interstitial space, decreases levels of factor VIII and von Willebrand factor (vWF), decreases the function of activated factor XIII, and inhibits platelet function [132]. These changes are more significant than those induced by crystalloid or colloid treatment [133]. The HES-induced coagulopathy can be reversed with fibrinogen and Factor XIII which together will improve fibrin polymerization. The use of HES in resuscitation is currently controversial, as meta-analyses of HES versus control fluids show adverse effects on renal function and trends toward increased mortality [134, 135].

Transfusion

Severe trauma often results in uncontrolled and noncompressible microvascular bleeding which can potentially lead to exsanguination. Resuscitation is a key component in trauma management, but trauma-associated coagulopathy is still seen in approximately 40 % of patient deaths [136]. So-called *damage control resuscitation* strategies target conditions that worsen hemorrhage in these patients [137]. In 2005, The US Army Institute of Surgical Research proposed a resuscitation strategy for severely injured military personnel which minimizes the use of crystalloids and colloids and matches RBC transfusions to FFP and PLT in an effort to treat and prevent ongoing coagulopathy [138]. A large study showed that patients with greater FFP: RBC ratios ($\geq$1:2) had a decrease in short-term and 30-day mortality without any increase in multi-organ failure [139].

Damage control resuscitation differs from conventional approaches by attempting to more aggressively correct coagulation and metabolic abnormalities in the assumption that coagulopathy is present early. This strategy includes the use of blood products over isotonic fluid for volume replacement, is permissive of some degree of hypotension, and provides early correction of coagulation disorders by using blood component therapy [140]. The goal of permissive hypotension is to achieve palpable radial pulses, with the caveat that patients with head injuries should maintain a systolic blood pressure of >110 mmHg [141, 142]. In addition, relative anemia is permitted in the early stages of resuscitation before hemostasis has been achieved.

Any extrapolation of data from non-pregnant trauma patients directly to pregnant trauma patients, or pregnant patients with massive hemorrhage (as occurs with placenta accreta) without taking into account the particular physiologic requirements of pregnancy should be viewed with caution, especially in light of the increased metabolic demands of pregnancy. In a study of postpartum patients admitted to an ICU with severe hemorrhagic shock, 51 % percent were found to have elevated serum levels of cardiac troponin I (cTnI) [143]. Factors associated with elevated troponins were hemoglobin of $\leq$6.0 g/dL on admission, systolic blood pressure of $\leq$88 mmHg or diastolic blood pressure of $\leq$50 mmHg, and transfusion of $\geq$9 units of RBC within 24 h. Electrocardiogram abnormalities have been noted in patients

Minimize early crystalloid administration
Early use of FFP with RBC in >1:2 ratio
Early use of platelets
Aggressive treatment of coagulopathy
  • antifibrinolytics–tranexamic acid
  • fibrinogen concentrate
  • prothrombin complex concentrate
  • recombinant Factor VIIa

Fig. 16.4 Damage control resuscitation strategies in the pregnant trauma patient

undergoing routine cesarean sections without massive hemorrhage [144].

In the event of urgent blood transfusion in pregnant patients, O-negative/Rh-negative blood should be used in order to prevent sensitization to Rho (D) factors and erythroblastosis fetalis in future pregnancies. Balanced administration of warmed RBCs, FFP, and PLT is warranted, guided by monitoring and treatment of the coagulation abnormalities often seen with massive hemorrhage. Frequent arterial blood gas sampling during transfusion is necessary to prevent acidosis and electrolyte abnormalities (see Fig. 16.4) [145].

The optimal dose and timing of FFP delivery to trauma patients remains controversial. Collective data indicate that an FFP:RBC ratio greater than 1:2 is associated with improved survival compared to one that is less than 1:2 [146–149]. Increased platelet administration to patients with massive hemorrhage has also been shown to increase survival [150].

Techniques which minimize the use of colloids and crystalloids to avoid dilutional coagulopathy and optimize the FFP:RBC:PLT ratio have been employed in the case of massively bleeding parturients with placenta accreta or extreme uterine atony. Considered together, 1 unit of RBC, one of FFP, and one pack of PLT have a hematocrit of 29 %, a platelet count of 85,000 cells/mL, and coagulation factor activity of 62 % [151]. Early use of cryoprecipitate and antifibrinolytic agents has also been advocated [152].

Massive transfusion is defined as the loss of more than half of the circulating blood volume in 3 h or an ongoing loss of 150 mL/min. If rapid transfusion devices are used to deliver blood products (such as the Belmont® Rapid Infuser

FMS 2000; Belmont Instrument Corporation, Billerica, MA which can deliver 1,000 mL/min, or the Level-1® H-1200 Fast Flow Fluid Warmer; Smiths-Medical, St. Paul, Minnesota), then point-of-care testing must be available to evaluate acidosis and electrolyte imbalances that can rapidly occur [151, 153].

Both RBC and FFP are stored in citrate-containing solutions. A healthy adult liver can metabolize the amount of citrate contained in 1 unit of RBCs administered every 5 min, but liver metabolism is adversely affected by hypotension and hypothermia. These rates of transfusion are often exceeded in the exsanguinating patient, and as a result the liver may be underperfused. Hypocalcemia, due to citrate toxicity, and hyperkalemia from RBCs can lead to cardiac arrest, and ionized calcium and potassium must be measured frequently during massive transfusion [145].

Other complications of large volume transfusion include acute respiratory distress syndrome (ARDS), transfusion-related acute lung injury (TRALI), and transfusion-associated circulatory overload (TACO), all of which are associated with FFP and PLT administration [154]. While there is compelling evidence supporting RBC and FFP in the early stages of damage control resuscitation, there are less data supporting the aggressive use of platelets in initial therapy. Evidence supporting blood replacement rather than using isotonic crystalloids is promising but not conclusive, and the optimal ratio for RBC:FFP:PLT is still under investigation [155–157]. Platelets should be administered if the platelet count falls below 50,000/µg L. In the case of traumatic brain injury or known platelet dysfunction, a platelet count of 100,000/µg L should be maintained [158].

Point of care viscoelastic coagulation monitoring, such as rotational thromboelastography (ROTEM®; Tem International, Munich, Germany) and thromboelastography (TEG®; Haemonetics, Braintree, MA), permits rapid assessment of clot formation, strength, and stability. This allows identification and guides treatment of specific deficits in the clotting cascade in order to reverse the effects of shock and endothelial dysfunction while improving coagulation function [159–161].

Trauma-Induced Coagulopathy

The extent of coagulation abnormalities in trauma patients is a significant predictor of their prognosis. The pathophysiology of trauma-induced coagulopathy (TIC) differs from that of disseminated intravascular coagulation (DIC). Blood loss, localized consumption of coagulation factors, and hypoperfusion are contributors in TIC [162]. Hypoperfusion induces coagulopathy through activation of anticoagulation and fibrinolytic pathways [163, 164].

Hypothermia independently contributes to coagulopathy by causing platelet dysfunction, reduced factor activity, and initiating fibrinolysis [165]. Active rewarming with heated blankets, warmed IV fluids and products, and body cavity lavage can more rapidly correct hypothermia than the use of fabric or forced warm-air blankets.

Antifibrinolytics

Tranexamic acid (TXA) is a synthetic derivative of lysine, which competitively inhibits the activation of plasminogen to plasmin by binding to sites on each molecule and preventing hyper-fibrinolysis. In a trauma coagulopathy model (using tissue plasminogen activator and tissue factor), TXA reversed hyperfibrinolysis and abnormal thromboelastogram findings induced by dilution with crystalloid, colloid, or HES [166].

TXA has been successfully used to minimize hemorrhage in a wide variety of operative settings. The randomized controlled CRASH-2 study of 20,000+ adult trauma patients found that administration of TXA reduced all-cause mortality and specifically reduced deaths due to bleeding [167]. A trial of TXA in patients with intracranial hemorrhage and traumatic brain injury was nested within CRASH-2. Investigators found no significant reduction in intracranial hemorrhage size, nor benefit or harm. Neither of these two studies found significant

increases in serious prothrombotic complications if TXA was administered within 3 h of injury [168]. A meta-analysis of the use of TXA in orthopedic surgery found significant reductions in blood loss and no increased risk of deep venous thrombosis [169].

TXA can be given orally in both the hospital and in damage control resuscitation in the field, and it has great potential to reduce postpartum hemorrhage worldwide [170]. The WOMAN Trial (World Maternal Antifibrinolytic Trial) is a double-blind placebo-controlled trial currently examining TXA for the treatment of postpartum hemorrhage [171]. There are as yet no specific reports of TXA treatment in pregnant trauma patients, although it has been used in cesarean section, postpartum hemorrhage, and metrorrhagia [172]. In a pregnant trauma patient, supplementation with tranexamic acid should be considered as part of efforts to reduce ongoing hemorrhage and coagulopathy.

Fibrinogen

Fibrinogen levels reach critically low levels (<100 mg/dL) before red cell transfusion is even necessary due to loss, dilution, increased breakdown, and insufficient synthesis. Small amounts of colloid administration (>1,000 mL) can impair fibrinogen polymerization [122]. There is evidence that fibrinogen supplementation helps manage trauma-induced coagulopathy. European recommendations call for fibrinogen repletion when levels reach 1.5–2.0 g/L [173]. Six units of FFP deliver roughly the same amount of fibrinogen as one bag of cryoprecipitate. As an alternative to cryoprecipitate, fibrinogen concentrate can be used and reconstituted with sterile water or saline.

Prothrombin Complex

The use of prothrombin complex concentrate (PCC) has also been examined in trauma resuscitation. PCC is a formula of vitamin K-dependent clotting factors (II, VII, IX, and X) that are essential for thrombin formation. Reduced thrombin formation generally occurs when blood losses exceed 150–200 % of estimated blood volume [174]. Experimental and clinical data suggest that PCC can be helpful in reversing trauma-induced coagulopathy. One study demonstrated that using fibrinogen concentrates with PCC in a goal-directed manner that was guided by thromboelastographic measurements from ROTEM® made it possible to treat coagulopathy without using FFP [175]. Should this finding be replicated in larger and randomized studies, it will allow resuscitation to be undertaken without the time delay associated with cross-matching, thawing, and transfusing FFP [176].

Recombinant Factor VIIa

The use of recombinant factor VIIa (rFVIIa, NovoSeven®; NovoNordisk, Copenhagen, Denmark) was shown to be safe and effective in reducing the amount of blood transfused in blunt trauma patients [177]. However, this two-armed double-blinded randomized placebo-controlled trial failed to show statistically significant differences in transfusion requirements for pelvic fractures or penetrating injuries. rFVIIa has been used to stem massive postpartum hemorrhage, prevent cesarean hysterectomy, and treat disseminated intravascular coagulation in pregnant patients [178–181]. As yet there are no robust data or guidelines for its broad use in obstetric patients. Existing hypothermia, acidosis, hypofibrinogenemia, and thrombocytopenia should be corrected before rFVIIa use is considered. It should not be used to compensate for inadequate transfusion and factor therapy, but may have a role to play along with timely and targeted coagulation factors, fibrinogen, and systematic antifibrinolytics in trauma-induced coagulopathy [182].

Anti-shock Garments

Anti-shock garments, such as Military Anti-Shock Trousers (MAST) or Pneumatic Anti-Shock Garment (PASG), are currently not recommended for massive antepartum hemorrhage due to concerns about restricting pelvic blood flow and uterine perfusion. If they are used in the undelivered pregnant patient, only the lower extremity portion should be inflated. They are considered a Class III intervention in non-pregnant patients and current indications are: (1) to splint and provide control of bleeding from pelvic fractures; and (2) to stabilize patients with intra-abdominal trauma and severe hypovolemia during transport [183]. Indications for using anti-shock devices include signs of severe hemorrhagic shock with systolic blood pressure <80 mmHg, unconsciousness, and absent or weak radial pulses after uterine displacement. Leg compartments should be inflated to 50 mmHg and the patient reassessed. Further inflation may be required if shock persists. Sequential deflation should occur only in a hospital setting after upper-extremity intravenous lines are secure and definitive management of the causes of hemorrhage has occurred.

Anti-shock garments can reduce uterine perfusion and increase cardiac workload, and they are poorly tolerated in patients with mitral stenosis, congestive heart failure, or pulmonary hypertension [4]. Use of MAST may delay transportation to trauma centers and worsen the outcomes of thoracic and abdominal injuries [183]. Anti-shock garments are relatively contraindicated in obstetric trauma, but in low resource setting they may be useful as adjuncts in controlling severe postpartum hemorrhage or in cases of ruptured ectopic pregnancies [184]. Non-pneumatic Anti-Shock Garments (NASG) may be used to stabilize hypovolemic shock in postpartum hemorrhage. Each light and washable neoprene device has three segments to cover each leg and one to cover the pelvis. A third segment is provided with a foam compression ball to cover the abdomen. Using Velcro® closures, the garment provides 20–40 mmHg circumferential counterpressure to shunt blood to core organs. Special training is not required for its use, and uterine and vaginal procedures can be performed with the NASG in place [185, 186]. They have been shown to reduce internal iliac

Complete maternal history and/or exam
- Mechanism of injury
- Medications/allergies
- Last menstrual period
- Presence or absence of contractions
- Abdominal pain/vaginal bleeding/rupture of membranes

Fetal Evaluation
- Fetal Movement
- Check fetal heart rate–continuous fetal heart rate after 23–24 weeks for minimum 4–6 hours
- Biophysical profile and/or middle cerebral artery Doppler

Focused Assessment with Sonography in Trauma (FAST)

Labs and Imaging

Fig. 16.5 Secondary survey in the pregnant trauma patient

blood flow, indicating a mechanism for stabilizing uterine hemorrhage when all three compartments are deployed [187].

Secondary Survey

After confirming the hemodynamic stability of the mother and fetus, the universal secondary survey should be performed, with particular attention given to pregnancy-related findings: fetal well-being and placental injury (see Fig. 16.5).

Information should be elicited about the mechanism of injury; for example, the type of weapon used (if any), the use of drugs or alcohol or the use of seatbelts in motor vehicle accidents. A past medical and obstetric history should include the last menstrual period, current or previous pregnancy complications, and estimated gestational age.

Using McDonald's rule for uterine growth, at approximately 23–24 weeks the fundus can be palpated at the umbilicus and an injury at this gestational age should prompt fetal monitoring which should be continued for at least 4–6 h [96]. Continuous fetal monitoring is more sensitive in detecting placental abruption than ultrasonography, Kleihauer-Betke testing, or physical examination. A decision to cease fetal monitoring should be made in consultation with obstetricians, and should take into account the presence of uterine contractions, fetal well-being, and plans for operative delivery.

Uterine monitoring should commence when gestational age is >20 weeks. Recurrent uterine contractions with cervical change suggest preterm labor. More than four contractions per hour may signal placental abruption.

The secondary survey should involve a sterile speculum exam to look for vaginal lacerations or bony fragments, which may indicate pelvic fracture. If fluid is present, its pH should be determined; pH 7.0 indicates amniotic fluid and pH 5.0 indicates normal vaginal secretions. Fluid can also be evaluated for nitrazine color-change, ferning, and the presence of fetal fibronectin. In addition, newer bedside tests for insulin-like growth factor-binding protein-1 (IGFBP-1) and placental alpha-microglobulin-1 (PAMG-1) can be considered; they may be more accurate in detecting membrane rupture [188, 189]. If vaginal bleeding is present in a second or third trimester trauma patient, a vaginal exam should be deferred until placenta previa can be excluded by ultrasound. The exam should be postponed until a double set-up for emergency cesarean section is available.

Maternal and Fetal Monitoring

Standard noninvasive monitoring of the pregnant trauma patient includes pulse oximetry, electrocardiography, blood pressure monitoring, temperature measurement, together with monitoring of the fetal heart rate and uterine tocodynamometry when necessary. An indwelling urinary catheter should be inserted to measure hourly urine output. Invasive arterial monitoring is indicated if there is persistent hypotension, hypoxia, or labile blood pressure; it provides a means for periodic arterial blood sampling and gas analysis. Pulmonary artery catheters are currently used less frequently in general critical care patients. In obstetric patients, they are more commonly used in those with pulmonary edema, known severe mitral or aortic stenosis, NYHA class III–IV disease in labor, intrapartum or intraoperative cardiac failure, shock or adult respiratory distress syndrome. In patients who are intubated, tidal volume, airway pressure, and end-tidal carbon dioxide should be monitored. If a volatile anesthetic agent is used, the end-tidal concentration should be observed. Monitoring of cardiac function through transesophageal echocardiography may also be useful.

The fetal heart rate tracing should be recorded in all pregnancies above 20 weeks and recorded continuously at viability. Fetal heart rate tracings which indicate distress (i.e., Category II or Category III [190]), or a low biophysical profile score should prompt suspicion of maternal hypovolemia, placental abruption, or fetomaternal hemorrhage.

Laboratory Tests

Initial laboratory tests in the pregnant trauma patient should include: complete blood count, basic metabolic panel with electrolytes and glucose, type and crossmatch, Rh status, coagulation profile, fibrinogen, liver function tests, blood lactate, toxicology screen, Kleihauer-Betke (KB) test, urinary protein, blood, bilirubin and glucose and urine osmolality or specific gravity. An arterial blood gas should be evaluated if respiratory function is compromised. All laboratory values should be measured against "normal" parameters for pregnant patients. Care must be taken in interpreting the results; for example, low platelets could be a sign of hypertensive diseases of pregnancy (see Fig. 16.6).

In the pregnant trauma patient, Rh typing is necessary. As little as 0.01 mL of fetal blood can cause sensitization in the Rh-negative mother [191]. The KB test can be used to quantify fetal hemoglobin in the maternal circulation. A positive KB test (>0.01 mL of fetal RBC) has been associated with significant fetomaternal hemorrhage and preterm labor. All Rh-negative women should be treated with Rh-immune globulin within 72 h (300 µg initially and an additional 300 µg for each 30 mL of estimated fetomaternal transfusion). A positive KB test should be repeated in 24–48 h to investigate ongoing hemorrhage. In the future, anti-fetal hemoglobin (anti-HbF) flow cytometry may prove to be a more reliable and easily standardized test [192, 193].

While the utility of KB testing in Rh-positive patients has been questioned, it has been found to be a reliable independent predictor of preterm labor after trauma and the test should be obtained in all patients. Fetal middle cerebral artery Doppler testing may be considered when significant fetomaternal hemorrhage is suspected [194]. Fetal anemia can be rapidly detected and treated in cases where immediate delivery is not anticipated and lethal fetal hydrops prevented.

Imaging

The ATLS recommends radiographs of the cervical spine, chest, and pelvis. Concern about effects of ionizing radiation should not prevent medically indicated maternal X-rays. During the period of organogenesis (4–10 weeks), ionizing radiation is most likely to cause congenital malformations. A fetus is most susceptible to radiation-induced developmental delay from 10 to 17 weeks. Non-cancer fetal injuries diminish with increasing gestational age. Theoretical risks associated with radiation exposure at any time during pregnancy include an increased incidence of childhood leukemia (absolute risk ~1:2,000). Exposure to less than 5 rad (50 mGy), however, has not been associated with an increase in fetal anomalies or pregnancy loss and this is deemed a safe level throughout the gestation.

If multiple diagnostic studies are performed, consultation with a radiologist should be considered for calculating the estimated fetal exposure. The uterus should be shielded as much as possible and using a posterior-anterior exposure can

Fig. 16.6 Initial laboratory evaluation of the pregnant trauma patient

- Blood type, cross–match, Rh status
- Complete blood count (hemoglobin, white blood cell count, platelet count)
- Coagulation profile (prothrombin and partial thromboplastin time)
- Fibrinogen concentration and fibrinogen split products (D–dimer)
- Serum electrolytes
- Serum glucose level
- Liver function tests
- Serum amylase
- Serum lactate and urate
- Toxicology screen
- Arterial blood gas (pH, PaO2, PaCO2, bicarbonate, base deficit)
- Kleihauer–Betke test
- Urinary protein, blood, bilirubin, and glucose
- Urine specific gravity or urine osmolality

increase the distance from the anterior uterus to the radiation source [195]. If computed tomography is necessary, it can be performed with fewer slices, reduced current, or increased pitch. The interventional radiologist can use several techniques to minimize fluoroscopy time, decrease the fluoroscopy frame rates, and minimize image magnification [196]. Lead shields and internal shielding (with barium) should be used as much as possible [197]. Magnetic resonance imaging (MRI) and ultrasonography during pregnancy have not been associated with any adverse effects and there is no evidence of teratogenicity with gadolinium, a paramagnetic ion administered for contrast definition in MRIs [198].

Focused abdominal sonography for trauma (FAST) can be useful in patients who have experienced blunt trauma. FAST provides evidence of free fluid in four areas: the subxiphoid, the right and left upper quadrants, and the suprapublic area. In pregnant patients, it has a sensitivity of 80–83 % and specificity of 98–100 % in detecting intraperitoneal fluid [199, 200]. It can also be used to establish the diagnosis of an unknown pregnancy [201]. FAST can often reduce the need for multiple radiographic imaging studies, but it is of limited use in detecting maternal injuries such as arterial hemorrhage [202].

Bedside ultrasound and rapid computed tomography scans have largely rendered diagnostic peritoneal lavage unnecessary. In resource-limited settings, however, these tests can be performed safely using a supra-umbilical open technique [203, 204].

Specific Management Issues

Traumatic Brain Injury

As indicated above, resuscitation with crystalloids instead of colloids is preferable in traumatic brain injury. Specific techniques to elevate the head and minimize head and neck flexion encourage venous drainage and decrease elevated intracranial pressure. In pregnant trauma patients, hypoventilation should be avoided because it can decrease uterine blood flow by decreasing maternal cardiac output and blood pressure and by causing uterine vasoconstriction. $PaCO_2$ should be maintained within the normal range for pregnancy with a baroprotective ventilation strategy. Aggressive resuscitation to prevent hypotension and hypoxia is necessary to maintain perfusion of the brain and other vital organs.

Spinal Cord Injuries

Traumatic injuries to the spinal cord have implications for pregnant patients. Of the 12,000 women of childbearing age who sustain spinal cord injuries per year, 2,000 become pregnant in any given year [205]. Roughly 14 % of these women will have at least one pregnancy after being injured [206]. Should the spinal injury occur above the T5-T6 level, the patient is at risk of developing autonomic dysreflexia (AD) or hyperreflexia. In patients with this condition, noxious stimuli below the level of injury result in unopposed sympathetic activity, piloerection, vasoconstriction, and pallor below the level of injury. Above the level of injury, unopposed parasympathetic activity can cause flushing, sweating, pupillary constriction, and nasal congestion. Without treatment, autonomic hyperflexia can lead to seizures, retinal hemorrhage, pulmonary edema, renal insufficiency, myocardial infarction, cerebral hemorrhage, and death [207].

A review of cases of spinal cord injury in pregnancy found rates for vaginal delivery, assisted vaginal delivery, and cesarean section were 37 %, 31 %, and 32 %, respectively [208]. Invasive hemodynamic monitoring may be indicated in these patients [209]. Initial management of autonomic dysreflexia includes elevating the head of the bed, loosening tight clothing, emptying bowel and rectum, and eliminating any triggering stimulus if possible [210]. Rapidly acting vasodilators, such as sublingual nitrates, oral clonidine, or topical nitropaste can be used in an outpatient setting and the medications can be changed to intravenous vasodilators or ganglionic blockers in an intensive care unit setting [211].

In labor and delivery, the pain of uterine contractions can be a stimulant for AD, which can be attenuated by administration of spinal, or epidural anesthesia. Further blood pressure management can be achieved with sodium nitroprusside or trinitroglycerin as needed [212, 213]. In most patients, confirmation of spinal anesthesia can be confirmed by the absence of a Babinski sign and the patellar tendon reflex and the loss of spasticity, although determining the exact level of block can be difficult [213]. Finally, additional care must be taken to prevent ascending urinary tract infections and thromboembolic events in pregnant women with spinal cord injuries [214].

[154]. The use of extracorporeal membrane oxygenation (ECMO) in acute lung injury remains controversial, and data on its benefits compared with conventional treatment are limited. The use of ECMO in trauma is hindered by concerns over hemorrhage during cannulation in the presence of trauma-induced coagulopathy, contraindications to anticoagulation, decreased venous return as a result of abdominal packing in damage-control surgery, and risk of iatrogenic intracranial hemorrhage [215].

A retrospective analysis of ten non-pregnant trauma patients who were treated with either high-flow ECMO or interventional lung assist in one center showed survival in six out of ten patients, indicating that extracorporeal gas exchange can be considered as rescue therapy in adult trauma patients. In another 10-year retrospective analysis of chest trauma patients treated with ECMO, the overall survival rate was 79 % [216].

There is only one case report of successful ECMO therapy in a pregnant trauma patient who developed ARDS [217]. However, pumpless and pump-driven extracorporeal lung support systems have been used to treat pregnant women with ARDS due to influenza and pneumonia, with successful maternal and neonatal outcomes [218–221]. ECMO has also been employed in cases of massive thromboembolism/ amniotic fluid embolism and peripartum cardiomyopathy [222–224]. Recognizing the need to maintain aortocaval blood flow during medical procedures, a technique for venous ECMO cannulation has been described for left uterine displacement during late pregnancy [225]. Extracorporeal lung support should be considered as salvage therapy in pregnant patients with severe thoracic trauma and acute lung injury.

Respiratory Failure and Extracorporeal Lung Support

Thoracic trauma and massive transfusion are independent risk factors for acute lung injury that may be refractory to conventional therapy. Approximately 4.6 % of all trauma patients develop adult respiratory distress syndrome

Analgesia

All pregnant trauma patients should receive adequate analgesia. Pain causes high levels of circulating catecholamines, which can reduce placental blood flow. Opioids cause a reduction in fetal heart rate variability and the obstetrician and neonatal team should be informed whenever they are given. Remifentanil, an ultra short-acting synthetic opioid rapidly metabolized by nonspecific plasma and tissue esterases, can be used if imminent delivery is suspected and avoidance of neonatal respiratory depression deemed is a priority.

Nonsteroidal anti-inflammatory medications should generally be avoided because of their effects on platelet and renal function. They are also relatively contraindicated late in gestation because of risk of fetal ductus arteriosus closure. Intravenous acetaminophen may be used to minimize total opiate doses. Regional anesthetic techniques can be used in cases where there are no coagulation abnormalities.

Thromboprophylaxis

Trauma patients in general are at risk of thrombotic events. Orthopedic injuries and immobility independently contribute to elevated risk for blood clots. Recent research indicates patients develop a hypercoagulable state 48 h after blunt injury to abdominal organs and that fibrinogen plays an important role in clot strength [226, 227]. Specific venous thromboembolic prophylaxis regimens have not been established in nonpregnant trauma patients and routine thromboprophylaxis after trauma remains debated. Coagulation changes of pregnancy, however, predispose women to thromboembolism even without injury. All pregnant trauma patients should receive thromboembolic prophylaxis after hemostasis is obtained. Unfractionated heparins and low molecular weight heparin are too large to cross the placenta and are safe for the fetus.

Antibiotic and Tetanus Prophylaxis

All patients with traumatic injuries should receive antibiotic prophylaxis. If emergency laparotomy is necessary, antibiotics should cover streptococcal, staphylococcal, clostridial, and polymicrobial infections [20]. If massive transfusion is required, care must be taken to administer antibiotics at intervals that are sufficient to maintain adequate tissue levels.

In addition to antibiotics, patients who have tetanus-prone wounds should be given 0.5 mL of tetanus toxoid if they have not received a booster dose within the past 5 years. If they have never been immunized with tetanus toxoid and have a high-risk injury, they should receive an additional 500 units of tetanus immunoglobulin intramuscularly [30]. A tetanus-prone wound is an injury or burn that requires surgical intervention due to a treatment delay greater than 6 h. Injuries with a significant degree of devitalized tissue, puncture-type injuries (particularly when contaminated with soil or manure, as might be found with farm equipment), and animal bites are also at risk. Wounds containing foreign bodies, compound fractures, and injuries in patients who have systemic sepsis are prone to tetanus infection.

Pregnancy-Related Management Issues

Hypertensive disease in pregnancy is typically marked by elevated blood pressure and proteinuria. A patient with preeclampsia may have a normal or an unexpectedly elevated blood pressure in the setting of significant blood losses related to injury. In a pregnant woman with trauma, a near normal blood pressure in association with proteinuria, abnormal liver enzymes, elevated serum uric acid and otherwise unexplained thrombocytopenia should suggest the possibility of underlying preeclampsia. Seizures after traumatic brain injury in a pregnant patient with the same findings should prompt consideration of eclampsia, and intravenous magnesium sulfate therapy should be initiated. In trauma patients with suspected preeclampsia, blood pressure should be supported at a level that maintains adequate uterine perfusion and relative hypotension should be avoided.

Fetal Delivery

Delivery of the fetus may be required in the setting of placental abruption, uterine rupture, maternal shock, or fetal intolerance to maternal trauma surgery. The fetal heart rate is a sensitive indicator of placental perfusion and a fetal heart rate tracing that is not reassuring (i.e., Category II or Category III) or does not recover with maternal resuscitation and uterine displacement should prompt immediate delivery. Continued maternal instability in the face of ongoing resuscitation or cardiac arrest is also an indication for fetal delivery. Relief of aortocaval compression by delivery will increase cardiac output by approximately 60–80 %, decrease oxygen requirements, improve ventilation, and make cardiopulmonary resuscitation more effective [228].

Cardiac Arrest and Perimortem Cesarean Delivery

The global incidence of maternal cardiac arrest is unknown due to lack of reliable reporting and differences in standards of perinatal care. Maternal cardiac arrest is rare, but it appears to have increased in incidence from 2.20 to 2.37 per 100,000 maternities according to the most recent data from the United Kingdom's Confidential Enquiry into Maternal Deaths [228]. Following cardiac arrest, the American Heart Association (AHA) recommends urgent operative delivery within 4 min. Perimortem cesarean section is defined as cesarean delivery initiated after maternal arrest [230].

In developing countries, hemorrhage and sepsis are the most frequent contributors to maternal cardiac arrest and death. Cardiac disease is now the most common cause of maternal arrest in developed countries, exceeding hemorrhage, thromboembolism, and sepsis. Direct causes of cardiac arrest include eclampsia, hemorrhage, thromboembolism, and amniotic fluid embolism. Indirect causes include underlying cardiac disease, sepsis, malignancy, and trauma. Anesthetic causes such as airway failure and local anesthetic toxicity may be contributing factors.

Resuscitation efforts during pregnancy should take into account the physiologic changes of pregnancy (see Fig. 16.7) [231]. Because aortocaval compression reduces cardiac output,

thoracic compressions need to be given with the uterus displaced 15–30°. Wedges, such as the Cardiff Resuscitation Wedge, have been designed to produce an adequate degree of tilt, but they are seldom available [232]. Manual displacement of the uterus may be superior to tilting the entire patient or raising the right hip to achieve left uterine displacement, and can be easily accomplished [233–236]. The force of compressions needs to be increased when the patient is no longer supine. When the body is tilted at 27° for uterine displacement, the force of adequate chest compressions is reduced to 80 % of that when the patient is flat. Chest compressions should be performed 2–3 fingers above the xiphoid in the midsternum to avoid injury to the uterine fundus, liver, or spleen.

Paddle placement for defibrillation must account for enlarged breasts, but thoracic impedance remains unchanged and normal defibrillator current settings can be used [237]. Similarly, standard doses of ACLS drugs should be used; the benefits of restoring maternal circulation outweigh the risk of uteroplacental vasoconstriction. However, the volume of drug distribution and drug metabolism differs in pregnancy, and higher doses should be considered if standard doses do not yield an adequate response [238].

In cases of cardiac arrest, cesarean delivery should be considered when the fetus is estimated to be beyond 20 weeks gestation and the uterus is palpable at the umbilicus. It is vital that CPR be continued during cesarean section. Fetal delivery during maternal arrest has been shown to improve overall maternal and fetal outcomes. Maternal and fetal survival rates have been reported to be 72 % and 45 %, respectively, in cases of non-traumatic maternal cardiac arrest [239]. A review of maternal cardiac arrests noted that 12 out of 20 mothers who experienced cardiac arrest had improved hemodynamics or a return to spontaneous circulation following urgent cesarean section [240]. Evacuation of the uterus relieves aortocaval compression, provides autotransfusion of the uterine blood, decreases maternal metabolic requirements, and improves ventilation.

Prompt delivery of the fetus increases the likelihood of intact neurologic function in

Chest compressions
- Hand placement mid–sternum, 2–3 finger–breadths higher
- Uterus displaced after 18–20 weeks with wedge, manual displacement, or tilted backboard

Defibrillation
- Paddle placement unchanged
- Current unchanged

Drugs
- Doses unchanged

Delivery
- Plan for perimortem cesarean delivery within 4 minutes

Fig. 16.7 Cardiopulmonary resuscitation

neonates [241, 242]. Data from patients who experienced cardiac arrest after amniotic fluid embolism show that 98 % of fetuses had intact neurologic function if delivered within 5 min, 83 % had intact neurologic function if delivered within 6–15 min, but none had neurologic function if delivered 36+ min after maternal amniotic fluid embolism [243]. Unfortunately, in cases of traumatic hypovolemic cardiac arrest, fetal outcomes are likely to be worse because the fetus has already suffered prolonged hypoxia prior to the maternal arrest.

An analysis of case reports of maternal cardiac arrest indicates that a 4-min time frame for emergency hysterotomy was not met in 93 % of cases, yet the neonatal survival rate was still 50 %, and this included cases in which the fetus was delivered 10 min after the arrest began [244]. This analysis also indicated that cesarean delivery during maternal arrest provided clear improvement in maternal hemodynamics in only 31.7 % of cases, which may reflect prolonged arrest times prior to initiation of cesarean section. Currently, one-third of women who die during pregnancy remain undelivered at time of death. It is unclear whether cesarean section during maternal arrest might increase the number of viable fetuses who would otherwise have remained undelivered [245].

Where cesarean delivery during arrest should be performed is subject to debate. In a mannequin-based study of simulated maternal arrest, maternal transport impaired the quality of the resuscitation [246]. During cardiac arrest, hemorrhage is minimal and definitive surgical hemostasis and antibiotic therapy can be completed in the operating room after spontaneous circulation is restored. If resources are available emergency cesarean sections should be performed where the arrest occurs.

In cases of maternal arrest with return to spontaneous circulation, therapeutic hypothermia may be considered if coagulation parameters are normal. The AHA recommends considering therapeutic hypothermia in the undelivered patient with continuous fetal monitoring [116]. Occasionally resuscitation is successful, but the patient has irreversible brain damage and remains undelivered. Several case reports show that such patients may deliver viable fetuses even though they sustained their injuries as early as the 15th week of pregnancy [247–249].

Anesthetic Management

The anesthetic care of the pregnant trauma patient combines the principles of trauma resuscitation with the anesthetic management of pregnant women undergoing non-obstetric surgery. Uteroplacental perfusion and maternal hemodynamics must be maintained in order to optimize maternal and fetal outcomes. The specific anesthesia techniques employed will depend on the nature of the patient's injuries.

Induction and Intubation

All pregnant trauma patients should receive antacid prophylaxis if possible prior to intubation.

After denitrogenation with 100 % oxygen, a rapid sequence induction with cricoid pressure is preferred, if conditions permit. Airway management in pregnancy and trauma poses increased risks and additional airway equipment should be available. Pregnant patients >18–20 weeks gestation should be placed in left uterine displacement to prevent aortocaval compression and optimize placental perfusion.

Most drugs for induction are considered safe for use in pregnant trauma patients. The choice of induction agents includes etomidate or ketamine. In hypotensive patients with ongoing hemorrhage, they provide better blood pressure support than thiopental or propofol. Ketamine should be avoided in patients with traumatic head injuries because it may increase intracranial pressure. It can also cause myocardial depression in patients with severe hypovolemia and in large doses it has caused increased uterine tone in pregnant ewes [250]. Opiates such as remifentanil or fentanyl can be used to supplement the induction agent. Neuromuscular blockade can be achieved with succinylcholine or rocuronium. Once endotracheal intubation has been achieved, an oro- or nasogastric tube should be passed to decompress the stomach. When muscle tone has recovered, muscle relaxation can be re-initiated and maintained with a nondepolarizing muscle relaxant guided by peripheral nerve monitoring.

Maintenance of Anesthesia

A balanced anesthetic technique using a volatile agent, opioids, and neuromuscular blockade is favored to maintain maternal hemodynamics during trauma surgery. If a volatile anesthetic is contraindicated because of hypotension, an opiate such as fentanyl and an antianxiolytic agent should be used until a volatile agent can be safely administered. Nitrous oxide should be limited in trauma cases in which there is a possibility of pneumothorax. In its absence, nitrous oxide can be considered to help minimize the use of volatile agents in postpartum patients, thus reducing the risk of uterine atony and ongoing hemorrhage.

If the fetus is between 20 and 23 weeks fetal heart rate should be evaluated prior to induction and after surgery is completed. If the fetus greater than 23 weeks, intraoperative fetal monitoring can detect fetal distress that might indicate a need for urgent cesarean section. Continuous fetal monitoring is contingent on adequate facilities, the availability of trained personnel to interpret the heart rate tracing in the operating room, and an obstetrical team that is immediately ready for cesarean delivery.

If a cesarean delivery is performed, uterotonic agents should be immediately available. An oxytocin infusion should be started after the fetus is delivered. A slow intravenous drip is preferred to a bolus dose because rapid infusion can cause vasodilation and hypotension. In order to minimize ongoing bleeding, high-concentrations of volatile anesthetic agents should be avoided. Additional uterotonic agents such as prostaglandin E1, prostaglandin F2 alpha, and methyl ergonovine may be used if oxytocin alone proves insufficient.

Intraoperative fluid therapy should be guided by the preoperative fluid status, preoperative and intraoperative blood losses, maternal hemodynamics, urine output, and additional information from transesophageal echocardiography (TEE), or central venous pressure monitoring. Early treatment of hemorrhage and coagulopathy is vital. If massive hemorrhage occurs, intraoperative red blood cell salvage can be achieved with a Cell Saver® (Haemonetics Corporation, Braintree, Massachusetts), with care to avoid collection of amniotic fluid. A rapid infuser should be used to assist transfusion management.

Conclusion

The global burden of trauma mortality is greater than the mortality burden attributed to HIV/AIDS, malaria, and tuberculosis combined. In the United States, maternal mortality from traumatic injury exceeds direct pregnancy-related causes of death.

Motor vehicle accidents and intimate partner violence remain leading causes of maternal trauma. Providing information on

Transport and stabilize in trauma center
- protect brain and spinal cord

Monitor maternal vital signs and fetal heart rate

Restore maternal tissue perfusion and oxygenation
- resuscitate with FFP and RBC transfusion in ratio > 1:2

Prevent and treat coaguloapthy
- prevent hypothermia
- early use of antifibrinolytics, fibrinogen concentrate, prothrombin complex, rFactorVIIa

Optimize uteroplacental blood flow and fetal well-being
- uterine displacement
- supplemental oxygen

Prevent preterm labor
- tocolysis

Prepare for emergency cesarean delivery
- Fetal deterioration with gestation > 23–24 weeks
- maternal deterioration with fetus > 23–24 weeks
- maternal arrest

Fig. 16.8 Management strategies for pregnant trauma patients

seatbelts during prenatal visits can help prevent injury related to absent or improper seat belt use. Similarly, routine questions about substance and alcohol use, and exposure to intimate partner violence can enable appropriate referral and assistance.

Maternal and fetal outcomes of trauma are often poor and fetal outcomes do not correspond with severity of maternal injury. All women of childbearing age who experience trauma should be evaluated for possible pregnancy. Pregnant women who are discharged following their initial injury should be considered high-risk patients for the remainder of their pregnancy.

Pregnancy involves significant alterations in maternal physiology that directly influence the evaluation and management of trauma (see Fig. 16.8). Cardiovascular and hematologic changes clinically compensate for hemorrhage, but can delay recognition of the extent of injury. Airway, cardiovascular, and respiratory changes affect the use of ATLS protocols. Uterine displacement to relieve aortocaval compression must be established for all patients with pregnancies of 18–20 weeks or greater.

Fluid resuscitation and blood transfusion should be guided by maternal needs and blood pressure supported at levels that optimize fetal well-being. All pregnant patients who require emergency transfusion should receive O-negative/Rh-negative blood to avoid Rho sensitization. Trauma-induced coagulopathies should be aggressive treated and may require use of tranexamic acid, fibrinogen, or prothrombin complex concentrate.

All pregnant women with trauma should be evaluated for fetomaternal hemorrhage. Rh immune globulin should be administered if fetomaternal hemorrhage is suspected. The fetal heart rate should be recorded for all pregnancies above 20 weeks. Continuous fetal heart rate monitoring should be initiated for pregnancies greater than 23–24 weeks and it should be maintained for at least 6 h during the trauma hospitalization.

If pregnant women require diagnostic imaging, care must be taken to shield the uterus. Following trauma, they should also receive thromboprophylaxis, antibiotics, and tetanus prophylaxis when indicated.

If a pregnant trauma patient suffers a cardiac arrest after 20 weeks gestation, chest compressions must be performed with uterine displacement. As soon as the arrest occurs, a cesarean section for fetuses >23–24 weeks should be initiated within 4 min. Cesarean delivery of nonviable or dead fetuses should also be considered as it can improve maternal hemodynamics and prompt return to spontaneous circulation.

Anesthesiologists may have more knowledge of the pregnant patient than other members of a trauma team. As such, they can play a critical role in integrating their understanding of the physiologic changes of pregnancy with the life support and trauma protocols needed to reduce morbidity and mortality in pregnant women who experience trauma.

References

1. Mirza FG, Devine PC, Gaddipati S. Trauma in pregnancy: a systematic approach. Am J Perinatol. 2010;22(7):579–86.
2. Pearlman MD. Motor vehicle crashes, pregnancy loss and preterm labor. Int J Gynaecol Obstet. 1997;57(2):127–32.
3. Ikossi DG, Lazar AA, Morabito D, et al. Profile of mothers at risk: an analysis of injury and pregnancy loss in 1,195 trauma patients. J Am Coll Surg. 2005;200:49–56.
4. Mattox KL, Goetzl L. Trauma in pregnancy. Crit Care Med. 2005;33(Suppl):S385–9.
5. El Kady D. Perinatal outcomes of traumatic injuries during pregnancy. Clin Obstet Gynecol. 2007;50:582–91.
6. Chames MC, Pearlman MD. Trauma during pregnancy: outcomes and clinical management. Clin Obstet Gynecol. 2008;51:398–408.
7. Aboutanos SB, Aboutanos MG, Dompkowski D, et al. Predictors of fetal outcome in pregnant trauma patients: a five-year institutional review. Am Surg. 2007;73:824–7.
8. Horon IL. Underreporting of maternal deaths on death certificates and the magnitude of the problem of maternal mortality. Am J Public Health. 2005;95:478–82.
9. Horon IL, Cheng D. Effectiveness of pregnancy check boxes on death certificates in identifying pregnancy-associated mortality. Public Health Rep. 2011;126:195–200.
10. Fildes J, Reed L, Jones N, et al. Trauma: the leading cause of maternal death. J Trauma. 1992;32:643–5.
11. Harper M, Parsons L. Maternal deaths due to homicide and other injuries in North Carolina: 1992–1994. Obstet Gynecol. 1997;90:920–3.
12. Dannenberg AL, Carter DM, Lawson HW, et al. Homicide and other injuries as causes of maternal death in New York City, 1987 through 1991. Am J Obstet Gynecol. 1995;172:1557–64.
13. Pearlman MD, Tintinalli JE, Lorenz RP. A prospective controlled study of outcome after trauma during pregnancy. Am J Obstet Gynecol. 1990;162:1502–7.
14. Schiff MA, Holt VL, Daling JR. Maternal and infant outcomes after injury during pregnancy in Washington state from 1989 to 1997. J Trauma. 2002;53:939–45.
15. Pak LL, Reece EA, Chan L. Is adverse pregnancy outcome predictable after blunt abdominal trauma? Am J Obstet Gynecol. 1998;179:1140–4.
16. El-Kady D, Gilbert WM, Anderson J, et al. Trauma during pregnancy: an analysis of maternal and fetal outcomes in a large population. Am J Obstet Gynecol. 2004;190:1661–8.
17. Schiff MA, Holt VL. Pregnancy outcomes following hospitalization for motor vehicle crashes in Washington state from 1989 to 2001. Am J Epidemiol. 2005;161:503–10.
18. Weiss HB, Songer TJ, Fabio A. Fetal deaths related to maternal injury. JAMA. 2001;286:1863–8.
19. Kuo C, Jamieson DJ, McPheeters ML, et al. Injury hospitalizations of pregnant women in the United States, 2002. Am J Obstet Gynecol. 2007;196:161. e1–6.
20. Hill C. Trauma in the obstetrical patient. Womens Health. 2009;5:269–85.
21. Hyde LK, Cook LJ, Olson LM, et al. The effect of motor vehicle crashes on adverse fetal outcomes. Obstet Gynecol. 2003;102:279–86.
22. Patteson SK, Snider CC, Meyer DS, et al. The consequence of high-risk behaviors: trauma during pregnancy. J Trauma. 2007;62:1015–20.
23. Gazmararian JA, Lazorick S, Spitz AM, et al. Prevalence of violence against pregnant women. JAMA. 1996;275:1915–20.
24. Tinker SC, Reefhuis J, Dellinger AM, et al. National Birth Defects Prevention Study. Epidemiology of maternal injuries during pregnancy in a population-based study, 1997–2005. J Womens Health (Larchmont). 2010;19:2211–8.
25. Fischer PE, Zarzaur BL, Fabian TC, et al. Minor trauma is an unrecognized contributor to poor fetal outcomes: a population-based study of 78,552 pregnancies. J Trauma. 2011;71:90–3.
26. Sperry JL, Casey BM, McIntyre DD, et al. Long-term fetal outcomes in pregnant trauma patients. Am J Surg. 2006;192:715–21.
27. Schiff MA, Holt VL. The injury severity score in pregnant trauma patients: predicting placental abruption and fetal death. J Trauma. 2002;53:946–9.

28. Biester EM, Tomich PG, Esposito TJ, et al. Trauma in pregnancy: normal revised trauma score in relation to other markers of maternofetal status–a preliminary study. Obstet Gynecol. 1997;176:1206–12.

29. Baerga-Varela Y, Zietlow SP, Bannon MP, et al. Trauma in pregnancy. Mayo Clin Proc. 2000;75:1243–8.

30. Tweddale CJ. Trauma during pregnancy. Crit Care Nurs Q. 2006;29:53–67.

31. Shah KH, Simons RK, Holbrook T, et al. Trauma in pregnancy: maternal and fetal outcomes. J Trauma. 1998;45:83–6.

32. American College of Obstetricians and Gynecologists. ACOG educational bulletin Obstetric aspects of trauma management. Number 251, September 1998 (replaces Number 151, January 1991, and Number 161, November 1991). Int J Gynaecol Obstet. 1999;64:87–94.

33. Romero VC, Pearlman M. Mortality due to trauma. Semin Perinatol. 2012;36:60–7.

34. Petrone P, Talving P, Browder T, et al. Abdominal injuries in pregnancy: a 155-month study at two level 1 trauma centers. Injury. 2011;42:47–9.

35. Theodorou DA, Velmahos GC, Souter I, et al. Fetal death after trauma in pregnancy. Am Surg. 2000;66:809–12.

36. Leggon RE, Wood GC, Indeck MC. Pelvic fractures in pregnancy: factors influencing maternal and fetal outcomes. J Trauma. 2002;53:796–804.

37. Aboutanos MB, Aboutanos SZ, Dompkowski D, et al. Significance of motor vehicle crashes and pelvic injury on fetal mortality: a five year institutional review. J Trauma. 2008;65:616–20.

38. Cannada LK, Pan P, Casey BM, et al. Pregnancy outcomes after orthopedic trauma. J Trauma. 2010;69:694–8.

39. El Kady D, Gilbert WM, Xing G, et al. Association of maternal fractures with adverse perinatal outcomes. Am J Obstet Gynecol. 2006;195:711–6.

40. Lavery JP, Staten-McCormick M. Management of moderate to severe trauma in pregnancy. Obstet Gynecol Clin North Am. 1995;22:69–90.

41. Tinker SC, Reefhuis J, Dellinger AM, et al. Epidemiology of maternal injuries during pregnancy in a population-based study, 1997–2005. J Womens Health. 2010;19:2211–8.

42. Kvarnstrand L, Milsom I, Lekander T, et al. Maternal fatalities, fetal and neonatal deaths related to motor vehicle crashes during pregnancy: a national population-based study. Acta Obstet Gynecol Scand. 2008;87:946–52.

43. Pearlman MD, Philips ME. Safety belt use during pregnancy. Obstet Gynecol. 1996;88:1026–9.

44. Schiff M, Albers L, McFeely P. Motor vehicle crashes and maternal mortality in New Mexico: the significance of seat belt use. West J Med. 1997;167:19–22.

45. Motozawa Y, Hitosugi M, Abe T, Tokudome S. Effects of seat belts worn by pregnant drivers during low-impact collisions. Am J Obstet Gynecol. 2010;203:62.e1–8.

46. Metz T, Abbott JT. Pregnancy after motor vehicle crashes with airbag deployment: a 30-case series. J Trauma. 2006;61:658–61.

47. Sirin H, Weiss HB, Sauber-Schatz EK, et al. Seat belt use, counseling and motor-vehicle injury during pregnancy: results from a multi-state population-based survey. Matern Child Health J. 2007;11:505–10.

48. Klinich KD, Flannagan CAC, Rupp JD, et al. Fetal outcome in motor-vehicle crashes: effect of crash characteristics and maternal restraint. Am J Obstet Gynecol. 2008;198:450.e1–9.

49. Astarita DC, Feldman B. Seat belt placement resulting in uterine rupture. J Trauma. 1997;42:738–40.

50. Fusco A, Kelly K, Winslow J. Uterine rupture in a motor vehicle crash with airbag deployment. J Trauma. 2001;51:1192–4.

51. Schultze PM, Stamm CA, Roget J. Placental abruption and fetal death with airbag deployment in a motor vehicle accident. Obstet Gynecol. 1998;92(Pt 2):719.

52. Schiff MA, Mack CD, Kaufman RP, et al. The effect of airbags on pregnancy outcomes in Washington State. Obstet Gynecol. 2010;115:85–92.

53. Mendez-Figueroa H, Dahlke JD, Vrees RA, et al. Trauma in pregnancy: an updated systematic review. Am J Obstet Gynecol. 2013;209:1–10.

54. Kady E, Gilbert WM, Xing G, et al. Maternal and neonatal outcomes of assaults during pregnancy. Obstet Gynecol. 2005;105:357–63.

55. Connolly AM, Katz VL, Bash KL, et al. Trauma and pregnancy. Am J Perinatol. 1997;14:331–6.

56. Schiff MA. Pregnancy outcomes following hospitalization for a fall in Washington state from 1987 to 2004. BJOG. 2008;115:1648–54.

57. Dunning K, Lemasters G, Bhattacharya A. A major public health issue: the high incidence of falls during pregnancy. Matern Child Health J. 2010;14:720–5.

58. Lymberly JK, Gilleard W. The stance phase of walking during late pregnancy; temporospatial and ground reaction force variables. J Am Podiatr Med Assoc. 2005;95:247–53.

59. Butler EE, Colon I, Druzing ML, et al. Postural equilibrium during pregnancy: decreased stability with an increased reliance on visual cues. Am J Obstet Gynecol. 2006;195:1104–8.

60. Fries EC, Hellebrandt FA. The influence of pregnancy on the location of the center of gravity, postural stability, and body alignment. Am J Obstet Gynecol. 1943;46:374–80.

61. McCrory JL, Chambers AJ, Daftary A, Redfern MS. Dynamic postural stability during advancing pregnancy. J Biomech. 2010;43:2434–9.

62. Palladino CL, Singh V, Campbell J, et al. Homicide and suicide during the perinatal period: findings from the National Violent Death Reporting System. Obstet Gynecol. 2011;118:1056–63.

63. Shadigian E, Bauer ST. Pregnancy-associated death: a qualitative systematic review of homicide and suicide. Obstet Gynecol Surv. 2005;60(3):183–90.

64. Krulewitch CJ, Pierre-Louis ML, de Leon-Gomez R, et al. Hidden from view: violent deaths among pregnant women in the District of Columbia, 1988–1996. J Midwifery Womens Health. 2001;46(1):4–10.

65. Sachs BP, Brown DA, Driscoll SG, et al. Maternal mortality in Massachusetts. Trends and prevention. N Engl J Med. 1987;316(11):667–72.

66. Ho EM, Brown J, Graves W, et al. Maternal death at an inner-city hospital, 1949–2000. Am J Obstet Gynecol. 2002;187(5):1213–6.

67. Thaden P, Thoennes N. Extent, nature and consequences of intimate partner violence: findings from the national violence against women survey. Washington, DC: US Department of Justice; 2000.

68. Truman JS. National criminal victimization survey: criminal victimization, 2010. Washington, DC: US Department of Justice, Bureau of Justice Statistics; 2011. http://www.bjs.gov/content/pub/pdf/cv10.pdf.

69. Ribe JK, Teggatz JR, Harvey CM. Blows to the maternal abdomen causing fetal demise: report of three cases and a review of the literature. J Forensic Sci. 1993;38:1092–6.

70. Dietz PM, Rochat RW, Thompson BL, et al. Differences in the risk of homicide and other fatal injuries between postpartum women and other women of childbearing age: implications for prevention. Am J Public Health. 1998;88:641–3.

71. Horon IL, Cheng D. Enhanced surveillance for pregnancy-associated mortality—Maryland, 1993–1998. JAMA. 2001;285:1455–9.

72. Lin P, Gill LR. Homicides of pregnant women. Am J Forensic Med Pathol. 2011;32:161–3.

73. Wiencrot A, Nannini A, Manning SE, et al. Neonatal outcomes and mental illness, substance abuse, and intentional injury during pregnancy. Matern Child Health J. 2012;16:979–88.

74. Chang J, Berg CJ, Saltzman LE, et al. Homicide: a leading cause of injury deaths among pregnancy and postpartum women in the United States, 1991–1999. Am J Public Health. 2005;95:471–7.

75. Ghandi SG, Gilbert WM, McElvy SS, et al. Maternal and neonatal outcomes after attempted suicide. Obstet Gynecol. 2006;107:984–90.

76. Schiff MA, Grossman DC. Adverse perinatal outcomes and risk for postpartum suicide attempt in Washington state, 1987-2001. Pediatrics. 2006;118:e669–75.

77. Maghsoudi H, Samnia R, Garadaghi A, et al. Burns in pregnancy. Burns. 2006;32:246–50.

78. Guo SS, Greenspoon JS, Kahn AM. Management of burn injuries during pregnancy. Burns. 2001;27:394–7.

79. Chama CM, Na'aya HU. Severe burn injury in pregnancy in northern Nigeria. J Obstet Gynaecol. 2002;22:20–2.

80. Van Haren RM, Thorsen CM, Valle EJ, et al. Hypercoagulability after burn injury. J Trauma Acute Care Surg. 2013;75:37–43, discussion 43.

81. Rode H, Millar AJ, Cywes S, et al. Thermal injury in pregnancy—the neglected tragedy. S Afr Med J. 1990;77:346–8.

82. Karimi H, Momeni M, Rahbar H. Burn injuries during pregnancy in Iran. Int J Gynaecol Obstet. 2009;104:132–4.

83. Roderique JD, Gebre-Giorgis AA, Stewart DH, et al. Smoke inhalation injury in a pregnant patient: a literature review of the evidence and current best practices in the setting of a classic case. J Burn Care Res. 2012;33:624–33.

84. Fatovich DM. Electric shock in pregnancy. J Emerg Med. 1993;11:175–7.

85. Einarson A, Bailey B, Inocencion G, et al. Accidental electric shock in pregnancy: a prospective cohort study. Am J Obstet Gynecol. 1997;176:678–81.

86. Rayburn W, Aronow R, DeLancey B, et al. Drug overdose during pregnancy an overview from a metropolitan poison control center. Obstet Gynecol. 1984;64:611–4.

87. Perrone J, Hoffman RS. Toxic injestions in pregnancy: abortifacient use in a case series of overdose patients. Acad Emerg Med. 1997;4:206–9.

88. Bailey B. Are there teratogenic risks associated with antidotes used in the acute management of the poisoned pregnant woman? Birth Defects Res A Clin Mol Teratol. 2003;67:133–40.

89. Hardt N, Wong TD, Burt MJ, et al. Prevalence of prescription and illicit drugs in pregnancy-associated non-natural deaths of Florida mothers, 1999–2005. J Forensic Sci. 2013. doi:10.1111/1556-4029.12219.

90. Brown SA, Seifert S, Rayburn WF. Management of envenomations during pregnancy. Clin Toxicol (Phila). 2013;51:3–15.

91. Brookfield KF, Gonzalez-Quintero VH, Davis JS, et al. Maternal death in the emergency department from trauma. Arch Gynecol Obstet. 2013;288(3):507–12. doi:10.1007/s00404-013-2772-5.

92. Crosby WM. Traumatic injuries in pregnancy. Clin Obstet Gynecol. 1983;26:902–12.

93. American College of Obstetricians and Gynecologists. Committee on Obstetric Practice Safety for Maternal-Fetal Medicine. Committee Opinion No. 573: magnesium sulfate use in obstetrics. Obstet Gynecol. 2013;122:727–8.

94. Doyle LW, Crowther CA, Middleton P, et al. Magnesium sulphate for women at risk of preterm birth for neuroprotection of the fetus. Cochrane Database Syst Rev. 2009;(1):Art. No.: CD004661. doi:10.1002/14651858.CD004661.pub3.

95. Ali J, Yeo A, Gana TJ, et al. Predictors of fetal mortality in pregnant trauma patients. J Trauma. 1997;42:782–5.

96. Barraco RD, Chiu WC, Clancy TV, et al. Practice management guidelines for the diagnosis and management of injury in the pregnant patient: the EAST practice management guidelines work group. J Trauma. 2010;69:211–4.

97. Pearlman M, Tintinalli J. Evaluation and treatment of the gravida and fetus following trauma during pregnancy. Obstet Gynecol Clin North Am. 1991;18(2):371–80.

98. Shah AJ, Kilcane BA. Trauma in pregnancy. Emerg Med Clin North Am. 2003;21:615–29.

99. Ellingsen CL, Eggebø TM, Lexow K. Amniotic fluid embolism after blunt abdominal trauma. Resuscitation. 2007;75:180–3.

100. Kramer JS, Rouleau J, Siu S, et al. Amniotic fluid embolism: incidence, risk factors and impact on perinatal outcomes. BJOG. 2012;119:874–9.

101. Rose G, Strohm P, Zuspan FP. Fetomaternal hemorrhage following trauma. Am J Obstet Gynecol. 1985;153:844–7.

102. Fujitani S, Baldisseri MR. Hemodynamic assessment in a pregnant and peripartum patient. Crit Care Med. 2005;33(10 Suppl):S354–61.

103. Pilkington S, Carli F, Dakin MJ, et al. Increase in Mallampati score during pregnancy. Br J Anaesth. 1995;74(6):638–42.

104. Collins JS, Lemmens HJ, Brodsky JB, et al. Laryngoscopy and morbid obesity: a comparison of the "sniff" and "ramped" positions. Obes Surg. 2004;14(9):1171–5.

105. El-Orbany M, Woehlck M, Salem MR. Head and neck position for direct laryngoscopy. Anesth Analg. 2011;113(1):103–9.

106. Robitaille A, Williams SR, Tremblay MH, et al. Cervical spine motion during tracheal intubation with manual in-line stabilization: direct laryngoscopy versus GlideScope® videolaryngoscopy. Anesth Analg. 2008;106:935–41.

107. Maruyama K, Yamada T, Kawakami R, et al. Randomized cross-over comparison of cervical-spine motion with the AirWay Scope or Macintosh laryngoscope with in-line stabilization: a video-fluoroscopic study. Br J Anaesth. 2008;101:563–7.

108. Yeatts DJ, Dutton RP, Hu PF, et al. Effect of video laryngoscopy on trauma patient survival: a randomized controlled trial. J Trauma Acute Care Surg. 2013;75:212–9.

109. Quinn AC, Milne D, Columb M, et al. Failed tracheal intubation in obstetric anaesthesia: 2 yr national case–control study in the UK. Br J Anaesth. 2013;110:74–80.

110. Gress Jr FC. Uterine vascular response to hemorrhage during pregnancy, with observations on therapy. Obstet Gynecol. 1966;27(4):549–54.

111. John PR, Shiozawa A, Haut ER, et al. An assessment of the impact of pregnancy on trauma mortality. Surgery. 2011;149:94–8.

112. Wilkening RB, Mescha G. Fetal oxygen uptake, oxygenation, and acid-base balance as a function of uterine blood flow. Am J Physiol. 1983;244(6): H749–55.

113. Advanced Trauma Life Support (ATLS) for doctors. Chicago: American College of Surgeons Committee on Trauma; 2012. http://www.facs.org/trauma/atls/index.html.

114. Shackford SR, Hollingworth-Fridlund P, Cooper GF, et al. The effect of regionalization upon the quality of trauma care as assessed by concurrent audit before and after institution of a trauma system: a preliminary report. J Trauma. 1986;26(9):812–20.

115. Sasser SM, Hunt RC, Faul M, et al. Center for Disease Control and Prevention (CDC). Guidelines for field triage of injured patients. Recommendations of the national expert panel on field triage, 2011. MMWR Recomm Rep. 2012;61(RR-1):1–20.

116. Brown JB, Stassen NA, Bankey PE, et al. Mechanism of injury and special consideration criteria still matter: an evaluation of the national trauma triage protocol. J Trauma. 2011;70:38–44, discussion 44–5.

117. Vanden Hoek TL, Morrison LJ, Shuster M, et al. Part 12: cardiac arrest in special situations: 2010 American heart association guidelines for cardiopulmonary resuscitation and emergency cardiovascular care. Circulation. 2010;122(18 Suppl 3): S829–61.

118. Siddiqui N, Goldszmidt E, Haque SU, Carvalho JCA. Ultrasound simulation of internal jugular vein cannulation in pregnant and nonpregnant women. Can J Anaesth. 2010;57:966–72.

119. Chatterjee DJ, Bukunola B, Samuels TL, et al. Resuscitation in massive obstetric haemorrhage using an intraosseous needle. Anaesthesia. 2011;66 (4):306–10.

120. NAMET. PHTLS Trauma First Response. St. Louis, MO: Mosby/JEMS; 2011.

121. Practice guidelines for perioperative blood transfusion and adjuvant therapies: an updated reported by the American Society of Anesthesiologists Task force on Perioperative Blood Transfusion and Adjuvant Therapies. Anesthesiology. 2006;105:198–208.

122. Mittermayr M, Streif W, Haas T, et al. Hemostatic changes after crystalloid or colloid fluid administration during major orthopedic surgery: the role of fibrinogen administration. Anesth Analg. 2007;105:905–17.

123. Thorsen K, Ringdal KH, Strand K, et al. Clinical and cellular effects of hypothermia, acidosis and coagulopathy in major surgery. Br J Surg. 2011;98:894–907.

124. Morgan TJ, Venkatesh B, Hall J. Crystalloid strong ion difference determines metabolic acid-base change during acute normovolaemic haemodilution. Intensive Care Med. 2004;30:1432–7.

125. Bulger EM, May S, Kerby JD, et al. Out-of-hospital hypertonic resuscitation after traumatic hypovolemic shock: a randomized controlled trial. Ann Surg. 2011;253:431–41.

126. Cooper DJ, Myles PS, McDermott FT, et al. Prehospital hypertonic saline resuscitation of patients with hypotension and severe traumatic

brain injury: a randomized controlled trial. JAMA. 2004;291:1350–7.

127. Myburgh JA, Mythen MG. Resuscitation fluids. N Engl J Med. 2013;369:1243–51.

128. Duke MD, Guidry C, Guice J, Stuke L, et al. Restrictive fluid resuscitation in combination with damage control resuscitation: time for adaptation. J Trauma Acute Care Surg. 2012;73:674–8.

129. The SAFE Study Investigators. A comparison of albumin and saline for fluid resuscitation in the intensive care unit. N Engl J Med. 2004;350:2247–56.

130. The SAFE Study Investigators. A comparison of albumin and saline for fluid resuscitation in the intensive care unit. Saline or albumin for fluid resuscitation in patients with traumatic brain injury. N Engl J Med. 2007;357:874–84.

131. Winstedt D, Hanna J, Schött U. Albumin-induced coagulopathy is less severe and more effectively reversed with fibrinogen than is synthetic colloid-induced coagulopathy. Scand J Clin Lab Invest. 2013;73(2):161–9.

132. Hartog CS, Kohl M, Reinert K. A systemic review of third-generation hydroxyethyl starch (HES 130/0.4) in resuscitation: safety not adequately addressed. Anesth Analg. 2011;112:635–45.

133. Caballo C, Escolar G, Diaz-Ricart M, et al. Impact of experimental haemodilution on platelet function, thrombin generation and clot firmness: effects of different coagulation factor concentrates. Blood Transfus. 2013;11:391–9.

134. Haase N, Perner A. Hydroxyethyl starch for resuscitation. Curr Opin Crit Care. 2013;19(4):321–5.

135. FDA Safety Communication: Boxed Warning on increased mortality and severe renal injury, and additional warning on risk of bleeding, for use of hydroxyethyl starch solutions in some settings. June 24, 2013. http://www.fda.gov/biologicsbloodvaccines/safetyavailability/ucm358271.htm.

136. Kauvar DS, Wade CE. The epidemiology and modern management of traumatic hemorrhage: US and international perspectives. Crit Care. 2005;9 Suppl 5:S1–9.

137. Duchesne JC, McSwain NE, Cotton BA, et al. Damage control resuscitation: the new face of damage control. J Trauma. 2010;69:976–90.

138. Holcomb JB, Hess JR. Early massive trauma transfusion: state of the art. J Trauma. 2006;60:1.

139. Holcomb JB, Wade CE, Michalek JE, et al. Increased plasma and platelet to red blood cell ratios improves outcome in 466 massively transfused civilian trauma patients. Ann Surg. 2008;248:447–58.

140. Holcomb JB, Jenkins D, Rhee P, et al. Damage control resuscitation: directly addressing the early coagulopathy of trauma. J Trauma. 2007;62:307–10.

141. Dries DH. Hypotensive resuscitation. Shock. 1996;6:311–6.

142. Doreide E, Deaken CD. Pre-hospital fluid therapy in the critically injured patient—a clinical update. Injury. 2005;35:1001–10.

143. Karpati PCJ, Rossignol M, Pirot M, et al. High incidence of myocardial ischemia during postpartum hemorrhage. Anesthesiology. 2004;100:30–6.

144. Palmer RM. Postpartum hemorrhage is not the only setting for maternal myocardial ischemia. Anesthesiology. 2004;101:1035–7.

145. Sihler KC, Napolitano NM. Complications of massive transfusion. Chest. 2010;137:209–20.

146. Duchesne JC, Hunt JP, Wahl G, et al. Review of current blood transfusion strategies in a mature level I trauma center: we were wrong for the last 60 years? J Trauma. 2008;65:272–6.

147. Teixeria PG, Inaba K, Shulman I, et al. Impact of plasma transfusion in massive transfused trauma patients. J Trauma. 2009;66:693–7.

148. Murad MH, Stubbs JR, Gandhi MJ, et al. The effect of plasma transfusion on morbidity and mortality: a systematic review and meta-analysis. Transfusion. 2010;50:1370–83.

149. Johansson PI, Oliveri R, Ostrowski SR. Hemostatic resuscitation with plasma and platelets in trauma. A meta-analysis. J Emerg Trauma Shock. 2012;5:120–5.

150. Holcomb JB, Zarzabal LA, Michalek JE, et al. Trauma Outcomes Group: increased platelet: RBC ratios are associated with improved survival after massive transfusion. J Trauma. 2011;71(2 Suppl 3):S318–28.

151. Ho KM, Leonard A. Concentration-dependent effect of hypocalcaemia on mortality of patients with critical bleeding requiring massive transfusion: a cohort study. Anaesth Intensive Care. 2011;39:46–54.

152. Snegovskikh D, Clebone A, Norwitz E. Anesthetic management of patients with placenta accreta and resuscitation strategies for associated massive hemorrhage. Curr Opin Anaesthesiol. 2011;24:274–81.

153. Ho KM, Leonard A. Risk factors associated with hypomagnesemia in massive transfusion. Transfusion. 2011;51(2):270–6.

154. Chaiwat O, Lang JD, Vavilala MS, et al. Early packed red blood cell transfusion and acute respiratory distress syndrome after trauma. Anesthesiology. 2009;110:351–60.

155. Stansbury LG, Dutton RP, Stein DM, et al. Controversy in trauma resuscitation: do ratios of plasma to red blood cells matter? Transfus Med Rev. 2009;23:255–65.

156. Allen SR, Kashuk JL. Unanswered questions in the use of blood component therapy in trauma. Scand J Trauma Resusc Emerg Med. 2011;19:5.

157. Nascimento B, Callum J, Rubenfeld G, et al. Clinical review: fresh frozen plasma in massive bleedings-more questions than answers. Crit Care. 2010;14:202.

158. Spahn DR, Cerny V, Coasts TJ. Management of bleeding following major trauma: a European guideline. Crit Care. 2007;11:R17.

159. Grasseto A, De Nardin M, Ganzerla B, et al. ROTEM® guided coagulation factor concentrate therapy in trauma: 2-year experience in Venice, Italy. Crit Care. 2012;16:428.

160. Schöchl H, Maegele M, Solomon C, et al. Early and individualized goal-directed therapy for trauma-induced coagulopathy. Scand J Trauma Resusc Emerg Med. 2012;20:15.
161. Schöchl H, Schlimp CJ. Trauma bleeding management: the concept of goal-directed primary care. Anesth Analg. 2013. doi:10.1213/ANE.0b013e318270a6f7.
162. Fries D, Innerhofer P, Schobersberger W. Time for changing coagulation management in trauma-related massive bleeding. Curr Opin Anaesthesiol. 2009;22:267–74.
163. Brohi K, Singh J, Heron M, et al. Acute traumatic coagulopathy. J Trauma. 2003;54:1127–30.
164. Brohi K, Cohen MH, Gantner MT, et al. Acute coagulopathy of trauma: hypoperfusion induces systemic anticoagulation and hyperfibrinolysis. J Trauma. 2008;65:1211–7.
165. Wolberg AS, Meng ZH, Monroe III DM, et al. A systematic evaluation of the effects of temperature on coagulation enzyme activity and platelet function. J Trauma. 2004;56:1221–8.
166. Kostousov V, Wang YW, Cotton BA, et al. Influence of resuscitation fluids, fresh frozen plasma and fibrinolytics on fibrinolysis in a thromboelastography-based, in-vitro, whole-blood model. Blood Coagul Fibrinolysis. 2013;24:489–97.
167. CRASH-2 Trial Collaborators. Effects of TXA on death, vascular occlusive events, and blood transfusion in trauma patients with significant haemorrhage (CRASH-2): a randomized placebo-controlled trial. Lancet. 2010;376:2–32.
168. CRASH-2 Trial Collaborators. Effect of TXA in traumatic brain injury: a nested randomized, placebo controlled trial. CRASH-2 Intracranial Bleeding Study. BMJ. 2011;343:d3795. doi:10.1136/bmj.d3795.
169. Huang F, Wu D, Ma G, et al. The use of tranexamic acid to reduce blood loss and transfusion in major orthopedic surgery: a metaanalysis. J Surg Res. 2014;186(1):318–27. doi:10.1016/j.jss.2013.08.020.
170. Rappold JF, Pusateri AE. Tranexamic acid in remote damage control resuscitation. Transfusion. 2013;53:96S–9.
171. Shakur H, Elbourn D, Gülmezoglu M, et al. The WOMAN Trial World Maternal Antifibrinolytic Trial: tranxexamic acid for post-partum haemorrhage: an international randomized, double blind placebo controlled trial. Trials. 2010;11:40. doi:10.1186/1745-6215-11-40.
172. Sentürk M, Cakmak Y, Yildiz G, et al. Tranexamic acid for cesarean section: a double-blind placebo-controlled randomized clinical trial. Arch Gynecol Obstet. 2013;287:641–5.
173. Levy JH, Szlam F, Tanaka KA, et al. Fibrinogen and hemostasis: a primary hemostatic target for the management of acquired bleeding. Anesth Analg. 2012;114:261–74.
174. Hiippala ST, Myllyla GJ, Vahtera EM. Hemostatic factors and replacement of major blood loss with plasma-poor red cell concentrates. Anesth Analg. 1995;81:360–5.
175. Sørensen B, Spahn DR, Innerhofer P, et al. Clinical review: prothrombin complex concentrates—evaluation of safety and thrombogenicity. Crit Care. 2011;15:201.
176. David JS, Godier A, Dargaud Y, et al. Case scenario: management of trauma-induced coagulopathy in a blunt trauma patient. Anesthesiology. 2013;119:191–200.
177. Boffard KD, Riou B, Warren B, et al. Recombinant factor VIIa as adjunctive therapy for bleeding control in severely injured trauma patients: two parallel randomized, placebo-controlled, double-blind clinical trials. J Trauma. 2005;58:8–15.
178. Kobayashi T, Nakabayashi M, Yoshioka A, et al. Recombinant activated factor VII (rFVIIA/NovoSeven®) in the management of severe postpartum haemorrhage: initial report of a multicentre case series in Japan. Int J Hematol. 2012;95:157–63.
179. Huber AW, Raio L, Alberio L, et al. Recombinant human factor VIIa prevents hysterectomy in severe postpartum hemorrhage: single center study. J Perinat Med. 2011;40:43–9.
180. Seoud M, Cheaib S, Birjawi G, et al. Successful treatment of severe retroperitoneal bleeding with recombinant factor VII in a woman with placenta percreata invading into the left broad ligament: unusual repeated antepartum intra-abdominal bleeding. J Obstet Gynaecol Res. 2010;36:183–6.
181. Nohira T, Osakabe Y, Suda S, et al. Successful management by recombinant activated factor VII in a case of disseminated intravascular coagulopathy caused by obstetric hemorrhage. J Obstet Gynaecol Res. 2008;34:623–30.
182. Fries D. The early use of fibrinogen, prothrombin complex concentrate, and recombinant-activated factor VIIIa in massive bleeding. Transfusion. 2013;53:91S–5.
183. Frank LR. Is MAST in the past? The pros and cons of MAST usage in the field. FEMS. 2000;25:38–41, discussion 44–5.
184. Pease CS, Magrina JF, Finely BE. The use of MAST suit in obstetrics and gynecology. Obstet Gynecol Surv. 1984;39:416–22.
185. Miller S, Martin HB, Moris JL. Anti-shock garment in post-partum haemorrhage. Best Pract Res Clin Obstet Gynecol. 2008;22(6):1057–74.
186. Sutherland T, Downing J, Miller S, et al. Use of the non-pneumatic anti-shock garment (NASG) for life-threatening obstetric hemorrhage: a cost-effectiveness analysis in Egypt and Nigeria. PLoS One. 2013;8(4):62282. doi:10.1371/journal.pone.0062282.
187. Lester F, Stenson A, Meyer C, et al. Impact of the Non-pneumatic Antishock Garment on pelvic blood flow in healthy postpartum women. Am J Obstet Gynecol. 2011;204:409.e1–5.
188. Abdelazin A. Fetal Fibronectin (Quick Check fFN test®) for detection of premature rupture of fetal

membranes. Arch Gynecol Obstet. 2013;287 (2):205–10.

189. van der Ham DP, van Teefelen AS, Mol BW. Prelabor rupture of membranes: overview of diagnostic methods. Curr Opin Obstet Gynecol. 2012;24 (6):408–12.

190. Macones GA, Hankins GD, Spong CY, et al. The 2008 National Institute of Child Health and Human Development workshop report on electronic fetal monitoring: update on definitions, interpretation, and research guidelines. Obstet Gynecol. 2008;112(3):661–6.

191. Muehnch MV, Baschat AA, Reddy UM, Mighty HE, Weinder CP, Scalea TM, Harman CR. Kleihauer-Betke testing is important in all cases of maternal trauma. J Trauma. 2004;57(5):1094–8.

192. Kim YA, Makar RS. Detection of fetomaternal hemorrhage. Am J Hematol. 2012;87(4):417–23.

193. Chambers E, Davies L, Evans S, et al. Comparison of haemoglobin F detection by the acid elution test, flow cytometry and high-performance liquid chromatography in maternal blood samples analyzed for fetomaternal haemorrhage. Transfus Med. 2012;22 (3):199–204.

194. Cosmi E, Rampon M, Saccardi C, Zanardo V, Litta P. Middle cerebral artery peak systolic velocity in the diagnosis of fetomaternal hemorrhage. Int J Gynaecol Obstet. 2012;117(2):128–30.

195. Nguyen CP, Goodman LH. Fetal risk in diagnostic radiology. Semin Ultrasound CT MRI. 2012;33:4–10.

196. Sadro C, Bittle M, O'Connell K. Imaging the pregnant trauma patient. Ultrasound Clin. 2011;6:97–103.

197. Yousefzadeh D, Ward M, Reft C. Internal barium shielding to minimize fetal irradiation in spiral CT: a phantom simulation experiment. Radiology. 2006;239:751–8.

198. Webb JA, Thomsen HS, Morcos SK. Members of Contrast Media Safety Committee of European Society of Urogenital Radiology (ESUR). The use of iodinated and gadolinium contrast media during pregnancy and lactation. Eur Radiol. 2005;15:1234–40.

199. Ma OJ, Mateer JR, DeBehnke DJ. Use of ultrasonography for the evaluation of pregnant trauma patients. J Trauma. 1996;40(4):665–8.

200. Goodwin H, Holmes JF, Wisner DH. Abdominal ultrasound examination in pregnant trauma patients. J Trauma. 2001;50:689.

201. Bochiocchio GV, Haan J, Scalea TM. Surgeon-performed focused assessment with sonography for trauma as an early screening tool for pregnancy after trauma. J Trauma. 2002;52(6):1125–8.

202. Sadro C, Bernstein MP, Kanal KM. Imaging of Trauma: part 2, abdominal trauma and pregnancy—a radiologist's guide to doing what is best for the mother and baby. AJR Am J Roentgenol. 2012;199:1207–19.

203. Rothenberger DA, Quattlebaum FW, Zabel J, et al. Diagnostic peritoneal lavage for blunt trauma in pregnant women. Am J Obstet Gynecol. 1977;129 (5):479–81.

204. Scorpio RJ, Esposito TJ, Smith LG, et al. Blunt trauma during pregnancy: factors affecting fetal outcome. J Trauma. 1992;32(2):213–6.

205. National Spinal Cord Injury Statistics Center. UAB spinal cord injury info sheet #15. Birmingham, AL: University of Alabama; 2009. https://www.nscisc.uab.edu/PublicDocuments/fact_figures_docs/Facts%202012%20Feb%20Final.pdf. Updated February 2012. Accessed 12 Oct 2013.

206. Ghidini A, Simonson MR. Pregnancy after spinal cord injury: a review of the literature. Top Spinal Cord Inj Rehabil. 2011;16(3):93–103.

207. Furlan JC. Autonomic dysreflexia—a clinical emergency. J Trauma Acute Care Surg. 2013;75:496–500.

208. Hughes SJ, Short DJ, Usherwood MM, et al. Management of the pregnant woman with spinal cord injuries. Br J Obstet Gynaecol. 1991;98(6):513–8.

209. Krassioukov A, Warburton DE, Teasell R, et al. A systematic review of the treatment of autonomic dysreflexia after spinal cord injury. Arch Phys Med Rehabil. 2009;90(4):682–95.

210. Katz VL, Thorp Jr JM, Cefalo RC. Epidural analgesia and autonomic hyperreflexia: a case report. Am J Obstet Gynecol. 1990;162(2):471–2.

211. Periera L. Obstetric management of the patient with spinal cord injury. Obstet Gynecol Surv. 2003; 58(10):678–87.

212. Owen MD, Stiles MM, Opper SE, et al. Autonomic hyperreflexia in a pregnant paraplegic patient. Case report. Reg Anesth. 1994;19(6):415–7.

213. Takatsuki A, Ohtsuka M. Clinical trial of a method for confirming the effects of spinal anesthesia in patients with spinal cord injury. J Anesth. 2012;26 (6):914–7.

214. Camune BD. Challenges in the management of pregnant women with spinal cord injury. J Perinat Neonatal Nurs. 2013;27(3):225–31.

215. Biderman P, Einav S, Fainblut M, et al. Extracorporeal life support in patients with multiple injuries and severe respiratory failure: a single-center experience. J Trauma Acute Care Surg. 2013;75:907–12.

216. Ried M, Bein T, Philipp A, et al. Extracorporeal lung support in trauma patients with severe chest injury and acute lung failure: a 10-year institutional experience. Crit Care. 2013;17:R110. http://ccforum.com/content/17/3/R110.

217. Plotkin JS, Shah JB, Lofland GK, et al. Extracorporeal membrane oxygenation in the successful treatment of traumatic adult respiratory distress syndrome: case report and review. J Trauma. 1994;37(1):127–30.

218. Cunningham JA, Devine PC, Jelic S. Extracorporeal membrane oxygenation in pregnancy. Obstet Gynecol. 2006;103:792–5.

219. King PT, Rosalion A, McMillan J, et al. Extracorporeal membrane oxygenation in pregnancy. Lancet. 2000;356:45–6.

220. Robertson LC, Allen SH, Konamme SP, et al. The use of extra-corporeal membrane oxygenation in the case of a pregnant woman with severe h1N1 2009 influenza complicated by pneumonitis and adult respiratory distress syndrome. Int J Obstet Anesth. 2010;19:443–7.

221. Grasselli G, Bombino M, Patroniti P, et al. Use of extracorporeal respiratory support during pregnancy: a case report and literature review. ASAIO J. 2012;58:281–4.

222. Ho CH, Chen KB, Liu SK, et al. Early application of extracorporeal membrane oxygenation in a patient with amniotic fluid embolism. Acta Anaesthesiol Taiwan. 2009;47(2):99–102.

223. Weinberg L, Kay C, Liskaser F, et al. Successful treatment of peripartum massive pulmonary embolism with extracorporeal membrane oxygenation and catheter-directed pulmonary thrombolytic therapy. Anaesth Intensive Care. 2011;39(3):486–91.

224. Smith IJ, Gillham MJ. Fulminant peripartum cardiomyopathy rescue with extra-corporeal membranous oxygenation. Int J Obstet Anesth. 2009;18 (2):186–8.

225. Ngatchou W, Ramadan AS, Van Nooten G, et al. Left tilt position for easy extracorporeal membrane oxygenation cannula insertion in late pregnancy patients. Interact Cardiovasc Thorac Surg. 2012;15: 285–7.

226. Chapman BC, Moore EE, Barnett C, et al. Hypercoagulability following blunt solid abdominal organ injury: when to initiate anticoagulation. Am J Surg. 2013;206:917–23. doi:10.1016/j.amjsurg.2013.07.024.

227. Harr JN, Moore EE, Ghasabyan A, et al. Functional fibrinogen assay indicates that fibrinogen is critical in correcting abnormal clot strength following trauma. Shock. 2013;39:459. doi:10.1097/SHK.0b013e3182787122.

228. Hill CC, Pickinpaugh J. Trauma and surgical emergencies in the obstetric patient. Surg Clin North Am. 2008;88:282–7.

229. Nelson-Piercy C. Chapter 9: Cardiac disease in Center for Maternal and Child Enquiries (CMACE). Saving mother's lives: reviewing maternal deaths to make motherhood safer: 2006–08. The eighth report on confidential enquiries into maternal deaths in the United Kingdom. BJOG. 2011;118:1–203.

230. Hui D, Morrison LJ, Windrim R, et al. The American Heart Association 2010 guidelines for the management of cardiac arrest in pregnancy: consensus recommendations on implementation strategies. J Obstet Gynaecol Can. 2011;33:858–63.

231. Morris S, Stacey M. Resuscitation in pregnancy. BMJ. 2003;327:1277–9.

232. Rees GA, Willis BA. Resuscitation in late pregnancy. Anaesthesia. 1988;43:347–9.

233. Mathur D, Leon SB. Perimortem caesarean section: a review of the anaesthetist's nightmare. Trends Anaesth Crit Care. 2013;3(6):327–30. http://x.doi.org/10/10/16/j.tacc.2013.05.002.

234. Jeejeebhoy FM, Zelop CM, Windrim R, et al. Management of cardiac arrest in pregnancy: a systematic review. Resuscitation. 2011;82:801–9.

235. Suresh MS, LaToya MC, Munnur U. Cardiopulmonary resuscitation and the parturient. Best Pract Res Clin Obstet Gynaecol. 2010;24:383–400.

236. Kundra P. Manual displacement of the uterus during Caesarean section. Anaesthesia. 2007;62:460–5.

237. Nanson J, Elcock D, Williams M, et al. Do physiological changes in pregnancy change defibrillation energy requirements? Br J Anaesth. 2001;87:237–9.

238. Farinelli CK, Hameed AB. Cardiopulmonary resuscitation in pregnancy. Cardiol Clin. 2012;30:453–61.

239. Morris Jr JA, Rosenbower TH, Jurkowich GJ, et al. Infant survival after cesarean section for trauma. Ann Surg. 1996;223:481–8.

240. DePace NL, Betesh JS, Kotler MN. "Postmortem" cesarean delivery with recovery of both mother and offspring. JAMA. 1982;248:971–3.

241. Katz VL, Dotters DH, Droegmueller W. Perimortem cesarean delivery. Obstet Gynecol. 1986;68:571–6.

242. Katz VL, Balderston K, DeFreest M. Perimortem cesarean delivery: were our assumptions correct? Am J Obstet Gynecol. 2005;192:1916–20.

243. Clark SL, Hankins GD, Dudley DA, et al. Amniotic fluid embolism: analysis of the national registry. Am J Obstet Gynecol. 1995;172(4 Pt 1):1158–67.

244. Einav S, Kaufman N, Sela HY. Maternal cardiac arrest and perimortem cesarean delivery: evidence or expert-based? Resuscitation. 2012;83:1191–200.

245. Center for Maternal and Child Enquiries (CMACE). Saving mother's lives: reviewing maternal deaths to make motherhood safer: 2006–08. The eighth report on confidential enquiries into maternal deaths in the United Kingdom. BJOG. 2011;118:1–203.

246. Lipman SS, Wong JY, Arafeh J, et al. Transport decreases the quality of cardiopulmonary resuscitation during simulated maternal cardiac arrest. Anesth Analg. 2013;116:162–7.

247. Bernstein IM, Watson M, Simmons GM, et al. Maternal brain death and prolonged fetal survival. Obstet Gynecol. 1989;74:734–77.

248. Mallampalli A, Powner DJ, Gardner MO. Cardiopulmonary resuscitation and somatic support of the pregnant patient. Crit Care Clin. 2004;20:747–61.

249. Field DR, Gates EA, Creasy RK, et al. Maternal brain death during pregnancy: medical and ethical issues. JAMA. 1988;260:816–22.

250. Craft Jr JB, Coaldrake LA, Yonekura ML, et al. Ketamine, catecholaimes, and uterine tone in pregnant ewes. Am J Obstet Gynecol. 1983;146(4):429–34.

Anesthesia for the Geriatric Trauma Patient

17

Walid Alrayashi

Background

As medical care continues to improve, more people are living longer. The average life expectancy has increased by almost a decade just in the last 50 years [1]. Currently, there are about 40 million people over the age of 65, but that is expected to increase to over 72 million people [2]. As a result, hospitals have seen a steady increase in the age of their inpatient population. In fact, older adults account for 25 % of all hospital trauma admissions and that number is expected to grow to 40 % by 2050 [3, 4]. These numbers are also reflected in the financial outcomes that they entail. Although geriatric patients account for only 15 % of the patients seen in the ED, they account for almost 50 % of the ICU admissions, and consume on average, 50 % more diagnostic resources than younger people. For all of these reasons, it becomes practically important for anesthesiologists and critical care providers to gain a deeper understanding of the patients they will be taking care of more often.

There is no uniformly understood definition of "elderly." According to the injury severity scale (ISS), there is an increase in mortality for patients over 70 years old. The traditional Advanced Trauma Life Support (ATLS) approach is to transport any patient over 55 years old to a trauma center, whereas the Eastern Association for the Surgery of Trauma (EAST) classifies anyone over 65 years as elderly [5, 6]. However, it is probably more accurate to define an "elderly patient" as an individual who has undergone a group of anatomical and physiological changes, which have diminished his/her ability to adapt and recover from various physical ailments compared to their younger counterparts. It is well known that elderly trauma patients, especially those over 80 years, have significantly higher rates of morbidity and mortality.

Etiology of Geriatric Trauma

There are several key conditions that place the geriatric population at increased risk for traumatic events and for delayed recovery. Some of these factors include visual loss, cognitive dysfunction, unsteady balance, slowed reaction time, and syncope. In addition, the elderly are also prone to generalized weakness and deconditioning from chronic illnesses (Table 17.1). Most of the time, these conditions are not even recognized prior to a trauma. Prior trauma also places patients at about a threefold increased risk for further trauma.

In terms of the mechanism of geriatric injury, blunt trauma is more common than the penetrating trauma seen in younger patients. Furthermore, falls account for about 70 % of the

W. Alrayashi, M.D. (✉)
Department of Anesthesiology, New York University
Medical Center, 550 First Avenue, New York, NY 10016,
USA
e-mail: Walid.alrayashi@nyumc.org; 1walid@gmail.com

C.S. Scher (ed.), *Anesthesia for Trauma*, DOI 10.1007/978-1-4939-0909-4_17,
© Springer Science+Business Media New York 2014

Table 17.1 Factors contributing to geriatric trauma

Visual loss	• Cataract formation
	• Impaired pupillary response
	• Decreased peripheral vision
Hearing loss	
Cognitive dysfunction	• May be seen in 35% of geriatric patients in ED, only recognized 6% of the time [7]
	• Memory impairments
	• Depression
	• Dementia
Unsteady balance and gait	• Proprioception and inner ear derangements
Slowed reaction time	
Syncope	• Usually caused by undiagnosed cardiac and neural derangements as well as inappropriate medication use

elderly trauma, while motor vehicle accidents (MVAs) account for about 25 % of the remaining injuries. Penetrating and other traumas fill the remaining 5 % of presenting injuries [8]. The overwhelming majority of falls occur from the standing position. Falls associated with concurrent cerebral damage and long bone fractures are associated with significant morbidity and mortality [9, 10]. Furthermore, there are significant costs associated, with each fall costing about $18,000, not including the post hospital rehabilitation and nursing care [11]. Those suffering MVAs frequently sustain rib fractures with flail chest and pulmonary contusions, leading to worsening cardiopulmonary disease such as ischemia, pneumonia, and respiratory failure [12]. The elderly are also more prone to burn injuries involving larger surface areas, attributable to their reduced olfactory, visual, and auditory senses [13].

Physiological Considerations in the Elderly

In order for the body to survive, it has to be able to respond to various physiological stressors in order to maintain a steady state of homeostasis. That flexibility is called functional reserve. As one ages, functional reserve decreases steadily

[14]. When sustaining a traumatic insult, recovery is usually slow and complicated by infections and multiple organ dysfunction syndromes. However, there is a significant amount of variability from one elderly person to another, partially due to lifestyle, environmental factors, genetics, and other systemic diseases [15]. Taking an organ-system approach, we will review the physiological changes of the elderly trauma patient and discuss the pertinent anesthetic considerations.

Cardiovascular

There are normal physiologic changes that the heart undergoes as one gets older (Fig. 17.1). These include an increase in fibrosis of the myocardium and media of the arterial vasculature. It is common to have a hypertrophied left ventricle and a stiffened aorta which results in increased afterload and manifests as elevated systolic blood pressures. The pressure increases lead to prolonged myocardial contraction and impaired relaxation, raising the risk of heart failure. In order to maintain the same stroke volume, the left ventricle becomes more dependent on the atrial contribution during diastole, from 10 % in young adults to 30 % in the elderly [16]. To accommodate for this, the atrium frequently enlarges, increasing its propensity for dysrhythmias like atrial fibrillation. Also, the fat and collagen deposition within the heart affects the conduction system and leads to a slower resting heart rate and likelihood of dysrhythmias [17].

Anesthetic Considerations

In summary, the changes described above lead to diminished cardiac reserve especially when determining fluid resuscitation in a trauma patient. Rapid fluid shifts are not well tolerated. When sudden blood loss occurs, the geriatric heart cannot compensate with a faster heart rate when a higher cardiac output is needed because of decreased response to circulating catecholamines and increased vagal tone. These patients are also frequently taking β-blockers, further impeding their sympathetic response to

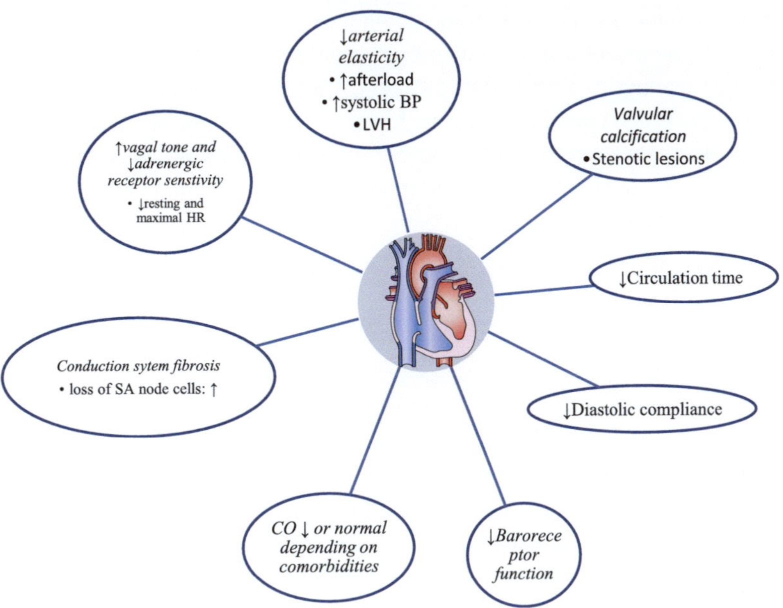

Fig. 17.1 Cardiovascular physiology in the elderly. *BP* blood pressure, *LVH* left ventricular hypertrophy, *CO* cardiac output, *HR* heart rate, and *SA* sinoatrial node, *downward arrow* decreased, *upward arrow* increased

hypovolemia and making heart rate a less reliable diagnostic tool. Conversely, sudden boluses of fluid or blood products are also not well tolerated as in patients with diastolic dysfunction. Although older patients have some degree of diastolic dysfunction, many have more significant disease especially those with hypertension, coronary artery disease, cardiomyopathy, and valvular heart disease. When there is a small change in the left ventricular volume, the end diastolic pressure increases drastically, leading to fluid overload among other things. Consequently, geriatric patients are more sensitive to Starling's forces and fluid management should be based on the type of surgery and the patients' comorbidities. Monitoring modalities such as echocardiography and systolic pressure variations SPVs should be used to guide fluid administration. SPV is the difference between the maximum and minimum systolic pressure following a positive pressure breath. When the difference is ≥10, this usually reflects a hypovolemic state.

The prolonged circulation time results in slowed onset of intravenous agents but faster induction of inhalational agents, however this is of minimal clinical significance. During induction there may be an exaggerated drop in blood pressure due to the diminished cardiac reserve and the fact that most anesthetic agents are negative inotropes with vasodilatory properties. These agents cause sympathetic blockade which the geriatric myocardium may be heavily reliant on for normal resting function.

Pulmonary

The prominent feature of geriatric pulmonary physiology is the decreased compliance of the chest wall and parenchymal lung tissue. While the chest wall muscles become more fibrotic and the costal cartilages calcify, the thorax becomes more barrel-shaped. The diaphragm also becomes flat. In combination, these features increase the amount of work needed for adequate ventilation and oxygenation. The alveoli end up becoming over distended while the small airways collapse, ultimately minimizing the overall alveolar surface area available for gas exchange. Both the anatomic and physiologic dead space increase. The vital capacity is decreased, but the functional residual capacity and closing capacity are increased. Ventilation and perfusion mismatching is more pronounced [18]. Geriatric patients have decreased pulmonary capillary blood volume and pulmonary membrane permeability. The alveolocapillary membrane thickens as well leading to a decreased oxygen diffusion capacity. When combined with the lower resting arterial oxygenation (see the Raine–Bishop equation below), these patients are also more prone to rapid hypoxemia [19].

clearance, but they produce less creatinine in general because of decreased muscle mass in the elderly, ultimately leaving serum creatinine within the low-normal range. However, the creatinine clearance is a good measure of kidney function which can be calculated using the Cockroft–Gault equation.

$$\text{GFR} = \frac{(140 - \text{age}) \times (\text{weight in kg}) \times (0.85 \text{ if female or } 1.0 \text{ if male})}{72 \times \text{Creatinine in mg/dL}}$$

Anesthetic Considerations

The described physiologic derangements, geriatric patients experience hypoxemia more rapidly when apneic. So denitrogenation (or preoxygenation) usually takes a longer period of time and induction of anesthesia usually causes more rapid desaturation. There are also important anatomical considerations in the elderly. They have decreased protective laryngeal reflexes making them prone to aspiration. Poor dentition and lack of teeth may make mask ventilation difficult. Patients may have limited range of motion of the neck and temporomandibular joint potentially making intubation difficult. One should recognize that the elderly are prone to cervical spine injuries, often requiring a neck collar until damage to vertebrae or ligaments is ruled out. Patients who undergo abdominal or thoracic surgery often have increased atelectasis due to splinting which often increases the elderly patient's already-elevated work of breathing. In addition, narcotic and benzodiazepine use further decrease the already low baseline response to hypoxia and hypercarbia; ultimately making these patients at higher risk for early respiratory failure.

Renal

At the anatomic level, elderly kidneys have a loss of both glomeruli and renal mass, up to 50 % less than their younger counterparts [19]. There is also a decreased renal blood flow due to fewer capillaries. Patients also have a lower creatinine

The kidneys are also unable to concentrate or absorb glucose as effectively. These changes usually result in a high incidence of previously unrecognized renal dysfunction. This is significant because acute renal failure contributes to a one in five deaths during the perioperative period of geriatric surgical patients [20]. The rennin–angiotensin–aldosterone system's ability to adapt to fluid and pressure changes is also decreased. The kidney's ability to regulate fluids and electrolytes is also impaired placing patients at risk for hypo or hypervolemia as well as deranged electrolyte levels. These effects may result in neurological or cardiovascular abnormalities like seizures and/or cerebral edema, or arrhythmias, respectively.

Anesthetic Considerations

Due to the altered concentrating ability and the possibility for inappropriate diuresis, urine output is not a reliable way to interpret renal function. Skin turgor is also a poor marker of fluid status as the elderly usually have a thinner dermis with loss of elasticity. Medications which need careful control of plasma levels should be titrated based on serum concentrations. Unfortunately, in trauma, an accurate assessment of a patient's renal function cannot occur until the postoperative period. Nonetheless, nephrotoxic medications and diagnostic agents like contrast dye, should be minimized. One should be mindful of using drugs which depend on renal clearance as their duration of action is usually prolonged [19, 20].

Central Nervous System

Geriatric cognitive function is mostly preserved, in the absence of cerebral diseases like Parkinson's or Alzheimer's. That being said, there is a high prevalence of all forms of dementia and other neurologic disorders. Short term memory is modestly decreased, while long term usually remains unchanged [21]. Anatomically, there is a decrease in brain mass with an appropriate decrease in cerebral blood flow according to an intact autoregulation curve. There is a considerable decrease in neuron mass, degree of synapses as well as the synthesis of neurotransmitters and their receptors [22]. At the cellular level, it is theorized that there is a reduction of certain proteins that promote new neuron growth like fibroblast growth factor-2, insulin-like growth factor-1, and vascular endothelial growth factor [23]. Physiologically, the elderly have impaired thermoregulation and a lower vasoconstriction threshold making them very sensitive to ambient temperature changes.

Anesthetic Considerations

One of the most important goals of intraoperative management is to maintain adequate cerebral perfusion. It is difficult to determine what "adequate perfusion" is because many geriatric patients have chronic hypertension which may or may not be controlled. Moreover, the autoregulation curve of the elderly is commonly shifted to the right. What this implies is that the limits of where the mean arterial pressures (MAP), and consequently cerebral perfusion pressure (CPP), should be maintained may be different than expected. It is widely accepted to maintain the MAPs within 20 % of the patient's baseline. It is also important to aggressively maintain normothermia in the geriatric population because of their impaired thermoregulation worsened further by general anesthesia. The value of maintaining a normal temperature cannot be overstated in a trauma patient because the lack of it places them at risk for coagulopathy, delayed wound healing, increased oxygen requirements, arrhythmias, and ischemic events.

The decreased cognitive reserve of the geriatric patient increases the likelihood of postoperative delirium and cognitive dysfunction. Post-op delirium, occurring in 5–50 % of the patients and up to 80 % in the critically ill; manifests as a transient fluctuating change in consciousness that happens after surgery. There are many possible causes, such as anemia, pain, sleep deprivation, electrolyte abnormalities, infection, and preexisting dementia. It has been demonstrated that the elderly brain is more sensitive to the peripheral inflammatory mediators released during trauma. In animal models, it has been shown that these inflammatory cytokines in particular interleukn-1 and 6 (IL-1 and IL-6) as well as tumor necrosis factor stimulate microglia to promote further neural inflammation. Ultimately, this inflammatory cascade in the brain leads to neurodegeneration of cholinergic neurons in the basal forebrain as well as the delayed progressive loss of dopaminergic neurons in the substantia nigra [24]. Postoperative cognitive dysfunction is a more persistent change in mental status which manifests as personality changes, unstable moods, as well as impaired focus and memory. Risk factors include age, years of formal education, duration of anesthetic, postoperative infection, and repeat surgery. It is frequently associated with longer hospitalization stays and healthcare costs.

Pharmacologic Considerations

There are specific physiologic changes in the elderly which have significant pharmacokinetic effects. There is decrease in total body water which means their central compartment in the three compartment model is decreased. This implies that the peak concentrations of drugs administered as a rapid infusion or bolus are much higher. With this in mind, it is better to calculate drug dosage by using lean body mass. However, older adults also have a lower lean body mass which decreases the second (rapid equilibrating) compartment and an increase in body fat which causes an increase in the third compartment (slow equilibrating) compartment. Together, these changes result in an increased volume of distribution that results in altered drug onset, peak, and duration that are sometimes difficult to predict.

During trauma, as the body undergoes shock, there are several unique changes. Protein-bound drugs are more readily available in circulation thereby amplifying their affect, whereas water-soluble drugs have an initial exaggerated effect because of the smaller overall volume of distribution (VD). The increased VD also causes the duration of fat-soluble drugs to be significantly prolonged. There is also an increased prevalence of drug–drug interactions because of the simple fact that the elderly take many more medications. When dosing drugs, it is important that the MAC of volatile agents may be significantly lower and that the rate of induction and emergence is slower. One must also reduce intravenous induction and narcotic drugs by up to 50%. In general, the aminosteroid muscle relaxants have a prolonged effect because of the high plasma concentration and slow elimination time due to reduced renal and hepatic clearance. However, there are no changes in onset and duration of the benzylisoquinolines.

Initial Assessment of the Geriatric Trauma Patient

When an elderly trauma patient first comes in, one may not be able to get a reasonable history. It may be necessary to just rely on collateral information from relatives or witnesses and on physical examination with careful attention to old scars. An attempt should be made to obtain a complete medication list, which may significantly affect diagnosis and treatment. Aging is associated with increased cardiovascular disease as so many of these patients are frequently taking anticoagulation therapies and/or β-blockers. Multiple studies have shown that head injury patients who were previously on warfarin have significantly worse outcomes, with a risk of mortality that is more than doubled compared to

those not taking them [25, 26]. The use of β-blocker may be an indicator to other coexisting diseases like diabetes, hypertension, hyperlipidemia, and renal failure. A retrospective study in a trauma center showed that β-blocker use in the elderly trauma patient conferred a twofold increased likelihood of mortality [27]. Normal appearing vital signs may actually be completely deranged. For example, tachycardia may be blunted by β-blockers and that what is a normal blood pressure may, in fact, be too low for a patient who has chronic hypertension. Failure to recognize these changes may delay diagnosis and treatment.

Triaging

Despite what we currently understand about the elderly and their overall decreased physiological reserve, many of these patients are under-triaged. One study that reviewed a trauma network of multiple hospitals showed that there were less trauma codes called for the elderly when compared to their younger counterparts with similar injuries [28]. On the contrary, when the elderly injured patients were quickly moved to a trauma center, they had improved outcomes with respect to infections, respiratory failure, and overall survival [29, 30]. There are several ways to identify patients who might benefit from aggressive resuscitation strategies. One of which is to use an anatomic scoring system which gives a global picture of a patient with multiple injuries, such as the Injury Severity Score (ISS). Several studies have demonstrated that this scoring system is a strong predictor of mortality [31].

Initial Management

Oxygenation and Ventilation

Initial management of the older trauma patient should follow standard ATLS guidelines, but with certain special considerations. Airway patency should be confirmed or established with endotracheal intubation, but that may prove challenging in a patient with direct head and neck injury, edema, or foreign bodies. The elderly are also more prone to poor dentition with loose teeth or they may have dentures, which should be removed prior to intubation. Edentulous patients may be difficult to mask ventilate. The elderly have reduced laryngeal reflexes because of a general atrophy of muscles and neural structures, making them prone to aspiration. Geriatric patients are also more prone to cervical neck injuries due to reduced bone density from osteoporosis, so neck stabilization should be maintained during intubation [32].

Chest injuries are very common with pulmonary contusions being the most common. Pulmonary contusions also deteriorate over time especially with excessive fluid resuscitation as many of these patients often require. The elderly are also more prone to rib fractures and flail chest due to the fragile bones secondary to osteoporosis. Thoracic epidural analgesia should be considered in these situations as they provide superior analgesia without the side effects of systemic opioids. Early chest tube placement should be done to relieve pneumothorax or hemothorax which would improve oxygenation and ventilation.

In establishing the airway, induction doses of certain drugs should be adjusted appropriately for the older adult in order to avoid severe hypotension, especially in light of hypovolemia. Sedative agents such as propofol, etomidate, benzodiazepines, and barbiturates should be decreased by up 20–50 % in order to attain the same electroencephalographic goals [33–35]. Finally, at induction, opioid doses should also be decreased, while neuromuscular blocking agent dosing should remain unchanged.

Cardiovascular Considerations

As discussed earlier, the elderly are prone to myocardial ischemic events as they are more likely to have previously undiagnosed atherosclerotic plaque in their coronaries. The myocardium is also less responsive to circulating catecholamines released after sustaining a trauma. This results in a reduced ability for the myocardium to compensate for shock physiology with an increased heart rate and cardiac output. These physiologic changes are further aggravated by β-blocking drugs. Therefore, a lower threshold should be used to assess an older patient. For example, when tachycardia is defined as a heart rate over 120 beats per minute (bpm) in a young adult (according to the ATLS protocols), a heart rate of 90 bpm in the elderly should raise equal concern [36]. Similarly, blood pressure may be deceiving as they may not indicate the true hemodynamic state of the patient. While a blood pressure less than 100–110 mmHg may be worrisome in a young patient, many studies have suggested that the threshold for older adults be increased to 120 mmHg for those aged 50–69 years and 140 mmHg for those over 70 years old [37].

Since vital signs may be misleading, it is important to assess tissue perfusion using serum levels of lactic acid and calculated base deficit. There have been many studies showing that elevated serum lactate levels are associated with increased mortality in patients who might otherwise be considered as having "normal" vital signs. A serum lactate level greater than 4 mmol/L was associated with a 12 % mortality in younger adults, but an astounding 40 % mortality in those older than 65 years [38].

The value in recognizing hypovolemia is that it often leads to hypoperfusion and tissue damage in the form of stroke, myocardial infarction, and acute renal failure. One should therefore establish adequate intravenous access and resuscitate with colloids, crystalloids, and blood in order to improve oxygen delivery. Patients on warfarin or clopidogrel may bleed excessively even with minor injuries. For these patients, aggressive correction with fresh frozen plasma (FFP) and platelets should be started early. Many trauma patients also suffer coagulopathy from shock secondary to their injuries, often necessitating replacement therapy with FFP, platelets, cryoprecipitate, fibrinogen, prothrombin complex concentrates, and recombinant factor VII.

Fig. 17.2 An algorithm for the initial resuscitation of the elderly trauma patient. *ISS* Injury Severity Score, *PACWP* pulmonary artery capillary wedge pressure, *PCWP* pulmonary capillary wedge pressure. Adapted from Surg Clin North Am, 74, Thi Santora TA, Schinco MA, Trooskin SZ, Management of TRAUMA in the elderly patient, pp. 163–85, Copyright 1994, with permission from Elsevier

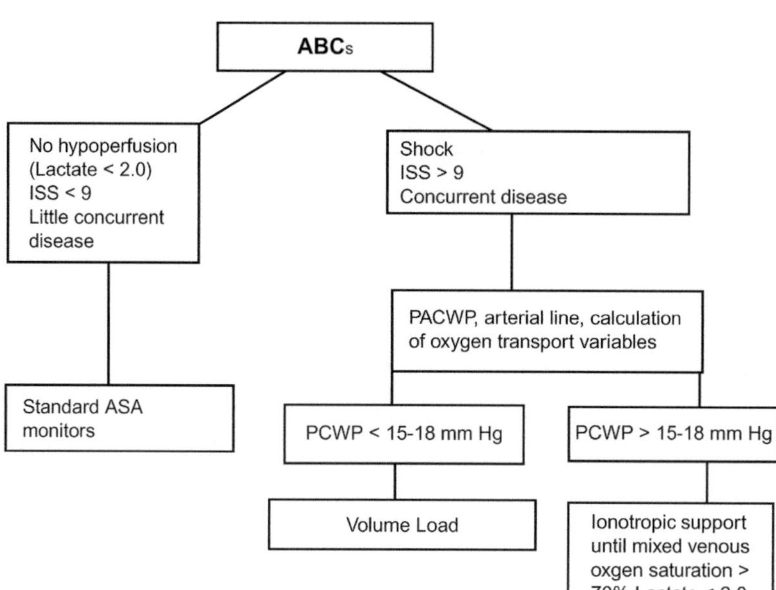

Temperature Considerations

Temperature regulation is an important and frequently overlooked factor in the management of the acute elderly trauma patient. Because they have less fat stores and subcutaneous tissue, they have less shivering and nonshivering thermogenesis. General anesthesia causes peripheral vasodilation which also exacerbates hypothermia. The complications of low core body temperatures are many and include worsening coagulopathy, platelet dysfunction, and metabolic acidosis. It is therefore important to aggressively warm patients in the operating room by increasing room temperature, using radiant and convective warming devices, and using fluid warmers.

Monitoring

Early invasive monitoring for guiding resuscitation was associated with improved survival in the geriatric trauma patient [39]. However, more recent data is showing that pulse pressure variation (PPV), SPV, and stroke volume variation (SVV) measurements to be very accurate indicators of volume status [40]. The concept behind invasive monitoring is to provide better diagnostic tools that would allow a more tailored approach in optimizing oxygen delivery. An algorithm that uses the ISS has been developed to guide initial resuscitation using invasive monitors (Fig. 17.2). After the initial assessment per ATLS guidelines, one can then determine if the injuries are minor or major by using an ISS of 9, lactate levels, or any other evidence of hypoperfusion. If the trauma is minor with no signs of shock, then standard American Society of Anesthesiologists (ASA) monitors can be used (inspired oxygen, arterial saturation, capnography, ECG, blood pressure, and temperature). However, if there are signs of hypovolemia, the patient has a high-risk mechanism of injury, uncertain cardiovascular status, or renal disease, then an arterial line and pulmonary artery catheter should be placed [41].

Anesthetic Concerns for Specific Injuries

Orthopedic Injuries

The elderly are prone to bone fractures due to the high incidence of osteoporosis. Many of these may be an isolated hip fracture or multiple fractures in a polytrauma. Many of these fractures are considered surgical emergencies because of the increased mortality, prolonged hospitalization, and precipitous decline in functional mobility associated with postponing fixation [42]. Several studies have shown that delaying the operative repair of these fractures more than 48 h confers a twofold increase in mortality in the first postoperative year [43]. One study found that in patients with up to two comorbidities had an increased mortality if their surgery was delayed for more than 24 h. However, that same study showed that those with three or more comorbidities had a decreased survival rate if operated on within that first 24 h [44]. Another study that adjusted for the severity of comorbid conditions showed no difference in mortality when surgery was delayed for 120 h [45]. It appears that those without other significant disease processes benefit the most from surgical intervention within 24–48 h. On the other hand, those with multiple comorbidities deserve a full multidisciplinary risk versus benefit analysis on the best time to proceed with surgery and how much optimization is necessary before going to the operating room.

Anesthetic choice between general versus regional has been an issue of debate. Older studies showed no differences between the two techniques in inpatient morbidity, 1-year mortality, or functional recovery [46, 47]. However, other prospective studies have shown a significant reduction in venous thromboembolism and intraoperative blood loss [48]. A more recent study in 2012 of inpatients with hip fractures showed a 29 % reduction in mortality and a 25 % decrease in pulmonary complications in those receiving regional compared to general anesthesia [49].

Head Injuries

Falls are the most common cause of head injuries in the elderly, frequently associated with a high incidence of intracranial bleeds [50]. Higher severity injuries, lower Glasgow Coma Scale (GCS) scores, and anticoagulation therapies are all associated with poorer neurologic outcomes in the geriatric patient. Unfortunately, the mortality of patients with severe brain injury is around 80 % in those over the age of 55 years compared to 38 % for all age groups [51]. The inpatient mortality for the geriatric patient with moderate to severe brain injury was 30 % and those with a GCS less than 9 had a mortality of 80 % [52].

Anesthetic management of patients with head injuries follows the same general principles. First, airway and ventilation should be established as neurologic injury is often associated with hypoventilation and hypoxia. The intubation is usually done with manual in-line stabilization as many of the elderly patients frequently have occult cervical instability [53]. Rapid sequence induction should be used, however cricoid pressure for prevention of aspiration is controversial especially since it has been shown that it may worsen cervical spine injuries [54]. Virtually all induction agents, except ketamine, are acceptable. Both etomidate and propofol decrease sympathetic stimulation to intubation, blunts intracranial pressure changes, and decreases the cerebral metabolic rate for oxygen [55].

Intraoperatively, the goal is to maintain adequate perfusion to the brain to avoid hypoxic injury. Cerebral autoregulation is often severely deranged in the acutely injured brain. Although there are no specific guidelines of where to maintain CPP according to age, it is commonly accepted to keep the CPP at least 60 mmHg [56]. See full chapter on head injuries for a more in depth discussion.

Thoracic Injuries

Although the elderly suffer from many thoracic injuries including blunt and penetrating cardiac, aortic, diaphragmatic, and intrathoracic airway injuries, the most common chest injury in this age group are rib fractures. They are associated with an increased risk of pneumonias, hemothorax, pneumothorax, contusions, respiratory failure, and death [57]. The most common mechanisms of injury in the elderly are falls (64 %) and MVAs (27 %) [58]. One study that evaluated the risk of death following blunt chest trauma, found that age over 65 years, three or more rib fractures, and pre-injury cardiopulmonary comorbidities increased mortality by 19 % per rib [59]. The major pathological processes include parenchymal hemorrhage, interstitial edema, and decreased surfactant production. Furthermore, these changes result in ventilation/perfusion mismatch, pulmonary shunting, and decreased lung compliance [60]. The signs and symptoms include tachypnea, hypoxemia, hypercarbia, and hemoptysis. Contusions usually do not manifest on chest X-ray in the early phases and are usually diagnosed on computerized tomography (CT) scan, but can also be seen with ultrasound.

The main goals in managing the elderly with these injuries revolve around maintaining oxygenation and ventilation. All modes of ventilation have been used including noninvasive, invasive, and high frequency ventilation as well as lung isolation, extracorporeal membrane oxygenation (ECMO), and surfactant [61]. One should use low tidal volumes, high positive end expiratory pressures (PEEP), and permissive hypercarbia strategies when managing patients with contusions to prevent further lung injury [62]. In order to optimize deep breathing and coughing, the patient should receive adequate pain control. Epidural analgesia should be used for patients with rib fractures and flail chest as it has been shown to reduce ventilator days, ICU length of stay, in-hospital days, and tracheostomy rates compared to patients receiving intravenous narcotic patient controlled analgesia (PCA) [63–65].

Summary

In summary, the elderly have unique physiology and experience trauma very differently at the anatomic and biochemical level compared to younger patients. The perioperative issues that arise significantly alter the anesthetic management approach of most of the procedures they undergo. Therefore, it is imperative that we continue expanding our understanding of the elderly, especially as the population of these patients continues to dramatically increase.

References

1. Center for Disease Control and Prevention National Center for Health Statistics. Life expectancy. http://www.cdc.gov/nchs/fastats/lifexpec.htm. Accessed June 20, 2013.
2. Federal Interagency Forum on Aging-Related Statistics. Older Americans 2010: key indicators of well-being. Washington, DC; 2010 July. http://www.agingstats.gov/agingstatsdotnet/Main_Site/Data/2010_Documents/Docs/OA_2010.pdf
3. Campbell JW, et al. In harm's way: moving the older trauma patient toward a better outcome. Geriatrics. 2009;64(1):8–13.
4. MacKenzie EJ, et al. Acute hospital costs of trauma in the United States: implications for regionalized systems of care. J Trauma. 1990;30(9):1096–101; discussion 101–3.
5. American College of Surgeons Committee on Trauma. Geriatric trauma. In: ATLS: student course manual. 8th edition. Chicago: ACLS; 2008. pp. 247–57.
6. The Eastern Association for the Surgery of Trauma. Geriatric trauma (update). http://www.east.org/resources/treatment-guidelines/geriatric-trauma. Accessed July 20, 2012.
7. Carpenter CR, DesPain B, Keeling TN, et al. The Six-Item Screener and AD8 patients. Ann Emerg Med. 2011;57(6):653–61.
8. Labib N, Nouh T, Winocour S, et al. Severely injured geriatric population: morbidity, mortality and risk factors. J Trauma. 2011;71:1908–14.
9. Thompson HJ, McCormick WC, Kagan SH. Traumatic brain injury in older adults: epidemiology, outcomes, and future implications. J Am Geriatr Soc. 2006;54:1590–5.
10. Keller JM, Sciadini MF, Sincalir E, et al. Geriatric trauma: demographics, injuries and mortality. J Orthop Trauma. 2012;26(9):e161–5.
11. Ganz DA, Bao Y, Shekelle PE, et al. Will my patient fall? JAMA. 2007;297:77–86.
12. Roudsari BS, Ebel BE, Corso PS, et al. The acute medical care costs of fall-related injuries among the US older adults. Injury. 2005;36:1316–22.
13. Linn BS. Age differences in the severity and outcome of burns. J Am Geriatr Soc. 1980;28:118–23.
14. Buckner RL. Memory and executive function in aging and AD: multiple factors that cause decline and reserve factors that compensate. Neuron. 2004;44:195–208.
15. Lewis MC, Karim A, Paniagua M. Geriatric trauma: special considerations in the anesthetic management

of the injured elderly patient. Anesthesiol Clin. 2007;25:75–90.

16. Geokas MC, Lakatta EG, Makinodan T, et al. The aging process. Ann Intern Med. 1990;113:455466.

17. Rooke GA. Autonomic and cardiovascular function in the geriatric patient. Anesthesiol Clin North America 2000;18:31,46, v–vi.

18. Raine JM, Bishop JM. A-a difference in O_2 tension and physiologic dead space in normal man. J Appl Physiol. 1963;18:284.

19. Varon A, Smith C, et al. Anesthetic management of geriatric trauma patient. In: Essentials of trauma anesthesia. Cambridge: Cambridge University Press; 2012. p. 275–87.

20. Muravchick S. Anesthesia for the elderly. In: Miller RM, editor. Anesthesia. 5th ed. Philadelphia: Churchill Livingstone; 2000. p. 2140–5.

21. Small SA. Age-related memory decline: current concepts and future directions. Arch Neurol. 2001;58:360–4.

22. Peters A. Structural changes that occur during normal aging of primate cerebral hemispheres. Neurosci Biobehav Rev. 2002;26:733–41.

23. Shetty AK, Hattiangady B, Shetty GA. Stem/progenitor cell proliferation factors FGF-2, IGF-1, and VEGF exhibit early decline during the course of aging in the hippocampus: role of astrocytes. Glia. 2005;51:173–86.

24. Steiner LA. Postoperative delirium. Part 1: pathophysiology and risk factors. Eur J Anesthesiol. 2011;28(9):628–36.

25. Franko J, Kish KJ, O'Connell BG, et al. Advanced age and preinjury warfarin anticoagulation increase the risk of mortality after head trauma. J Trauma. 2006;61:107–10.

26. Lavoie A, Ratte S, Clas D, et al. Preinjury warfarin use among elderly patients with closed head injuries in a trauma center. J Trauma. 2004;56:802–7.

27. Neideen T, Lam M, Brasel KJ. Preinjury beta blockers are associated with increased mortality in geriatric trauma patients. J Trauma. 2008;65:1016–20.

28. Lambert DA, Sattin RW. Death from falls, 1978-1984. MMWR CDC Surveill Summ. 1998;37:S21–6.

29. Finelli FC, Jonsson J, Champion HR, et al. A case control study for major trauma in geriatric patients. J Trauma. 1989;29:541–8.

30. Phillips S, Rond PC, Kelly SM, et al. The failure of triage criteria to identify geriatric patients with trauma: results from the Florida Trauma Triage Study. J Trauma. 1996;40:278–83.

31. Baker SP, O'Neill B, Haddon W, et al. The injury severity score: a method for describing patients with multiple injuries and valuating emergency care. J Trauma. 1974;14:187–96.

32. Lomoschitz FM, Blackmore CC, Mirza SK, et al. Cervical spine injuries in patients 65 years old and older: epidemiologic analysis regarding the effects of age and injury mechanism on distribution, type, and stability of injuries. Am J Roentgenol. 2002;178:573–7.

33. Arden JR, Holley FO, Stanski DR. Increased sensitivity to etomidate in the elderly: initial distribution versus altered brain response. Anesthesiology. 1986;65:9–27.

34. Homer TD, Stanski DR. The effect of increasing age on thiopental disposition and anesthetic requirement. Anesthesiology. 1985;62:714–24.

35. Reves JG, Fragen RJ, Vinik HR, et al. Midazolam: pharmacology and uses. Anesthesiology. 1985;62:310–24.

36. Heffernan DS, Thakkar RK, Monaghan SF, et al. Normal presenting vital signs are unreliable in geriatric blunt trauma victims. J Trauma. 2010;69:813–20.

37. Martin J, Alkhoury F, O'Connor J, et al. 'Normal' vital signs belie occult hypoperfusion in geriatric trauma patients. Am Surg. 2010;76:65–9.

38. Callaway DW, Shapiro NI, Donnino MW, et al. Serum lactate and base deficit as predictors of mortality in normotensive elderly blunt trauma patients. J Trauma. 2009;66:1040–4.

39. Jacobs DG, Plaisier BR, Barie PS, et al. Practice management guidelines for geriatric trauma: the EAST practice management guidelines work group. J Trauma. 2003;54:391–416.

40. Marik PE, Cavallazzi R, Vasu T, et al. Dynamic changes in arterial waveform derived variables and fluid responsiveness in mechanically ventilated patients: a systematic review of the literature. Crit Care Med. 2009;37:2642–7.

41. Santora TA, Schinco MA, Trooskin SZ. Management of TRAUMA in the elderly patient. Surg Clin North Am. 1994;74:163–85.

42. Siegmeth AW, Gurusamy K, Parker MJ. Delay to surgery prolongs hospital stay in patients with fractures of the proximal femur. J Bone Joint Surg Br. 2005;87:1123–6.

43. Zuckerman JD, Skovron ML, Koval KJ, et al. Postoperative complications and mortality associated with operative delay in older patients who have a fracture of the hip. J Bone Joint Surg Am. 1995;77:1551–6.

44. Sexson SB, Lehner JT. Factors affecting hip fracture mortality. J Orthop Trauma. 1987;1:298–305.

45. Vidan MT, Sanchez E, Gracia Y, et al. Causes and effects of surgical delay in patients with hip fracture: a cohort study. Ann Intern Med. 2011;155:226–33.

46. Koval KJ, Aharonoff GB, Rosenberg AD, et al. Functional outcome after hip fracture: effect of general versus regional anesthesia. Clin Orthop Relat Res. 1998;348:37–41.

47. Gilbert TB, Hawkes WG, Hebel JR, et al. Spinal anesthesia versus general anesthesia for hip fracture repair: a longitudinal observation of 741 elderly patients during 2-year follow-up. Am J Orthop. 2000;29:25–35.

48. Valentin N, Lomholt B, Jensen JS, et al. Spinal or general anesthesia for surgery of the fractured hip? A prospective study of mortality in 578 patients. Br J Anaesth. 1986;58:284–91.

49. Neuman MD, Silber JH, Elkassabany NM, et al. Comparative effectiveness of regional versus general anesthesia for hip fracture surgery in adults. Anesthesiology. 2012;117:72–92.
50. Pentland B, Hutton LS, Jones PA. Late mortality after head injury. J Neurol Neurosurg Psychiatry. 2005;76:395–400.
51. Tornetta III P, Mostafavi H, Riina J, et al. Morbidity and mortality in elderly trauma patients. J Trauma. 1999;46:702–6.
52. Utomo WK, Gabbe BJ, Simpson PM, et al. Predictors of in-hospital mortality and 6-month functional outcomes in older adults after moderate to severe traumatic brain injury. Injury. 2011;40:973–7.
53. Irvine DH, Foster JB, Newell DJ. Prevalence of cervical spondylosis in a general practice. Lancet. 1965;22 (14):1089–92.
54. Donaldson 3rd WF, Towers JD, Doctor A, et al. A methodology to evaluate motion of the unstable spine during intubation techniques. Spine. 1993;18:2020–3.
55. Unni VK, Johnston RA, Young HS, et al. Prevention of intracranial hypertension during laryngoscopy and endotracheal intubation. Br J Anaesth. 1984;56:1219–23.
56. Bratton SL, Chestnut RM, Ghajar J, et al. Guidelines for the management of severe traumatic brain injury. IX. Cerebral perfusion thresholds. J Neurotrauma. 2007;24:S59–64.
57. Battle CE, Hutchings H, Evans PA. Risk factors that predict mortality in patients with blunt chest wall trauma: a systematic review and meta-analysis. Injury. 2012;43:8.
58. Gowing G, Jain MK. Injury patterns and outcomes associated with elderly trauma victims in Kingston, Ontario. Can J Surg. 2007;50(6):437–44.
59. Bulger EM, Arneson MA, Mock CN, Jurkovich GJ. Rib fractures in the elderly. J Trauma. 2000;48:1040.
60. Cohn S. Pulmonary contusion: review of the clinical entity. J Trauma. 1997;42:973–9.
61. Cordell-Smith JA, Roberts N, Peek GJ, Firmin RK. Traumatic lung injury treated by extracorporeal membrane oxygenation (ECMO). Injury. 2006;37:29–32.
62. ARDSnet. Ventilation with lower tidal volumes as compared with traditional tidal volumes for acute lung injury and acute respiratory distress syndrome. N Engl J Med. 2000;342:1301–8.
63. Ullman DA, Wimpy RE, Fortune JB, et al. The treatment of patients with multiple rib fractures using continuous thoracic epidural narcotic infusions. Reg Anesth. 1989;14:43–7.
64. John AD, Sieber FE. Age associated issues: geriatrics. Anesthesiol Clin North America. 2004;22:45–58.
65. Bickel H, Gradinger R, Kochs E, Forstl H. High risk of cognitive and functional decline after postoperative delirium. A three-year prospective study. Dement Geriatr Cogn Disord. 2008;26:26–31.

Trauma Critical Care

18

J. David Roccaforte

Introduction

In a typical urban trauma system, severely injured patients may spend 10–20 min being treated by paramedics in the field and during transport, then 20–40 min in the trauma resuscitation area while the primary and secondary surveys of advanced trauma life support (ATLS®) are performed. If patients are hemodynamically unstable and a damage control procedure is indicated, they will be in the operating room for 45 min to an hour. Critical care has begun.

For the subsequent 1–3 days that patients may spend between the operating room and the post-anesthesia recovery unit (PACU) during the damage control sequence, critical care medicine is being practiced. Once the definitive surgical and interventional procedures are completed, patients are then formally transferred to an intensive care unit, where they may remain for the next 2–3 weeks or even longer, if they survive. This is not to minimize the importance of properly executed pre-hospital care and ATLS®, but from the time of injury to hospital discharge, most of the severely injured trauma victim's time is clearly spent as a critical care patient.

Comprehensive management of trauma victims is a team effort, and nowhere is this more apparent than in the operating room. While the surgeons are focused on the operative repair of injuries, the anesthesiologists are managing all other aspects of an unstable patient in shock. Upwards of 90 % of what constitutes critical care for trauma patients is what anesthesiologists are providing for them in the operating room and subsequently in the PACU.

In most European countries, critical care training and certification is part of every anesthesiologist's credentialing. In the United States and some other countries, the critical care subspecialty requires an additional year of fellowship training. Regardless, the value of anesthesiologists' expertise and collaborative participation in the critical care of the severely injured trauma patient cannot be overstated.

In the critical care management of the severely injured trauma patient, there is significant overlap in expertise between surgical and anesthesiology-trained intensivists. Indeed, the unique capabilities of each are complementary, and close collaboration yields a complete spectrum of necessary expertise (see Table 18.1).

Increasingly, traumatic injuries are treated non-operatively, with or without interventional radiology, or with a staged, damage control approach. An integral component to all of these management strategies is a significant amount of time spent in the PACU or the intensive care unit (ICU) for close monitoring, continued resuscitation, and correction of coagulation and metabolic abnormalities. At a minimum, for PACU management, all anesthesiologists must

J.D. Roccaforte, M.D. (✉)
Department of Anesthesiology, New York University, Bellevue Hospital, 1st Avenue, 27th Street, New York, NY 10016, USA
e-mail: jdavidr@mail.com

C.S. Scher (ed.), *Anesthesia for Trauma*, DOI 10.1007/978-1-4939-0909-4_18,
© Springer Science+Business Media New York 2014

Table 18.1 Expertise required to manage severely injured trauma patients

Unique to surgeons	Shared by intensivists	Unique to anesthesiologists
Expeditiously diagnosing life-threatening traumatic injuries	Fluid resuscitation from hemorrhagic shock	Enabling unstable trauma patients to tolerate surgery without pain
Repairing damage surgically	Advanced hemodynamic monitoring	Maintaining intraoperative physiologic homeostasis
Advanced bedside procedures	Invasive line placement	Advanced airway management
Wound care	Basic pain management and sedation	Advanced pain management
	Management of elevated ICP, spinal cord injury	
	Assessing chronic and acute medical issues (stroke, MI, DM, etc.)	
	Managing coagulation	
	Ventilator management and weaning	
	Diagnosing and treating infection	
	Performing bronchoscopy, basic echocardiography	
	Providing adequate nutrition	
	Supporting renal function	
	Providing family communication and social support	

be familiar with the critical care issues of the severely injured trauma patient, and ideally anesthesiologists can contribute their expertise as fully integrated members of the trauma team.

Intensivist-led critical care (closed ICU) appears to confer both process efficiencies, as well as survival benefits when compared to an open-ICU model of care [1], especially with respect to the elderly [2]. From the patient's perspective there is not a surgical team, ICU team, nursing team, physical therapy team, etc.—there is only one, multidisciplinary team. Once the time-dependent acute care has transitioned into the longer-term critical care phase, patients benefit from collaborative care, where all providers are able to offer and discuss their recommendations and priorities based on their perspectives, experience, and expertise. From the ensuing negotiations and compromises, the best care plan emerges. Ultimately, the plan must be unified and deliberate, and that is the responsibility of the intensivist, regardless of his or her primary specialty [3].

Critical care issues commonly encountered in the severely injured trauma patient span resuscitation, procedural, damage control, subacute, and occasionally end-of-life phases of the patient's hospital course. Specific considerations will be addressed for each phase.

Resuscitation and Intraoperative Phase

Acute trauma (especially penetrating) can be described as the uncontrolled start to a surgical procedure, where the incision has been made, but anesthetic care has yet to begin. Whenever possible, even when not formally required to respond to a trauma activation, a member of the anesthesia and/or intensive care service should make an effort to be present when trauma patients arrive at the hospital, if for no other reason than to anticipate and communicate staffing and operating room needs. Apart from airway management issues, tremendous value is derived from their presence by providing early access to anesthesia-related and critical care services.

All stable patients eventually destined for the operating room (e.g., open ankle fractures) should be screened for significant comorbidities, potential difficult airway issues, or any other obvious anesthetic concerns. Patients may be conscious initially, or family members, friends, or colleagues may be present who can be queried about medical conditions, allergies, etc. While the primary and secondary surveys are directed at quickly diagnosing trauma-related injuries, it is of benefit to have someone assessing the patient with a different perspective. Occasionally a traumatic injury from a vehicular crash or a fall is precipitated by syncope secondary to a medical condition such as an arrhythmia, or hypoglycemia. Although not the first priority when significant injuries are present, these aspects of history and observation may often have critical implications later in the patient's course.

Early anesthesiologist/intensivist participation also provides an opportunity for observing a patient on arrival, which can present with a very different picture than 18 h later, when the same patient is intubated, unconscious, edematous, has eyes taped closed, and may have an open abdomen.

For unstable patients who require rapid transfer to the operating room (OR) or to interventional radiology (IR), immediate and continuous bedside anesthesia and critical care management can be initiated. This may include airway management, vascular access, arterial line placement, resuscitation and transfusion, sedation and analgesia. If time allows, a more thorough preoperative evaluation, and anesthesia consent may be obtained and documented. The anesthesiologist/intensivist can then assist in the safe transport of the unstable patient to the IR suite or the OR, and facilitate a safe transfer of care to the anesthesiologists who will take over the case.

When chronic or acute medical conditions such as a permanent pacemaker, an automated implantable cardioverter-defibrillator, chronic heart failure, diabetes, anticoagulation, renal dysfunction, electrolyte abnormalities, or arrhythmias are identified, they should be managed as soon as possible.

If the anesthesiologist/intensivist is involved in the resuscitation, clear communication with the trauma surgeon is paramount. Anesthesiologists are tremendously capable of maintaining a patient's vital signs near normal with fluids, blood products and/or pressors. It must be appreciated that some of the surgeon's decision-making acumen is contingent on an accurate assessment of the patient's hemodynamic stability. Examples of this are whether to move the patient to radiology to perform a diagnostic study or to proceed to the OR directly, or to attempt limb salvage versus performing an amputation. If a patient's vital signs are maintained only with ongoing resuscitation or with pressors, this does NOT reflect hemodynamic stability and MUST be communicated to the surgeon as such.

During the acute resuscitation and operative phase of the patient's course, the most immediate threats to life are uncontrolled hemorrhage, and brainstem herniation. Infection is generally a low-priority concern. However, this is the phase where contamination and microbial exposure occur, and to successfully save a patient's life in the operating room, only to have them succumb to sepsis 2 weeks later can be devastating. Consequently, all lines placed in the field or those placed in the hospital using less-than-ideal sterile technique must be removed and replaced as soon as possible. Additionally, standard antibiotic prophylaxis must be administered [4], and in the setting of a massive resuscitation, repeated as appropriate.

In the operating room, having a clear vision of future ICU issues can suggest possible early interventions. For example, a patient with a high lower extremity amputation with perineal involvement might benefit from a diverting colostomy to help maintain clean wound care. To help prevent decubitus ulcers, back boards must be removed, using log-rolling to protect the spine, and hard-padded extrication cervical immobilizing collars from the field must be replaced with those designed for longer-term use such as the Miami-J or Philadelphia collar. Anticipating frequent painful dressing changes might suggest the placement of a peripheral catheter for the regional infusion of local anesthetic or an epidural if the neuraxial spine has been cleared.

Early tracheostomy and enteral feeding access can often be accomplished safely during the first operative procedure. While the merits of these interventions performed early can be debated [5], often the reason that they were not done is that the clinical focus at the time was on immediate injuries, not subsequent ICU issues.

Patients with baseline renal insufficiency, those receiving copious amounts of intravenous (IV) contrast media, or those with massive crush injuries with rhabdomyolysis may benefit from early initiation of renal prophylaxis using enteral *N*-acetylcysteine (NAC) and intravenous sodium bicarbonate hydration as per published protocols [6]. In addition, dialysis access may be placed sterilely in the operating room and arrangements made for renal replacement therapy.

How blood products are managed in a massive transfusion scenario can have implications for the subsequent critical care phase. The priorities in an exsanguinating patient are to control bleeding surgically, to anticipate and avoid severe hypovolemia, anemia, and coagulopathy. However, once bleeding is controlled, subsequent transfusions should aim to treat specific objective abnormalities, not to "catch up" to an arbitrary packed red blood cell (PRBC):fresh frozen plasma (FFP):platelet ratio. Transfusions of blood products have been independently associated with the systemic inflammatory response syndrome, multi-organ system failure, immunosuppression, infection, acute respiratory distress syndrome (ARDS), and increased mortality [7]. There is often an opportunity to conserve blood using cell-saver autologous transfusion, especially with thoracic trauma [8].

For patients with an anticipated critical illness of greater than 5 days, early erythropoietin, 40,000 units weekly should be considered. In a 2002 prospective, placebo-controlled, randomized trial, this intervention demonstrated a decreased ICU transfusion exposure for anemia due to phlebotomy and suppressed endogenous erythropoiesis [9]. However, a follow-up study published in 2007 failed to demonstrate significantly decreased PRBC transfusions, although for trauma patients specifically mortality was reduced, despite having thrombotic complications significantly increased overall [10]. Erythropoietin is discontinued on discharge from the intensive care unit. Thrombotic complications associated with chronic erythropoietin reported in oncology and renal failure

patients [11] do not appear to occur with similar frequency in the trauma ICU population [12].

Family communication and ethical issues surrounding surrogate decision-making, advanced directives, futility, and organ procurement often present first during the resuscitation and operative phase of care. While the eventual resolution of these issues can require hours of meetings and discussion, it is important to be attentive to the brief discussions that occur at this early phase, as they will set the tone for further interactions during the rest of the patient's hospital stay.

Damage Control Phase

During the damage control phase of care, all of the critical care objectives described in the Resuscitation and Intraoperative phase remain in effect. The strategy of damage control refers to the acute operative management of an unstable trauma patient with the following objectives [13]:

- Abbreviated laparotomy and/or resuscitative thoracotomy
- Provisional control of arterial bleeding
- Provisional control of fecal spillage
- Packing of venous bleeding
- Fracture stabilization (ex-fix or splint only)
- Angio-embolization as required
- PACU or ICU for resuscitation
- Staged return to OR for definitive procedures

Definitive repair of vascular and abdominal injuries is deferred until the patient's physiologic and metabolic abnormalities can be corrected. Therefore, "damage control resuscitation" has been described, in addition to "damage control surgery," with the objectives being restoration of intravascular volume, red cell mass, coagulation functionality, and normothermia [14]. In a retrospective analysis, the combination of damage control surgical and resuscitation strategies was associated with improved survival [15].

In between a patient's damage control and each definitive operation, it is important to lighten sedation in the PACU or ICU and to confirm a basic neurologic exam. Any focal deficits should prompt thorough evaluation. Generally, patients remain sedated, intubated, and ventilated during this period. Prophylactic antibiotics should be re-dosed, and a tetanus booster given if not already done [16]. For patients at risk of renal failure, all medications should be dose-adjusted to estimated creatinine clearance.

Once the patient is no longer in shock, initiation of enteral feeding at trophic rates should be considered. Animal data suggests that bowel edema may be minimized by providing enterocytes with access to directly absorbed energy [17]. Obviously, patients with bowel injury or a severe ileus may become distended, and in these cases full enteral nutrition must unfortunately be deferred.

If the abdominal fascia has been left open, abdominal compartment syndrome is unlikely to occur. However if closed, the combination of decreased urine output, hypotension, and tachycardia despite elevated central venous pressure, a rising serum lactate, and elevated airway pressures should trigger objective measurement of bladder pressure which is a surrogate of intra-abdominal pressure [18].

In patients with head trauma, a repeat head CT is often obtained after the initial damage control procedure. Senior anesthesia or critical care personnel should accompany the patient, as transport represents a vulnerable period when tubes, lines, drains, and monitors may be inadvertently and tragically dislodged [19].

Intracranial pressure may need to be actively managed. Ideally an intracranial pressure monitor will have been placed in the operating room, which will allow cerebral perfusion pressure to be optimized when coupled with central venous and arterial pressure monitoring. The comprehensive guidelines for managing traumatic brain injury published by the Brain Trauma Foundation should be followed [20].

Subacute Phase

The longer a patient remains in the hospital, the more likely they are to suffer from nosocomial infections [21], iatrogenic complications, and from their chronic medical conditions. A comprehensive treatment of all possible critical care issues is beyond the scope of this chapter, which will focus on the most common conditions faced by trauma patients in the ICU, and the pitfalls to treatment faced by their providers.

Neurologic Issues

Frequently severely injured trauma patients are unconscious. It is incumbent on the intensivist to differentiate residual (or intentional) sedation from pathologic coma. A daily wake-up, i.e., a sedation holiday, should be initiated in all but a few select patients. Daily wake-up testing has been associated with less time spent mechanically ventilated [22], but it also allows for a neurologic examination. Caution should be exercised when interrupting sedation in patients with elevated intracranial pressure [23].

The prognosis for functional outcome after traumatic and anoxic brain injury is not the same [24]. For anoxic brain injury without improvement, it is possible with a high degree of certainty to state that the condition will be chronic after only a few days in a vegetative state. In contrast, following traumatic brain injury, generally only 6 months after the acute medical issues such as ARDS or renal failure have resolved can families be counseled that the patient's condition is unlikely to improve [25].

Even for patients without structural damage visible on a head CT, injuries resulting in loss of consciousness or other evidence of concussion may have neurologic sequelae [26] such as dizziness, inattention, or personality changes, that are difficult to detect without objective neuropsychiatric testing, or a close, personal knowledge of the patient.

The relationship of sedation and analgesia to delirium is complex [27]. Benzodiazepine use is associated with delirium [28]. Delusional memories of delirious ICU episodes [29] appear to be a risk factor for post-traumatic stress disorder [30], especially if pain is undertreated [31]. On the other hand, deep sedation, especially with benzodiazepines induces amnesia of the ICU stay, and post-traumatic stress disorder risk is minimal [32]. Ideally we should be able to keep patients comfortable, interactive, and free from psychic trauma and delirium [33]. Various techniques such as dexmedetomidine [34] and bispectral index (BIS) monitors [35] have been studied, though a reliable recipe to accomplish those objectives remains to be described.

The mere presence of a patient in an ICU has been suggested as a cause of delirium, an "intensive care unit syndrome," [36] even though a simple dose-response relationship does not exist. The delirium is probably multifactorial—with factors like mild head injury, electrolyte abnormalities, mild hepatic dysfunction, and systemic inflammation all contributing. In managing the delirious ICU patient it is important not to overlook a treatable condition such as alcohol withdrawal, while at the same time keeping the patient safe.

Phantom limb and chronic pain syndromes are common following traumatic amputation [37]. It might seem that a dense nerve block with a regional or epidural catheter would mitigate the development of these syndromes. Paradoxically, however, this may render patients more susceptible by blocking inhibitory pathways.

Brain death is a diagnosis that is equivalent to death. It represents an irreversible condition of no blood flow to the brain or brain stem [38]. Protocols for evaluating and declaring brain death should only be implemented in patients with a known diagnosis that can explain the condition [39]. Validated trauma centers will have standing relationships with organ procurement organizations.

Cardiac Support

Typical cardiac issues with trauma patients are new-onset atrial fibrillation (AF) or supraventricular tachycardia (SVT), non-ST-segment myocardial infarction (MI) or subclinical troponin leaks, blunt cardiac injury, heart failure, and cardiomyopathy.

Acute AF or SVT can be problematic, especially when relative contraindications exist for therapeutic anticoagulation, such as traumatic subarachnoid hemorrhage. The increased sympathetic tone provoking the arrhythmia is usually transient, and provided the patient is volume resuscitated and has normal baseline cardiac function, aggressive beta blockade is usually sufficient for rate control. This allows spontaneous conversion to sinus rhythm to occur in greater than 50 % of patients at 48 h. Calcium channel blockers can potentially inhibit conversion to sinus rhythm [40], and should be reserved for rate control in a patient who has an intracardiac thrombus, or who has committed to long-term anticoagulation and rate control. Digoxin would be the rate-control agent of choice for a patient with baseline cardiac dysfunction.

After 24 h, if sinus rhythm is not restored, an anti-arrhythmic agent such as procainamide or amiodarone can be given, and if at 48 h the AF/SVT persists, then cardioversion may be attempted. If successful, short-term therapeutic anticoagulation should then be initiated, unless contraindicated. If cardioversion is unsuccessful and AF/SVT persists, then long-term anticoagulation will have to be implemented to decrease the risk of stroke [41]. The risk of long-term anticoagulation may be higher in the trauma population given that a good predictor of future traumatic injury is past trauma [42].

Blunt cardiac injury [43], non-ST-wave MI, and subclinical troponin leak are all treated supportively with monitoring. An invasive procedure should be considered only if symptoms occur, or if heart failure manifests. The value of routine echocardiography in these settings remains controversial. Acute coronary interventions are rarely indicated. Conventionally, if a patient has remained hemodynamically stable, without arrhythmias for 24 h post-injury, further ICU telemetry monitoring may not be necessary.

If heart failure develops, either as a consequence of baseline pathology, or from blunt cardiac injury, or (rarely) from a tachycardia-induced cardiomyopathy, prognosis is poor, especially if this is accompanied by multi-organ failure following blunt polytrauma. Echocardiography may be employed to assist in diagnosing cardiac dysfunction. Supra-normal cardiac indices are associated with improved outcomes, however elevating cardiac output exogenously with inotropes, or increasing oxygen delivery with transfusions does not appear to improve outcome. It is simply that those who can elevate their cardiac function to meet the increased metabolic demands following trauma are more likely to survive than those who cannot [44].

Respiratory Support

The criteria for securing a trauma patient's airway are more liberal than with the typical medical patient [45]. Patients are frequently intoxicated [46] and may not cooperate with diagnostic studies, thereby delaying care during the golden hour. Other early indications for respiratory support include pneumothorax, aspiration pneumonitis, pulmonary contusions or lacerations, multiple rib fractures, cervical spinal cord injury, and fat embolism syndrome. Respiratory failure or hypoxia occurring later in the trauma patient's course can be from pneumonia, congestive heart failure (CHF), transfusion-related acute lung injury (TRALI), or ARDS.

Recruitment maneuvers can cure atelectasis [47]. Ventilator management is supportive, and should follow an open-lung, lung-protective strategy such as that described in the ARDSnet trial [48]. Typical settings would be volume-control or pressure support with 6 mL/kg tidal volume, respiratory rate high enough to maintain normal pCO_2, limited by evidence of air-trapping and auto-peep, in which case elevated pCO_2 would be tolerated with increased sedation and rarely neuromuscular blockade. FIO_2 and positive end-expiratory pressure (PEEP) are titrated to maintain pO_2 above 55, as per the ARDnet protocol [49] (see Table 18.2).

Novel modes of ventilation such as high-frequency oscillation [50], or airway-pressure-release ventilation (APRV) [51], may be used as rescue modes, but none have proved to improve survival compared to the ARDSnet protocol.

Indications for bronchoscopy include diagnostic evaluation for penetrating injury or foreign body aspiration, and therapeutic removal of

Table 18.2 FIO_2 and PEEP combinations for ARDS-net protocol ventilator settings [48]

FIO_2	PEEP
0.30	5
0.40	5
0.40	8
0.50	8
0.60	10
0.70	10
0.70	12
0.80	14
0.90	14
0.90	16
1.0	18
1.0	20–24

mucous plugging refractory to straight-catheter suctioning. Bronchoscopy need not be employed routinely for percutaneous tracheostomy, though it may be appropriate for select patients such as those in cervical fixation devices, with known difficult airway anatomy, the obese, or those with high FIO_2 requirements [52].

Respiratory failure due to pain and splinting from multiple rib fractures, flail chest, or pulmonary contusion [53] is best treated with a thoracic epidural catheter. If that is contraindicated because of spinal injury or anticoagulation, intercostal nerve blocks are an alternative [54].

Ventilator support should be weaned continuously, and discontinued as early as possible.

Renal Support

Renal prophylaxis has been discussed, and should be implemented whenever exposure to IV contrast is anticipated, especially if baseline creatinine is elevated [55]. Oral NAC, intravenous hydration and sodium bicarbonate are low-cost, low-risk interventions which may benefit and are unlikely to cause harm in a monitored patient [56].

For patients requiring renal replacement therapy, continuous veno-venous hemofiltration (CVVH) offers a hypothetical advantage by causing less hemodynamic instability as compared to conventional intermittent hemodialysis (HD).

A prospective randomized trial comparing the two modes failed to demonstrate a survival benefit of CVVH [57]. The study randomized all ICU patients requiring renal replacement to receive CVVH or HD. However, since ICU mortality in most patients rarely depends on the mode of dialysis, it is unlikely that the study as designed could reveal improved survival for CVVH. A properly designed study would enroll only those patients who were unable to tolerate conventional HD, and randomize them to receive CVVH or to continue with HD, but this would be unethical. CVVH availability must therefore be justified, despite the lack of class I evidence and, given its increased expense, staffing requirements, and resource utilization, should be reserved for patients who do not tolerate conventional HD.

Infectious Disease and Antibiotic Issues

Fever in the ICU has a poor signal to noise ratio [58]. Trauma patients are often febrile from their inflammatory response to soft-tissue injury, as a consequence of central dysregulation following traumatic brain injury, or from an immunologic reaction to transfusions or medications. The specter of infection cannot, however, be dismissed merely because a noninfectious explanation can be provided. When evaluating a patient for fever, source control is the top priority [59]. A thorough head-to-toe examination will identify most soft-tissue infections and disclose an intra-abdominal source. Culture specimens should be promptly collected from blood, sputum, and urine as per established guidelines [60], as well as from any other suspected source, as indicated by the patient's history. Broad-spectrum antibiotics should be initiated as soon as possible [61], ideally after cultures are obtained. Antibiotics should then be narrowed or discontinued depending on the culture results and the patient's condition.

Nutrition, Electrolytes, and Prophylaxis

All patients should receive adequate nutrition. The consequences of malnutrition and starvation begin to manifest as organ system dysfunction after 2 weeks, continuing to irreversible damage by 3 or 4 weeks, and ultimately ending in death [62]. No prospective randomized trial has ever been performed attempting to demonstrate the survival benefit of starvation. There are, in contrast, innumerable examples worldwide and throughout history associating starvation with death [63].

The ideal route for nutrition is the digestive tract. When the gut is unavailable, parenteral nutrition is acceptable, and while it has associated complications [64], it can sustain life for years [65]. Caloric needs of trauma patients are greater than those of the uninjured [66]. Burn [67] and head injuries [68] increase metabolic demands, and additional calories and protein should be provided. Overfeeding can manifest as respiratory failure from increased CO_2 production, elevated liver function enzymes from fatty liver, and diarrhea from the increased osmotic load [69]. In general, underfeeding is the bigger concern. In studies observing prescribed vs. delivered calories, on average, only 75 % of nutritional goals are met [70]. For ICU patients scheduled for an operative procedure, tube feeding need not be interrupted if the airway is protected with an endotracheal tube, and the surgery does not involve the aero-digestive tract.

Refeeding syndrome, which initially presents with hypophosphatemia, can be lethal if untreated [71]. While in starvation mode, the body defers many cellular functions, and once nutrition becomes available the backlog of cellular maintenance accelerates. This requires ATP, which requires phosphate. The body's store of phosphate is vast, however release from bone occurs relatively slowly. Initially during refeeding, serum phosphate can become depleted, and an acute ATP deficit develops. As a consequence, any cells requiring ATP as an energy source (i.e., all cells) are subject to dysfunction or failure. Late manifestations include rhabdomyolysis, hemolysis, diffuse intravascular coagulopathy, renal failure, cardiomyopathy, arrhythmias, liver failure, and death [72].

Hypophosphatemia must be treated aggressively when detected [73], and if refractory, nutrition must be held until serum phosphate levels can be restored to normal.

Other electrolytes are supplemented or restricted based on laboratory values. Sodium abnormalities are common, though rarely of consequence provided the levels change slowly [74].

Several prophylactic interventions have been associated with improved outcomes and cost-benefit to patients in the ICU. These include head of bed elevation to decrease ventilator-associated pneumonia, gastric acid suppression to prevent stress ulcers and anticoagulation and/or sequential compression devices to prevent deep vein thrombosis. Specific recommendations and guidelines are frequently updated [75].

The placement of an inferior vena cava (IVC) filter is clearly indicated for only a minority of cases, such as a patient with a known lower extremity DVT. Other ongoing risk factors include a baseline hypercoagulable syndrome and immobility, lower extremity fractures, poor respiratory reserve, right heart strain, and a contra-indication to anticoagulation or thrombolysis, like a recent subarachnoid hemorrhage. In most patients, however, the risks and benefits are equivocal. IVC filters are mildly effective protection from massive pulmonary thromboembolus for only a few weeks, after which time collateral veins dilate, and the risk of PE returns to baseline. The potential complications of the in situ filter, however, persist. Retrievable filters would seem to be a good compromise, however, the retrieval rate is very low [76].

Palliative Care and End-of-Life Issues

Despite tremendous advances in trauma surgery, damage control, and critical care, immortality remains elusive [77]. Early recognition of the dying patient can offer opportunities for open, realistic discussions with family members regarding their loved one's wishes given the circumstances, and allow for meaningful interactions during the patient's remaining time alive. Various organ-system-failure and acuity grading methodologies like APACHE-2 [78] can be utilized to provide some perspective on prognosis, but an experienced intensivist can both recognize and compassionately communicate to the family that the patient's condition is deteriorating despite maximum critical care.

Having expertise in providing palliative care and comfort measures is invaluable in these circumstances. Traumatic injuries generally affect a younger, more active population, and as a rule they are sudden and unanticipated. When trauma patients die it can be incredibly emotional for families and care providers alike [79]. Being able to advise and counsel families and staff through this period can be both a difficult and rewarding aspect of critical care [80].

Conclusion

From the moment a trauma patient arrives to the hospital, anesthesiologists have ample expertise and opportunity to provide critical care. A thorough understanding of critical care issues and principles enables seamless care as severely injured patients transition from the trauma resuscitation area to the operating room, to the PACU and eventually to the ICU.

References

1. Nathens AB, Rivara FP, MacKenzie EJ, Maier RV, Wang J, Egleston B, Scharfstein DO, Jurkovich GJ. The impact of an intensivist-model ICU on trauma-related mortality. Ann Surg. 2006;244(4):545–54.
2. Petitti D, Bennett V, Chao Hu CK. Association of changes in the use of board-certified critical care intensivists with mortality outcomes for trauma patients at a well-established level I urban trauma center. J Trauma Manag Outcomes. 2012;6:3.
3. Matsushima K, Goldwasser ER, Schaefer EW, Armen SB, Indeck MC. The impact of intensivists' base specialty of training on care process and outcomes of critically ill trauma patients. J Surg Res. 2013;184 (1):577–81.
4. Goldberg SR, Anand RJ, Como JJ, Dechert T, Dente C, Luchette FA, Ivatury RR, Duane TM, Eastern Association for the Surgery of Trauma. Prophylactic antibiotic use in penetrating abdominal trauma: an Eastern Association for the Surgery of Trauma practice management guideline. J Trauma Acute Care Surg. 2012;73(5 Suppl 4):S321–5.
5. Gomes Silva BN, Andriolo RB, Saconato H, Atallah AN, Valente O. Early versus late tracheostomy for critically ill patients. Cochrane Database Syst Rev. 2012;3, CD007271.

6. Brown JR, Block CA, Malenka DJ, O'Connor GT, Schoolwerth AC, Thompson CA. Sodium bicarbonate plus N-acetylcysteine prophylaxis: a meta-analysis. JACC Cardiovasc Interv. 2009;2(11):1116–24.

7. Sihler KC, Napolitano LM. Complications of massive transfusion. Chest. 2010;137(1):209–20.

8. Salhanick M, Corneille M, Higgins R, Olson J, Michalek J, Harrison C, Stewart R, Dent D. Auto-transfusion of hemothorax blood in trauma patients: is it the same as fresh whole blood? Am J Surg. 2011;202(6):817–21; discussion 821–2.

9. Corwin HL, Gettinger A, Pearl RG, Fink MP, Levy MM, Shapiro MJ, Corwin MJ, Colton T, EPO Critical Care Trials Group. Efficacy of recombinant human erythropoietin in critically ill patients: a randomized controlled trial. JAMA. 2002;288(22):2827–35.

10. Corwin HL, Gettinger A, Fabian TC, May A, Pearl RG, Heard S, An R, Bowers PJ, Burton P, Klausner MA, Corwin MJ, EPO Critical Care Trials Group. Efficacy and safety of epoetin alfa in critically ill patients. N Engl J Med. 2007;357(10):965–76.

11. Lippi G, Franchini M, Favaloro EJ. Thrombotic complications of erythropoiesis-stimulating agents. Semin Thromb Hemost. 2010;36(5):537–49.

12. Luchette FA, Pasquale MD, Fabian TC, Langholff WK, Wolfson M. A randomized, double-blind, placebo-controlled study to assess the effect of recombinant human erythropoietin on functional outcomes in anemic, critically ill, trauma subjects: the Long Term Trauma Outcomes Study. Am J Surg. 2012;203(4):508–16.

13. Waibel BH, Rotondo MF. Damage control in trauma and abdominal sepsis. Crit Care Med. 2010;38(9 Suppl):S421–30.

14. Sagraves SG, Toschlog EA, Rotondo MF. Damage control surgery—the intensivist's role. J Intensive Care Med. 2006;21(1):5–16.

15. Duchesne JC, Kimonis K, Marr AB, Rennie KV, Wahl G, Wells JE, Islam TM, Meade P, Stuke L, Barbeau JM, Hunt JP, Baker CC, McSwain Jr NE. Damage control resuscitation in combination with damage control laparotomy: a survival advantage. J Trauma. 2010;69(1):46–52.

16. Talan DA, Abrahamian FM, Moran GJ, Mower WR, Alagappan K, Tiffany BR, Pollack Jr CV, Steele MT, Dunbar LM, Bajani MD, Weyant RS, Ostroff SM. Tetanus immunity and physician compliance with tetanus prophylaxis practices among emergency department patients presenting with wounds. Ann Emerg Med. 2004;43(3):305–14.

17. Moore-Olufemi SD, Padalecki J, Olufemi SE, Xue H, Oliver DH, Radhakrishnan RS, Allen SJ, Moore FA, Stewart R, Laine GA, Cox Jr CS. Intestinal edema: effect of enteral feeding on motility and gene expression. J Surg Res. 2009;155(2):283–92.

18. Kirkpatrick AW, Roberts DJ, De Waele J, Jaeschke R, Malbrain ML, De Keulenaer B, Duchesne J, Bjorck M, Leppaniemi A, Ejike JC, Sugrue M, Cheatham M, Ivatury R, Ball CG, Reintam Blaser A, Regli A, Balogh ZJ, D'Amours S, Debergh D, Kaplan M, Kimball E, Olvera C, Pediatric Guidelines Sub-Committee for the World Society of the Abdominal Compartment Syndrome. Intra-abdominal hypertension and the abdominal compartment syndrome: updated consensus definitions and clinical practice guidelines from the World Society of the Abdominal Compartment Syndrome. Intensive Care Med. 2013;39(7):1190–206.

19. Parmentier-Decrucq E, Poissy J, Favory R, Nseir S, Onimus T, Guerry MJ, Durocher A, Mathieu D. Adverse events during intrahospital transport of critically ill patients: incidence and risk factors. Ann Intensive Care. 2013;3(1):10.

20. Brain Trauma Foundation, American Association of Neurological Surgeons; Congress of Neurological Surgeons. Guidelines for the management of severe traumatic brain injury. J Neurotrauma. 2007;24 Suppl 1:S1–106.

21. Glance LG, Stone PW, Mukamel DB, Dick AW. Increases in mortality, length of stay, and cost associated with hospital-acquired infections in trauma patients. Arch Surg. 2011;146(7):794–801.

22. Mehta S, Burry L, Cook D, Fergusson D, Steinberg M, Granton J, Herridge M, Ferguson N, Devlin J, Tanios M, Dodek P, Fowler R, Burns K, Jacka M, Olafson K, Skrobik Y, Hébert P, Sabri E, Meade M, SLEAP Investigators, Canadian Critical Care Trials Group. Daily sedation interruption in mechanically ventilated critically ill patients cared for with a sedation protocol: a randomized controlled trial. JAMA. 2012;308(19):1985–92.

23. Helbok R, Kurtz P, Schmidt MJ, Stuart MR, Fernandez L, Connolly SE, Lee K, Schmutzhard E, Mayer SA, Claassen J, Badjatia N. Effects of the neurological wake-up test on clinical examination, intracranial pressure, brain metabolism and brain tissue oxygenation in severely brain-injured patients. Crit Care. 2012;16(6):R226.

24. Cullen NK, Park YG, Bayley MT. Functional recovery following traumatic vs non-traumatic brain injury: a case-controlled study. Brain Inj. 2008;22(13–14):1013–20.

25. Attia J, Cook DJ. Prognosis in anoxic and traumatic coma. Crit Care Clin. 1998;14(3):497–511.

26. Reuben A, Sampson P, Harris AR, Williams H, Yates P. Postconcussion syndrome (PCS) in the emergency department: predicting and pre-empting persistent symptoms following a mild traumatic brain injury. Emerg Med J. 2014;31(1):72–7.

27. Devlin JW, Fraser GL, Ely EW, Kress JP, Skrobik Y, Dasta JF. Pharmacological management of sedation and delirium in mechanically ventilated ICU patients: remaining evidence gaps and controversies. Semin Respir Crit Care Med. 2013;34(2):201–15.

28. Micek ST, Anand NJ, Laible BR, Shannon WD, Kollef MH. Delirium as detected by the CAM-ICU predicts restraint use among mechanically ventilated medical patients. Crit Care Med. 2005;33(6):1260–5.

29. Jones C, Griffiths RD, Humphris G, Skirrow PM. Memory, delusions, and the development of acute

posttraumatic stress disorder-related symptoms after intensive care. Crit Care Med. 2001;29(3):573–80.

30. Svenningsen H. Associations between sedation, delirium and post-traumatic stress disorder and their impact on quality of life and memories following discharge from an intensive care unit. Dan Med J. 2013;60(4):B4630.

31. Wade D, Hardy R, Howell D, Mythen M. Identifying clinical and acute psychological risk factors for PTSD after critical care: a systematic review. Minerva Anestesiol. 2013;79(8):944–63.

32. Weinert CR, Sprenkle M. Post-ICU consequences of patient wakefulness and sedative exposure during mechanical ventilation. Intensive Care Med. 2008;34 (1):82–90.

33. Ethier C, Burry L, Martinez-Motta C, Tirgari S, Jiang D, McDonald E, Granton J, Cook D, Mehta S, Canadian Critical Care Trials Group. Recall of intensive care unit stay in patients managed with a sedation protocol or a sedation protocol with daily sedative interruption: a pilot study. J Crit Care. 2011;26(2):127–32.

34. Riker RR, Shehabi Y, Bokesch PM, Ceraso D, Wisemandle W, Koura F, Whitten P, Margolis BD, Byrne DW, Ely EW, Rocha MG, SEDCOM (Safety and Efficacy of Dexmedetomidine Compared With Midazolam) Study Group. Dexmedetomidine vs midazolam for sedation of critically ill patients: a randomized trial. JAMA. 2009;301(5):489–99.

35. Nasraway Jr SASA, Wu EC, Kelleher RM, Yasuda CM, Donnelly AM. How reliable is the bispectral index in critically ill patients? A prospective, comparative, single-blinded observer study. Crit Care Med. 2002;30(7):1483–7.

36. McGuire BE, Basten CJ, Ryan CJ, Gallagher J. Intensive care unit syndrome: a dangerous misnomer. Arch Intern Med. 2000;160(7):906–9.

37. Halbert J, Crotty M, Cameron ID. Evidence for the optimal management of acute and chronic phantom pain: a systematic review. Clin J Pain. 2002;18(2):84–92.

38. Wijdicks EF, Varelas PN, Gronseth GS, Greer DM, American Academy of Neurology. Evidence-based guideline update: determining brain death in adults: report of the Quality Standards Subcommittee of the American Academy of Neurology. Neurology. 2010;74(23):1911–8.

39. Hassan T, Mumford C. Guillain-Barré syndrome mistaken for brain stem death. Postgrad Med J. 1991;67 (785):280–1.

40. Balser JR, Martinez EA, Winters BD, Perdue PW, Clarke AW, Huang W, Tomaselli GF, Dorman T, Campbell K, Lipsett P, Breslow MJ, Rosenfeld BA. Beta-adrenergic blockade accelerates conversion of postoperative supraventricular tachyarrhythmias. Anesthesiology. 1998;89(5):1052–9.

41. Bradley D, Creswell LL, Hogue Jr CW, Epstein AE, Prystowsky EN, Daoud EG, American College of Chest Physicians. Pharmacologic prophylaxis: American College of Chest Physicians guidelines for the prevention and management of postoperative atrial fibrillation after cardiac surgery. Chest. 2005; 128(2 Suppl):39S–47.

42. Poole GV, Griswold JA, Thaggard VK, Rhodes RS. Trauma is a recurrent disease. Surgery. 1993;113 (6):608–11.

43. Clancy K, Velopulos C, Bilaniuk JW, Collier B, Crowley W, Kurek S, Lui F, Nayduch D, Sangosanya A, Tucker B, Haut ER, Eastern Association for the Surgery of Trauma. Screening for blunt cardiac injury: an Eastern Association for the Surgery of Trauma practice management guideline. J Trauma Acute Care Surg. 2012;73(5 Suppl 4):S301–6.

44. Velmahos GC, Demetriades D, Shoemaker WC, Chan LS, Tatevossian R, Wo CC, Vassiliu P, Cornwell 3rd EE, Murray JA, Roth B, Belzberg H, Asensio JA, Berne TV. Endpoints of resuscitation of critically injured patients: normal or supranormal? A prospective randomized trial. Ann Surg. 2000;232(3):409–18.

45. Mayglothling J, Duane TM, Gibbs M, McCunn M, Legome E, Eastman AL, Whelan J, Shah KH, Eastern Association for the Surgery of Trauma. Emergency tracheal intubation immediately following traumatic injury: an Eastern Association for the Surgery of Trauma practice management guideline. J Trauma Acute Care Surg. 2012;73(5 Suppl 4):S333–40.

46. Kowalenko T, Burgess B, Szpunar SM, Irvin-Babcock CB. Alcohol and trauma–in every age group. Am J Emerg Med. 2013;31(4):705–9.

47. Constantin JM, Futier E, Cherprenet AL, Chanques G, Guerin R, Cayot-Constantin S, Jabaudon M, Perbet S, Chartier C, Jung B, Guelon D, Jaber S, Bazin JE. A recruitment maneuver increases oxygenation after intubation of hypoxemic intensive care unit patients: a randomized controlled study. Crit Care. 2010;14(2):R76.

48. Ventilation with lower tidal volumes as compared with traditional tidal volumes for acute lung injury and the acute respiratory distress syndrome. The Acute Respiratory Distress Syndrome Network. N Engl J Med. 2000;342(18):1301-8.

49. Kilickaya O, Gajic O. Initial ventilator settings for critically ill patients. Crit Care. 2013;17(2):123.

50. Briggs S, Goettler CE, Schenarts PJ, Newell MA, Sagraves SG, Bard MR, Toschlog EA, Rotondo MF. High-frequency oscillatory ventilation as a rescue therapy for adult trauma patients. Am J Crit Care. 2009;18(2):144–8.

51. Maung AA, Schuster KM, Kaplan LJ, Ditillo MF, Piper GL, Maerz LL, Lui FY, Johnson DC, Davis KA. Compared to conventional ventilation, airway pressure release ventilation may increase ventilator days in trauma patients. J Trauma Acute Care Surg. 2012;73(2):507–10.

52. Jackson LS, Davis JW, Kaups KL, Sue LP, Wolfe MM, Bilello JF, Lemaster D. Percutaneous tracheostomy: to bronch or not to bronch—that is the question. J Trauma. 2011;71(6):1553–6.

53. Simon B, Ebert J, Bokhari F, Capella J, Emhoff T, Hayward 3rd T, Rodriguez A, Smith L, Eastern Association for the Surgery of Trauma. Management of

pulmonary contusion and flail chest: an Eastern Association for the Surgery of Trauma practice management guideline. J Trauma Acute Care Surg. 2012;73(5 Suppl 4):S351–61.

54. Simon BJ, Cushman J, Barraco R, Lane V, Luchette FA, Miglietta M, Roccaforte DJ, Spector R, EAST Practice Management Guidelines Work Group. Pain management guidelines for blunt thoracic trauma. J Trauma. 2005;59(5):1256–67.

55. Guru V, Fremes SE. The role of N-acetylcysteine in preventing radiographic contrast-induced nephropathy. Clin Nephrol. 2004;62(2):77–83.

56. Wu MY, Hsiang HF, Wong CS, Yao MS, Li YW, Hsiang CY, Bai CH, Hsu YH, Lin YF, Tam KW. The effectiveness of N-acetylcysteine in preventing contrast-induced nephropathy in patients undergoing contrast-enhanced computed tomography: a meta-analysis of randomized controlled trials. Int Urol Nephrol. 2013;45(5):1309–18.

57. Lins RL, Elseviers MM, Van der Niepen P, Hoste E, Malbrain ML, Damas P, Devriendt J, SHARF Investigators. Intermittent versus continuous renal replacement therapy for acute kidney injury patients admitted to the intensive care unit: results of a randomized clinical trial. Nephrol Dial Transplant. 2009;24(2):512–8.

58. Laupland KB, Shahpori R, Kirkpatrick AW, Ross T, Gregson DB, Stelfox HT. Occurrence and outcome of fever in critically ill adults. Crit Care Med. 2008;36 (5):1531–5.

59. Marik PE. Fever in the ICU. Chest. 2000;117(3):855–69.

60. O'Grady NP, Barie PS, Bartlett JG, Bleck T, Carroll K, Kalil AC, Linden P, Maki DG, Nierman D, Pasculle W, Masur H, American College of Critical Care Medicine, Infectious Diseases Society of America. Guidelines for evaluation of new fever in critically ill adult patients: 2008 update from the American College of Critical Care Medicine and the Infectious Diseases Society of America. Crit Care Med. 2008;36(4):1330–49.

61. Gaieski DF, Mikkelsen ME, Band RA, Pines JM, Massone R, Furia FF, Shofer FS, Goyal M. Impact of time to antibiotics on survival in patients with severe sepsis or septic shock in whom early goal-directed therapy was initiated in the emergency department. Crit Care Med. 2010;38(4):1045–53.

62. Altun G, Akansu B, Altun BU, Azmak D, Yilmaz A. Deaths due to hunger strike: post-mortem findings. Forensic Sci Int. 2004;146(1):35–8.

63. Spear S, Sim V, Moore FA, Todd SR. Just say no to intensive care unit starvation: a nutrition education program for surgery residents. Nutr Clin Pract. 2013;28(3):387–91.

64. Maroulis J, Kalfarentzos F. Complications of parenteral nutrition at the end of the century. Clin Nutr. 2000;19(5):295–304.

65. Kawakami C, Fujiwara C. Experiences of parents' with children receiving long-term home parenteral nutrition. Pediatr Int. 2013;55(5):612–8.

66. Frankenfield D. Energy expenditure and protein requirements after traumatic injury. Nutr Clin Pract. 2006;21(5):430–7.

67. Rousseau AF, Losser MR, Ichai C, Berger MM. ESPEN endorsed recommendations: Nutritional therapy in major burns. Clin Nutr. 2013;32(4):497–502.

68. Foley N, Marshall S, Pikul J, Salter K, Teasell R. Hypermetabolism following moderate to severe traumatic acute brain injury: a systematic review. J Neurotrauma. 2008;25(12):1415–31.

69. Reid C. Frequency of under- and overfeeding in mechanically ventilated ICU patients: causes and possible consequences. J Hum Nutr Diet. 2006;19(1):13–22.

70. Kim H, Stotts NA, Froelicher ES, Engler MM, Porter C. Why patients in critical care do not receive adequate enteral nutrition? A review of the literature. J Crit Care. 2012;27(6):702–13.

71. Skipper A. Refeeding syndrome or refeeding hypophosphatemia: a systematic review of cases. Nutr Clin Pract. 2012;27(1):34–40.

72. Marinella MA. Refeeding syndrome and hypophosphatemia. J Intensive Care Med. 2005;20(3):155–9.

73. French C, Bellomo R. A rapid intravenous phosphate replacement protocol for critically ill patients. Crit Care Resusc. 2004;6(3):175–9.

74. Roccaforte JD. Electrolyte abnormalities. In: Atchabahian A, Gupta R, editors. The anesthesia guide. 1st ed. New York: McGraw-Hill; 2013. p. 128–42.

75. Dellinger RP, Levy MM, Rhodes A, Annane D, Gerlach H, Opal SM, Sevransky JE, Sprung CL, Douglas IS, Jaeschke R, Osborn TM, Nunnally ME, Townsend SR, Reinhart K, Kleinpell RM, Angus DC, Deutschman CS, Machado FR, Rubenfeld GD, Webb SA, Beale RJ, Vincent JL, Moreno R, Surviving Sepsis Campaign Guidelines Committee including the Pediatric Subgroup. Surviving sepsis campaign: international guidelines for management of severe sepsis and septic shock: 2012. Crit Care Med. 2013;41(2):580–637.

76. Sarosiek S, Crowther M, Sloan JM. Indications, complications, and management of inferior vena cava filters: the experience in 952 patients at an academic hospital with a level I trauma center. JAMA Intern Med. 2013;173(7):513–7.

77. World Death Rate Holding Steady At 100 Percent. The Onion, Issue 31.02 Jan 22, 1997. Available at http://www.theonion.com/articles/world-death-rate-holding-steady-at-100-percent,1670/ last accessed June, 2013.

78. Ho KM. Combining sequential organ failure assessment (SOFA) score with acute physiology and chronic health evaluation (APACHE) II score to predict hospital mortality of critically ill patients. Anaesth Intensive Care. 2007;35(4):515–21.

79. Curtis JR. Communicating about end-of-life care with patients and families in the intensive care unit. Crit Care Clin. 2004;20(3):363-80, viii.

80. Mercadante S, Giarratano A. The anesthesiologist and end-of-life care. Curr Opin Anaesthesiol. 2012;25 (3):371–5.

Trauma Simulation

19

Lynn Choi and Corey S. Scher

Introduction

Trauma is the leading cause of death for people 1–44 years old and the fourth leading cause of death in the western world [1, 2]. Despite the widespread recognition of basic principles of trauma resuscitation, the applications of these principles remain sporadic in many trauma centers. This is partly secondary to a culmination of changes in medical education. With the reduction in resident work hours, rapid introduction to new medical technologies and medical knowledge, the need to assure patient safety in a dynamic environment becomes increasingly difficult. The main objectives of a trauma team is to rapidly resuscitate and stabilize the patient, determine the nature and extent of injuries, prioritize the management of injuries, and prepare the patient for transfer to the site of definitive care. Successful trauma resuscitation not only requires highly trained medical professionals, but it also requires a multidisciplinary team from a variety of subspecialties including anesthesia, emergency medicine, surgery, nursing, and support staff to work together cohesively and function as an integrated team (Table 19.1).

L. Choi, M.D. (✉)
Department of Anesthesiology, Bellevue Hospital—NYU,
462 First Avenue, New York, NY 10010, USA
e-mail: Lynn.choi@nyumc.org

C.S. Scher, M.D.
Department of Anesthesiology, NYU/Bellevue Hospital
Center, 462 First Avenue, New York, NY 10016, USA

While intended to achieve the best possible outcome for patients, this diversity of team members has posed a major challenge in regard to medical errors resulting from poor communication skills and lack of cohesiveness [3]. The advantage of simulation is that it allows for a controlled and safe practice environment outside of the clinical setting and may reduce medical errors and increase patient safety. In the past, most surgery, emergency, and anesthesiology-related curriculum devoted little attention to team-training exercises or emphasis on effective team function in the context of trauma care delivery. As more emphasis on the importance of communication and teamwork is made, simulation technology has played a major role in improving team-training exercises.

Brief History of Simulation

Simulation training in medical education is perhaps the most notable innovation over the past 15 years. The heightened interest in simulation is evident by events such as the creation of an academic society dedicated to simulation, the inauguration of a simulation journal, and the proliferation of simulation-based research [4]. Many medical centers and health care professional training hospitals have either simulation centers or simulation-based education (Fig. 19.1).

Simulation training has been used in a variety of different settings including aviation, military, and medical training. Flight simulation was first

C.S. Scher (ed.), *Anesthesia for Trauma*, DOI 10.1007/978-1-4939-0909-4_19,
© Springer Science+Business Media New York 2014

Table 19.1 Composition of a trauma team

Core trauma team members	– Trauma surgeon
	– Anesthesiologist
	– Emergency medicine physician
	– Reparatory therapist
	– Radiographer
	– Nurses
Additional staff	– Scribe
	– Blood bank
Surgical subspecialties (optional)	– Neurosurgeon
	– Thoracic surgeon
	– Plastic surgeon
	– Radiologist

developed to train military personnel in preparation for World War I. A meta-analysis study on flight simulation found that more than 90 % of experimental comparisons favored simulator and aircraft training over aircraft training alone [5]. It was recognized early on that those errors that occur in aircrafts stem largely from failures in communication, teamwork, and decision-making rather than from technical deficiencies. As a result, the aviation industry introduced Crew Resource Management (CRM) training in order to enhance the performance of nontechnical skills by providing a set of preventable outcomes. CRM training emphasizes seven key elements: command, leadership communication, situational awareness, workload management, resource management, and decision-making. The medical profession adopted these concepts in order to reduce medical errors.

Medical simulation as an instrument to enhance the development of technical, behavioral, and cognitive skills was first introduced in the 1950s. Anesthesiologists were the first to implement the core ideas of CRM training by the use of simulated operation rooms. Two anesthesiologists, Dr. Peter Safar and Dr. Bjorn Lind, introduced the mannequin simulator [6]. The first training mannequin was known as Resusci-Annie and was developed in a toy factory by Dr. Lind. It was designed to accurately simulate human anatomic landmarks and respiratory system to facilitate training. In the 1960s, Dr. Stephen Abrahamson presented the advantage of using a full-scale,

computer-controlled human patient simulator (HPS) to train anesthesiology residents [7]. By the 1980s, realistic mannequin simulators that could replicate the human physiologic responses were developed [8] (Fig. 19.2). Dr. David M. Gaba of Stanford University, a pioneer of simulation, began the use of computer-controlled mannequins for educational and trauma purposes to simulate various anesthetic crisis scenarios with the goal of reducing anesthetic complications [9].

Simulation can be divided into five categories: verbal, standardized patient, part-task trainers, computer trainers, and electronic trainers [8]. Verbal simulation is a form of simple verbal exercises or role-playing with or without the use of a passive mannequin. Standardized patients are trained actors who are assigned to play a simulated patient role and are utilized to evaluate bedside manner, professionalism, and history-taking skills of the trainee. Due to ethical constraints, invasive procedures and therapeutic interventions are not performed on standardized patients. Part-task trainers are anatomic mock-up devises that are made from synthetic material to represent human full and partial body parts. They are used to replicate a certain portion of a patient or specific task so that trainees can practice invasive procedures and interventions (Fig. 19.3). Computer trainers are a more cost-effective means to achieve the same goals as standardized patients. The most interactive and comprehensive form of simulators is the electronic patient.

What Is Trauma Simulation?

Trauma simulation differs from Advance Trauma Life Support (ATLS) in that it emphasizes team dynamics, leadership, and communication as important skills for successful management of acutely injured patients. ATLS is an effective teaching program that demonstrates crucial aspects of acute trauma management but is focused on training a single practitioner rather than a multidisciplinary team. It is a simplified and standardized approach to managing trauma patients and includes didactic lectures, sessions

Fig. 19.1 Simulator mannequin. The mannequin provides a voice-linked speaker to allow the instructor to speak to the participants during the case scenario

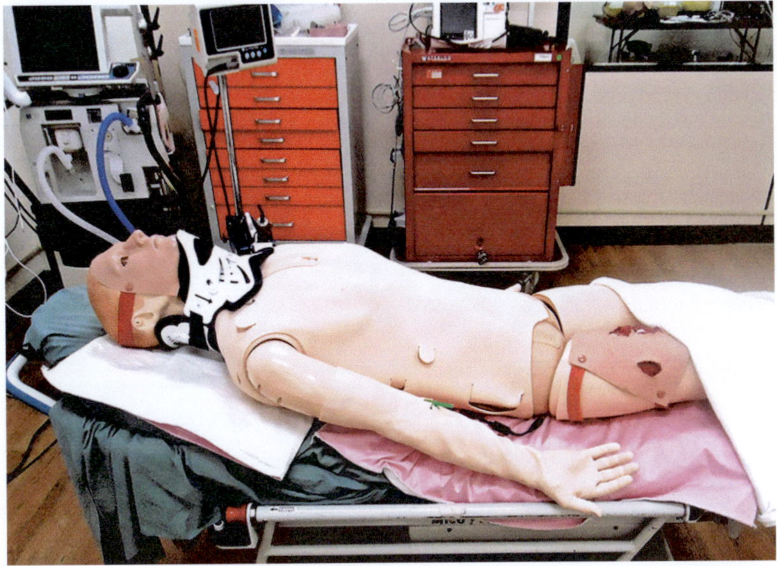

Fig. 19.2 Computer-generated vital signs appear on the display monitor, including respiratory rate, blood pressure, heart rate, and capnography. Vital signs are programmed on a laptop computer by an operator before the mock scenario

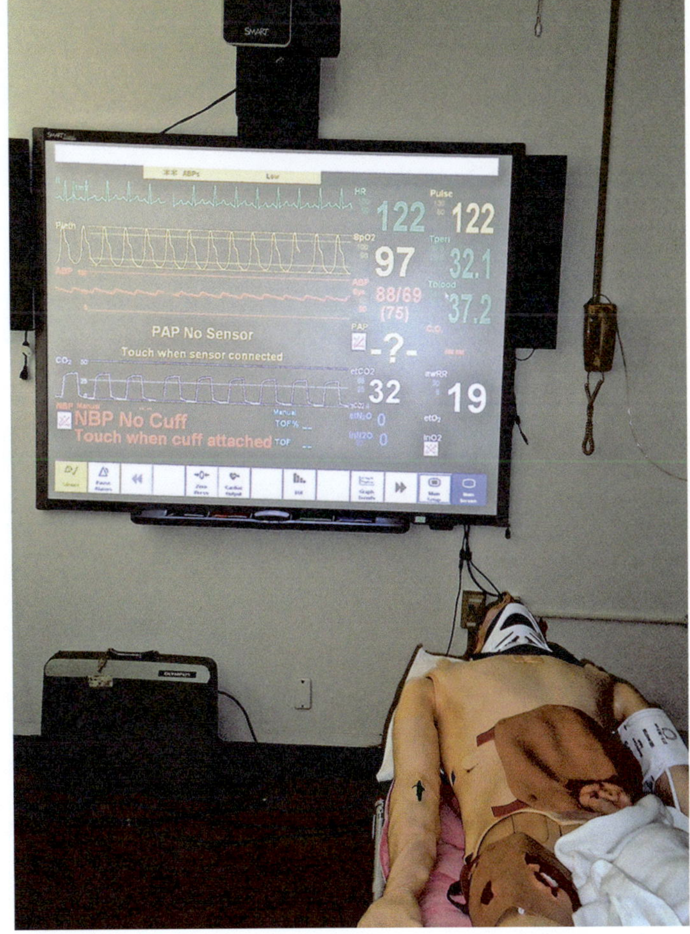

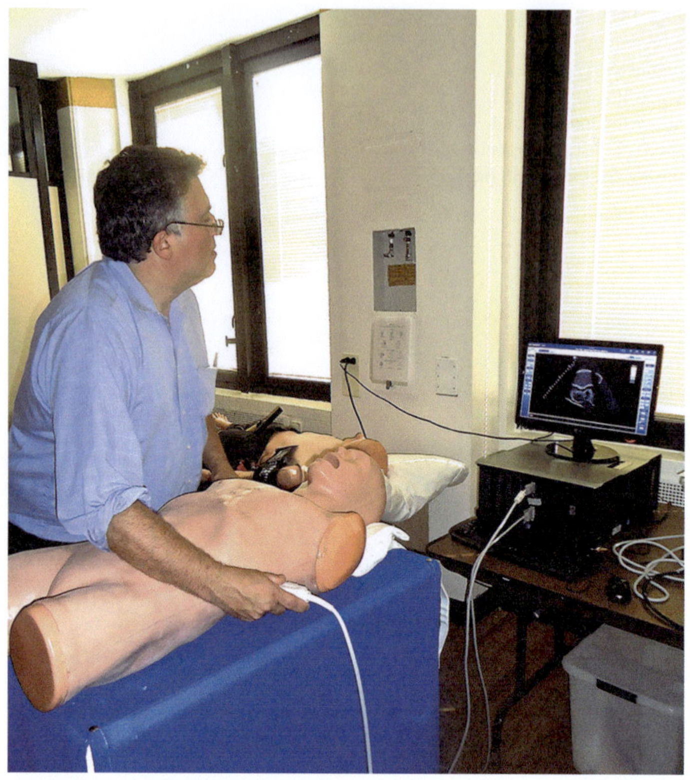

Fig. 19.3 FAST exam simulator. The FAST simulator is a learning tool devised to read a FAST (focused assessment with sonography for trauma) exam. This diagnostic ultrasound training system allows the participants to learn key landmarks on the body to understand and become familiar with the various views of the exam

for technical skills development, and trauma scenarios with mock patients. Courses such as Simulated Trauma and Resuscitation Team Training (STARTT), which uses principles from ATLS in conjunction with group dynamics, stresses the emphasis on communication and leadership skills, effective utilization of resources, problem solving, and situational awareness.

The use of HPSs and recreating realistic mock scenarios with members of different medical specialties has allowed for exposure to group dynamics and leadership roles. Identifying each group member's roles and understanding the expectations of a group leader are major goals of trauma simulation. Mock trauma scenarios that span a broad range of topics are created to reflect trauma scenarios that are frequently encountered. Each teaching scenario should include a description of the expected care of the mock trauma patient so that members of the trauma team can be appropriately evaluated.

Mock patients simulators are then programmed to fit the age and sex of the patient with physical signs and symptoms consistent with the injured patient. Pre-programmed monitors that display real-time physiologic data are set to correspond according to treatment modalities, to enhance the experience (Fig. 19.4).

Several studies have advocated the use of videotape recordings of mock scenarios to critique and analyze group members and identify methods to improve group dynamics at the conclusion of each scenario [3, 10]. Perhaps the most challenging aspects of trauma simulation is recognizing one's role in the group and communicating effectively with other members. The trauma team leader is usually a resident physician from the emergency department or trauma surgery service. The team leader must be able to assign tasks to each team member in a clear and concise manner, and make critical decisions for the critically injured patient.

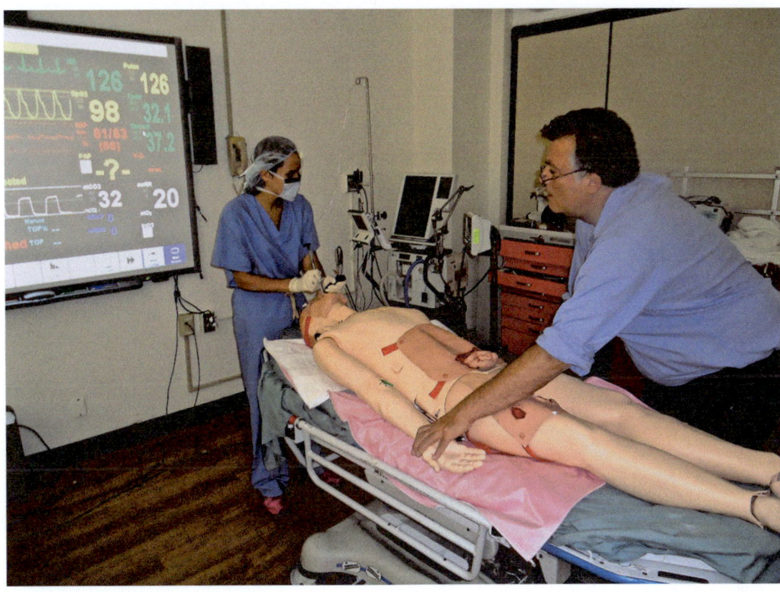

Fig. 19.4 Computer-based clinical display. With realistic anatomy and clinical functionality, mannequins provide simulation-based education to challenge and test clinical skills during realistic patient care scenarios. Participants are able to practice the emergency treatment of patients including nasal and oral intubation techniques

Fig. 19.5 Trauma simulation assessment

Goals and Assessment of Trauma Team Simulation
• Team leader is clearly identified
• Each team member recognizes his/her role
• Team members actively verbalize activities to each other in a clear and concise manner
• Team members repeat back orders to team leader to verify hearing the correctly
• All team members call attention to actions that might result in complications

Anesthesiologists play a critical role in trauma resuscitation. Because of the extensive training in clinical physiology, anesthesiologists have a key role in successful resuscitation of trauma patients. In most trauma centers, anesthesiologists are present in the trauma bay for all major trauma cases. Their primary role is to provide airway management, cardiac and pulmonary resuscitation, advance life support, and stabilize the patient for emergency surgery when indicated. Effective communication and cooperation between the anesthesia and surgical teams are key qualities for successful trauma care.

As emphasis on the use of simulation and teamwork training to improve trauma care become increasingly evident, methods for evaluating team performance are important aspects in determining the effectiveness of simulation training (Fig. 19.5). Designing an objective method to measure performance during actual trauma resuscitation has been a challenge. Measureable actions that are considered crucial in trauma resuscitation include assuring prompt intubation when indicated, calling out difficult airway findings, ordering blood product transfusions, and recognizing the need for emergent surgery, head CT, or pelvic embolization. Rosen et al. categorized team performance measurement and evaluation into three groups: observational rating scales, team self-assessment, and the event-based approach [11]. Observational rating scales are objective measurement protocols in which observers are asked to rate and record team behavior. Teamwork self-assessment is a tool that allows team members to individually assess themselves and react to the training program. Event-based assessment is a rating tool used to assess complex simulation scenarios in which raters are informed of behaviors that should occur depending on a pre-determined scenario. Different approaches to evaluating teamwork in simulations have associated pros and cons, and a combined approach can help obtain a compete assessment of team performance [11]. To be able to fully assess the range of team dynamics and performance, a measurement tool that involves multiple approaches should be implemented.

Example of Trauma Simulation Scenario: Penetrating Chest Trauma

Case Description

The emergency department nurse tells the ED attending, "a patient is being brought in by EMS after being stabbed in the chest." According to EMS, the patient was hemodynamically stable. The trauma team consists of 1–3 nurses, the ED attending and resident, and a medical student. The role of the medical student is to record the history and physical and other major events. As the case proceeds, anesthesia and surgery attending and resident will be called.

The paramedic provides the following report: This is a 25-year-old man who was stabbed in the chest in his apartment from a drug-related dispute. His stab wound appears to be just right to his sternum. There is minimal bleeding and the patient is responsive and appropriate to questions. At the scene, he was initially tachycardic, but his heart rate was within normal limits. Currently the patient is hemodynamically stable. Vitals are: BP 120/67 HR 98 RR 16 SpO_2 98% on room air. He has one large bore IV and has received 1 L of balanced salt solution. He states he has past medical history and has never had surgery in the past. He has no allergies.

During the case, the patient will develop a moderate pneumothorax and severe pericardial effusion as a result of an unrecognized second stab wound in the patient's left axilla.

Learning Objectives

The entire trauma team should understand how to obtain the primary and secondary surveys. In the primary survey, which focuses on the initial assessment of the patient, Beck's triad of hypotension, neck vein distension, and muffle heart sounds should be recognized. Possible causes including cardiac tamponade, tension pneumothorax, myocardial dysfunction, and system air embolism should be considered. Once the patient develops cardiac tamponade, the need for immediate pericardiocentesis should be recognized. When a pneumothorax develops, the resident should be able to recognize the physical and physiological signs (seen on the simulated monitors) and place a chest tube of a size 28 or greater. He should also call for the anesthesia and surgical teams to secure the airway and take back to the operating room without performing unnecessary diagnostic studies.

The secondary survey is focused history and physical exam. The medical staff should adhere to ATLS and obtain full exposure to complete the physical exam. Once the patient is fully exposed, the resident should be able to identify the axillary would missed by the paramedics (this will be visible on the mannequin simulator).

After the case scenario and debriefing, participants should develop basic multidisciplinary team skills.

Simulation Environment

The trauma simulation lab is set up as a trauma bay of an emergency department. The computer mannequin has one large bore IV in the right arm and one small puncture wound on the right side of the chest with evidence of minimal bleeding, and another larger wound in the left axilla which should only be visible by extending the mannequin arm. Other props that are present in the room are pericardiocentesis tray, chest tube tray, pleurovac, airway box with equipment for intubation, ventilator, and monitors demonstrating active EKG, blood pressure, and saturations which correlate to the patient's current status.

Case Narrative

The case narrative describes the scenario that the trauma providers will be experiencing during the simulation. Initially, the patient will be able to communicate and is able to verbalize his chest pain. Initially the patient will have a relatively normal physical exam aside from a puncture wound on the right side of his sternum. The trauma team will have to complete the secondary exam in order to recognize the second stab wound in his left axilla. As the pericardial tamponade develops, the blood pressure begins to drop and his mental status diminishes. The vital signs on the monitor should rapidly decompensate as the patient becomes unresponsive. The emergency medicine physician should call for the anesthesia and surgical teams. The resident should listen to the mannequin's chest and note that there are decreased breath sounds on the left side.

If the traumatic pericardial effusion/tamponade is appropriately treated with pericardiocentesis, the patient's blood pressure will transiently stabilize but he will remain moderately hypoxic with oxygen saturations in the high 80s. This hypoxia, as a result of the developing pneumothorax will not resolve unless a chest tube is placed by either the emergency or surgery resident. If the left-sided pneumothorax is not discovered, or if the decision was made to intubate the patient without placing the chest tube, then a tension pneumothorax will develop. The patient will stabilize only after pericardiocentesis and tube thoracostomy are performed.

Debriefing

Debriefing can be done in a group setting while reviewing a video of the scenario that took place.

The discussion should focus on the participants' performances and lessons that can be learned from the simulations session. After viewing the video, participants should comment on ways to improve teamwork and communication in order to act more efficiently.

What Is the Evidence?

It is estimated that 90,000 fatalities occur each year in the United States as a result of medical errors, resulting in a cost of 29 billion dollars [12]. If medical errors were included as a category, it would be the sixth leading cause of death in America [13]. The combination of unstable patients, unknown medical histories, time-critical decisions, simultaneous tasks, and involvement of various medical specialties are all risk factors in trauma for medical errors [14]. Trauma simulation has been utilized in many teaching hospitals across the country and studies have assessed the effectiveness of trauma simulation in improving trauma care.

Marshal et al. was among the first to evaluate the use of HPSs in ACLS courses for surgery interns. In the study, trauma management skills were evaluated in three areas critical-treatment decisions, potential for adverse outcomes, and team behavior. After participating in HPS trauma scenarios, subjects completed a self-confidence questionnaire. Results showed significant improvement in all criteria but were most notable in team behavior, which increased by 50 % over the control group [15]. Holcomb et al. assessed trauma team performance using HSP for resuscitation training. He evaluated ten 3-person military resuscitation teams at the arrival and completion of a 28-day rotation at a civilian trauma center. Performance was measured using a human performance assessment tool that utilized both scored and timed task that were considered essential in the initial assessment of trauma patients. They found significant improvement in scores by all ten teams at the conclusion of the rotation with scores approaching that of expert teams [15]. Ali et al. described a study on fourth-year medical students and their experience with a simulated trauma patient teaching module [16]. Results concluded that the students demonstrated improvement in trauma knowledge as well as trauma skills with the use of the simulator [16].

Knudson et al. studied the role of simulation in mid-level surgery residents. They evaluated the residents on initial trauma evaluation/treatment skills (Part I) and crisis-management skills (Part II), which included teamwork, decision-making, and situational awareness [17]. Utilizing a five-part scenario-based trauma curriculum, residents were randomized to receiving didactic lectures or HPS. They found that scores were similar in the initial evaluation/treatment skills but found a significant improvement in crisis-management skills in the human performance simulator group.

Drawbacks of Medical Simulation

The efficacy of simulation, while not definitively positive, does suggest that it is an important addition for educational purposes. Trauma simulation allows for medical personnel to engage in interactive training through the use of HPSs and offers a more hands-on approach to learning. Teamwork, management, and communications skill that are difficult to convey in a lecture setting can be practiced and cultivated in a simulated environment. The result is that medical residents can act more efficiently and become prepared for all aspects of providing care in an emergency setting.

Whether or not simulation truly enhances performance in real-life trauma situations remains to be discovered. Measuring the effectiveness of team behavior is a challenge that requires several approaches. In theory, practice makes perfect. However, mock scenarios, which are created to simulate a highly intense situation, have its obvious drawbacks. There is no alternate for the human body and as with any devise, there are drawbacks to medical simulation. A simulated scenario can never substitute for a real-life experience. The more real-life trauma experiences a person gains through his or her career is likely to be the most effective way to enhance performance in trauma situations. A trauma curriculum that includes the use of human performance simulators may be useful for trauma team training, but only if it can be demonstrated to enhance performance in practical trauma situations.

References

1. The Center for Disease Control. Ten leading causes of death and injury. http://www.cdc.gov/injury/wisqars/leadingcauses.html. Assessed July 5, 2013.
2. National confidential enquiry into patient outcomes and death: Trauma: who cares. 2007 http://www.ncepod.org.uk/2007t.htm. Last assessed July 5, 2013.
3. Hamilton N, Freeman BD, Woodhouse J, et al. Team behavior during trauma resuscitation: a simulation-based performance assessment. J Grad Med Educ. 2009;1(2):253–9.
4. Passiment M, Sacks H, Huang G. Medical simulation in medical education: results of an AAMC Survey. Sept 2009.
5. Hays RT, Jacobs JW, Prince C et al. Flight simulator training effectiveness: a meta-analysis. Mil Psychol. 2009
6. Marshall RL, Smith JS, Gorman PJ, Krummel TM, Haluck RS, Cooney RN. Use of a human patient simulator in the development of resident trauma management skills. J Trauma. 2001;51:17–21.
7. Abrahamson S, Denson JS, Wolf RM. Effectiveness of a simulator in training anesthiesology residents. J Med Educ. 1969;44:515–9.
8. Cooper JB, Taqueti VR. A brief history of the development of mannequin simulators for clinical education and training. Qual Saf Health Care. 2004;13 Suppl 1:i11–8.
9. Helmreich RL. Managing human error in aviation. Sci Am. 1997;276:62–7.
10. Barsuk D, Ziv A, Lin G. Using advanced simulation for recognition and correction of gaps in airway and breathing management skills in prehospital trauma care. Anesth Analg. 2005;100:803–9.
11. Rosen MA, Weaver SJ, Lazzara EH, et al. Tools for evaluating team performance in simulation-based training. J Emerg Trauma Shock. 2010;3(4):353–9.
12. Weingart SN, Wilson RM, Gibberd RW, et al. Epidemiology of medical error. BMJ. 2000;7237:774–7.

13. Deaths/Mortality, 2005, National Center for Health Care Statistics at the Centers for Disease Control. http://www.cdc.gov/nchs/ats/deaths.htm. Last assessed June 30, 2013.
14. Gruen RL, Jurkovich GJ, McIntyre LK, et al. Patterns of errors contributing to trauma mortality: lessons learned from 2594 death. Ann Surg. 2006;244:371–80.
15. Holcomb JB, Dumaire RD, Crommett JW, et al. Evaluation of trauma team performance using an advanced human patient simulator for resuscitation training. J Trauma. 2002;52:1078–86.
16. Ali J, Adam RU, Sammy I, et al. The simulated trauma patient teaching module—does it improve student performance? J Trauma. 2007;62:1416–20.
17. Knudson MM, Khaw L, Gaba D, et al. Teamwork in the trauma bay (ACS/APDS surgical skills curriculum). http://elearning.facs.org. Accessed June 28, 2013.

Civilian Trauma Systems

20

J. David Roccaforte

Trauma medicine is both one of the oldest and the most recent medical specialties. Egyptian hieroglyphs and ancient Greek texts record a history of wound management, including fractures, amputations, dislocations, lacerations, and penetrating trauma [1]. Worldwide, the care of the wounded has advanced as a consequence of military conflicts throughout history. However, formal Trauma Surgery fellowship training and guidelines for civilian trauma systems have only been established since the 1970s in the United States, and even more recently elsewhere.

Wide disparities exist in the availability of high-level civilian trauma care, especially between rural and populated areas [2]. Average field-to-hospital transport times can range from several hours in remote locations, to 10 min in urban centers [3]. Additional disparities in trauma care in the United States have been associated with racial background and insurance coverage [4]. Despite the influx of experienced military physicians and nurses into the civilian trauma system [5], recent reports describe an impending critical shortage of adequately trained trauma personnel [6].

Different regions manage trauma patients differently, particularly with respect to pre-hospital care, but also with in-hospital organization. In some systems, primarily European, the initial strategy is to bring the hospital to the patient [7]. Specially trained physicians staff ambulances and endeavor to stabilize trauma victims in the field utilizing advanced medications, monitoring, and procedures, and then accompany patients during transport to the most appropriate hospital.

In other locales, typically in North America and the UK, the goal is to bring the patient to the hospital as quickly as possible. Emergency medical technicians perform basic first-aid only and paramedics are ACLS trained, but the primary goal for both is to expedite transport to the nearest trauma-designated hospital for definitive care, the so-called scoop and run directive.

The debate regarding which pre-hospital strategy is superior may be unnecessary. Although direct comparisons are difficult due to the complex nature of comprehensive trauma care, either system appears to yield similar outcomes when applied capably [8]. Given the chaotic nature of trauma, any system is better than an improvized and disorganized approach. Patients benefit from a well-planned and competently implemented trauma system [9], which clearly will always perform better than a poorly planned, ineffectively implemented system.

In regions where "scoop and run" is the prevailing strategy of pre-hospital trauma management, urban trauma victims are able to be transported more quickly than rural victims [10]. For equivalent injury severity, mortality increases as transport times become longer. However, if a rural trauma victim survives an

J.D. Roccaforte, M.D. (✉)
Department of Anesthesiology, New York University,
Bellevue Hospital Surgical Intensive Care Unit,
1st Avenue at 27th Street, New York, NY 10016, USA
e-mail: JDavidR@mail.com

C.S. Scher (ed.), *Anesthesia for Trauma*, DOI 10.1007/978-1-4939-0909-4_20,
© Springer Science+Business Media New York 2014

403

extended transport and arrives alive at a designated trauma center, subsequent survival is nearly equivalent to those transported rapidly from an urban area [3].

Once at the hospital, there may be differences in the prevailing system and organization of services. In some systems, patients are admitted to a specialty Trauma Service whose surgeons are trained to perform nearly every relevant procedure from orthopedic repairs to simple neurosurgical decompression. Other systems admit patients to a dedicated Trauma Service [11] where they are managed by trauma-fellowship trained general surgeons who manage and coordinate overall care, and perform most intra-abdominal procedures, simple amputations, and wound debridements, but consult specialists (who often operate concurrently) for neurosurgery, complex orthopedic, thoracic, ENT, vascular, and plastic surgical procedures. In yet other systems, patients are admitted to an established non-trauma surgical or even a medical service, depending on the patient's primary issue (e.g., orthopedics or neurosurgery), and the trauma service provides consultant advice. Outcomes appear to favor a trauma service being an admitting, rather than consultative service [12].

The American College of Surgeons (ACS) Committee on Fractures and Other Trauma was established in 1939 by merging two existing committees: the Committee on Fractures, which was notable for standardizing emergency splinting in the field, and the Committee on Industrial Medicine and Traumatic Surgery. In 1950 the name was changed to the Committee on Trauma (COT). In 1954, with the emphasis still on managing fractures, the committee published the manual *Early Care of Soft Tissue Injuries*, which was maintained with revisions until 1972, when it was replaced with the manual *Early Care of the Injured Patient*. The first version specifically directed at hospital trauma centers was *Optimal Hospital Resources for Care of the Injured Patient*, which was released in 1976. In 1980 the "Advanced Trauma Life Support®" course was introduced, with revisions every 4 years to date. Trauma Center verification was first offered in 1987, and the National Trauma Data Bank® was initiated in 1989.

As originally formulated, the focus of the ACS/COT was training physicians to manage acute trauma, and specifying for hospitals the resources necessary for managing trauma patients. Over time the emphasis has broadened, with the objectives of developing comprehensive, inclusive trauma systems and coordinating resources and training to encompass pre-hospital treatment, transport, triage, acute and subacute in-patient management, and rehabilitation. Community education, injury prevention, research, and quality improvement are also important.

Over 60 countries utilize guidelines and specifications set out by the ACS/COT for the acute management of trauma patients, certification of trauma centers, and organization of trauma systems. ACS/COT publishes and revises a manual of standards for trauma care, *Resources for Optimal Care of the Trauma Patient*. In the United States, ACS/COT verifies regional hospitals in most states for trauma center designation and certification. In some regions, state or local officials verify trauma centers. Typically, their requirements are similar to those specified by the ACS/COT [13].

Adherence to the outlined standards appears to affect survival. In a retrospective study evaluating trauma care compliance at a Level-1 center using 25 evidence-based or expert consensus panel recommendations, for each 10 % increase in compliance a 14 % reduction in risk-adjusted in-hospital mortality was observed [14].

The ACS/COT describes four levels of adult and pediatric trauma centers: Level I—most resources to Level IV—least resources. There are separate requirements for burn centers. In the most recent revision of standards, with emphasis placed on trauma systems organization, separate considerations are given for rural and urban systems. In an urban region with adequate Level I capacity, numerous Level II centers may not be necessary.

A Level IV hospital is always located in a rural or remote area. It must provide 24 h physician coverage and initial resuscitation and assessment prior to transfer to a higher-level facility.

Well-defined collaborations with higher-level trauma centers, including expedited transfer protocols, are critical.

Level III facilities are typically rural and, like Level IV, must have active collaboration and transfer agreements with higher-level facilities. A Level III facility would be considered capable of assessing, stabilizing, and treating a majority of traumatic injuries. General surgeons must be available 24 h/day, and able to be at the patient's bedside within 30 min of the patient's arrival. A Level III trauma service must have a surgical director, and maintain a Performance Improvement and Patient Safety (PIPS) program. Level III centers are not required to have available advanced radiology, blood bank, laboratory, orthopedic, or neurosurgical services.

Level II and Level I centers are nearly identical in terms of the resources available to trauma patients. The main difference is in how immediately certain resources are available. In addition, Level I centers perform research, and serve a leadership role in the regional trauma system, providing organization, and education.

Despite similarly available resources, outcomes for equivalent trauma appear to be better at Level I centers, compared to Level II centers. In a multivariate-adjusted retrospective analysis of the National Trauma Data Bank® statistics, patients suffering the most severe injuries were more likely to survive if treated at a Level I center compared to a Level II center. Even among survivors, those treated at Level II centers had worse functional outcomes. The same study investigated the effect of trauma volume on outcomes. Interestingly, there was no survival benefit for patients brought to high-volume centers at either Level [15].

A Level II trauma center in an urban area may be a complementary facility to a nearby Level I center, transferring high-acuity patients to the Level I facility for interventional radiology, advanced orthopedic, vascular, thoracic, neurosurgical, or intensive care when these are needed, and accepting lower acuity patients from the Level I facility if the Level I capacity is overwhelmed. In a rural area without nearby Level I care, a Level II trauma center may function as the regional leadership facility of the rural system of Level III and IV centers, providing organization and education [16].

Highlights of features common to Level II and I trauma centers include:

- A trauma surgeon on call at all times.
- All general surgeons and Emergency Medicine physicians on the trauma team are ACLS® certified.
- Trauma team members fulfill trauma-related Continuing Medical Education (CME).
- Neurosurgical care is promptly and continuously available.
- Orthopedic care is promptly and continuously available.
- Attending physicians involved in trauma care are board certified in their specialties.
- Radiographs and CT scans are available at all times.
- Catheter angiography and sonography are available at all times.
- Critical care services are available for trauma patients
- Intracranial pressure monitoring is available.
- Respiratory therapists are available at all times.
- Laboratory and Blood bank services are available at all times.
- Social workers, and Rehabilitation Medicine are available.
- Speech, Physical, and Occupational therapy are available.
- A trauma registry is maintained and submitted to the NTDB®.
- The center has an active PIPS program.
- The center engages in public and professional education, including injury prevention.
- The trauma center is prepared for disasters.
- The trauma center is able to procure organs for transplant.

Additional requirements for a Level I trauma center include:

- A general surgery residency program with a trauma rotation.
- Cardiac surgery and cardiopulmonary bypass capabilities.
- Microvascular and replant capabilities.
- In-house CT technician always available.

- MRI available.
- Acute hemodialysis always available.
- Operating room and personnel immediately available at all times.
- A surgical ICU physician in-house at all times.
- A surgically directed and staffed ICU service.
- $\geq$1,200 trauma admissions/year.
- $\geq$240 patients, or >35 patients/surgeon per year with Injury Severity Score (ISS) > 15.
- Ongoing research with academic peer-reviewed publication.
- Extramural presentations at educational or research conferences.
- Participation in ATLS® training.

Separate requirements in *Resources for Optimal Care of the Trauma Patient* are specified for Pediatric trauma and Burn centers.

Requirements Specifically Related to Anesthesiologists

At all levels of trauma centers, an anesthesiologist is designated as a liaison to the trauma service. This individual should have experience in trauma anesthesia, and a commitment to education and performance improvement. The anesthesiology representative to the trauma program must attend at least 50 % of the multidisciplinary peer review meetings.

Furthermore, at all levels of trauma centers, anesthesia services must be promptly available for all emergency operations and for managing airway problems. Responsibilities assumed by anesthesiologists extend beyond the operating room and may include invasive monitoring, line placement, resuscitation, and pain management.

At Level III centers, a CRNA may be the sole on-call provider, while at Level I and II centers the anesthesiologist of record must be a board-certified attending. For Level I centers, anesthesiology providers must be in-house 24 h/day. When a senior resident or CRNA fulfills the availability requirements at Level I or II facilities, a board-certified staff anesthesiologist on-call must be immediately advised, promptly available, and present for all operations.

At Level I trauma centers, an operating room must be adequately staffed and immediately available at all times. This may be accomplished by reserving a designated operating room or by staggering A.M. starting times so that a rotating room is free at all times. If the primary operating room is occupied at a Level I or II center, there must be a mechanism for providing additional staff to open a second room.

Full operating room equipment must be available at all centers, and this must include rapid infusers, bronchoscopes, thermal control equipment, and resuscitation fluids [16].

At all Trauma center levels, the Post-Anesthesia Care Unit (PACU) must be available and staffed 24 h/day. The PACU must be capable of monitoring with pulse oximetry, end-tidal carbon dioxide detection, intra-arterial pressure monitoring, pulmonary artery pressure monitoring, patient rewarming, and intracranial pressure monitoring.

The development, implementation, verification, and continuing improvement of civilian trauma systems is an ongoing process and has been in evolution since before recorded history. Improved survival benefit to trauma victims is possible is contingent on sound evidence-based protocols and guidelines, on seamless collaboration and coordination among many disparate groups of providers, and on continuous and ongoing training, research, and education. But most of all, it is dependent on a deep and profound commitment to excellent care.

References

1. Pikoulis EA, Petropoulos JC, Tsigris C, Pikoulis N, Leppäniemi AK, Pavlakis E, Gavrielatou E, Burris D, Bastounis E, Rich NM. Trauma management in ancient Greece: value of surgical principles through the years. World J Surg. 2004;28(4):425–30.
2. MacKenzie EJ, Hoyt DB, Sacra JC, Jurkovich GJ, Carlini AR, Teitelbaum SD, Teter Jr H. National inventory of hospital trauma centers. JAMA. 2003;289(12):1515–22.
3. Fatovich DM, Phillips M, Langford SA, Jacobs IG. A comparison of metropolitan vs rural major trauma in Western Australia. Resuscitation. 2011;82(7):886–90.

4. Haider AH, Weygandt PL, Bentley JM, Monn MF, Rehman KA, Zarzaur BL, Crandall ML, Cornwell EE, Cooper LA. Disparities in trauma care and outcomes in the United States: a systematic review and meta-analysis. J Trauma Acute Care Surg. 2013;74 (5):1195–205.

5. Eastridge BJ, Jenkins D, Flaherty S, Schiller H, Holcomb JB. Trauma system development in a theater of war: experiences from Operation Iraqi Freedom and Operation Enduring Freedom. J Trauma. 2006;61(6):1366–72, discussion 1372–3.

6. Cohn SM, Price MA, Villarreal CL. Trauma and surgical critical care workforce in the United States: a severe surgeon shortage appears imminent. J Am Coll Surg. 2009;209(4):446–52.

7. Leppäniemi A. Trauma systems in Europe. Curr Opin Crit Care. 2005;11(6):576–9.

8. Nathens AB, Brunet FP, Maier RV. Development of trauma systems and effect on outcomes after injury. Lancet. 2004;363(9423):1794–801. Erratum in: Lancet. 2005;366(9499):1772.

9. MacKenzie EJ, Rivara FP, Jurkovich GJ, Nathens AB, Frey KP, Egleston BL, Salkever DS, Scharfstein DO. A national evaluation of the effect of trauma-center care on mortality. N Engl J Med. 2006;354 (4):366–78.

10. Grossman DC, Kim A, Macdonald SC, Klein P, Copass MK, Maier RV. Urban-rural differences in prehospital care of major trauma. J Trauma. 1997;42 (4):723–9.

11. Ursic C, Curtis K, Zou Y, Black D. Improved trauma patient outcomes after implementation of a dedicated trauma admitting service. Injury. 2009;40(1):99–103.

12. Wong TH, Lumsdaine W, Hardy BM, Lee K, Balogh ZJ. The impact of specialist trauma service on major trauma mortality. J Trauma Acute Care Surg. 2013;74 (3):780–4.

13. Bailey J, Trexler S, Murdock A, Hoyt D. Verification and regionalization of trauma systems: the impact of these efforts on trauma care in the United States. Surg Clin North Am. 2012;92(4):1009–24, ix–x.

14. Shafi S, Rayan N, Barnes S, Fleming N, Gentilello LM, Ballard D. Moving from "optimal resources" to "optimal care" at trauma centers. J Trauma Acute Care Surg. 2012;72(4):870–7.

15. Demetriades D, Martin M, Salim A, Rhee P, Brown C, Chan L. The effect of trauma center designation and trauma volume on outcome in specific severe injuries. Ann Surg. 2005;242(4):512–7, discussion 517–9.

16. American College of Surgeons Committee on Trauma. Resources for optimal care of the trauma patient. Chicago, IL: American College of Surgeons; 2006.

Modern Military Trauma

Aaron M. Fields

Modern military trauma began for the United States with Operation Iraqi Freedom (OIF) and continues today with the Global War on Terrorism. To date there have been over 58,000 casualties from OIF, Operation New Dawn, and Operation Enduring Freedom (OEF). The ratio of killed in action (KIA) to wounded in action (WIA) is between 8.48 and 11.4 % (Defense). This unprecedented survivability is due to a host of changes in the way that war casualties are handled. This chapter will be broken into three categories: Pre Hospital Treatment, Hospital Treatment, and Aeromedical Evacuation.

Pre-hospital Treatment

While there is little evidence to support it "The Golden Hour" is a much discussed period of time in which adequate treatment can greatly influence whether a casualty moves into the KIA category [1]. "The Platinum 10" is being taught to medics as the 10 min after injury for control of bleeding [2]. Adequate body armor has significantly decreased the severity of injuries in modern military trauma.

In 2006, Peleg and colleagues used a national trauma registry and retrospectively analyzed injury from firearms in those protected by body armor and those that were not. Those with body armor had statistically significantly lower injury severity scores (ISS), less intensive care unit (ICU) stays, and half the inpatient mortality. Those with traumatic brain injury from a firearm had no difference in mortality whether they were wearing body armor or not. Overall, lower rates of head, brain, chest, and abdominal injuries were seen and the severity of injury to the chest and abdomen were decreased [3].

In mechanized (i.e., "mounted") divisions, injury patterns were slightly different. Most of the injuries were from improvised explosive devices (IEDs) and mines, with only 3 % of injuries in one study from gunfire. Torso injuries were relatively minor due to body armor, as was lower extremity injury due to protection from the vehicle [4]. Enemy tactics also changed from gunshot wounds (5 %) to fragmentation munitions (95 %) [5].

In 2005, Xydakis et al. analyzed the data from several military databases and concluded that Kevlar helmets and vests were very effective at preventing intracranial and intrathoracic penetration of shrapnel and bullets, and that solid armored plates warn in addition to Kevlar prevented most projectiles from entering the chest and abdomen. Additionally, emerging enemy tactics led to new patterns of combat injuries such that the majority of wounds were limited to the extremities which are easily tourniqueted [6].

The healthcare provider must be knowledgeable in the safe removal of body armor and the

A.M. Fields, M.D. (✉)
Department of Surgery, Tripler Army Medical Center,
1 Jarrett White Road, Honolulu, HI 96859, USA
e-mail: Aaron.fields.1@us.af.mil

C.S. Scher (ed.), *Anesthesia for Trauma*, DOI 10.1007/978-1-4939-0909-4_21,
© Springer Science+Business Media New York 2014

safe storage of weapons and ordinance often found on patients presenting to military trauma centers [7]. However, CT imaging is feasible with Kevlar helmets and soft body armor as well as ceramic plate armor in place if advantageous [8].

Tourniquet: In Operation Desert Storm, the predominant cause of death for patients treated at Seventh Corps Hospitals was exsanguination from extremity wounds [5]. This led the military to issue tourniquets to all soldiers. A tourniquet was soon described as an "instrument of the devil that sometimes saves a life" [9]. At the time it was thought that most extremity hemorrhage could be controlled with direct pressure and that they led to more ischemic complications and unnecessary amputations than lives saved. Additionally, there was fear that tourniquets "cause venous rather than arterial occlusion and often increase rather than decrease hemorrhage" and that "tourniquets should be prohibited" [10] However, retrospective analysis in Israel showed that tourniquets were safe, effective, and had a high success rate. There were almost no complications (5.5 %) despite ischemic times out to 305 min. There were no deaths from uncontrolled limb hemorrhage with 550 injured during this 4-year retrospective analysis. This is in contrast to 10 % of all deaths in the Vietnam War attributed to limb hemorrhage [11]. Civilian trauma centers also reported deaths due to extremity exsanguination [12]. By 2005, more than 275,000 Combat Application Tourniquets (CAT-1) had been sent to Iraq [13] and by 2008 every soldier carried a tourniquet [14]. Early reports in 2006 showed that these were very effective and had few adverse outcomes [15] and it was soon called "the leading lifesaving device available to soldiers in the field" [16]. By 2012, vascular injury in modern combat was five times that reported in previous wars, but survivability was up to 99.1 % for those receiving treatment for vascular injuries [17].

Animal data showed that hemostatic bandages improved survival. A large-scale military conflict provided the testing ground for hemostatic agents and bandages. While a few had been tested, most only had animal data and some were later shown to be no better than regular bandages. One that has continued to be used is QuckClot (QC) manufactured by Z-Medica (Newington, CT) and contains (Mineral Zeolite molecular sieve). It became Federal Drug Administration (FDA) approved in 2002 and at the time only cost about $10/packet. The greatest risk of this agent was thought to be thermal injury to the surrounding tissue as its reaction with blood is highly exothermic as it absorbs water and concentrates the cells and factors [18]. By 2006, several products were FDA approved or available commercially. Their cost varied widely ($8–$1,000/dose), and they were often developed using funding from the US Army. The FDA approved these products based on randomized animal data or the dressings were sent to troops in Afghanistan and Iraq under investigational new drug protocols. Those that were FDA approved at the time were only approved for external application. Additional information was becoming available on the exothermic reactions taking place application of QC. There was a direct correlation between the volume of blood the product was exposed to and the maximum temperature attained at the wound. Large volumes of blood generated temperatures in excess of 100° C [19]. The solution was to impregnate the hemostatic agent into gauze mesh pouch so that it could be applied at the wound site without the compound washing away. Additionally, the manufacturer pre-hydrated the solution to decrease the heat produced [20]. This made less debris in the wound and decreased the exothermic reaction. In 2009 a retrospective analysis showed that QuickClot Bandages were saving lives but continued to occasionally cause burns [21]. Cost was $25/device and is the current teaching for prehospital medics in the United States [23]. In one retrospective analysis, it worked in 100 % of prehospital uses [24]. Work continues to find an even better product, but few reach statistically significant improvement over the current standard of care, QuickClot Combat Gauze (Z-Medica, Wallingford, CT) [25].

For decades, conventional wisdom was to fluid resuscitate hemorrhagic shock as quickly and aggressively as possible. However, new data has shown that low volume resuscitation, just adequate enough to maintain radial pulses improve mortality in patients with uncontrolled or ongoing bleeding [26]. The first prospective human trial showed increased survivability to hospital discharge despite some problems with the study [27]. Subsequent trials have failed to show a difference [28], but hetastarch transfusion to palpable radial pulse (1 L maximum) remains the teaching for prehospital military medics [22, 29]. This is mirrored in the Israeli Defense Force Protocols where they infuse 500 mL boluses of crystalloid until radial pulses, HR < 130, or SBP > 80 [30].

The lethal triad consists of hypothermia, metabolic acidosis, and hypercoagulability [31]. Treatment of acidosis and coagulopathy is beyond the scope of most prehospital providers. However, treatment and prevention of hypothermia can have profound changes in outcomes. Eastridge and colleagues showed that hypothermia on presentation was associated with increased blood product utilization and mortality [32]. Current military doctrine teaches the use of the Hypothermia Prevention Management Kits (HPMKs) (North American Rescue Products, Greer, SC) [22]. It consists of an exothermic chemical powder containing blanket and a reflective shell which includes a hood. This device was superior to both passive and other active heating devices including electrical heaters [33].

Bleeding that is quickly controlled in a patient without signs of shock are often treated with oral fluid replacement to prevent dehydration. However, intravenous (IV) fluid resuscitation is often necessary in modern military trauma. However, even under ideal circumstances, peripheral IV (PIV) access can be challenging. A recent prospective randomized controlled trial (RCT) showed that intraosseous (IO) catheter placement had better first attempt success rate and shorter time to good flow than both PIV and central line placement [34]. Many drugs have been demonstrated to be safely administered via IO [35]. Additionally, several studies have shown that medications given via sternal IO catheters reach the central circulation faster than other IO sites [36, 37]. Prehospital medics currently are trained

on the EZ-IO mechanical sternal insertion kit (Vidacare Corporation Shavano Park, Texas, USA) [22].

As late as the 1993 Mogadishu action, prehospital antibiotics were not being given. Additionally, there was an average of 15 h between injury and definitive hospital treatment. As a result, four of the five open fractures from gunshot wounds became infected. Moxifloxacin is available in oral form and has been shown to be very efficacious against a wide variety of gram positive and negative bacteria as well as anaerobic and aerobic bacteria [38, 39]. This training has led to increased adherence with timely antibiotic administration reaching nearly 80 % [40]. Increased adherence has led to infection rates as low as 26.6 % including pneumonia [41]. All soldiers are deployed with a foil pack containing Meloxicam 15 mg, Acetaminophen ER 650 mg, two caplets, Moxifloxacin 400 mg and instructed to take all four capsules in the event of an open wound.

Hospital Treatment

Damage control surgery (DCS) is when rapid control of hemorrhage is intraoperative obtained and the patient is quickly moved to the ICU for further warming, resuscitation, correction of electrolyte abnormalities, and coagulopathy. Only when these have taken place is the patient then taken back to the operating room (OR) for more surgery [42]. DCS prevents extensive procedures on unstable patients [31]. This strategy appears to be very effective when examined retrospectively: 99.1 % survival with 84 % amputation-free survival [17]. While there have been no RCT with regard to DCS versus immediate and definitive repair in patients with major abdominal surgery or vascular surgery, the retrospective data supports increased survivability and decreased blood product utilization [43].

Fresh whole blood (FWB) administration has been one of the more controversial treatments used in modern military trauma. It was first described in 1667, but did not gain widespread acceptance until World War II when 2,000 units of stored whole blood were shipped to US military hospitals during peak usage in 1945 [44]. It has been used in every combat operation since World War I [45]. Between March 2003 and July 2007 over 6,000 units of warm FWB were transfused. Current military guidelines indicate the FWB should be given when there is life-threatening hemorrhage and component therapy is not available [46]. In one retrospective analysis, FWB was associated with a higher 24 h ($p = 0.018$) and 30 day ($p = 0.002$) survival rate [47]. In a recent Norwegian study, soldiers were tested on several physical fitness tests and a marksmanship test. They then performed phlebotomy on each other removing 450 mL of whole blood. The physical fitness tests and marksmanship tests were then repeated. Finally, the soldiers placed a sternal intraosseous device and reinfused the FWB. Physical fitness and marksmanship were unaffected by the phlebotomy, all soldiers were able to perform phlebotomy and all were able to place the intraosseous device [48].

The ratio of component blood products has changed over the course of the recent conflicts. In 2007, Borgman published a retrospective analysis of the ratio of packed red blood cells (PRBC) to fresh frozen plasma (FFP) in patients receiving a massive transfusion defined as ≥ 10 units of PRBC in 24 h. The patients were divided into three groups correlating to the ratio of FFP received. In the low ratio group the FFP to PRBC ratio was 1:8, medium was 1:2.5, and high was 1:1.4. Mortality was 65 %, 34 %, and 19 %, respectively, and hemorrhage mortality rates were 92.5 %, 78 %, and 37 %. A prospective RCT is underway (ClinicalTrials.gov Identifier: NCT00945542), but more recent retrospective trials have shown decreased mortality with increased early administration of FFP [49, 50]. The ability to predict who will need massive transfusion allows the clinician to begin FFP earlier, and several factors have been shown to be predictive. They are hemoglobin ≤ 11 g/dL, International Normalized Ration >1.5, and a penetrating mechanism [51].

In 2005, Boffard and colleagues demonstrated that recombinant Factor VIIa (rFVIIa) was safe and effective for both blunt and penetrating trauma in two separate prospective RCTs [52]. This led to widespread use in the Iraq and Afghanistan conflicts. However, concerns soon developed that it was being used too frequently, in acidotic patients [53], its high cost and risk of thromboembolic events. After an Army whistleblower lawsuit was settled, Novo Nordisk, the makers of rFVIIa, paid $25 million for violating the False Claims act [54]. More recent studies have failed to show a decrease in mortality [55, 56].

Thromboelastography has been shown to be beneficial in trauma and has been used with increasing frequency in modern military trauma to provide point of care and real-time assessment of hypercoagulopathy [57] or the need for blood products [58].

New pain control modalities are being used in modern military trauma. Low dose ketamine infusion for neuropathic pain commonly associated with limb amputation has been shown to be safe and effective in reducing both pain and opiate use [59]. Training has led to increased administration of prehospital pain medication [60]. For those unable to tolerate oral medications and without intravenous access, oral transmucoscal fentanyl citrate has been shown to be safe and significantly reduce pain [61]. Continuous peripheral nerve blocks are being used more and more frequently and an RCT is currently underway [62].

Aeromedical Evacuation

The ability to aeromedically (AE) evacuate patients from the battlefield to stateside hospitals in a matter of days has revolutionized trauma and burn treatment. During the Vietnam War, it took weeks to evacuate patients to Army burn Centers [63, 64]. In Iraq and Afghanistan, the United States pushed surgical teams far forward with advanced treatment capabilities but poor ability to hold patients for long periods of time. This made AE a crucial capability. Intensive Care requires a large logistical footprint, and it became clear that it was easier to move the patient back from the front lines using US Air Force Critical Care Air Transport Team (CCATT). This team consists of an ICU capable physician (Anesthesiologist, Emergency Medicine Physician, or a Pulmonary/Critical Care Physician), an ICU qualified nurse, and a cardiopulmonary technician. They are capable of caring for 3 intubated patients or 6 critical but not intubated patients for up to 24 h. They carry with them medications, ventilators, a defibrillator, monitors, suction, iSTAT point-of-care testing devices, and the ability to place central lines, chest tubes, endotracheal tubes, and arterial lines to support these patients. In addition to their training for ground-based patients, they are given additional instruction on the unique environment of flight. This includes the effects of decreased barometric pressure and temperature at altitude [65]. The most common aircraft used are C-130, KC-135, and C-17. Retrospective analysis shows that CCATT is safe and capable of responding to rapid and potentially deadly physiological changes in the patients. Of 656 patients examined in one study, there were no deaths [66]. In a smaller study of 133 patients, there were also no deaths [67]. Hyptotension and hemoglobin desaturation were the most common adverse events in the previous two studies, but retrospective study found that fever occurred in 41 % of CCATT patients and found no en route deaths of the 248 included.

Dr. Renz and colleagues looked at burn patients admitted to the US Army Institute of Surgical Research. 540 patients were admitted, the mean time from injury to admission in San Antonio, Texas was 4 days over a distance of 8,600 km. About 1/3 of the patients required in flight ventilatory support, and about 1/3 of them were transported by CCATT. There were no inflight deaths [68].

Conclusion

From point of injury and prehospital care to hospital treatment and aeromedical evacuation, modern military trauma is influencing the way trauma is treated in civilian practice and around the world.

References

1. Lerner EB, Moscati RM. The golden hour: scientific fact or medical "urban legend"? Acad Emerg Med. 2001;8:758–60. doi:10.1111/j.1553-2712.2001.tb00201.x.
2. Bukowski MCW. The Platinum 10. Infantry 2006; 11–15.
3. Peleg K, Rivkind A, Aharonson-Daniel L. Does body armor protect from firearm injuries? J Am Coll Surg. 2006;202:643–8. doi:10.1016/j.jamcollsurg.2005.12.019.
4. Gondusky JS, Reiter MP. Protecting military convoys in Iraq: an examination of battle injuries sustained by a mechanized battalion during Operation Iraqi Freedom II. Mil Med. 2005;170:546–9.
5. Carey ME. Analysis of wounds incurred by U.S. Army Seventh Corps personnel treated in Corps hospitals during Operation Desert Storm, February 20 to March 10, 1991. J Trauma. 1996;40:S165–9.
6. Xydakis MS, Fravell MD, Nasser KE, Casler JD. Analysis of battlefield head and neck injuries in Iraq and Afghanistan. Otolaryngology Head Neck Surg. 2005;133:497–504. doi:10.1016/j.otohns.2005.07.003.
7. Starnes BW. Peacekeeping and stability operations: a military surgeon's perspective. Surg Clin North Am. 2006;86:753–63. doi:10.1016/j.suc.2006.02.008.
8. Harcke HT, Schauer DA, Harris RM, Campman SC, Lonergan GJ, et al. Imaging body armor. Mil Med. 2002;167:267–71.
9. Navein J, Coupland R, Dunn R. The tourniquet controversy. J Trauma. 2003;54:S219–20. doi:10.1097/01.TA.0000047202.16935.E9.
10. Husum H, Gilbert M, Wisborg T, Pillgram-Larsen J. Prehospital tourniquets: there should be no controversy. J Trauma. 2004;56:214–5. doi:10.1097/01.TA.0000104494.62175.2F.
11. Lakstein D, Blumenfeld A, Sokolov T, et al. Tourniquets for hemorrhage control on the battlefield: a 4-year accumulated experience. J Trauma. 2003;54:S221–5. doi:10.1097/01.TA.0000047227.33395.49.
12. Dorlac WC, DeBakey ME, Holcomb JB, et al. Mortality from isolated civilian penetrating extremity injury. J Trauma. 2005;59:217–22. doi:10.1097/01.TA.0000173699.71652.BA.
13. Beekley AC. United States military surgical response to modern large-scale conflicts: the ongoing evolution of a trauma system. Surg Clin North Am. 2006;86:689–709. doi:10.1016/j.suc.2006.02.007.
14. Hess JR, Holcomb JB. Transfusion practice in military trauma. Transfus Med (Oxford, England). 2008;18:143–50. doi:10.1111/j.1365-3148.2008.00855.x.
15. Sebesta J. Special lessons learned from Iraq. Surg Clin North Am. 2006;86:711–26. doi:10.1016/j.suc.2006.03.002.
16. Mabry RL. Tourniquet use on the battlefield. Mil Med. 2006;171:352–6.

17. Dua A, Patel B, Kragh JF, et al. Long-term follow-up and amputation-free survival in 497 casualties with combat-related vascular injuries and damage-control resuscitation. J Trauma Acute Care Surg. 2012;73: 1517–24. doi:10.1097/TA.0b013e31827826b7.

18. Wortham L. Hemorrhage control in the battlefield: role of new hemostatic agent. Mil Med. 2005;170:ii, author reply ii, 1004.

19. Pusateri AE, Holcomb JB, Kheirabadi BS, et al. Making sense of the preclinical literature on advanced hemostatic products. J Trauma. 2006;60:674–82. doi:10.1097/01.ta.0000196672.47783.fd.

20. Achneck HE, Sileshi B, Jamiolkowski RM, et al. A comprehensive review of topical hemostatic agents: efficacy and recommendations for use. Ann Surg. 2010;251:217–28. doi:10.1097/SLA. 0b013e3181c3bcca.

21. Cox ED, Schreiber MA, McManus J, et al. New hemostatic agents in the combat setting. Transfusion. 2009;49 Suppl 5:248S–55. doi:10.1111/j.1537-2995. 2008.01988.x.

22. Defense UD of casualty report. www.defense.gov/news/casualty.pdf. Accessed 13 Aug 2013.

23. Defense UD of tactical combat casualty care. 2013. http://www.health.mil/Education_And_Training/TCCC

24. Rhee P, Brown C, Martin M, et al. QuikClot use in trauma for hemorrhage control: case series of 103 documented uses. J Trauma. 2008;64:1093–9. doi:10.1097/TA.0b013e31812f6dbc.

25. Rall JM, Cox JM, Songer AG, et al. Comparison of novel hemostatic dressings with QuikClot combat gauze in a standardized swine model of uncontrolled hemorrhage. J Trauma Acute Care Surg. 2013;75:S150–6. doi:10.1097/TA. 0b013e318299d909.

26. Stern SA. Low-volume fluid resuscitation for presumed hemorrhagic shock: helpful or harmful? Curr Opin Crit Care. 2001;7:422–30.

27. Bickell WH, Wall MJ, Pepe PE, et al. Immediate versus delayed fluid resuscitation for hypotensive patients with penetrating torso injuries. N Engl J Med. 1994;331:1105–9. doi:10.1056/NEJM199410273311701.

28. Dutton RP, Mackenzie CF, Scalea TM. Hypotensive resuscitation during active hemorrhage: impact on in-hospital mortality. J Trauma. 2002;52:1141–6.

29. Rhee P, Koustova E, Alam HB. Searching for the optimal resuscitation method: recommendations for the initial fluid resuscitation of combat casualties. J Trauma. 2003;54:S52–62. doi:10.1097/01.TA. 0000064507.80390.10.

30. Lipsky AM, Ganor O, Abramovich A, et al. Walking between the drops: Israeli defense forces' fluid resuscitation protocol. J Emerg Med. 2013;44:790–5. doi:10.1016/j.jemermed.2012.08.029.

31. Cirocchi R, Montedori A, Farinella E, et al. Damage control surgery for abdominal trauma. Cochrane Database Syst Rev. 2013;(3):CD007438. doi:10.1002/14651858.CD007438.pub3.

32. Eastridge BJ, Owsley J, Sebesta J, et al. Admission physiology criteria after injury on the battlefield predict medical resource utilization and patient mortality. J Trauma. 2006;61:820–3. doi:10.1097/01.ta. 0000239508.94330.7a.

33. Allen PB, Salyer SW, Dubick MA. Preventing hypothermia: comparison of current devices used by the US Army in an in vitro warmed fluid model. J Trauma. 2010;69 Suppl 1:S154–61. doi:10.1097/TA.0b013e3181e45ba5.

34. Paxton JH, Knuth TE, Klausner HA. Proximal humerus intraosseous infusion: a preferred emergency venous access. J Trauma. 2009;67:606–11. doi:10.1097/TA.0b013e3181b16f42.

35. Paxton JH. Intraosseous vascular access: a review. Trauma. 2012;14:195–232. doi:10.1177/1460408611430175.

36. Hoskins SL, do Nascimento P, Lima RM, et al. Pharmacokinetics of intraosseous and central venous drug delivery during cardiopulmonary resuscitation. Resuscitation. 2012;83:107–12. doi:10.1016/j.resuscitation.2011.07.041.

37. Carness JM, Russell JL, M e Lima R, et al. Fluid resuscitation using the intraosseous route: infusion with lactated Ringer's and hetastarch. Mil Med. 2012;177:222–8.

38. Mather R, Karenchak LM, Romanowski EG, Kowalski RP. Fourth generation fluoroquinolones: new weapons in the arsenal of ophthalmic antibiotics. Am J Ophthalmol. 2002;133:463–6.

39. Butler F, O'Connor K. Antibiotics in tactical combat casualty care 2002. Mil Med. 2003;168:911–4.

40. Tribble DR, Lloyd B, Weintrob A, et al. Antimicrobial prescribing practices following publication of guidelines for the prevention of infections associated with combat-related injuries. J Trauma. 2011;71: S299–306. doi:10.1097/TA.0b013e318227af64.

41. Tribble DR, Conger NG, Fraser S, et al. Infection-associated clinical outcomes in hospitalized medical evacuees after traumatic injury: trauma infectious disease outcome study. J Trauma. 2011;71:S33–42. doi:10.1097/TA.0b013e318221162e.

42. Fox CJ, Gillespie DL, Cox ED, et al. The effectiveness of a damage control resuscitation strategy for vascular injury in a combat support hospital: results of a case control study. J Trauma. 2008;64:S99–106; discussion S106–7. doi:10.1097/TA.0b013e3181608c4a.

43. Cotton BA, Gunter OL, Isbell J, et al. Damage control hematology: the impact of a trauma exsanguination protocol on survival and blood product utilization. J Trauma. 2008;64:1177–82. doi:10.1097/TA. 0b013e31816c5c80. discussion 1182–3.

44. Hess JR, Thomas MJG. Blood use in war and disaster: lessons from the past century. Transfusion. 2003;43: 1622–33.

45. Kauvar DS, Holcomb JB, Norris GC, Hess JR. Fresh whole blood transfusion: a controversial military practice. J Trauma. 2006;61:181–4. doi:10.1097/01. ta.0000222671.84335.64.

46. Spinella PC. Warm fresh whole blood transfusion for severe hemorrhage: U.S. military and potential civilian applications. Crit Care Med. 2008;36:S340–5. doi:10.1097/CCM.0b013e31817e2ef9.

47. Spinella PC, Perkins JG, Grathwohl KW, et al. Warm fresh whole blood is independently associated with improved survival for patients with combat-related traumatic injuries. J Trauma. 2009;66:S69–76. doi:10.1097/TA.0b013e31819d85fb.

48. Strandenes G, Skogrand H, Spinella PC, et al. Donor performance of combat readiness skills of special forces soldiers are maintained immediately after whole blood donation: a study to support the development of a prehospital fresh whole blood transfusion program. Transfusion. 2013;53:526–30. doi:10.1111/j.1537-2995.2012.03767.x.

49. Zink KA, Sambasivan CN, Holcomb JB, et al. A high ratio of plasma and platelets to packed red blood cells in the first 6 hours of massive transfusion improves outcomes in a large multicenter study. Am J Surg. 2009;197:565–70; discussion 570. doi:10.1016/j.amjsurg.2008.12.014.

50. Mitra B, Mori A, Cameron PA, et al. Fresh frozen plasma (FFP) use during massive blood transfusion in trauma resuscitation. Injury. 2010;41:35–9. doi:10.1016/j.injury.2009.09.029.

51. Schreiber MA, Perkins J, Kiraly L, et al. Early predictors of massive transfusion in combat casualties. J Am Coll Surg. 2007;205:541–5. doi:10.1016/j.jamcollsurg.2007.05.007.

52. Boffard KD, Riou B, Warren B, et al. Recombinant factor VIIa as adjunctive therapy for bleeding control in severely injured trauma patients: two parallel randomized, placebo-controlled, double-blind clinical trials. J Trauma. 2005;59:8–18. doi:10.1097/01.TA.0000171453.37949.B7.

53. Fries D. The early use of fibrinogen, prothrombin complex concentrate, and recombinant-activated factor VIIa in massive bleeding. Transfusion. 2013;53 Suppl 1:91S–5. doi:10.1111/trf.12041.

54. Christenson S, Finley D. Drug firm's wooing made whistleblower suspicious|FAIR. In: FAIR. 2011. http://fairwhistleblower.ca/content/drug-firms-wooing-made-whistleblower-suspicious. Accessed 16 Aug 2013.

55. Hauser CJ, Boffard K, Dutton R, et al. Results of the CONTROL trial: efficacy and safety of recombinant activated factor VII in the management of refractory traumatic hemorrhage. J Trauma. 2010;69:489–500. doi:10.1097/TA.0b013e3181edf36e.

56. Dutton RP, Parr M, Tortella BJ, et al. Recombinant activated factor VII safety in trauma patients: results from the CONTROL trial. J Trauma. 2011;71:12–9. doi:10.1097/TA.0b013e31821a42cf.

57. Park MS, Martini WZ, Dubick MA, et al. Thromboelastography as a better indicator of hypercoagulable state after injury than prothrombin time or activated partial thromboplastin time. J Trauma. 2009;67:266–75; discussion 275–6. doi:10.1097/TA.0b013e3181ae6f1c.

58. Da Luz LT, Nascimento B, Rizoli S. Thrombelastography (TEG®): practical considerations on its clinical use in trauma resuscitation. Scand J Trauma Resusc Emerg Med. 2013;21:29. doi:10.1186/1757-7241-21-29.

59. Polomano RC, Buckenmaier CC, Kwon KH, et al. Effects of low-dose IV ketamine on peripheral and central pain from major limb injuries sustained in combat. Pain Med (Malden, Mass). 2013;14:1088–100. doi:10.1111/pme.12094.

60. Bowman WJ, Nesbitt ME, Therien SP. The effects of standardized trauma training on prehospital pain control: have pain medication administration rates increased on the battlefield? J Trauma Acute Care Surg. 2012;73:S43–8. doi:10.1097/TA.0b013e3182606148.

61. Wedmore IS, Kotwal RS, McManus JG, et al. Safety and efficacy of oral transmucosal fentanyl citrate for prehospital pain control on the battlefield. J Trauma Acute Care Surg. 2012;73:S490–5. doi:10.1097/TA.0b013e3182754674.

62. Hunter JG. Managing pain on the battlefield: an introduction to continuous peripheral nerve blocks. J R Army Med Corps. 2010;156:230–2.

63. Allen BD, Whitson TC, Henjyoji EY. Treatment of 1,963 burned patients at 106th general hospital, Yokohama, Japan. J Trauma. 1970;10:386–92.

64. Treat RC, Sirinek KR, Levine BA, Pruitt BA. Air evacuation of thermally injured patients: principles of treatment and results. J Trauma. 1980;20:275–9.

65. Johannigman JE. Critical care aeromedical teams (Ccatt): then, now and what's next. J Trauma. 2007;62:S35. doi:10.1097/TA.0b013e31806540f3.

66. Lairet J, King J, Vojta L, Beninati W. Short-term outcomes of US Air Force Critical Care Air Transport Team (CCATT) patients evacuated from a combat setting. Prehosp Emerg Care. 2013. doi:10.3109/10903127.2013.811564.

67. Mason PE, Eadie JS, Holder AD. Prospective observational study of United States (US) Air Force Critical Care Air Transport team operations in Iraq. J Emerg Med. 2011;41:8–13. doi:10.1016/j.jemermed.2008.06.032.

68. Renz EM, Cancio LC, Barillo DJ, et al. Long range transport of war-related burn casualties. J Trauma. 2008; 64:S136–44; discussion S144–5. doi:10.1097/TA.0b013e31816086c9.

Disaster Preparedness

22

J. David Roccaforte

That which does not kill us makes us stronger.
(Friedrich Nietzsche)

Disasters have been an unpredictable and interminable affliction challenging human civilization since the dawn of time. Historically, the typical pattern of preparedness has been reactive and auto-extinguishing. Consider an infrequent disaster such as a wildfire. A community finds itself unprepared, and suffers greatly. Herculean efforts are undertaken at great expense to prepare for the next wildfire, which statistically won't recur for over 50 years. In the interim, memories fade, concern wanes, and community priorities shift. Wildfire preparedness therefore deteriorates and before the next wildfire even arrives, the area is devastated by a flood [1].

Recognizing this recurring pattern, a great deal of effort has gone into escaping the paradigm. The field of disaster preparedness has grown to be well funded, drawing a pool of highly motivated bureaucrats, administrators, and clinicians who have elucidated vulnerabilities and suggested solutions [2], but who, at the same time, have created what can sound like a foreign language to those unfamiliar with the field. A body of scholarly work has emerged that requires familiarity with equal parts of data, strategy, and vocabulary.

J.D. Roccaforte, M.D. (✉)
Department of Anesthesiology, New York University,
Bellevue Hospital, 1st Avenue at 27th Street, New York,
NY 10016, USA
e-mail: JDavidR@mail.com

Definitions

All-hazards approach: A strategy of general preparations which are easily adaptable to a wide variety of disasters. The all-hazards approach is best-suited for regional and hospital administrative issues which are applicable to all disasters such as managing media communications, hospital security, the information technology system, or maintaining a list of redundant vendors for critical supplies. The clinical resources necessary for different disaster scenarios, however, may be quite diverse and specific as, for instance, in treating the victims of a tornado vs. those of an anthrax attack.

Hospital Incident Command System (HICS): A general template plan for hospital administrative organization which is implemented during a disaster incident. HICS provides no direction or guidelines for the medical or surgical management of casualties [3].

Definitive Care Area (DCA): Locations in a hospital and the resources required to acutely treat life-threatening injuries and illnesses, i.e., operating rooms (ORs), interventional radiology (IR) suites, recovery room (PACU), and intensive care unit (ICU) beds.

Triage: From the French "to sort." The screening and sorting of patients, attempting to match a patient's injury or illness with appropriate care.

Rationing: The process by which scarce resources are distributed, ideally in a prioritized manner to those who need them the most.

C.S. Scher (ed.), *Anesthesia for Trauma*, DOI 10.1007/978-1-4939-0909-4_22,
© Springer Science+Business Media New York 2014

Worried well: People presenting to a hospital after a disaster event with no injury or illness. Also known as psychological casualties.

Walking wounded: Ambulatory victims from a disaster arriving at a hospital with minor injuries, often bypassing Emergency Medical Services (EMS) field triage.

Critically injured: Trauma victims with an Injury Severity Score (ISS) $\geq$ 15.

Critically ill: Disaster or pandemic victims with an Acute Physiology And Chronic Health Evaluation (APACHE) II score $\geq$ 25.

Overtriage: Patients evaluated by the triage system who ultimately have no severe injury or serious illness.

Undertriage: Patients in whom triage screening has missed detecting severe injury or serious illness.

Critical mortality: Death rate among the critically injured with ISS $\geq$ 15. Critical mortality increases as overtriage rate increases.

Surge: The maximum number of casualties presenting to a hospital in the shortest period of time.

Multiple Casualty Incident (MCI): A large number of casualties, generated over a short period of time, which can be appropriately managed with existing or extended resources.

Mass Casualty Event (MCE): A major medical disaster that destroys organized community support mechanisms and results in overwhelming casualties.

Internal disaster: An event affecting hospital infrastructure or facilities. For example, fire, electrical disruption, hospital building flood, or collapse.

External disaster: An event occurring in the community which leaves hospital functionality unaffected.

Slowly evolving event: A predicted and anticipated disaster that unfolds over a period of days to weeks. For example, pandemics, hurricanes, radiation fallout. Allows for a proactive response. Civilian evacuation and/or mobilization of resources in advance of the surge is generally possible.

Rapidly evolving event: A disaster that occurs suddenly or explosively over a period of minutes to hours. Also known as a no-notice event. Requires a reactive response. For example, earthquakes, terrorist bombings.

Explosive energy: An estimation of the force imparted by a rapidly evolving event. Useful in predicting the dead:injured ratio and, given the population density of the disaster location, in anticipating the number of casualties of each triage type—mild, moderate, and severely injured. Natural disasters such as earthquakes and tornados release tremendous amounts of energy, an open-air terrorist bomb less so. When an explosion occurs in an enclosed space, the energy is amplified, and if a building collapse is also involved, the explosive energy of the bomb is further augmented.

Dead:injured ratio: The greater the concentration of explosive energy to which victims are exposed, the higher the dead:injured ratio. As a consequence, as the size and energy imparted during an explosive event increases, the number of dead increases, while the number of surviving injured plateaus or even decreases (see Fig. 22.1).

Dead:injured ratio in military combat is typically 1:3. That ratio may be reversed with high-energy events such as enclosed-space explosions with building collapse [4], or natural disasters such as tornados (see Table 22.1).

Process inventory: An analysis of all resources normally utilized to provide definitive care. The results of this analysis will identify all parties required to participate in table-top exercises for disaster preparedness planning.

Hazard Vulnerability Analysis: Evaluation of the disaster scenarios most likely to be encountered given local risks.

Surge resources: Alternate equipment, locations, and personnel that can be utilized in the treatment of additional patients while maintaining the standard of care. Also known as conventional resources.

Surge capacity: The total number of patients that can be managed by a facility with both normal and surge resources.

Overflow resources: Alternate equipment, locations, and personnel that can be utilized in the treatment of additional patients, but with compromised standard of care.

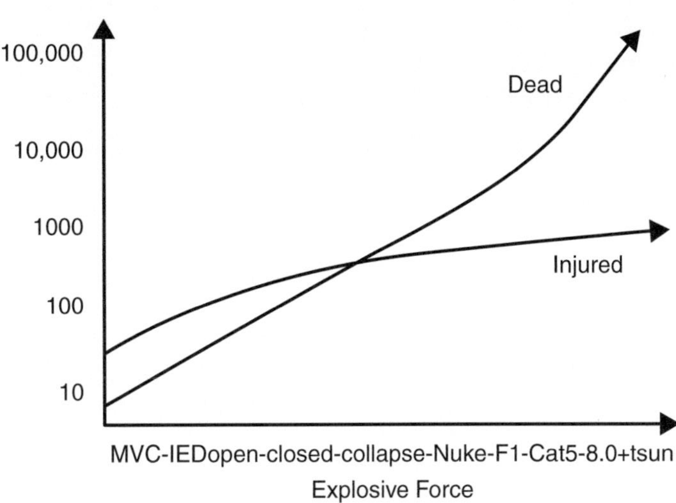

Fig. 22.1 Dead:Injured vs. explosive energy released. *MVC* multiple motor vehicle crash, *IEDopen* improvized explosive device open air, *Closed* IED enclosed explosion, *Collapse* explosion with building collapse, *Nuke* first generation nuclear warhead (20 kiloton TNT equivalent), *F1* Force 1 tornado, *Cat5* category 5 hurricane, *8.0* Richter magnitude 8 earthquake, *+tsun* earthquake + widespread tsunami

Table 22.1 Dead: injured ratios

	Dead	Injured
Typical urban trauma center	1	20
Terrorist bombings	1	5–20
Conventional war	1	3–5
1983 Beirut marine barracks	3	1
Natural disasters	3–20	1
9/11 WTC attack	10	1

Overflow capacity: The total number of patients that can be managed by a facility with normal, surge, and overflow resources.

Care-limiting resource: The resource in the lowest supply that limits capacity to care for patients. This resource becomes the focus of capacity expansion.

Table-top Exercises: Planned rehearsals of MCIs or MCEs, organized to challenge the facility personnel involved in the management of patients during a disaster, and to identify surge, overflow, and care-limiting resources.

Overwhelmed scenario: An MCE, which creates a condition where demands exceed resources. Care rationing must be employed, and evacuation becomes a priority.

Each time the news brings us images of disaster, from a tsunami in the Indian Ocean to a terrorist bombing attack, many people think about what they would do if they found themselves in the midst of a comparable scenario. For most, this thought experiment is quickly abandoned by concluding either that the probability is so low, or the consequences so overwhelming, that disaster preparedness of any kind is either a waste of time or ultimately futile. The result, unfortunately, is a lack of readiness to adequately respond to disasters when they do occur [5, 6].

Reviewing historical disaster responses and outcomes, it is quickly apparent that much of what happens following a disaster is very different from standard operating procedure. Often the most appropriate strategy is counterintuitive [7]. Our ability to predict and anticipate the difficulties we may face is generally poor. Consequently, a reflexive or improvized reaction will yield worse outcomes than a pre-planned response.

The spectrum of disaster preparedness spans elements of public education, infrastructure upgrades, computer modeling, public health, and beyond. From a clinical perspective however, the final common pathway for the critically injured and ill victims of any disaster from any cause will be DCAs. These areas are typically operating rooms (ORs) and ICUs.

The victims of a disaster, especially one of sudden onset, will in decreasing order of severity fall into one of the four categories: (1) those immediately killed, (2) those destined to die regardless of any care they receive, (3) those whose survival depends on timely and appropriate medical care, and (4) those who will live even without medical attention.

In most disasters, the third category is the smallest in number. However, as anesthesiologists, surgeons, and intensivists, it is our biggest concern and becomes the focus of our attention. This is with good reason: the final event mortality rate will be determined by our ability to expand and protect DCAs in order to deliver care to these sickest victims. Saving their lives is the immediate objective of the clinical disaster response.

Beyond the first 48–72 h following an event, any remaining untreated casualties in the third category will have slipped into the second category (destined to die regardless of any care they receive), and beyond 96 h, the priority of disaster response becomes the continued provision of public health needs: food, water, shelter, etc. [8].

The goal of this chapter is to provide a conceptual framework for DCA-specific disaster preparedness for anesthesiologists, surgeons, and intensivists, to be used for rational development of strategies for both expanding and protecting surgical and critical care resources during these events.

Before disaster planning can take place, it is important to understand the relevant characteristics of disaster victims, events, and resources and how they interrelate. Once these concepts are understood, the process of developing plans via the use of table-top exercises will be described.

Victim Characteristics

The key characteristic of disaster victims relevant to those who manage DCAs is whether their status is critical or not.

As one follows the path of the victim from the scene to field evacuation, to a casualty collection area, to transportation to a medical facility, through the diagnostic areas, and finally to transfer to an operating room or ICU, an ongoing process of triage takes place (see Fig. 22.2).

Triage & Rationing

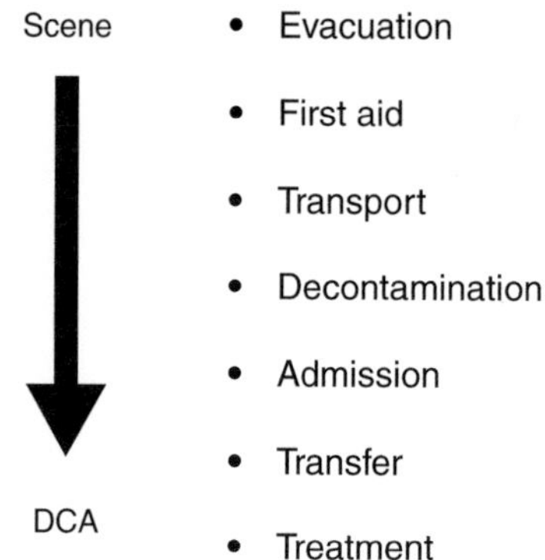

Fig. 22.2 Triage and rationing

The decisions surrounding triage are highly situational. Triage attempts to match a patient's injury or illness severity with appropriate care [9]. Triage, by considering both the types of resources that an individual patient requires, as well as the availability of those resources, performs two functions: routing and rationing [10].

During normal circumstances, triage functions simply to properly route patients to appropriate areas for clinical care. When resources are inadequate to meet needs, triage performs a second function: rationing. Rationing is the process by which scarce resources are distributed, ideally in a prioritized manner to those most in need of them. Rationing is a charged topic in the US health care debate, but is a long recognized function of triage, routinely practiced in military medicine, though seldom invoked in the civilian setting since resources are rarely unavailable [11].

Rationing decisions may occur at each of multiple points between the disaster scene and the DCA: Evacuation, First-aid, Transport, Decontamination, Admission, Transfer, and Treatment. If resources at each step are adequate, no rationing takes place; however, in a disaster the closer to the scene one evaluates resources relative to needs, the more likely that rationing must take place [12].

The consequence of this for a DCA is that triage decisions upstream serve to screen and select from the many casualties those who will benefit from surgery and/or critical care [13]. Thus, rationing of care at the level of the DCA should be assiduously avoided, as that will deny care to precisely those patients whom the entire triage system has identified as standing to benefit the most. Provision of uncompromised care without rationing is the goal of DCA disaster preparedness planning.

During rapidly evolving events, in the field, during transit, or on arrival to the hospital, a triage officer will attach a color-coded classification tag to each victim (see Fig. 22.3).

Black designates dead or moribund. Victims with serious injuries requiring immediate treatment are tagged red. Those with yellow tags will eventually require treatment. Green signifies ambulatory patients with minor injuries. In addition, most casualties arrive from the scene untagged and with no obvious injury; they may require decontamination and counseling. They have been called the "worried well," but now are more appropriately identified as psychological casualties. They are terrified and cannot simply be sent home. Finally, there is everyone else arriving to the hospital untagged: media, family, bystanders, well-meaning volunteers, and, following a terrorist event, potentially those with nefarious intent.

The absolute and relative numbers of each victim type triaged for any event will vary. The biggest variability in urban explosive events is the untagged mass, which will mainly depend on how many people are present, the location, and the time of day. Different mechanisms generate reproducible patterns of death, injury, and illness. Examples include closed-space vs. open-air explosions [14] and food-borne [15] vs. airborne infectious agents [16]. Familiarity with different patterns enables clinicians to anticipate types, timing, acuity, and treatment needs of victims [17].

The immediate focus should be on the red- and yellow-tagged victims. These are the victims whose lives hang in the balance; with timely diagnosis and appropriate treatment most will live, without this most will die. These are the

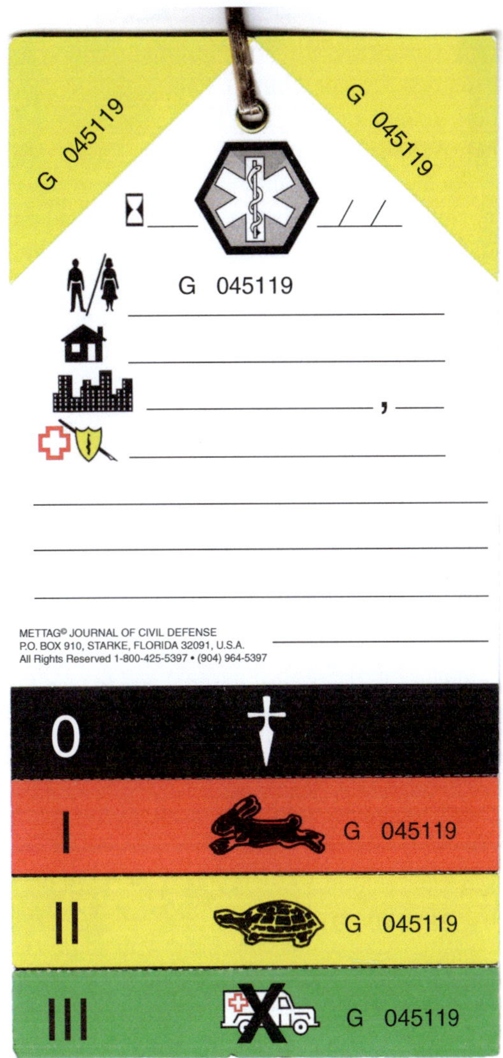

Fig. 22.3 Triage tag

lives at risk, and as anesthesiologists, surgeons, and intensivists, they will be under our care.

Once the triage system identifies a victim as critical but with potential to survive, and then delivers her or him to a DCA, triage ceases to function as routing; ORs and ICUs are the acme of what the hospital has to offer clinically. In a DCA, rationing must be employed only as a last resort. It may be appropriate to offer less than optimal care to green-tagged victims, i.e., lightly injured; they can be triaged to a cafeteria or gymnasium for observation and delayed treatment. The impact on their short- and long-term outcomes will be minimal, but when resources are compromised or withheld from those routed to ORs and ICUs, mortality will increase [18].

For the management of casualties from physical injury under routine circumstances, the American College of Surgeons [19] recommends that trauma centers maintain a 50 % "overtriage" rate. That is, 50 % of all those activating a full trauma response should have an ISS [20] of less than 15 after work-up, signifying no serious injuries. This is believed to ensure capture of all serious injuries, yielding a low "undertriage" rate (defined as missed severe injuries among all those screened) of less than 5 %.

Thus, triage officers intentionally employ a strategy of controlled overtriage while screening patients, which is both acceptable and desirable. In contrast, during a disaster most victims refer themselves to the nearest hospital and bypass the established, official triage screening system, thus creating an uncontrolled and excessive overtriage situation [21]. In normal circumstances, the only adverse outcome associated with overtriage is additional expense due to screening and evaluating victims who eventually prove to have no serious injury. During a disaster, however, excessive overtriage is associated with additional mortality [22].

On October 23, 1983, Lieutenant Erik Frykberg, a general surgeon, was the chief medical officer on board the USS Iwo Jima. With two ORs and two ICU beds, Frykberg, along with an orthopedic surgeon, an anesthesiologist, and a CRNA, managed the 112 survivors injured by the Beirut marine barracks terrorist bombing. His observations and subsequent analysis of his experience initiated an academic interest in disaster management, which continued throughout his life. The explosion generated 346 casualties, 234 of whom were immediately killed. Of the 112 survivors, 96 were injured. Only 19 of the survivors were critical, with an ISS of ≥ 15, indicating severe trauma. The 77 lightly injured survivors with ISS <15 created an "overtriage" rate (77/96) of 80 %. Among the 112 initial survivors, there were seven additional

deaths, all among the 19 critically injured. Frykberg realized that the overall mortality of survivors (7/112 or 6.3 %) did not tell the whole story. He concluded that a better gauge of the medical response in a disaster would be the "critical mortality," or those deaths occurring among the critically injured as a proportion of all critically injured. Because all seven late deaths in the Beirut bombing occurred among those with ISS ≥ 15, the critical mortality was 7/19 or 37 %, a statistic undiluted by the majority of survivors without significant injury. Of note, within this definition, moribund victims with non-survivable injuries are not counted as initial survivors.

Frykberg began an exhaustive review of terrorist bombing events and noted an interesting relationship. As overtriage for an event increased, so did critical mortality. He published these observations in 1988 [23] and updated them with additional data in 2002 [24], and again in 2008 [22]. The association between overtriage and critical mortality carries a linear correlation coefficient (r) of 0.92. In more modern MCIs, the curve is shifted to the right, indicating improved critical mortality for any given degree of overtriage, but the relationship remains intact (see Fig. 22.4).

The explanation for this relationship is twofold. First is the "needle in the haystack" concept. Sorting through 500 victims as opposed to 50, in order to find the few critically injured, takes valuable time. Second is that even when the critically injured patients are properly routed, the burden placed on the facility by the mass of those with minor injuries and those who are uninjured effectively prevents the DCA from functioning optimally. Predictably [25], radiology becomes a bottleneck [26], lab results are lost or delayed, computers crash, phone lines are overloaded, clinicians cannot respond to pages, medications are not properly dispensed, charts are incomplete, and staff become stressed and tired. Although those working in the ORs and ICUs believe they are providing appropriate care, the result of all these seemingly inconsequential inadequacies is to conspire to increase the mortality of those patients whose lives hang in the balance, those victims for whom every

Fig. 22.4 Relationship of overtriage rate to critical mortality rate in 10 (1969–1995) vs. 4 (2001–2007) terrorist events. Note shift of curve to right. *GP* Guildford pubs, *CA* Craigavon, *OC* Okalhoma City bombing, *TL* Tower of London, *BP* Birmingham pubs, *Bol* Bologna, *AMIA* Buenos Aires, *OB* Old Bailey, *CC* Cu Chi, *BE* Beirut, *VT* 2007 Virginia Tech shooting. From John H. Armstrong, Jeffrey Hammond, Asher Hirshberg, and Erik R. Frykberg, Is overtriage associated with increased mortality? The evidence says "yes," Disaster Medicine and Public Health Preparedness, 2(1), 2008. Reprinted with the permission of Cambridge University Press

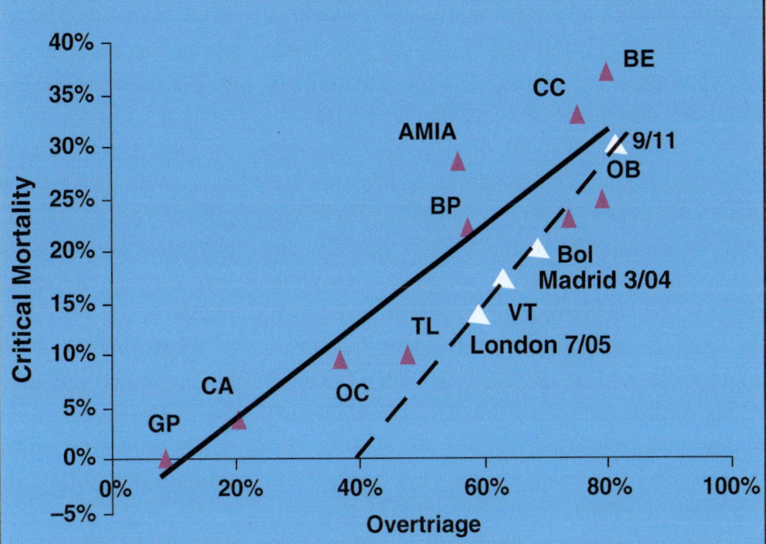

detail of the cumulative clinical response in a DCA must be perfect for them to survive.

While the treatment of non-critically ill or injured victims is not the direct responsibility of a DCA, their presence in the facility therefore significantly impacts the success of efforts to care for the critical victims. During a disaster, a "siege mentality" sets in: the insidious distractions and delays attributable to overtriage are not overtly obvious to those working in the ORs and ICUs, and virtually incomprehensible to those local officials, hospital administrators, pre-hospital providers, and emergency physicians who are largely responsible for the management of the disaster response upstream from DCAs. Regional plans must therefore include a mechanism to decompress non-critical victims away from the facility charged with managing the critically injured and ill in DCAs or, alternatively, to rapidly transport the critically ill and injured to other less-stressed facilities. It is imperative that DCA clinicians with an understanding of this phenomenon participate in regional and upstream planning.

Event Characteristics

The key characteristics of disaster events relevant to those who manage DCAs are the relative size (small, medium, large, or extra-large), type (internal, external, or both), and timing (slowly or rapidly evolving).

In 2001, Hirshberg, Holcomb and Mattox [27] differentiated MCIs from MCEs. By their definitions, the absolute numbers of victims are not as relevant as how demands reconcile with the capacity of the receiving facility. They defined an MCI as a large number of casualties, generated over a short period of time, which can be appropriately managed with existing or extended resources. An MCE in contrast is larger: a major medical disaster that destroys organized community support mechanisms and results in overwhelming casualties. These are useful concepts for planning. The goal is thus not to plan for an MCE, which is impossible since it is overwhelming by definition. Instead, the goal is to organize and extend resources appropriately after an MCI, in order to avoid what would otherwise be an overwhelming major medical disaster.

The size of an event must always be placed in the context of the medical facility's normally available resources. A small event is defined as one that generates a casualty load that can be managed by the involved facility using normal resources. The absolute numbers will be quite different for a freestanding, rural surgi-center than for a large, urban, university-affiliated trauma center. At the opposite end of the event size spectrum, is an extra-large event, defined as one that overwhelms the facility by generating a casualty load that cannot be accommodated even utilizing overflow resources. Neither small, nor extra-large events can benefit from DCA planning. Small events are routinely managed with available resources [28], and extra-large MCEs are overwhelming by definition (see Table 22.2).

A truly overwhelming MCE mandates a triage strategy that involves rationing access, including access to definitive care. Rationing entails difficult ethical decisions [29]. The priority becomes saving as many victims as possible, given the available resources. The military has the most experience in these types of situations, since they commonly occur on battlefields. The experience is much less in the civilian sector [30, 31]. How to render care in austere circumstances is not this author's area of expertise nor within the scope of this chapter; suffice it to say that difficult clinical and ethical decisions must be made until outside assistance arrives. Contingency planning for an overwhelming scenario does not fall on individual departments or hospitals but rather is performed regionally, and is the responsibility of government and nongovernmental assistance organizations [32].

Plans developed at the clinical DCA level are designed to prevent, or at least postpone, being overwhelmed. If that does happen, clinicians will have to do their best with what is available until outside help arrives. If overwhelmed, care providers should plan on providing only basic first-aid and rationing access to definitive care resources.

Regarding an overwhelming event, public health needs will quickly supercede in priority the treatment of critically injured victims. These needs include provisions for food, shelter, proper sanitation facilities, and clean water.

In 2012, The National Institute of Medicine published a 520-page report which is comprehensive in describing a systematic approach to developing and implementing "Crisis Standards of Care" for catastrophic disasters when demands exceed resources [33]. Fortunately, clinical DCA planning efforts are much simpler, focusing only on medium and large MCIs. Medium events are those in which the critically ill or injured can be managed while maintaining standard of care with surge capacity resources. Large events can be handled only by utilizing auxiliary, substandard overflow capacity.

Internal disaster events, i.e., fire, electrical failure, and flooding, affect hospital infrastructure. The clinical response is to maintain ongoing patient care. For the most part, protocols for internal disasters are already in place (see Fig. 22.5).

The challenges during solitary internal disasters are largely administrative and logistic. The HICS lends itself well to these types of events. The major decision facing facilities during an internal disaster (as with slowly evolving disasters) is whether or not to evacuate [34, 35]. As far as clinical planning, every anesthesiologist and most intensivists have contemplated what their contingencies would be if they had to render care without electricity [36]: battery back-

Table 22.2 Implications anticipated from event size

Status	Normal	Multiple casualty incident (MCI)		Mass casualty event (MCE)
Event size	Small	Medium	Large	Extra-large
Resources	Normal	Red and Yellow: Surge resources Green: Overflow	Overflow resources for all casualty types	Overwhelmed situation
Rationing	None	Red and Yellow: No rationing Green: Ration time to treat (OK to delay)	Compromise standards of care	Ration access to care
		Typical numbers of victims for an urban Trauma Center:		
Red	2	5	15	(Large + 1)
Yellow	4	10	30	(Large + 1)
Green	8	20	60+	(Large + 1)
Untagged	10–30	30–300	100–2,000	2,000+

Fig. 22.5 Typical fire-response protocol

In Case of FIRE: RACE

R =	Rescue	Move patients to safety
A =	Alarm	Activate nearest fire alarm
C =	Contain	Close fire doors
E =	Extinguish or Evacuate	As appropriate

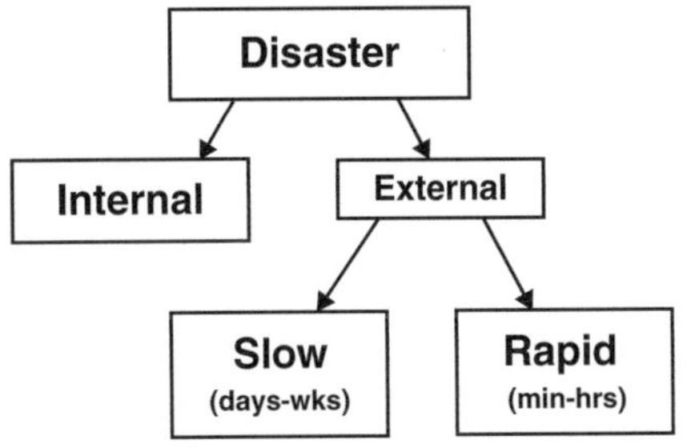

Fig. 22.6 Disaster location and timing

up, emergency generator, etc. Plans for internal disasters and evacuation must be protocol based, formulated in advance, activated automatically, and drilled periodically (see Fig. 22.6).

Slowly evolving events include infectious epidemics, radiologic contamination, and hurricanes. With Severe Acute Respiratory Syndrome (SARS), for example, the worldwide surge of patients was clearly delayed, peaking at 56 days following the initial outbreak (see Fig. 22.7) [37].

In addition, the surge of SARS patients was dispersed; victims were not all treated at the same facility, emphasizing that the planning and response for slowly evolving events (as with extra-large events, or MCEs) must be coordinated at a regional level by federal or regional relief agencies such as the Red Cross, WHO, or U.S. Centers for Disease Control and Prevention (CDC). These plans need not be automatic and protocol based. The delayed surge of victims typical of an infectious epidemic or any slowly evolving event such as a hurricane, allows planners the opportunity to gauge the time available to relocate patients, or to expand DCA capacity by mobilizing resources.

Combined internal/external disasters present especially difficult challenges [38]. In rapidly evolving disasters, external or combined (earthquakes, tornados, bombings, etc.) inadequate planning will leave the seriously injured and critically ill most vulnerable [39].

The timing of victims' arrival to the DCAs can be predicted based on historical data. The CDC has published simple models to predict the distribution of triage types (1/3 critical, 2/3 non-

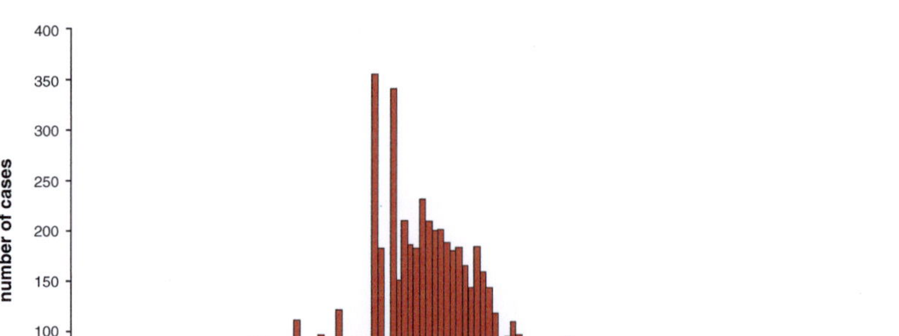

Fig. 22.7 Probable cases of SARS by date of report worldwide ($n = 7,588$), 1 March–10 July 2003. From Epidemic curves—Severe Acute Respiratory Syndrome (SARS), Global Alert and Response (GAR), World Health Organization, n.d. Web page. Last accessed Dec. 22, 2013. http://www.who.int/csr/sars/epicurve/epiindex/en/index2.html

critical) [40], as well as for surge timing [41]. Per the CDC, approximately half of all casualties will arrive at the hospital within a 1-h window which begins when the first casualty arrives at the hospital (see Fig. 22.8). To predict the total number of casualties the hospital can expect, double the number of casualties the hospital receives in the first hour.

This basic model can be augmented with data from observations published by investigators following actual explosive events. From a series of terrorist bombings in Israel, Shamir, et al. reported that the surge of patients undergoing surgical procedures was approximately 3–4 h following the explosion (see Fig. 22.9) [42].

Reports following the 2005 bombing in London indicate the timing of the surge of victims arriving in operating rooms and to ICUs (see Fig. 22.10) [43].

Because disaster events are infrequent, it is crucial for those involved in managing patients in DCAs to publish accounts of their experience, including validated data on the nature of injuries, over- and under-triage rates, critical mortality, types and timing of interventions, and an assessment of the response and lessons learned [44–52].

Resource Characteristics

The key characteristic of medical resources relevant to those who manage DCAs is whether they can or cannot maintain normal standard of care.

Resource categorization focuses on the ability to maintain standard of care, and meshes with victim triage categorization and event characteristics (above). The types of resources are divided into: normal, surge, and overflow. *Normal resources* are those used conventionally on a daily basis to care for patients in DCAs. These resources are identified with a process inventory, and define optimal standard of care.

Surge resources are alternate equipment, locations, and personnel not normally used, but available for the treatment of additional patients while maintaining normal standard of care, for instance using a modern anesthesia machine to provide ventilator support to an ICU patient. In contrast, *overflow resources* include equipment, locations, and personnel that can be utilized in the treatment of additional patients, but which compromise the standard of care, for example, using an ambu bag and a family

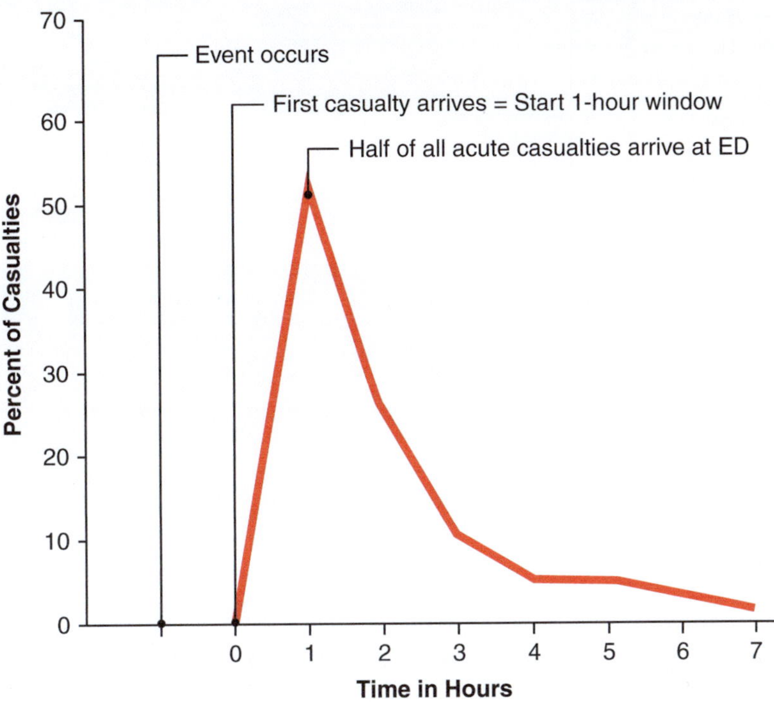

Fig. 22.8 Surge timing for explosive events. From U.S. Centers for Disease Control and Prevention. Predicting Casualty Severity and Hospital Capacity; Predicting Triage Severity World Wide Web URL: http://www.bt.cdc.gov/masscasualties/predictor.asp Last accessed June 24, 2013

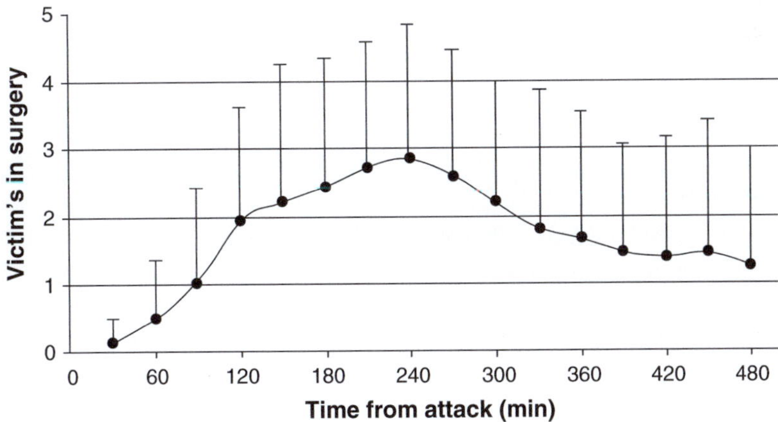

Fig. 22.9 OR surge timing for terrorist bombing events. From Shamir MY, Weiss YG, Willner D, Mintz Y, Bloom AI, Weiss Y, Sprung CL, Weissman C, Multiple casualty terror events: the anesthesiologist's perspective, Anesth Analg. 2004 Jun;98(6):1746-52

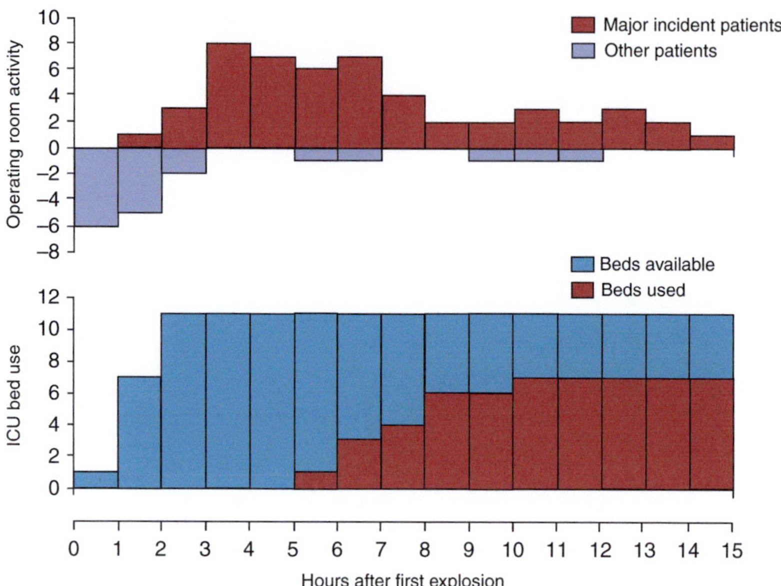

Fig. 22.10 2005 London bombing surge. Reprinted from Lancet, 368(9554), Aylwin CJ, König TC, Brennan NW, Shirley PJ, Davies G, Walsh MS, Brohi K, Reduction in critical mortality in urban mass casualty incidents: analysis of triage, surge, and resource use after the London bombings on July 7, 2005, pp. 2219-25, Copyright 2006, with permission from Elsevier

member to provide ventilatory support to an ICU patient [53].

As casualty loads increase, normal, then surge, then overflow resources are engaged, and eventually exhausted. Once all overflow resources are consumed, the system is overwhelmed, and at this point either evacuation or rationing victims' access to definitive care must take place. Explosive disasters with large numbers of casualties (Oklahoma City [54], Atlanta Olympics [55], World Trade Center [39], Madrid [56], London [43], Boston [57]) have repeatedly demonstrated that without proper organization, the hospital with the nearest geographic proximity reproducibly becomes burdened with a massive demand (and overtriage) that threatens to or actually overwhelms its capacity. This phenomenon establishes the identity of the "Ground Zero Hospital" for a given disaster event.

The *surge capacity* of a facility is defined simply as the total number of patients that can be managed with only surge (and normal) resources. *Overflow capacity* is likewise defined as the absolute number of patients that can be accommodated with the addition of overflow resources. In reality, during a disaster, as casualty loads increase, not all resources will be exhausted while treating the same number of patients. Thus each resource (ventilators, monitors, nursing staff, etc.) has its own normal, surge, and overflow capacity. For the purposes of planning, once a single resource of the next level must be employed, the patient should be considered as being treated within the next level's capacity. For instance, to manage a critically ill patient in the PACU (surge resource) with a 1:4 nursing care ratio (overflow strategy) would be considered as utilizing the hospital's DCA overflow capacity [58].

The rationale behind distinguishing these types of resources is to clarify resource management in the face of escalating needs. From this perspective, the system can be considered to be continuously in some version of "disaster mode," which ranges along a spectrum from normal to surge to overflow to overwhelmed. Many institutions utilize their surge capacity on a regular basis, for example, by holding patients overnight in the PACU because the ICUs are full [59].

Once surge resources are consumed, substandard, compromised resources must be utilized to accommodate additional patients [60]. These overflow resources are acceptable and appropriate to treat the large numbers of non-critical victims of any disaster, and may be necessary even for critical victims in extreme circumstances. However, if additional surge capacity (maintaining standard of care) for critically ill and injured victims can be pre-identified and quickly mobilized, the greater will be the impact on overall survival from the event.

Response Sequence

All disasters share similar components or phases: Recognition, Triage, Treatment, and Mass Relocation—also called a surge if patients are arriving to the hospital, and evacuation if they are being moved away. The sequence is as follows for each type of disaster (see Fig. 22.11):

For an internal disaster such as a fire, for example, patients are already being treated. Someone smells smoke, pulls the alarm—Recognition, the disaster plan is activated, patients are triaged for evacuation. Planning and response must be immediate, automatic, and protocol based. Fortunately, as noted, plans are generally in place for most internal disasters.

For slowly evolving events such as a covert biological release, index cases begin to present one at a time to numerous facilities. Astute clinicians [61] notify public health officials and alone or together, they make a diagnosis—Recognition. Treatment begins as victims arrive. As the infection spreads over the subsequent days to weeks, the surge of victims peaks. They may need to be evacuated as individual facilities reach capacity; otherwise, if resources are inadequate, victims are triaged, to ensure that those most likely to survive obtain treatment. Planning here can be general, and responses can be adapted and modified in real time. There is sufficient opportunity to adequately prepare patients for safe transfer, or to bring in additional resources and staff to keep up with the demand. The responsibility for managing these resources does not fall upon individual DCAs, but is rather the role of federal or international relief agencies. The threshold for becoming overwhelmed regionally during a slowly evolving event is quite high.

Response Sequence

Internal	Slow	Rapid
Treatment	Recognition	Recognition
Recognition	Treatment	Surge
Triage	Surge/Evac	Triage
Evacuation	Triage	Treatment

Fig. 22.11 Response sequence

For rapidly evolving events, for example, an explosion with possible chemical release, where patients arrive at the hospital from an auditorium a few blocks away coughing with burning eyes, EMS calls ahead and reports they have a possible chemical event—Recognition, the surge of victims quickly starts to arrive both on their own and by ambulance. Patients are triaged according to acuity, and treatment begins with decontamination. Like internal disasters, planning and response for rapidly evolving events must be immediate, automatic, and protocol based.

Table-Top Exercises

Table-top exercises [62] are performed by appropriate clinical, support, and administrative leadership identified via a process inventory for definitive care. Table-top exercises are the fundamental mechanism by which surge and overflow capacity planning occurs. First considered is the highest probability disaster scenario (from a Hazard Vulnerability Analysis [63]). The process begins by identifying all the components necessary to provide care to a typical victim (process inventory). Once normal resources are identified, participants then conceptualize potential surge and overflow resources. For each level of care (normal, surge, overflow), the care-limiting resource is identified. Participants then explore ways to expand that specific limitation to uncover the next limited resource. The process continues by reassessing the subsequently exposed care-limiting resources, and then the exercise is repeated, assessing the next most likely scenario and the next and so on. When this process is complete, the group will have generated an inventory of all resources needed to provide each level of care in the ORs and ICUs, i.e., normal, surge, and overflow. Within each category, a sequence of resource utilization is defined. For instance, the sequence of locations where emergency major trauma surgery can be performed (with hypothetical capacity in parentheses) might look like this:

Surgery normally performed in ORs (15) →
Then surge to: Day surgery (2), then OB (3) →
Then overflow to:

Cystoscopy suites (2)

Angiography suites (2), PACU (12), ICU (18)

It is imperative to involve all clinical services and areas in these exercises to anticipate problems where surge resources may overlap. An anesthesia machine in a cystoscopy suite cannot serve to expand ICU ventilator capacity at the same time that surgeons are planning on using that room to perform an overflow trauma procedure.

In addition, it is critical that all clinical support services (radiology, blood bank, laboratory services, pharmacy, dietary, sterile supply, etc.) collaborate in these iterative table-top exercises. Frequently process and systems vulnerabilities can be anticipated.

This practice of continuously identifying the capacity- or care-limiting resource is crucial. Expansion planning then can focus on that weak link. It makes no sense to devote time and energy to expanding one resource like OR availability, when its usage will be limited by lack of sterile instruments.

The advantage of defining relevant aspects of victims, events, and resources as described, and of adopting the table-top system for developing limited resource expansion, is that the resulting plans can be considered to be in use on a daily basis. It is likely that several times per year, surge, and even overflow resources may need to be utilized simply because of the normal variations in admissions and acuity. Incorporating disaster preparedness vernacular and algorithms into daily clinical usage maintains preparedness at a continuously high level.

A number of concepts have been presented regarding the clinical DCA response to disaster. The goals here are threefold. First is to define an understandable vocabulary and to create a usable framework to simplify and focus planning of the tasks at hand. The second goal is to provide tools and strategies to use in developing plans for a clinical response to disaster. The final goal is to present some of the remaining challenges such as overtriage, which seriously threaten the ability to care for patients in DCAs, and which have major consequences on overall mortality following any given event. By exposing these challenges, anesthesiologists who routinely manage trauma patients may be inspired to become involved in departmental, hospital, and regional disaster planning.

References

1. Curran MP, et al. Large-scale erosion and flooding after wildfires: understanding the soil conditions. BC Ministry of Forests and Range, Research Branch, Victoria. BC Technical Report 030. 2006. http://www.for.gov.bc.ca/hfd/pubs/Docs/Tr/Tr030.htm
2. Rubinson L, Hick JL, Hanfling DG, Devereaux AV, Dichter JR, Christian MD, Talmor D, Medina J, Curtis JR, Geiling JA; Task Force for Mass Critical Care. Definitive care for the critically ill during a disaster: a framework for optimizing critical care surge capacity: from a Task Force for Mass Critical Care summit meeting, January 26–27, 2007, Chicago, IL. Chest. 2008;133(5 Suppl):18S–31S.
3. Hospital Incident Command System. HICS IV August 2006. California Emergency Medical Services Authority Web site. http://www.emsa.ca.gov/HICS/. Accessed 23 June 2013.
4. Arnold JL, Halpern P, Tsai MC, Smithline H. Mass casualty terrorist bombings: a comparison of outcomes by bombing type. Ann Emerg Med. 2004;43(2): 263–73.
5. Champion HR, Mabee MS, Meredith JW. The state of US trauma systems: public perceptions versus reality–implications for US response to terrorism and mass casualty events. J Am Coll Surg. 2006;203(6): 951–61.
6. Christian MD, Devereaux AV, Dichter JR, Geiling JA, Rubinson L. Definitive care for the critically ill during a disaster: current capabilities and limitations: from a Task Force for Mass Critical Care summit

meeting, January 26-27, 2007, Chicago, IL. Chest. 2008;133(5 Suppl):8S–17.

7. Auf der Heide E. The importance of evidence-based disaster planning. Ann Emerg Med. 2006;47(1):34–49.

8. Bame SI, Parker K, Lee JY, Norman A, Finley D, Desai A, Grover A, Payne C, Garza A, Shaw A, Bell-Shaw R, Davis T, Harrison E, Dunn R, Mhatre P, Shaw F, Robinson C. Monitoring unmet needs: using 2-1-1 during natural disasters. Am J Prev Med. 2012; 43(6 Suppl 5):S435–42.

9. Mitchell GW. A brief history of triage. Disaster Med Public Health Prep. 2008;2 Suppl 1:S4–7.

10. Repine TB, Lisagor P, Cohen DJ. The dynamics and ethics of triage: rationing care in hard times. Mil Med. 2005;170(6):505–9.

11. Sprung CL, Zimmerman JL, Christian MD, Joynt GM, Hick JL, Taylor B, Richards GA, Sandrock C, Cohen R, Adini B, European Society of Intensive Care Medicine Task Force for Intensive Care Unit Triage during an Influenza Epidemic or Mass Disaster. Recommendations for intensive care unit and hospital preparations for an influenza epidemic or mass disaster: summary report of the European Society of Intensive Care Medicine's Task Force for intensive care unit triage during an influenza epidemic or mass disaster. Intensive Care Med. 2010;36(3):428–43.

12. Bostick NA, Subbarao I, Burkle Jr FM, Hsu EB, Armstrong JH, James JJ. Disaster triage systems for large-scale catastrophic events. Disaster Med Public Health Prep. 2008;2 Suppl 1:S35–9.

13. Kahn CA, Schultz CH, Miller KT, Anderson CL. Does START triage work? An outcomes assessment after a disaster. Ann Emerg Med. 2009;54(3):424–30, 430.

14. Kluger Y, Peleg K, Daniel-Aharonson L, Mayo A, Israeli Trauma Group. The special injury pattern in terrorist bombings. J Am Coll Surg. 2004;199:875–9.

15. Todd EC. Epidemiology of foodborne diseases: a worldwide review. World Health Stat Q. 1997; 50(1–2):30–50.

16. Iskander J, Strikas RA, Gensheimer KF, Cox NJ, Redd SC. Pandemic influenza planning, United States, 1978–2008. Emerg Infect Dis. 2013;19(6):879–85.

17. Roccaforte JD, Cushman JG. Disaster preparation and management for the intensive care unit. Curr Opin Crit Care. 2002;8:607–15.

18. Simchen E, Sprung CL, Galai N, et al. Survival of critically ill patients hospitalized in and out of intensive care units under paucity of intensive care unit beds. Crit Care Med. 2004;32:1654–61.

19. American College of Surgeons Committee on Trauma. Resources for optimal care of the trauma patient. Chicago, IL: American College of Surgeons; 2006.

20. Baker SP, O'Neill B, Haddon W, Long WB. The injury severity score: a method for describing patients with multiple injuries and evaluating emergency care. J Trauma. 1974;14:187–96.

21. Gutierrez de Ceballos JP, Turégano Fuentes F, Perez Diaz D, Sanz Sanchez M, Martin Llorente C, Guerrero Sanz JE. Casualties treated at the closest hospital in the Madrid, March 11, terrorist bombings. Crit Care Med. 2005;33(1 Suppl):S107–12.

22. Armstrong JH, Hammond J, Hirshberg A, Frykberg ER. Is overtriage associated with increased mortality? The evidence says "yes". Disaster Med Public Health Prep. 2008;2(1):4–5, author reply 5–6.

23. Frykberg ER, Tepas III JJ. Terrorist bombings: lessons learned from Belfast to Beirut. Ann Surg. 1988;208:569–76.

24. Frykberg ER. Medical management of disasters and mass casualties from terrorist bombings: how can we cope? J Trauma. 2002;53:201–12.

25. Abir M, Davis MM, Sankar P, Wong AC, Wang SC. Design of a model to predict surge capacity bottlenecks for burn mass casualties at a large academic medical center. Prehosp Disaster Med. 2013; 28(1):23–32.

26. Körner M, Krötz M, Kanz KG, Pfeifer KJ, Reiser M, Linsenmaier U. Development of an accelerated MSCT protocol (Triage MSCT) for mass casualty incidents: comparison to MSCT for single-trauma patients. Emerg Radiol. 2006;12(5):203–9.

27. Hirshberg A, Holcomb JB, Mattox KL. Hospital trauma care in multiple-casualty incidents: a critical view. Ann Emerg Med. 2001;37:647–52.

28. Ball CG, Kirkpatrick AW, Mulloy RH, Gmora S, Findlay C, Hameed SM. The impact of multiple casualty incidents on clinical outcomes. J Trauma. 2006; 61(5):1036–9.

29. Daniel M. Bedside resource stewardship in disasters: a provider's dilemma practicing in an ethical gap. J Clin Ethics. 2012;23(4):331–5.

30. Okie S. Dr. Pou and the hurricane—implications for patient care during disasters. N Engl J Med. 2008;358: 1–5.

31. Pou AM. Hurricane Katrina and disaster preparedness. N Engl J Med. 2008;358(14):1524.

32. Levin D, Cadigan RO, Biddinger PD, Condon S, Koh HK, Joint Massachusetts Department of Public Health-Harvard Altered Standards of Care Working Group. Altered standards of care during an influenza pandemic: identifying ethical, legal, and practical principles to guide decision making. Disaster Med Public Health Prep. 2009;3 Suppl 2:S132–40.

33. Crisis standards of care: a systems framework for catastrophic disaster response. Washington, DC: National Academies Press; 2012.

34. Powell T, Hanfling D, Gostin LO. Emergency preparedness and public health: the lessons of Hurricane Sandy. JAMA. 2012;308(24):2569–70.

35. Hassol A, Biddinger P, Zane R. Hospital evacuation decisions in emergency situations. JAMA. 2013; 309(15):1585–6.

36. Klein KR, Rosenthal MS, Klausner HA. Blackout 2003: preparedness and lessons learned from the

perspectives of four hospitals. Prehosp Disaster Med. 2005;20(5):343–9.

37. World Health Organization. Epidemic curves—severe acute respiratory syndrome (SARS). Geneva, Switzerland: World Health Organization; 2003. World Wide Web URL: http://www.who.int/csr/sars/epicurve/epiindex/en/. Accessed 24 June 2013.

38. McSwain Jr NE. Disaster response. Natural disaster: Katrina. Surg Today. 2010;40(7):587–91.

39. Cushman JG, Pachter HL, Beaton HL. Two New York city hospitals' surgical response to the September 11, 2001, terrorist attack in New York city. J Trauma. 2003;54:147–55.

40. U.S. Centers for Disease Control and Prevention. Predicting casualty severity and hospital capacity; predicting triage severity. World Wide Web URL: http://www.bt.cdc.gov/masscasualties/capacity.asp. Accessed 24 June 2013.

41. U.S. Centers for Disease Control and Prevention. Predicting casualty severity and hospital capacity; predicting triage severity. World Wide Web URL: http://www.bt.cdc.gov/masscasualties/predictor.asp. Accessed 24 June 2013.

42. Shamir MY, Weiss YG, Willner D, et al. Multiple casualty terror events: the anesthesiologist's perspective. Anesth Analg. 2004;98:1746–52.

43. Aylwin CJ, König TC, Brennan NW, Shirley PJ, Davies G, Walsh MS, Brohi K. Reduction in critical mortality in urban mass casualty incidents: analysis of triage, surge, and resource use after the London bombings on July 7, 2005. Lancet. 2006;368(9554):2219–25.

44. Raiter Y, Farfel A, Lehavi O, Goren OB, Shamiss A, Priel Z, Koren I, Davidson B, Schwartz D, Goldberg A, Bar-Dayan Y. Mass casualty incident management, triage, injury distribution of casualties and rate of arrival of casualties at the hospitals: lessons from a suicide bomber attack in downtown Tel Aviv. Emerg Med J. 2008;25(4):225–9.

45. Kellermann AL, Peleg K. Lessons from Boston. N Engl J Med. 2013;368(21):1956–7.

46. Murakawa M. Anesthesia department preparedness for a multiple-casualty incident: lessons learned from the Fukushima earthquake and the Japanese nuclear power disaster. Anesthesiol Clin. 2013;31(1):117–25.

47. Hartmann EH, Creel N, Lepard J, Maxwell RA. Mass casualty following unprecedented tornadic events in the Southeast: natural disaster outcomes at a Level I trauma center. Am Surg. 2012;78(7):770–3.

48. Brevard SB, Weintraub SL, Aiken JB, Halton EB, Duchesne JC, McSwain Jr NE, Hunt JP, Marr AB. Analysis of disaster response plans and the aftermath of Hurricane Katrina: lessons learned from a level I trauma center. J Trauma. 2008;65(5):1126–32.

49. Postma IL, Weel H, Heetveld MJ, van der Zande I, Bijlsma TS, Bloemers FW, Goslings JC. Mass casualty triage after an airplane crash near Amsterdam. Injury. 2013;44(8):1061–7.

50. Bhandarwar AH, Bakhshi GD, Tayade MB, Borisa AD, Thadeshwar NR, Gandhi SS. Surgical response to the 2008 Mumbai terror attack. Br J Surg. 2012;99(3):368–72.

51. Wild J, Maher J, Frazee RC, Craun ML, Davis ML, Childs EW, Smith RW. The Fort Hood Massacre: lessons learned from a high profile mass casualty. J Trauma Acute Care Surg. 2012;72(6):1709–13.

52. Gaarder C, Jorgensen J, Kolstadbraaten KM, Isaksen KS, Skattum J, Rimstad R, Gundem T, Holtan A, Walloe A, Pillgram-Larsen J, Naess PA. The twin terrorist attacks in Norway on July 22, 2011: the trauma center response. J Trauma Acute Care Surg. 2012;73(1):269–75.

53. Branson RD, Johannigman JA, Daugherty EL, Rubinson L. Surge capacity mechanical ventilation. Respir Care. 2008;53(1):78–88.

54. Hogan DE, Waeckerle JF, Dire DJ, Lillibridge SR. Emergency department impact of the Oklahoma City terrorist bombing. Ann Emerg Med. 1999;34:160–7.

55. Feliciano DV, Anderson Jr GV, Rozycki GS, et al. Management of casualties from the bombing at the centennial olympics. Am J Surg. 1998;176:538–43.

56. Gutierrez de Ceballos JP, Fuentes FT, et al. Casualties treated at the closest hospital in the Madrid, March 11, terrorist bombings. Crit Care Med. 2005;33:S107–12.

57. Biddinger PD, Baggish A, Harrington L, d'Hemecourt P, Hooley J, Jones J, Kue R, Troyanos C, Dyer KS. Be prepared–the Boston Marathon and mass-casualty events. N Engl J Med. 2013;368(21):1958–60.

58. Kiekkas P, Poulopoulou M, Papahatzi A, Androutsopoulou C, Maliouki M, Prinou A. Workload of postanaesthesia care unit nurses and intensive care overflow. Br J Nurs. 2005;14(8):434–8.

59. Ziser A, Alkobi M, Markovits R, Rozenberg B. The postanaesthesia care unit as a temporary admission location due to intensive care and ward overflow. Br J Anaesth. 2002;88(4):577–9.

60. Rubinson L, Hick JL, Curtis JR, Branson RD, Burns S, Christian MD, Devereaux AV, Dichter JR, Talmor D, Erstad B, Medina J, Geiling JA; Task Force for Mass Critical Care. Definitive care for the critically ill during a disaster: medical resources for surge capacity: from a Task Force for Mass Critical Care summit meeting, January 26–27, 2007, Chicago, IL. Chest. 2008;133(5 Suppl):32S–50S.

61. Subbarao I, Johnson C, Bond WF, Schwid HA, Wasser TE, Deye GA, Burkhart KK. Symptom-based, algorithmic approach for handling the initial encounter with victims of a potential terrorist attack. Prehosp Disaster Med. 2005;20(5):301–8.

62. Henning KJ, Brennan PJ, Hoegg C, O'Rourke E, Dyer BD, Grace TL. Health system preparedness for bioterrorism: bringing the tabletop to the hospital. Infect Control Hosp Epidemiol. 2004;25(2):146–55.

63. Campbell P, Trockman SJ, Walker AR. Strengthening hazard vulnerability analysis: results of recent research in Maine. Public Health Rep. 2011;126(2):290–3.

Ethan O. Bryson

Introduction

Addiction is characterized by the repeated use or compulsive seeking of mood altering substances despite the adverse psychological, physical, or social consequences associated with doing so [1]. It is significantly prevalent in our society, so much so that up to 15 % of the population will at some point meet the criteria for alcohol use disorder and up to 8 % for substance use disorder [2, 3]. Substance abuse is not limited to illicit substances and many over the counter or prescription medications have significant abuse potential. According to the National Institute on Drug Abuse (NIDA), the misuse of prescription drugs is an increasing significant public health concern. These agents can cause tolerance, physical dependence, and result in withdrawal when the user stops taking them. Studies into the trends associated with substance abuse have shown an increase in reports of nonmedical use of prescription medications, and the rates of addiction to prescription pain medication are increasing [4]. More and more frequently trauma patients present with injuries associated with substance abuse, necessitating that the trauma anesthesiologist be facile with the management of acute intoxication and withdrawal syndromes in addition to acute trauma.

E.O. Bryson, M.D. (✉)
Department of Anesthesiology and Psychiatry, The Icahn
School of Medicine at Mount Sinai, 1 Gustave L.
Levy Place, New York, NY 10029, USA
e-mail: Ethan.bryson@mountsinai.org

Trauma in the Intoxicated Patient

The majority of trauma patients with injuries necessitating surgery arrive in a condition which may make the taking of a careful history or the performing of a complete physical examination difficult at best. Laboratory evaluations and ancillary studies are often required to establish or confirm the diagnosis of acute intoxication and identify the substance abused.

Many trauma patients, especially those who abuse drugs, may be unconscious, reluctant, or medically unable to give a reliable history. Informed consent may be difficult to obtain. In the awake and cooperative patient, it is helpful to maintain privacy and confidentiality. Be sure to reassure the patient that his/her drug use history will not negatively impact the care but emphasize that not revealing any prior use could be extremely dangerous, especially under anesthesia. Make every attempt to identify what drug(s) was (were) used, how much, and by what route. Remember that many patients will have consumed more than one drug, often from different drug classes. When performing the physical examination take careful note of the patient's mental status and vital signs, paying close attention to pupil size and the presence or absence of nystagmus. An accurate core temperature is essential as intoxicated patients often present with impaired thermoregulation. Look closely at the patients' skin for stigmata of intravenous drug use such as track marks or soft tissue

C.S. Scher (ed.), *Anesthesia for Trauma*, DOI 10.1007/978-1-4939-0909-4_23,
© Springer Science+Business Media New York 2014

infection or for the presence of medication patches that must be removed. Remember that the drug abusing trauma patient is at high risk for pulmonary complications such as alveolar hypoventilation, aspiration pneumonitis, or noncardiogenic pulmonary edema [5, 6] As with all patients, universal precautions should be strictly observed. Chronic infection with blood-borne viruses such as hepatitis B and C as well as HIV is common in addicts who administer drugs intravenously.

Most trauma patients with suspected intoxication will have urinalysis and blood sent for toxicology, though there is considerable debate surrounding the need for these tests [7, 8]. Despite concerns that these tests can be expensive and time consuming, unless the clinical diagnosis is clear it would seem reasonable to document the specific drug ingested. A basic metabolic panel can reveal hypoglycemia or electrolyte disturbances in the dehydrated patient and arterial blood gas analyses (ABG) is often helpful in the obtunded and hypoventilating patient. Do not forget the routine urine pregnancy test for any woman of childbearing age.

In the following section specific drugs of abuse, their mechanism of action, toxidromes, and potential for interaction with anesthetic agents are discussed along with management guidelines for the trauma patient intoxicated with such agents.

Specific Drugs

Alcohol

Alcohol (ethanol) has been consumed by humans throughout history and has played a significant role in many cultures. It is part of some religious rituals, and has been both revered and condemned. Since it is legal for adults in the USA to purchase and consume, alcohol remains ubiquitous, as does its use. Although acute intoxication with alcohol is rarely the primary reason for presentation to the emergency department, it is extremely common in patients requiring emergent care [9]. Excessive alcohol consumption

Table 23.1 Signs and symptoms of acute alcohol intoxication

• Nystagmus
• Slurred speech
• Unsteady gait
• Dis-coordination
• Emotional lability, aggressive behavior
• Impaired judgment and memory
• Hypotension
• Hypothermia
• Respiratory depression
• Stupor, coma, death

From Schwartz A, Knez D. Anesthesia and alcohol addiction. In Bryson EO, Frost EAM Editors, Perioperative Addiction. Springer Science and Business Media, NY: New York, 2011, used with permission

leading to drunkenness has long had a recognized association with increased risk for trauma-related injuries. These patients are more likely to fall, be involved in motor vehicle accidents, and be the victim of assault or homicide. It is estimated that uncomplicated alcohol intoxication is responsible for upwards of 600,000 emergency room visits in the USA per year [10].

Alcohol functions as a multi-action central nervous system (CNS) depressant. Ethanol enhances γ-amino butyric acid a-type (GABA$_A$), serotonin (5-HT3), glycine, and nicotinic acetylcholine receptor activity while antagonizing the major CNS excitatory neurotransmitter, glutamate at N-methyl-D-aspartate (NMDA) receptors. Alcohol also acts directly through physical binding to a pocket on a G protein-gated inwardly rectifying potassium (GIRK) channel which subsequently dampens neuronal chemical communication [11]. An increase in the activity of inhibitory systems coupled with a simultaneous decrease in the activity of excitatory neurotransmission produces the clinical effects of nystagmus, slurred speech, unsteady gait, and decreased coordination, as well as difficulty with memory, impaired judgment, and increased emotional labiality typically seen in the alcohol-intoxicated patient. Specific signs and symptoms associated with acute ethanol intoxication are listed in Table 23.1.

Treatment of the acutely ethanol-intoxicated trauma patient is mainly supportive. As blood alcohol levels increase, the degree of autonomic dysfunction worsens. Eventually the patient becomes hypotensive, hypothermic, stuporous, and may become entirely unresponsive. Often fluid resuscitation with balanced salt solutions is required to treat hypotension related to volume depletion or blood loss from trauma. In addition to fluids, these patients should receive parenteral thiamine to prevent Wernicke's encephalopathy. Respiratory depression and loss of protective airway reflexes accompany stupor and the threshold for intubation in the unresponsive patient should be very low. Lack of ability to protect the airway requires emergent intubation and mechanical ventilation. Rapid sequence induction is generally advised as with all trauma patients, but additionally the chronic alcohol abusing patient commonly has delayed gastric emptying and gastro-esophageal reflux disease.

Though the blood alcohol concentration (BAC) cannot be directly correlated with the degree of intoxication, it can be used for diagnosis and to direct treatment and should be obtained along with blood glucose levels and a basic metabolic panel. Other laboratory tests such as mean corpuscular volume (MCV), gamma-glutamyl transpeptidase (GGT), and carbohydrate-deficient transferrin (CDT) may also be useful but must be correlated with history and physical examination as none is sufficiently sensitive to establish the diagnosis of chronic alcohol abuse alone.

The issue of informed consent for surgery and other procedures may present a problem in the acutely intoxicated patient. Often these patients are either aggressive or violent and may pose a threat to healthcare professionals involved in their treatment. If they are confused and unable to give consent, they must be treated as lacking capacity to make decisions. If it is possible, surgical interventions should be delayed until the patient recovers from acute intoxication.

While the response to anesthesia is exaggerated in acute ethanol intoxication, the chronic abuser will likely exhibit an increased requirement for anesthetic agents secondary to cross-tolerance or metabolic tolerance resulting from induction of P-450 system enzymes. These patients may be at increased risk for awareness

Table 23.2 Medical problems associated with chronic alcohol abuse

Central nervous system
• Psychiatric disorders
• Nutritional disorders (Wernicke–Korsakoff syndrome)
• Alcohol withdrawal syndrome
• Cerebellar degeneration
• Cerebral atrophy
Cardiovascular
• Dilated cardiomyopathy
• Dysrhythmias
• Hypertension
Gastrointestinal and hepatobiliary
• Esophagitis
• Gastritis
• Pancreatitis
• Liver cirrhosis (portal hypertension manifested as esophageal varices or hemorrhoids)
Skin and musculoskeletal
• Spider angiomas
• Myopathy
• Osteoporosis
Endocrine and metabolic
• Decreased plasma testosterone
• Decreased gluconeogenesis
• Ketoacidosis
• Hypoalbuminemia
• Hypomagnesemia
Hematologic
• Thrombocytopenia
• Leukopenia
• Anemia

From Schwartz A, Knez D. Anesthesia and alcohol addiction. In Bryson EO, Frost EAM Editors, Perioperative Addiction. Springer Science and Business Media, NY: New York, 2011, used with permission

under anesthesia. Despite the potential for exaggerated drug responses due to decreased hepatic metabolism, decreased plasma protein binding and increased volume of distribution for medications secondary to hypoalbuminemia in patients with cirrhosis, most routine medications for the practice of general anesthesia are well tolerated. Medical problems commonly encountered in the chronic alcohol abuser which should be considered when treating the acutely ethanol-intoxicated trauma patient are listed in Table 23.2.

The ethanol-intoxicated trauma patient presents up to a fivefold risk for perioperative complications. Does this need a reference? Of primary concern to the trauma anesthesiologist are problems with hemostasis related to advanced liver disease and the intraoperative hemodynamic consequences of underlying cardiac disease. Poorly treated underlying cardiac disease in the chronic alcohol abusing patient may limit the ability of the heart to meet increased demands from either trauma-related injury or the stress of surgery itself. Chronically increased catecholamine levels contribute to a hyperdynamic state with an increased risk for a variety of cardiac rhythm disturbances including ventricular fibrillation and atrial dysrhythmias. Chronic alcohol abuse causes structural and functional damage of the left ventricle leading to concentric left ventricular hypertrophy even in patients asymptomatic for cardiac disease [12]. Alcoholic cardiomyopathy is characterized by a dilated left ventricle and decreased ejection fraction.

Cocaine

A pharmacologically diverse drug with local anesthetic, CNS stimulant, and sympathomimetic properties, cocaine has been used and abused for over 5,000 years [13]. Its use has risen steadily since the 1980s and as recently as 2008 almost 1 % of all adults and almost 2 % of adults between the ages of 18 and 25 reported using cocaine on a regular basis [14]. Cocaine is responsible for more drug-related deaths than any other abused substance. These deaths are usually related to problems with the cardiopulmonary system but cocaine also impacts the CNS, the hematological system, and the kidneys [15]. Of note, the trauma surgery patient is particularly likely to have recently used cocaine: one study reports that 38 % of such patients tested positive [16].

Cocaine exerts its effects by blocking reuptake of the sympathomimetic neurotransmitters dopamine (DA), norepinephrine (NE), and serotonin at postsynaptic nerve terminals leading to prolonged adrenergic stimulation. It effectively blocks catecholamine-binding sites, allowing free catecholamines, such as NE, to continue to stimulate the cardiovascular system [17]. This results in a sustained increase in systolic, diastolic, and mean arterial blood pressure (BP), heart rate (HR), and body temperature. The increased risk for coronary artery vasospasm resulting in ischemia-induced cardiac arrhythmias associated with cocaine use results from sympathetic stimulation secondary to increased plasma levels of NE [18]. The vast majority of morbidity and mortality associated with cocaine-induced myocardial infarction is seen within 3 h of use and can be directly linked to uptake and degree of bioavailability [19, 20].

Anesthetic management of the cocaine-intoxicated trauma patient should focus on minimizing hemodynamic extremes and avoiding ischemic consequences of vasospasm. It is difficult to predict how these patients will respond to general anesthesia. The minimum alveolar concentration (MAC) may be decreased because of the depletion of catecholamines (in chronic cocaine users) or increased secondary to acute elevation of catecholamine concentration (in acute cocaine intoxication) [21]. Cocaine-induced vasoconstriction may result in hypovolemia similar to what is typically seen in the chronic hypertensive patient, making it particularly difficult to manage the acutely intoxicated patient with increased MAC requirements [22]. Hypertension can be treated with the α-adrenergic blocking agent phentolamine, or nitroglycerin with or without a calcium channel-blocking agent [19, 23]. β-blocking agents, even mixed β-1 and β-2 receptor antagonist, should not be used in the setting of cocaine-induced hypertension or ischemia due to the possibility of precipitating a hypertensive crisis secondary to unopposed α-receptor activity [24]. Bronchospasm may be common during periods of light anesthesia, even in patients who do not snort or smoke cocaine, and pulmonary edema or pulmonary hypertension may complicate management. Treatment guidelines for the anesthetic management of the trauma patient intoxicated with cocaine are summarized in Table 23.3.

Table 23.3 Summary of management recommendations for the cocaine-intoxicated patient

Anxiolysis	Benzodiazepines or dexmedetomidine
Induction	RSI with propofol or thiopental and rocuronium
Maintenance	Isoflurane, sevoflurane, or desflurane
Hypertension	Benzodiazepines, nitroglycerin, phentolamine, $\pm$ verapamil, $\pm$ dexmedetomidine
Ischemia	Antihypertensives, aspirin
Arrhythmias	Sodium bicarbonate, $\pm$ACLS

From Kaye AD and Weinkauf JL. The Cocaine-Addicted Patient. In Bryson EO, Frost EAM Editors, Perioperative Addiction. Springer Science and Business Media, NY: New York, 2011, used with permission

Methamphetamine

Called speed, meth, crystal, crank, ice and glass, methamphetamine, a synthetic derivative of amphetamine, is a schedule II drug with a high abuse potential, similar to that of cocaine [25]. Methamphetamine is a white, odorless, bitter-tasting crystalline powder that easily dissolves in water or alcohol and can be snorted, smoked, swallowed, or taken intravenously [26]. The half-life of this drug varies from formulation to formulation but averages 12 h. Though it is not a catecholamine, the systemic effects of methamphetamine are sympathetic nervous system activation due to both increased release of and decreased reuptake of endogenous catecholamines [27]. As a result, heart rate and blood pressure increase and appetite and fatigue are suppressed as the fight-or-flight response is activated.

It should be assumed that the trauma patient who is high on methamphetamine will behave physiologically as a chronic, poorly controlled hypertensive. Methamphetamine can cause left ventricular hypertrophy and the affected individual will likely have decreased cardiac compliance and diastolic dysfunction, and may even present with heart failure [28]. Key anesthetic considerations in this setting are primarily related to control of heart rate (tachyarrhythmias are common) and maintenance of blood pressure in light of what may be compromised cardiovascular function. Smoking methamphetamine may put the user at the same increased risk for intraoperative bronchospasm as the heavy tobacco smoker. Airway management is often complicated by loose teeth, and oral abscesses. Malnutrition leading to hypoalbuminemia can affect both protein binding and drug metabolism. Hyperthermia and electrolyte imbalance may be associated with overdose.

MDMA

MDMA (3,4-methylenedioxymethamphetamine), more commonly known as ecstasy, is a psychostimulant drug which is structurally similar to both the hallucinogen mescaline and the stimulant amphetamine. First developed as an appetite suppressant in 1914 by Merck Pharmaceuticals, it was briefly used as a psychotherapeutic drug before being classified by the Drug Enforcement Administration (DEA) as a Schedule I drug in the 1980s [29–32]. Since the classification of MDMA as a Schedule I drug, there have been no available commercial preparations and it is now entirely produced illegally with variable purity and little quality control [33]. MDMA is prepared as a fine white powder which can be taken orally in the form of a capsule, snorted or dissolved for injection [34]. MDMA produces effects similar to methamphetamine including mild cardiovascular stimulation, autonomic effects (dry mouth, sweating, restlessness, tremor, jaw clenching, and restlessness) as well as euphoria, happiness stimulation, and a general sense of well-being [35]. Like cocaine, MDMA increases the release and decreases reuptake of dopamine, norepinephrine, and serotonin [36, 37]. The drug directly interacts with membrane transporters involved with the uptake and storage of these neurotransmitters [38] and has been shown to have both direct agonist properties at serotonergic and dopaminergic receptors as well as mild inhibition of monoamine oxidase (MAO) [39].

The trauma patient acutely intoxicated with MDMA is at increased risk for adverse effects under anesthesia specifically related to hyperthermia and electrolyte disturbances. Disruption of the hypothalamic thermoregulatory center can result in hyperthermia [40–43]. This can be compounded by sustained muscular activity and decreased fluid intake [44, 45]. Hypo- or hyponatremia and other electrolyte disturbances have been reported as well as acute liver failure [46]. Anesthetic management should include maintaining normothermia and replacing fluid volume with appropriate balanced salt solutions based on frequent blood gas measurements. The risks for wide variations in blood pressure and heart rate are considerably less than in the patient intoxicated with stimulants such as cocaine or methamphetamines, but MAC requirements may be altered.

Synthetic Cathinones

Currently known as "bath salts," synthetic cathinones are a group of novel psychoactive substance (NPS) drugs derived from any number of chemically similar sympathomimetic compounds isolated from *Catha edulis* (khat). Cathinone is a drug with high abuse potential and no legitimate medical use; it has been classified by the DEA as a schedule I drug since the 1970s [47]. Bath salts are manufactured as a dry powder that is typically snorted nasally, swallowed orally, inserted rectally, injected, or smoked [48]. Bath salts formulations vary by manufacturer but typically contain one or a combination of the three major synthetic cathinones: mephedrone (1-(4-methylphenyl)-2-methylaminopropan-1-one), MDPV (3,4-methylenedioxypyrovalerone), or methylone (3,4-methylenedioxymethcathinone). These compounds are structurally related to and chemically similar to ephedrine and other amphetamines and provide the user with a subjective experience similar to that provided by MDMA and cocaine by stimulating the release of and preventing the reuptake of dopamine from CNS dopaminergic nerve terminals [49, 50]. Hypertension results from stimulation of peripheral alpha-adrenergic receptors and tachycardia from activation of beta-adrenergic receptors, similar to that of methamphetamine [51]. In addition to euphoria and psychomotor agitation, users may experience auditory or visual hallucinations and become violent, injuring themselves or others [52, 53].

The patient intoxicated with "bath salts" is at significant increased risk for injury resulting in the need for hospital admission and trauma surgery [54]. Anesthetic management should focus on appropriate fluid repletion as electrolyte derangements similar to what was reported with MDMA use in the early 1990s have been reported [55] and encephalopathy due to hyponatremia can occur secondary to excessive thirst [56]. Our experience administering anesthesia to patients intoxicated with these drugs is limited but given the similarities between the synthetic cathinones and cocaine it would seem prudent to treat hypertension in a similar manner, avoiding β-blocking agents in favor of nitroglycerine or calcium channel-blocking drugs. Anxiety, agitation, paranoid delusions, and hallucinations, typically of a violent nature with threatening intruders and a feeling of intense fearfulness, have resulted in high-profile violent episodes involving law enforcement. These drugs have a high potential for abuse [57] and it is likely that as use becomes more widespread trauma centers will see an increasing number of patients admitted with injuries related to "bath salts" intoxication and overdose.

Synthetic Cannabinoid Receptor Agonists

Synthetic cannabinoids are compounds which were designed to stimulate human cannabinoid receptors much in the same way that delta-9 tetrahydrocannabinol (THC) does. Most commercial preparations contain one of the two compounds, either JWH 018 (developed by Clemson University) or CP 47,497 (developed by Pfizer), which are typically sprayed on inert dried vegetable matter and sold with names such as "Arctic Spice," "K2," or "Herbal Incense" [58]. These preparations are either smoked or eaten like naturally occurring marijuana and produce effects similar to the effects of THC. Psychological and CNS effects peak in 15 min and may persist for 12–24 h depending on the dose [59]. Users report feelings of euphoria, heightened sensory perception, and a distortion of space and time [60], anxiety and distress [61], and aggravation of psychotic states [62]. The synthetic cannabinoids are structurally different than THC and though they bind to the same receptors they do so with different affinities. Since they have not yet been tested in humans, it is unclear what long-term effects these drugs may have.

The trauma patient who has ingested synthetic cannabinoid receptor agonists will likely exhibit effects of acute intoxication similar to those of cannabis intoxication but more pronounced and for a longer period of time. Anesthetic management of these patients can be complicated by persistent refractory hypertension and tachycardia. As well, there is an increased potential for postsurgical agitation, insomnia, withdrawal syndrome, and other psychiatric effects which can persist for days [63].

depend on the amount of the substance added to the marijuana; often multiple additives are combined, and the user may not even know that he/she has ingested something other than marijuana. When the user is aware of these alterations and can name the product, knowledge of the terminology used may allow the healthcare practitioner to identify the substance being abused and anticipate any complications which may arise due to acute intoxication or chronic abuse.

Chronic exposure to embalming fluid (formaldehyde, methanol, ethyl alcohol or ethanol, phenol, ethylene glycol, glutaraldehyde, and other solvents) causes bronchitis, chronic inflammatory changes of the upper airway, impaired coordination, and brain damage [64]. The trauma patient who has smoked a dipped marijuana cigarette may present with hyperthermia, myocardial infarction, rhabdomyolysis leading to renal damage, acute on chronic lung damage, and brain damage leading to seizures, coma, and death [65]. If PCP has been added to the marijuana cigarettes, the patient may present with hallucinations, impaired motor coordination, depression, anxiety, or aggressive behavior. In this dissociative state the agitated patient does not experience pain and may be very difficult to subdue [66].

Chemically Altered Cannabis

Even naturally occurring marijuana can be chemically altered through the addition of agents designed to intensify the experience of the user. Called "A-bombs," "Wack," or "Woola" (when laced with heroin or opium), "51" or "3750," "Bazooka," "Primo," or "Torpedo" (if rolled with crack cocaine), "Candy Sticks," "Champagne," "Coco Puffs," or "Dirties" (when smoked with powder cocaine) and "Chips," "Dips," or "Happy Sticks" (when combined with phencyclidine (PCP)), or "Amp," "Clicker," "Fry," "Fry Stick," "Water-water," and "Wet daddies" (when dipped in formaldehyde or embalming fluid), chemically altered cannabis presents a unique problem in the trauma patient. The effects of such additives are variable and

Inhaled Volatile Compounds

The recreational inhalation of volatile household items such as air freshener, nail polish remover, model glue, and even mothballs has the potential to directly result in trauma, usually from falls due to acute intoxication [67–69]. Some of these easy to obtain items (inexpensive, legal, and with legitimate use) are listed in Table 23.4. Once inhaled, these volatile agents interact with gamma-aminobutyric acid (GABA)-gated chloride channels [70] and 5-hydroxytryptamine type 3 (%-HT3) receptors [71], and exhibit nonselective actions on a number of ion channels in much the same manner as volatile anesthetics [72]. At lower concentrations, peripheral vasodilatation occurs resulting in hypotension and compensatory tachycardia. At higher concentrations,

Table 23.4 Commonly abused household products

Cigarette lighter fluid	(Butane, an aliphatic hydrocarbon)
Model glues and rubber cement	(Hexane, an aliphatic hydrocarbon)
Mothballs	(Naphthalene, an aromatic hydrocarbon)
Toilet bowl freshener	(An aromatic hydrocarbon)
Resins and lacquers	(Benzene, an aromatic hydrocarbon)
Adhesives and paint thinner	(Toluene, an aromatic hydrocarbon)
Room air freshener	(Butyl-isobutyl nitrate, an alkyl nitrate)
Nail polish remover	(Acetone, a ketone)
Paints	(Methyl *n*-butyl ketone)
Spray paint	(Methyl isobutyl ketone and toluene, an aromatic hydrocarbon)

From Bryson EO, Frost EAM. Marijuana, Nitrous Oxide and other inhaled drugs. In Bryson EO, Frost EAM Editors, Perioperative Addiction. Springer Science and Business Media, NY: New York, 2011, used with permission

bradycardia combines with hypotension to decrease cardiac output. Occasionally death occurs due to malignant arrhythmia induced by an acute catecholamine surge in a patient whose myocardium has been sensitized to epinephrine by hydrocarbon inhalation [73].

The trauma patient who has abused volatile agents may have telltale traces of the agent (paint or glue) around the mouth and nose. The chronic abuser may develop a rash around the mouth and nose, and present with rhinitis, epistaxis, or a chronic cough and interference with the ability of the anesthetic gas analyzer to accurately measure end-tidal anesthetic concentrations has been reported [74]. These patients should be assumed to have sustained an acute lung injury until proven otherwise. Bronchospasm can occur in patients in chronic abusers, even with no history of reactive airway disease. Inhaled vapors may displace oxygen within the alveoli leading to asphyxiation. Elevated carboxyhemoglobin levels (15 % can reduce the availability of oxygen by up to 25 %) increase the risk for hypoxia and decreases oxygen delivery to tissues. There is some evidence to suggest an interaction (additive effects in the acutely intoxicated patient and cross-tolerance in the chronic smoker) between cannabinoids and anesthetic agents [75]. There is also an increased risk for laryngospasm and bronchospasm and these patients should be managed as though they were brittle asthmatics [76]. When possible, avoid the use of histamine releasing agents, use humidified fresh gas through the

breathing circuit and maintain a heightened awareness for signs of trouble such as increased peak airway pressures due to an obstructive mucus plug in the endotracheal tube.

Heroin and Other Opioids

Either as naturally occurring compounds or synthetic and semisynthetic derivatives, opioids have been available for recreational and medicinal use for thousands of years. These drugs can be used orally, nasally, subcutaneously, or intravenously and produce varying degrees of analgesia and euphoria depending on the preparation [77]. Opioids produce euphoria and other alterations in mood result from stimulation of the release of dopamine from presynaptic nerve terminals [78]. Drug-seeking behavior is quickly reinforced and drug cravings and withdrawal occur after only a few doses causing the user to seek out more of the drug [79]. Though all opioids have significant abuse potential, those with a rapid onset and increased intensity of effect carry an extremely high risk for abuse and the development of addiction [80]. Heroin is a semi-synthetic derivative of naturally occurring opioids which has recently enjoyed resurgence as it is increasingly available in a more pure form allowing addicts to obtain a satisfactory effect with nasal insufflation [81]. There is a wide range of cutting agents used to reduce the purity of heroin (sugar, starch, acetaminophen, procaine,

Table 23.5 Suggested doses for adjuvant therapy in the opioid-addicted trauma patient

• Ketamine 0.1–0.5 mg/kg IV bolus pre-incision followed by 0.1–0.5 mg/kg/h infusion
• Clonidine 0.3 μ/kg IV bolus pre-incision followed by 0.3 μ/kg/h infusion
• Clonidine 1 μg/mL added to local anesthesia for epidural or peripheral nerve block
• Celecoxib (Celebrex®) 400 mg initially, followed by an additional 200 mg dose if needed on the first day. On subsequent days, the recommended dose is 200 mg twice daily as needed
• Ketorolac (Toradol®) 30 mg IV every 6 h as needed
• Acetaminophen (Tylenol®) 650 mg PO every 4–6 h as needed. Reduce dose if acetaminophen containing opioid analgesics are also administered
• Pregabalin (Lyrica®) 75–150 mg PO twice daily or 50–100 mg PO three times daily

From Bryson EO, The anesthetic implications of illicit opioid abuse, International Anesthesiology Clinics, 49 (1): 67–78, 2011, used with permission

Note: The use of NSAIDs perioperatively may increase risk for bleeding and the decision to use should be made after discussion with the surgical team

benzocaine, quinine, steroids, clenbuterol, or even fentanyl [82–84]) any number of which may cause unanticipated problems encountered in the heroin abusing trauma patient. Higher purity heroin is now available and many users either snort or smoke heroin, reducing but not eliminating the prevalence of syringe-borne diseases, such as HIV and hepatitis [85, 86]. As tighter controls are placed on controlled prescription opioids due to the epidemic of prescription opioid abuse, opioid addicts are increasingly turning to heroin as a cheaper and more available alternative [87].

Anesthetic management of the trauma patient who is intoxicated with opioids presents several potential problems. Because of the highly addictive nature of these agents, chronic use is common and these patients often have developed tolerance to other opioids and related drugs. When intoxicated, these patients should be considered to be "pre-medicated" and may require a lower dose per weight of opioid anesthetics. However, because of their tolerance, many of these patients will require a greater amount of opioid anesthetics than the opioid naive patient [81]. If these patients have developed opiate hyperalgesia or hyperesthesia, they may become hypersensitive to surgical and other stimuli and may require even higher doses of anesthetic agents than would be expected from tolerance alone. In refractory cases, consider using non-opioid adjuncts such as ketamine, NSAIDS, COX-2 inhibitors. Table 23.5 outlines suggested doses for adjuvant therapy in the opioid-addicted trauma patient.

Identification and Treatment of Withdrawal

The clinical presentation of withdrawal varies by type of drug, with each class characterized by a discrete withdrawal syndrome. It is important for those involved with the treatment of the trauma patient to be familiar with symptoms specific to withdrawal from different classes of drugs so that when they occur they are not confused with symptoms related to underlying injuries or pathophysiology, possibly resulting in inappropriate treatment.

Identification and treatment of alcohol withdrawal syndrome (AWS) is essential. AWS occurs in upwards of 25 % of alcohol-dependent patients and carries with it a mortality rate as high as 15 % if untreated. Even treated patients have a 2 % chance of dying [88]. If it is not possible to delay surgical intervention assume that the acutely intoxicated patient is at increased risk for developing AWS. Institute stresses inhibition with low dose morphine (15 μg/kg/h) prior to induction and for 3 postoperative days or postoperative ethanol (0.5 g/kg/day) [89]. Administer parenteral thiamine as soon as possible and continue for 5 postoperative days to prevent Wernicke's encephalopathy and Korsakoff's syndrome. Use long acting benzodiazepines to prevent withdrawal delirium and use clonidine or haloperidol intraoperatively to prevent postoperative hallucinations and autonomic instability [90].

The patient in opioid withdrawal will experience body aches, fatigue, chills, flu-like symptoms, nausea, vomiting, diarrhea, and autonomic hyperactivity [91]. These symptoms may begin to occur either during surgery, in which case autonomic instability may be the only presenting sign, or depending on the half-life of the opioid, while in the postanesthesia care unit. Because of its extremely long half-life, patients who are maintained on methadone have about 24–48 h before the withdrawal syndrome begins, but it may last for days. Even given the frequent need to manage pain with opioids in the acutely injured trauma patient, opioid withdrawal can still present a significant issue when the patient has developed tolerance. Consider reintroduction and gradual tapering of an opiate agonist such as methadone, or an agonist–antagonist such as buprenorphine, with or without clonidine. Symptomatic management of pain with non-opioid agents such as NSAIDS, ketorolac, anxiety with hydroxyzine or benzodiazepines, nausea with ondansetron or phenergan, and diarrhea with loperamide can alleviate both the discomfort and potentially harmful effects of opioid withdrawal.

The patient who has abused stimulants such as cocaine and amphetamines will experience a withdrawal picture characterized by profound dysphoria, somnolence, and lethargy. Occasionally these patients will develop depression with suicidal ideation and a psychiatric consult may be appropriate. For these patients management is generally supportive, and while the depressive syndrome usually remits after several days, persistent substance-induced mood disorder or underlying major depression may require additional pharmacologic treatment or psychiatric care. Chronic abuse of amphetamines (i.e., methamphetamine, methylphenidate, methyledioxymethamphetamine and related drugs) can result catecholamine depletion that is evident even when the person is not actively using these drugs [92]. Long-term use of amphetamines and cocaine warrant concern for cardiac dysrhythmias, even when not acutely intoxicated. These patients might benefit from a focused cardiovascular assessment and diagnostics as appropriate [93].

Treatment Options and Referral Sources

Drug abuse in the trauma patient is a problem that needs to be addressed at several levels. Trauma resulting from unsafe activity while under the influence often brings the substance abusing patient to the attention of medical personnel, providing the opportunity for intervention before further injury occurs. For the acutely injured patient, this hospitalization represents an opportunity to break the cycle of continued drug use. The treatment of addiction in this population involves an initial phase of detoxification from the drug of abuse, followed by longer term treatment with the aim of addressing underlying issues and attempting to prevent relapse into patterns of abuse and dangerous, risk-taking behavior [94]. Coordination between all members of the medical team with addiction providers is essential, especially in high risk populations such as veterans with war injuries, patients with post-traumatic stress disorder (PTSD), and those with chronic pain. Early identification and treatment of psychiatric disorders coupled with psychosocial interventions, cognitive and behavioral approaches and referral to 12 step programs such as Alcoholics Anonymous (AA) or Narcotics Anonymous (NA) should be made prior to discharge from the hospital. For the patient with an identified substance use disorder, it is essential to optimize the use of non-opiate-based pain control regimens such as TENS, massage, physical therapy, acupuncture, and pharmacotherapy with various nonaddictive agents to reduce exposure to triggering agents.

Conclusion

The anesthetic management of the trauma patient presents many challenges to the anesthesia care provider, but when the patient is under the influence of a drug of abuse, the picture is that much more complicated. In this setting normal physiology is altered, the patients' response to interventions and anesthetic agents is unpredictable, and the presence of withdrawal may cloud the presentation.

Given the propensity for intoxicated persons to experience trauma, the anesthesia care provider must possess a solid working knowledge of the different toxidromes associated with specific drugs of abuse and maintain a high index of suspicion for substance abuse in this population.

References

1. Aloysi AS, Bryson EO. Prescription drugs: implications for the chronic pain patient. In: Bryson EO, Frost EAM, editors. Perioperative addiction. New York, NY: Springer Science and Business Media; 2011.

2. Regier DA, Boyd JH, Burke Jr JD. One month prevalence of mental disorders in the United States: based on five epidemiologic catchment area sites. Arch Gen Psychiatry. 1988;45:977–86.

3. Substance Abuse and Mental Health Services Administration. Results from the 2008 national survey on drug use and health: national findings (Office of Applied Studies, NSDUH Series H-36, HHS Publication No. SMA 09-4434), Rockville, MD; 2009.

4. Gilson AM, Kreis PG. The burden of the nonmedical use of prescription opioid analgesics. Pain Med. 2009; 10(2):S89–100.

5. Sporer K, Dorn E. A case series. Heroin-related noncardiogenic pulmonary. Chest. 2001;120:1628–32.

6. Cygan J, Trunsk M, Corbridge T. Inhaled heroin-induced status asthmaticus: five cases and a review of the literature. Chest. 2000;117:272–5.

7. Nafziger AN, Bertino Jr JS. Utility and application of urine drug testing in chronic pain management with opioids. Clin J Pain. 2009;25(1):73–9.

8. Moeller KE, Lee KC, Kissack JC. Urine drug screening: practical guide for clinicians. Mayo Clin Proc. 2008;83(1):66–76.

9. Schwartz A, Knez D. Anesthesia and alcohol addiction. In: Bryson EO, Frost EAM, editors. Perioperative addiction. New York, NY: Springer Science and Business Media; 2011.

10. Pletcher MJ, Maselli J, Gonzales R. Uncomplicated alcohol intoxication in the emergency department; an analysis of the National Hospital Ambulatory Medical Care Survey. Am J Med. 2004;117:863.

11. Aryal P, Hay D, Senyon C, Slesinger PA. A discrete alcohol pocket involved in GIRK channel activation. Nat Neurosci. 2009;12:988–96.

12. Spies CD, Sander M, Stangl K, Fernandez-Sola J, Preedy V, Rubin E, Andreasson S, Hanna EZ, Kox WJ. Effects of alcohol on the heart. Curr Opin Crit Care. 2001;7:337–43.

13. Kaye AD, Weinkauf JL. The cocaine-addicted patient. In: Bryson EO, Frost EAM, editors. Perioperative addiction. New York, NY: Springer Science and Business Media; 2011.

14. US Department of Health and Human Services. National survey on drug use and health. Washington, DC: US Department of Health and Human Services; 2008. Figures 2.1, 2.6.

15. Feinstein L, Schmidt K. Cocaine users present unique anesthetic challenges: part 1. Anesthesiol News. 2010;36–2:8–9.

16. Brookoff D, Campbell EA, Shaw LM. The underreporting of cocaine-related trauma: drug abuse warning network reports vs hospital toxicology tests. Am J Public Health. 1993;83(3):369–71.

17. Hertting G, Axelrod J, Whitby LG. Effect of drugs on the uptake and metabolism of H3-norepinephrine. J Pharmcol Exp Ther. 1961;134:146–53.

18. Jatlow PI. Drug of abuse profile: cocaine. Clin Chem. 1987;33:66B–71.

19. Lange RA, Hillis LD. Cardiovascular complications in cocaine use. N Engl J Med. 2001;345(5):351–8.

20. Hollander JE, Hoffman RS. Cocaine-induced myocardial infarction: an analysis and review of the literature. J Emerg Med. 1992;10:169–77.

21. Chestnut DH. "Substance abuse". Obstetric anesthesia: principle and practice. 3rd ed. New York: Elsevier Mosby; 2004.

22. Birnbach DJ, Stein DJ. The substance-abusing parturient: implications for analgesia and anesthesia management. Baillieres Clin Obstet Gynaecol. 1998;12:443–60.

23. Kuckowski KM. The cocaine abusing parturient: a review of anesthetic considerations. Obstetrical and pediatric anesthesia. Can J Anaesth. 2004;51 (2):145–54.

24. Hoffman RS. Cocaine and beta-blockers: should the controversy continue? Ann Emerg Med. 2008;51 (2):127–9. Epub 2007 Sep 24.

25. National Institute on Drug Abuse. Methamphetamine abuse and addiction: what is methamphetamine? NIDA research report series, NIH publication 98-4210. Bethesda, MD: National Institute of Health; 1998.

26. Bryson EO. Spotlight on methamphetamine. In: Bryson EO, Frost EAM, editors. Perioperative addiction. New York, NY: Springer Science and Business Media; 2011.

27. Yu Q, Montes S, Larson D, Watson RR. Effects of chronic methamphetamine exposure on heart function in uninfected and retrovirus-infected mice. Life Sci. 1995;75:29–43.

28. Karch SB, Stephens BG, Ho CH. Methamphetamine related deaths in San Francisco; demographic, pathologic and toxicologic profiles. J Forensic Sci. 1999; 44:359–68.

29. Suarez RV, Riemersma R. "Ecstasy" and sudden cardiac death. Am J Forensic Med Pathol. 1988;9:339–41.

30. Shulgin AT. The background and chemistry of MDMA. J Psychoactive Drugs. 1986;18:291–304.

31. Greer GR, Tolbert R. A method of conducting therapeutic sessions with MDMA. J Psychoactive Drugs. 1998;30(4):371–9.

32. Greer G, Tolbert R. Subjective reports of the effects of MDMA in a clinical setting. J Psychoactive Drugs. 1986;18:319–27.

33. Wolff K, Hay AWM, Sherlock K, Conner M. Contents of "ecstasy". Lancet. 1995;346:1100–1.

34. DeMaria Jr S. Club drugs: methylenedioxymethamphetamine, flunitrazepam, ketamine hydrochloride, and gamma-hydroxybutyrate. In: Bryson EO, Frost EAM, editors. Perioperative addiction. New York, NY: Springer Science and Business Media; 2011.

35. de la Torre R, Farre M, Roset PN, Pizarro N, Abanades S, Segura M. Human pharmacology of MDMA: pharmacokinetics, metabolism, and disposition. Ther Drug Monit. 2004;26:137–44.

36. Morgan MJ. Ecstasy (MDMA): a review of its possible persistent psychological effects. Psychopharmacology (Berl). 2000;152:230–48.

37. Morton J. Ecstasy: pharmacology and neurotoxicity. Curr Opin Pharmacol. 2005;5:79–86.

38. De la Torre R, Yubero-Lahoz S, Pardo-Lozano R, Farre M. MDMA, methamphetamine, and CYP2D6 pharmacogenetics: what is clinically relevant? Front Genet. 2012;3:235.

39. Battaglia G, Yeh SY, De Souza EB. MDMA-induced neurotoxicity: parameters of degeneration and recovery of brain serotonin neurons. Pharmacol Biochem Behav. 1988;29(2):269–74.

40. Hall AP. "Ecstasy" and the anaesthetist. Br J Anaesth. 1997;79:697–8.

41. Milroy CM, Clark JC, Forrest ARW. Pathology of deaths associated with "Ecstasy" and "Eve" misuse. J Clin Pathol. 1996;49:149–53.

42. Schmidt CJ, Black CK, Abbate GM, Taylor VL. MDMA induced hyperthermia and neurotoxicity are independently mediated by 5-HT2 receptors. Brain Res. 1990;529:85–90.

43. Logan ASC, Stickle B, O'Keefe N, Hewitson H. Survival following 'Ecstasy' ingestion with a peak temperature of 42°C. Anaesthesia. 1993;48:1017–8.

44. Nimmo SM, Kennedy BW, Tullett WM, Blyth AS, Dougall JR. Drug-induced hyperthermia. Anaesthesia. 1993;48(10):892–5.

45. Benowitz NL. Amphetamines. In: Olson KR, editor. Poisoning and drug overdose. 3rd ed. Stamford, CT: Appleton & Lange; 1999. p. 68–70.

46. Henry JA, Hill IR. Fatal interaction between ritonavir and MDMA. Lancet. 1998;352:1751–2.

47. Advisory Council on the Misuse of Drug. Consideration of cathinones. http://www.namsdl.org/documents/ACMDCathinonesReport.pdf. Accessed 18 Nov 2012.

48. Motbey CP, Hunt GE, Bowen MT, Artiss S, McGregor IS. Mephedrone (4-methyl-methycathinone, 'meow'): acute behavioural effects and distribution of Fos expression in adolescent rats. Addict Biol. 2012;17:409–22.

49. Kehr J, Ichinose F, Yoshitake S, Goiny M, Sievertsson T, Nyberg F, Yoshitake T. Mephedrone, compared with MDMA (ecstasy) and amphetamine, rapidly increases both dopamine and 5-HT levels in nucleus accumbens of awake rats. Br J Pharmacol. 2011;164:1949–58.

50. Schifano F, Albanese A, Fergus S, Stair JL, Deluca P, Corazza O, Davey Z, Corkery J, Siemann H, Scherbaum N, Farre' M, Torrens M, Demetrovics Z, Ghodse AH. Mephedrone (4-methyl-methycathinone; 'meow meow'): chemical and pharmacological and clinical issues. Psychopharmacology (Berl). 2011;214:593–602.

51. Baumann MH, Ayestas Jr MA, Partilla JS. The designer methcathinon analogs, mephedrone and methylone, are substrates for monoamine transporters in brain tissue. Neuropsychopharmacology. 2012;37:1192–203.

52. Hadlock GC, Webb KM, McFadden LM, Chu PW, Ellis JD, Allen SC, Andrenyak DM, Vieira-Brock PL, German CL, Hanson GR, Flecknstein AE. 4-Methyl-methycathinone (mephedrone): neuropharmacological effects of a designer stimulant of abuse. J Pharmacol Exp Ther. 2011;339:530–6.

53. Winstock A, Mitcheson L, Ramsey J, Davies S, Puchnarewicz M, Marsden J. Mephedrone: use, subjective effects and health risks. Addiction. 2011;106:1991–6.

54. Borek HA, Holstege CP. Hyperthermia and multiorgan failure after abuse of 'bath salts' containing 3,4-methylenedioxypyrovalerone. Ann Emerg Med. 2012;60:103–5.

55. DeMaria Jr S, Bryson EO, Frost EA. Anesthetic implications of acute methylenedioxymethamphetamine intoxication in a patient with traumatic intracerebral hemorrhage. Middle East J Anesthesiol. 2009;20(2):281–4.

56. Sammler EM, Foley PL, Lauder GD, Wilson SJ, Goudie AR, O'Riordan JI. A harmless high? Lancet. 2010;376:742.

57. Spiller HA, Ryan ML, Weston RG, Jansen J. Clinical experience with and analytical confirmation of 'bath salts' and 'legal highs' (synthetic cathinones) in the United States. Clin Toxicol. 2011;49:499–505.

58. Bryson EO, Frost EAM. Marijuana, nitrous oxide and other inhaled drugs: spotlight on chemically altered cannabis. In: Bryson EO, Frost EAM, editors. Perioperative addiction. New York, NY: Springer Science and Business Media; 2011.

59. Simmons JR, Skinner CG, Williams J, Kang CS, Schwartz MD, Willis BK. Intoxication from smoking "spice". Ann Emerg Med. 2011;57:187–8.

60. Schifano F, Corazza O, Deluca P. Psychoactive drug or mystical insence? Overview of the online available information on spice products. J Cult Ment Health. 2009;2:137–44.

61. Canning J, Ruha A, Pierce R, Torrey M, Reinhart S. Severe GI distress after smoking JWH-018. Clin Toxicol. 2010;48:618.

62. Hurst D, Loeffler G, McLay R. Psychosis associated with synthetic cannabinoid agonists: a case series. Am J Psychiatry. 2011;168:1119.

63. Zimmermann US, Winkelmann PR, Pilhatsch M, Nees JA, Spanagel R, Schulz K. Withdrawal

phenomena and dependence syndrome after the consumption of "spice gold". Dtsch Arztebl Int. 2009;106 (27):464–7.

64. Bardana EJ, Montanaro A. Formaldehyde: an analysis of its respiratory, cutaneous, and immunologic effects. Ann Allergy. 1991;66:441–52.

65. State of Connecticut, Department of Public Health and Addiction Services. Illy contains embalming chemicals that will poison you! Brochure, Hartford, CT; 1994.

66. Yago KB, Pitts FN, Burgoyne RW, Aniline O, Yago LS, Pitts AF. The urban epidemic of phencyclidine (PCP) use: clinical and laboratory evidence from a public psychiatric hospital emergency service. J Clin Psychiatry. 1981;42:193–6.

67. Kong JT, Schmiesing C. Concealed mothball abuse prior to anesthesia: mothballs, inhalants, and their management. Acta Anaesthesol Scand. 2005;49: 113–6.

68. Kurtzman TL, Otsuka KN, Wahl RA. Inhalant abuse by adolescents. J Adolesc Health. 2001;28:170–80.

69. Perron BE, Howard MO, Vaughn MG, Jarman CN. Inhalant withdrawal as a clinically significant feature of inhalant dependence disorder. Med Hypotheses. 2009;73:935–7.

70. MacIver BM. Abused inhalants enhance GABA-mediated synaptic inhibition. Neuropsychopharmacology. 2009;34:2296–304.

71. Lopreato GF, Phelan R, Borghese CM, Beckstead MJ, Mihic SJ. Inhaled drugs of abuse enhance serotonin-3 receptor function. Drug Alcohol Depend. 2003;70:11–5.

72. Bieda MC, Su H, MacIver MB. Anesthetics discriminate between tonic and phasic gamma-aminobutyric acid receptors on hippocampal CA1 neurons. Anesth Analg. 2009;108:484–90.

73. Bass M. Sudden sniffing death. JAMA. 1970;212: 2075–9.

74. Sicinski M, Kadam U. Monitoring of the anesthetic volatile agent may be impaired in hydrocarbon abusers. Anesthesia. 2002;57:510–1.

75. Flisberg P, Paech MJ, Shah T, Ledowski T, Kurowski I, Parsons R. Induction dose of propofol in patients using cannabis. Eur J Anaesthesiol. 2009;26:192–5.

76. Pertwee RG. Neuropharmacology and therapeutic potential of cannabinoids. Addict Biol. 2000;5:37–46.

77. Yaksh TL, Wallace MS. Chapter 18. Opioids, Analgesia, and Pain Management. In: Brunton LL, Chabner BA, Knollmann BC. eds. *Goodman & Gilman's The Pharmacological Basis of Therapeutics, 12e.* New York, NY: McGraw-Hill; 2011. http://accessmedicine.mhmedical.com/content.aspx? bookid=374&Sectionid=41266224. Accessed May 27, 2014.

78. Becerra L, Harter K, Gonzalez RG, Borsook D. Functional magnetic resonance imaging measures of the effects of morphine on central nervous system circuitry in opioid-naive healthy volunteers. Anesth Analg. 2006;103:208–16.

79. Lewis M, Souki F. The anesthetic implications of acute opioid intoxication and dependence. In: Bryson EO, Frost EAM, editors. Perioperative addiction. New York, NY: Springer Science and Business Media; 2011.

80. Roset P, Farre M, de la Torre R, et al. Modulation of rate of onset and intensity of drug effects reduces abuse potential in healthy males. Drug Alcohol Depend. 2001;64:285–98.

81. Bryson EO. The anesthetic implications of illicit opioid abuse. Int Anesthesiol Clin. 2011;49(1):67–78.

82. Koushesh HR, Afshari R, Afshari R. A new illicit opioid dependence outbreak, evidence for a combination of opioids and steroids. Drug Chem Toxicol. 2009;32(2):114–9.

83. Wingert WE, Mundy LA, Nelson L, Wong SC, Curtis J. Detection of clenbuterol in heroin users in twelve postmortem cases at the Philadelphia medical examiner's office. J Anal Toxicol. 2008;32(7):522–8.

84. Ojanperä I, Gergov M, Rasanen I, Lunetta P, Toivonen S, Tiainen E, Vuori E. Blood levels of 3-methylfentanyl in 3 fatal poisoning cases. Am J Forensic Med Pathol. 2006;27(4):328–31.

85. Substance Abuse and Mental Health Services Administration. Results from the drug and alcohol services information system report: heroin: changes in how it is used: 1995–2005; 2007.

86. Broz D, Ouellet LJ. Prevalence and correlates of former injection drug use among young noninjecting heroin users in Chicago. Subst Use Misuse. 2010; 45(12):2000–25.

87. Substance Abuse and Mental Health Services Administration. Results from the 2008 national survey on drug use and health: national findings (Office of Applied Studies, NSDUH Series H-36, HHS Publication No. SMA 09-4434), Rockville, MD. 2009. http://www.oas.samhsa.gov/nsduh/2k8nsduh/2k8Results.pdf. Accessed 24 Nov 2012.

88. Hines RL, Marschall KE. Psychiatric disease/substance abuse/drug overdose. In: Hines RL, Marschall KE, Stoelting RK, editors. Anesthesia and co-existing disease. 5th ed. Philadelphia: Churchill Livingstone; 2008.

89. Tonnesen H, Nielsen PR, Lauritzen JB, Moller AM. Smoking and alcohol intervention before surgery: evidence for best practice. Br J Anaesth. 2009; 102:297–306.

90. Kork F, Neumann T, Spies C. Perioperative management of patients with alcohol, tobacco and drug dependency. Curr Opin Anaesthesiol. 2010;23: 384–90.

91. Tetrault JM, O'Connor PG. Substance abuse and withdrawal in the critical care setting. Crit Care Clin. 2008;24(4):767–88, viii. Review. PubMed PMID: 18929942.

92. Klein M, Kramer F. Rave drugs: pharmacological considerations. AANA J. 2004;72:61–7.

93. Hamza H. Anesthetic considerations for the addicted patient in recovery. In: Bryson EO, Frost EAM, editors. Perioperative addiction. New York, NY: Springer Science and Business Media; 2011.

94. Denisco RA, Chandler RK, Compton WM. Addressing the intersecting problems of opioid misuse and chronic pain treatment. Exp Clin Psychopharmacol. 2008; 16(5):417–28. Review. PubMed PMID: 18837638.

Index